Revolutionizing Metabolic Medicine With Artificial Intelligence

Pranav Kumar Prabhakar
Nagaland University, India

Ashok K. Sah
https://orcid.org/0000-0002-7762-4351

A' Sharqiyah University, Oman

IGI Global
Scientific Publishing
Publishing Tomorrow's Research Today

Vice President of Editorial	Melissa Wagner
Director of Acquisitions	Mikaela Felty
Director of Book Development	Jocelynn Hessler
Production Manager	Mike Brehm
Cover Design	Jose Rosado

Published in the United States of America by
IGI Global Scientific Publishing
701 East Chocolate Avenue
Hershey, PA, 17033, USA
Tel: 717-533-8845 | Fax: 717-533-7115
Website: https://www.igi-global.com E-mail: cust@igi-global.com

Library of Congress Cataloging-in-Publication Data

LCCN: 2025019813 (CIP Data Pending)
ISBN: 9798337331966
eISBN: 9798337331980
British Cataloguing in Publication Data
A Cataloguing in Publication record for this book is available from the British Library.

Table of Contents

Detailed Table of Contents

Chapter 1

Mamta Verma, UPUMS, India
Shubham Gupta, Parul Institute of Paramedical Health Sciences, India
Megha Yadav, NAMO College of Allied Health Sciences, India

Early diagnosis and risk prediction are changing as a result of artificial intelligence's (AI) incorporation into healthcare systems, which has the potential to revolutionize a variety of clinical paths. This study examines how artificial intelligence driven technologies, such as machine learning algorithms, deep learning models, and natural language processing, are being used to identify people at high risk before clinical symptoms appear and to diagnose diseases in their earliest stages. AI can find small patterns and correlations in large datasets from genomes, imaging studies, wearable technology, and electronic health records that are frequently missed by conventional diagnostic methods. The use of AI reduces the burden of disease and improves patient outcomes by increasing diagnostic accuracy, clinical decision-making, and individualized preventive efforts. Early intervention will become the standard rather than the exception in the future as AI develops and is incorporated into healthcare.

Chapter 2

Ankur Vashishtha, Sharda University, Greater Noida, India
Anshu Kumar Singh, Subharti College of Allied and Healthcare, Meerut,
    India
Gaurav Kaushik, Sharda University, Greater Noida, India
Prigya Sharma, Sharda University, Greater Noida, India
Vivek Kumar, IIMT University, Meerut, India
Salender Singh, N.C. Medical College, Haryana, India
Ashok K. Sah, A' Sharqiyah University, Oman

Artificial intelligence (AI) is a disruptive computer science that has the potential to revolutionize medical practice and healthcare delivery. Its uses include patient diagnosis, medication research, improved communication, document transcription, and remote patient care. AI algorithms have lately acquired accuracies comparable to human expertise in medical research, and others believe that humans will be fully displaced in several disciplines. AI also helps with microbial research, including microbe categorization and functional annotation. Machine learning enhances microbial taxonomy accuracy by exposing functional properties and metabolic pathways. AI-driven protein design has the potential to create enzymes with increased catalytic activity and stability. AI systems can anticipate protein shapes, functions, and interactions, allowing for more logical application design. AI technologies are already being utilized in clinical microbiology laboratories to automate susceptibility testing and identification. Microbiological practitioners will increasingly rely on AI for preliminary screening, freeing them to concentrate on diagnostic concerns and sophisticated technical interpretation. The COVID-19 pandemic has boosted AI usage in telemedicine and chatbots, hence enhancing accessibility and medical education. AI-powered techniques offer the potential to better comprehend microbial ecosystems, accelerate drug development, and stimulate new medical cures.

Chapter 3

   Himansu, Amity Institute of Biotechnology, India
   Tushar Joshi, Amity Institute of Biotechnology, India
   Hina Bansal, Amity University, Noida, India

Metabolic disorders—including diabetes, weight problems, excessive blood pressure, etc, are getting increasingly more common in today's quick-moving, challenging world. These ailments don't arise instantly. Often, some subtle signs and vulnerabilities accumulate over time, however, they pass neglected till it is too overdue. Conventional checkout frameworks depend closely on inflexible criteria and obstacles, which can overlook the hidden systems. Artificial intelligence, however, is transforming this approach. With its capability to examine extensive information pools, computational intelligence is aiding healthcare providers in identifying threats earlier, tailoring therapy, and even foreseeing health deterioration. The essence of this chapter is to explore the developing function of artificial intelligence in determining metabolic disorders, emphasizing forecasting, predictive analysis, and risk assessment. We shall explore the most recent studies, AI models, current systems, tangible issues, and the personal consequences of these innovations, both now and in the future.

Chapter 4

Leena Arya, Koneru Lakshmiah Education Foundation, India
Ravi Rastogi, JIMS Engineering Management Technical Campus, India
Mandalapu Sivaparvathi, MAM Women's Engineering College, India
Rajesh Babu Yallamanda, Koneru Lakshmiah Education Foundation,
India
Latha Banda, JIMS Engineering Management Technical Campus, India
Venkata Rajani Katuri, Keshav Memorial Institute of Technology, India
Devendra Gautam, JIMS Engineering Management Technical Campus,
India
Mourad Elloumi, Bisha University, Saudi Arabia
Nimisha Tiwari, UIT, Pajiv Gandhi Proudyogiki Vishwavidyalay, India
Shalaka Tyagi, School of Computing Science and Engineering, Sharda
University, India

By enabling continuous, individualized, and predictive care, the incorporation of artificial intelligence (AI) into telemedicine has completely transformed the management of metabolic health. To treat metabolic disorders such as diabetes, obesity, and cardiovascular disease, a revolutionary model that integrates gut microbiome analysis with AI-powered telemedicine is examined. Real-time physiological and microbial data are recorded, analysed, and converted into valuable insights by utilizing wearable sensors, mobile health platforms, and cloud-based analytics. Risk stratification, dietary customization, and early intervention are made possible by artificial intelligence (AI) techniques like machine learning, deep learning, and natural language processing. In parallel, functional biomarkers of disease progression and treatment response are revealed by microbiome profiling. The chapter discusses ethical, legal, and technical challenges while presenting successful case studies. This convergence facilitates closed-loop, adaptive systems that maximise results and empower patients.

Chapter 5

Farhat Nazneen, Amity University, Kolkata, India
Arisha Ansari, Amity University, Kolkata, India
Joyeta Ghosh, Amity University, Kolkata, India

The rising burden of metabolic syndrome—obesity, insulin resistance, hypertension, and dyslipidemia—calls for personalized prevention. Precision nutrition, which tailors diets based on genetic, biological, lifestyle, and environmental data, shows promise, especially with AI integration. Advances in digital health, genomics, and metabolomics allow AI to analyze complex data and provide individualized dietary plans. In clinics, AI supports nutrition care by interpreting health records and biomarkers, improving outcomes. In public health, it helps detect dietary trends and optimize programs. AI also integrates multi-omics data to discover biomarkers and customize therapies for metabolic syndrome, obesity, cardiovascular disease, and diabetes. However, challenges like data privacy, bias, and inequality remain. Despite these, AI-powered precision nutrition offers a transformative path for predictive, personalized care—requiring ongoing research, ethics, and collaboration.

Chapter 6

Wasswa Shafik, Dig Connectivity Research Laboratory (DCRLab), Uganda

This chapter examines the transformative impact of Artificial Intelligence (AI) on the management of diabetes and obesity, two prevalent and interrelated chronic health conditions. It examines how AI-driven technologies, including machine learning, predictive analytics, and digital health tools, enable personalised and data-driven approaches to glucose regulation, weight control, and lifestyle interventions. The chapter discusses the application of AI in continuous glucose monitoring, insulin dosing, and the development of customized weight management programs. Furthermore, it highlights the integration of wearable devices, mobile health (mHealth) applications, and remote patient monitoring systems to enhance patient engagement and clinical outcomes. Ethical considerations, data privacy, and the challenges of AI adoption in healthcare systems are also addressed. This chapter highlights the potential of AI to enhance the prevention, diagnosis, and treatment of diabetes and obesity, ultimately supporting sustainable and effective management of chronic diseases.

Chapter 7

Harmanpreet Kaur, Chitkara University, India
Gurwinder Singh, Panjab University, India

Artificial Intelligence (AI) is revolutionizing the world of computer science with its power and disruptive potential of completely changing the ways medical profession serves the humanity and healthcare sector. The use of AI in medicine has already begun changing the way the prevention, diagnosis, treatment, amelioration, and other physical and mental impairments are done. We may anticipate much more revolutionary developments as technology develops, which will significantly change the field of medical imaging and artificial intelligence in the years to come. The main goal addressed in this chapter is to acquaint researchers with the capacities of AI and its medical applications, as well as with the dangers that may lie ahead.

This chapter presents recent advancements in the use of AI in healthcare, outlines challenges, legal/ethical considerations and future implications of AI in healthcare for creating safe and successful AI systems. In general, researchers might utilize the study as a reference manual for continuing advancements in research in pertinent realms of applications.

*Santhosh Kumar Veeramalla, BVRIT HYDERABAD College of
    Engineering for Women, India*
Roshan Bodile, National Institute of Technology, Jalandhar, India
B. Jailsingh, National Institute of Technology, Calicut, India

This study presents a secure image encryption method designed specifically for grayscale and color medical images, aimed at maintaining security and integrity during transmission and storage. The system utilizes a hybrid encryption method that integrates symmetric and asymmetric cryptography alongside image processing techniques. A specialized preprocessing step, optimized for medical image characteristics, improves both speed and encryption quality. The method facilitates the processing of color images via color space transformation, maintaining diagnostic integrity after decryption. A secure key management protocol effectively addresses the challenges associated with key generation and distribution. The system will undergo testing across various medical image datasets, assessing encryption and decryption speed, key sensitivity, attack resistance, and computational efficiency. This study enhances secure medical image processing applicable to telemedicine, cloud diagnostics, and electronic health record systems.

Shubham Gupta, Parul University, India
Vishnu Vinod, NAMO College of Allied Health Sciences, India

Artificial intelligence (AI) and radiomics are fundamentally transforming the future of medical imaging by uncovering therapeutically significant information that traditional interpretation methods often overlook. This chapter delves into their expanding roles in healthcare, radiology, and metabolic medicine, highlighting how AI-driven radiomic analysis can be seamlessly integrated into clinical workflows to enhance diagnostic precision. Radiomics enables predictive modeling and personalized diagnostics by extracting and analyzing subtle imaging features and complex patterns from common modalities such as CT, MRI, and PET. Utilizing advanced AI techniques to decode microscopic textural variations, metabolic activity trends, and early indicators of disease progression, radiologists are evolving into sophisticated data interpreters. The chapter explores the revolutionary impact of AI in improving diagnostic accuracy, stratifying patient risk, and tailoring treatment strategies—especially critical in metabolic diseases where early detection is vital for effective intervention.

Kunj Bihari Meena, Jaypee University of Engineering and Technology, Guna, India

Kunal Kumar Singh, Jaypee University of Engineering and Technology, Guna, India

Manan Jain, Jaypee University of Engineering and Technology, Guna, India

Shreyash Sundarrao Dhande, Jaypee University of Engineering and Technology, Guna, India

Vipin Tyagi, Jaypee University of Engineering and Technology, Guna, India

Metabolic syndrome involves abdominal adiposity, raised blood pressure, and lipid abnormalities. Early detection is essential, as timely intervention reduces future cardiometabolic risk. However, conventional diagnosis depends on structured clinical data, which is slow to collect and often incomplete. This chapter presents an AI-based prediction system that identifies metabolic syndrome from free-text patient descriptions. The approach uses NLP to convert symptom narratives into structured medical features. The pipeline includes preprocessing, feature engineering, named entity recognition, clinical term mapping, and classification using logistic regression, random forest, and XGBoost. Model performance was evaluated using accuracy and AUC-ROC. XGBoost achieved the best results, with 0.8732 accuracy and 0.9608 AUC.

Richa Singh, Lovely Professional University, India
Lovleen Marwaha, Lovely Professional University, India

However, AI has greatly changed the way that healthcare proceeds, making it possible to detect disease early and predict the risk of happening. Blood tests, MRI's, CT scans, X-rays and any other clinical, genetic and imaging data is used along with machine learning and deep learning models to detect diseases before the symptoms show up. For diseases such as cancer, cardiovascular and neurological etc., CNNs and NLP techniques help analyze scans, pathology slides, electronic health records.

Risk models based on the patient's history, lifestyle or genetics are evaluated using AI technology. Despite this, they face ethical and validation issues, risks regarding data privacy, and validation needs. To bring guaranteed and proper AI solutions, effective collaboration between medical professionals, AI researchers and policymakers is pivotal. This chapter focuses on the discussion of AI's applications, advantages and restrictions, future potential, for the benefit of clinicians and researchers to optimize patient outcomes and advance precision medicine.

Chapter 12

*Vishal Jain, Kuala Lumpur University of Science and Technology,
Malaysia & Vivekananda Institute of Professional Studies, New
Delhi, India*
Sachin Jain, Ajay Kumar Garg Engineering College, Ghaziabad, India
Danish Ather, Amity University, Tashkent, Uzbekistan
*Golnoosh Manteghi, Kuala Lumpur University of Science and
Technology, Malaysia*
*Abu Bakar Abdul Hamid, Kuala Lumpur University of Science and
Technology, Malaysia*

The healthcare industry is undergoing significant upheaval as more businesses use distributed edge computing. Better real-time data processing, simpler access, and more individualised patient care are just a few benefits of this shift. Security concerns with distributed edge-based healthcare systems are covered in this chapter. It looks at the bigger attack surface, the different kinds of features that devices can offer, and how hard it is to manage data in all of its forms (in use, at rest, and in motion). It carefully talks about HIPAA, other countries' data protection laws, and industry standards. Behavioral analytics, edge-based breach detection, and incident response in distributed settings are also talked about in this chapter. It focuses on risk management and governance models such as threat modelling, managing vulnerabilities, and making security better. These security rules are shown in a detailed case study on safe telemedicine implementation. Post-quantum cryptography, AI-powered security, and blockchain make up the last part of the chapter.

Chapter 13

Dolly Yumnam, Department of Optometry, UIAHS, Chandigarh
University, Mohali, India
Laxmi Oinam, Department of Optometry, UIAHS, Chandigarh
University, Mohali, India
Sachitanand Singh, Department of Optometry, UIAHS, Chandigarh
University, Mohali, India
Krishnasri Padamandala, Department of Optometry, School of Allied
and Health Care Sciences, Malla Reddy University, Hyderabad,
India
Sanskriti Singh, Department of Nursing, UIN, Chandigarh University,
Mohali, India

Abstract Metabolic diseases, such as diabetes, obesity, and dyslipidemia, are growing in complexity, and are increasingly seen across the globe where they are demanding a significant burden on health systems. Traditional methods continue to under-utilize the vast amount of health information available in Electronic Health Records (EHRs). Artificial intelligence (AI) is a powerful solution as it can study complex amounts of data to identify patterns and generate actionable insights. This AI-powered decision making benefits precision medicine because it creates opportunities for early diagnosis, tailored treatment, and long-term monitoring, when used with EHRs. This chapter explores the ways in which artificial intelligence (AI) can provide real-world guidance to clinicians making decisions in metabolic disease, specifically how it can use EHR sources of information to help with diagnosis, risk stratification and treatment decision making.

Chapter 14

C. Selvamurugan, Dhaanish Ahmed Institute of Technology, India
K. G. Parthiban, Aalim Muhammed Salegh College of Engineering,
India
J. Tharik Raja, Dhaanish Ahmed Institute of Technology, India
K. Lakshmikandhan, CMS College of Engineering and Technology,
India
M. Santhiya, Dhaanish Ahmed Institute of Technology, India
A. Munirathinam, Dhaanish Ahmed Institute of Technology, India

Artificial Intelligence (AI) has emerged as a transformative force in the field of metabolic medicine, offering innovative solutions to complex challenges. This paper delves into the pivotal role of AI in advancing metabolic medicine by exploring case studies and real-time applications. It highlights the integration of machine learning models, predictive analytics, and personalized medicine in diagnosing, monitoring, and treating metabolic disorders. The study emphasizes the successes achieved in areas such as diabetes management, obesity control, and lipid metabolism disorders. However, it also addresses the challenges faced, including ethical considerations, data privacy concerns, and the need for robust validation methods. Furthermore, this work envisions future directions, focusing on the potential of AI-driven precision medicine, enhanced patient care through real-time analytics, and interdisciplinary collaboration. By bridging existing gaps, this paper aims to foster innovation and provide a roadmap for the next phase of AI adoption in metabolic medicine.

Preface

Metabolic diseases including diabetes, obesity, cardiovascular dysfunction, and a broad spectrum of genetic or lifestyle-related disorders represent one of the most urgent global health challenges of the 21st century. Their rising prevalence, complex etiologies, and often-silent progression demand innovative solutions capable of transforming both prevention and clinical management. Artificial intelligence (AI), with its unmatched capacity to analyze vast datasets, detect invisible patterns, and support individualized decision-making, is rapidly emerging as the cornerstone of next-generation metabolic medicine.

Revolutionizing Metabolic Medicine With Artificial Intelligence brings together leading researchers, clinicians, data scientists, and technologists to explore how AI is reshaping metabolic health across diagnostics, therapeutics, monitoring, security, and systems-level care delivery. This edited volume provides a comprehensive, interdisciplinary view of AI's expanding role from early diagnosis and precision nutrition to medical imaging, drug repurposing, telemedicine, and secure data ecosystems.

The chapters offer not only scientific insight and technical depth but also practical perspectives, ethical considerations, and real-world case studies. Collectively, they illustrate an evolving paradigm in which AI enables proactive rather than reactive care, empowering clinicians, improving patient outcomes, and paving the way for personalized metabolic medicine.

We extend our deepest gratitude to all contributing authors for their dedication and expertise, and to the readers, researchers, clinicians, students, and innovators whose work will continue advancing this transformative field.

CHAPTER OVERVIEW

Chapter 1: AI at the Frontline—Enhancing Early Diagnosis and Risk Prediction Across Clinical Pathways

This chapter explores how machine learning, deep learning, and natural language processing are revolutionizing early detection by uncovering subtle risk indicators across multimodal datasets. It highlights AI's potential to identify pre-symptomatic disease patterns, enhance clinical decision-making, and shift healthcare toward preventive intervention.

Chapter 2: AI in Early Diagnosis & Risk Prediction

Building on the first chapter, this contribution examines AI applications across oncology, neurology, cardiology, and ophthalmology. It emphasizes design considerations, regulatory challenges, and the need for interdisciplinary frameworks to ensure accurate, ethical, and clinically integrated diagnostic tools.

Chapter 3: AI-Driven Diagnostics in Metabolic Disorders—Predictive Analytics and Risk Assessment

Focusing on metabolic disorders such as diabetes, obesity, and hypertension, this chapter demonstrates how AI addresses the limitations of conventional diagnostic systems. It discusses predictive analytics, emerging models, and real-world implementations that allow earlier intervention and personalized care planning.

Chapter 4: AI Integration in Telemedicine for Metabolic Monitoring and Gut Microbiome Analysis

This chapter presents a forward-looking convergence of AI, telemedicine, and microbiome science. It shows how real-time physiological and microbial monitoring enables adaptive metabolic care systems, and it discusses challenges related to ethics, data integration, and scalability.

Chapter 5: AI-Powered Precision Nutrition in Metabolic Syndrome Management

Addressing the growing metabolic syndrome crisis, this chapter illustrates how AI integrates genomics, metabolomics, lifestyle data, and clinical biomarkers to deliver personalized nutrition strategies. It also highlights public-health applications and the challenges of ensuring equity and data security.

Chapter 6: AI in Diabetes Management, Obesity, and Weight Control

A comprehensive examination of AI-based glucose monitoring, insulin dosing, weight-management algorithms, mHealth tools, and wearable-integrated systems. Ethical considerations and barriers to adoption are addressed alongside future opportunities for sustainable disease management.

Chapter 7: Role of Artificial Intelligence in Medical Imaging

A broad overview of AI's growing influence in medical imaging, covering emerging algorithms, clinical applications, challenges, and policy considerations. It serves as a foundational reference for imaging researchers and clinicians adopting AI-based workflows.

Chapter 8: Advanced Image Encryption Framework for Securing Gray and Color Medical Images

Centered on the security of diagnostic imaging, this chapter introduces a hybrid cryptographic system designed to protect medical images in telemedicine and cloud environments while preserving diagnostic integrity.

Chapter 9: Decoding the Invisible—AI and Radiomics for Predictive and Personalized Imaging

Here, the authors highlight how radiomics and AI reveal hidden imaging biomarkers to enhance predictive modeling and personalized care, particularly in metabolic conditions where early detection is crucial.

Chapter 10: Healthcare Text Mining to Detect Metabolic Syndrome from User-Entered Symptoms

This chapter describes an NLP-based system that converts free-text patient symptom descriptions into structured clinical features and accurately predicts metabolic syndrome, demonstrating the power of language-based diagnostics.

Chapter 11: Transforming Preventive Medicine through Artificial Intelligence

Covering multi-modal diagnostics including imaging, genetics, and EHR analysis, this chapter offers insights into AI's ability to detect disease before symptoms arise. It also addresses ethical constraints and emphasizes the role of collaboration in developing trustworthy AI solutions.

Chapter 12: Securing Patient Data in Distributed Healthcare Systems

The authors examine the heightened cybersecurity risks of distributed, edge-based healthcare environments, offering frameworks for threat modeling, secure telemedicine deployment, and emerging technologies such as blockchain and post-quantum cryptography.

Chapter 13: Integration of AI with Electronic Health Records

This chapter outlines how AI unlocks the full diagnostic and predictive potential of EHR data, supporting precision medicine approaches to metabolic disease. It focuses on clinical decision support, risk stratification, and long-term care optimization.

Chapter 14: Challenges and Future Directions—Case Studies and Real-Time Applications in AI-Based Metabolic Medicine

The concluding chapter synthesizes key learnings through real-world case studies, highlighting success stories in diabetes, obesity, and lipid metabolism management while addressing remaining challenges and paving the way for AI-driven precision care.

Together, these chapters provide a panoramic and authoritative overview of how AI is revolutionizing metabolic medicine—scientifically, clinically, technically, and ethically. We hope this book serves as a catalyst for continued innovation and collaboration across disciplines, ultimately improving lives worldwide.

Chapter 1
AI at the Frontline:
Enhancing Early Diagnosis and Risk Prediction Across Clinical Pathways

Mamta Verma
https://orcid.org/0009-0009-2513-6389
UPUMS, India

Shubham Gupta
https://orcid.org/0000-0003-1202-2779
Parul Institute of Paramedical Health Sciences, India

Megha Yadav
https://orcid.org/0009-0006-1842-9501
NAMO College of Allied Health Sciences, India

ABSTRACT

Early diagnosis and risk prediction are changing as a result of artificial intelligence's (AI) incorporation into healthcare systems, which has the potential to revolutionize a variety of clinical paths. This study examines how artificial intelligence driven technologies, such as machine learning algorithms, deep learning models, and natural language processing, are being used to identify people at high risk before clinical symptoms appear and to diagnose diseases in their earliest stages. AI can find small patterns and correlations in large datasets from genomes, imaging studies, wearable technology, and electronic health records that are frequently missed by conventional diagnostic methods. The use of AI reduces the burden of disease and improves patient outcomes by increasing diagnostic accuracy, clinical decision-

DOI: 10.4018/979-8-3373-3196-6.ch001

making, and individualized preventive efforts. Early intervention will become the standard rather than the exception in the future as AI develops and is incorporated into healthcare.

1 INTRODUCTION

1.1 Contextualizing the Role of AI in Modern Healthcare

Clinical prediction is a crucial tool in modern healthcare, involving the systematic analysis of historical and current medical data to anticipate future health outcomes. This process enhances diagnostic accuracy, guides personalized treatment plans, and enables early disease detection and prevention. The integration of artificial intelligence (AI) is central to this advancement, enabling rapid and precise analysis of vast and complex datasets. AI algorithms can uncover patterns and relationships that may go unnoticed by human clinicians, and their predictive capabilities continually improve as they learn from new data. This chapter explores the role of clinical prediction and AI in transforming healthcare decision-making and patient management. AI, including machine learning, deep learning, and natural language processing, is a rapidly advancing branch of computer science that enables systems capable of performing tasks traditionally requiring human intelligence (Lecun et al., 2015)

1.2 The Urgency for Early Diagnosis and Proactive Risk Prediction

Early detection is crucial for managing medical conditions, especially progressive ones like cancer, heart disease, and neurological disorders. These conditions often show mild or vague symptoms in their early stages, making them easy to overlook or misinterpret. Delays in diagnosis can lead to more serious conditions, making treatment more difficult and less effective. Regular breast cancer screenings can reduce mortality rates, while identifying individuals at risk of stroke early on allows for preventive steps. Early detection also benefits the healthcare system by reducing the need for hospitalizations and intensive treatments for late-stage diseases. Proactive risk prediction uses advanced data analysis tools like artificial intelligence and machine learning to estimate a person's likelihood of developing certain health conditions before symptoms appear. This information allows healthcare providers to take targeted preventive actions, such as dietary changes, vaccines, or early screenings, based on each person's risk profile. AI-driven models improve the accuracy and speed of these predictions, helping clinicians prioritize care and use healthcare resources more efficiently (Jansson et al., 2022)

1.3 Overview of Clinical Pathways and Decision-Making Challenges

Clinical pathways, also known as care paths or care maps, are structured plans that outline the key steps in treating patients with specific medical conditions. They aim to improve patient outcomes, reduce care variations, and create consistency in treatment approaches (D'Addario; 2025). These pathways streamline treatment, promote best practices, and improve communication among healthcare professionals. They also serve as valuable tools for staff training and quality improvement efforts within healthcare organizations.

Healthcare decision-making is a complex process influenced by clinical evidence, patient preferences, ethical considerations, and resource availability. Integrating early diagnosis and proactive risk prediction adds complexity. Challenges include interpreting and using predictive data effectively, as accuracy depends on data quality and completeness. Clinicians must rely on professional judgment when interpreting data and making decisions. Allocating resources is another challenge, as early diagnostic tools and predictive technologies require significant investment in equipment and training. Artificial intelligence can reduce long-term healthcare costs by preventing serious illnesses, but health systems must balance initial investment with projected long-term benefits. The chapters will explore AI applications in clinical contexts, overcome obstacles for safe and equitable use, and envision a collaborative, AI-augmented healthcare future where technology augments human touch.

2 FOUNDATIONS OF ARTIFICIAL INTELLIGENCE IN HEALTHCARE

Artificial Intelligence (AI) is revolutionizing healthcare, fundamentally transforming how diagnostics, treatment planning, patient monitoring, and administrative processes are carried out. AI is no longer a futuristic concept, as it is already embedded in today's medical practice, research and healthcare delivery systems. This chapter explores the historical evolution of AI in medicine, outlines the core technologies that drive its capabilities, and examines the diverse data sources that fuel AI applications. It also critically analyses the ethical challenges and regulatory frameworks that guide the safe and responsible integration of AI into healthcare. (Becker et al., 2022; Mohsen et al., 2022)

2.1 Historical Evolution of AI in Medical Diagnostics

The integration of artificial intelligence and medicine began in the mid-20th century with the development of the MYCIN system at Stanford University. This early rule-based expert system, which used "if-then" rules to diagnose bacterial infections, was found to be on par with human medical experts. However, it was never implemented in clinical practice due to legal liability concerns and challenges in integrating it into existing hospital workflows.

In the 1990s and early 2000s, machine learning (ML) approaches replaced conventional expert systems, making them more flexible and scalable. The growing use of digital health information and advances in medical imaging have made training algorithms easier. Methods like support vector machines, decision trees, and Bayes networks were used for disease classification and prediction. A new era of data-driven healthcare emerged when machine learning models helped diagnose diabetic eye disease from retina images and predicted cancer treatment results. In the 2010s, deep learning models made significant progress in applications like image identification and natural language processing, with applications in radiology, dermatology, and pathology widely adopting convolutional neural networks (CNNs). DeepMind Health, developed by Google, was able to diagnose eye conditions from retinal scans with an accuracy level on par with skilled ophthalmologists by 2016 (Jansson et al., 2022; Yu et al., 2018).

2.2 Core AI Technologies: Machine Learning, Deep Learning, NLP, Computer Vision

Machine Learning (ML) is a fundamental component of Artificial Intelligence (AI), which uses algorithms to make informed predictions or decisions from data. It is divided into three primary categories: supervised learning, unsupervised learning, and reinforcement learning. ML forms the foundation for predictive models in healthcare, supporting tasks such as disease risk assessment, forecasting hospital readmissions, and evaluating potential treatment outcomes (Jansson et al., 2022)

Deep Learning (DL) is transforming early diagnosis and risk prediction in healthcare by enabling the analysis of vast and complex datasets with exceptional accuracy. DL models are particularly effective in processing high-dimensional inputs, such as medical imaging, to detect subtle anomalies, often surpassing human diagnostic performance. Beyond image analysis, DL enhances risk stratification by integrating heterogeneous data sources, such as electronic health records (EHRs), genomic data, and real-time metrics from wearable devices. This holistic approach allows for the prediction of various clinical conditions with improved precision (Lecun et al., 2015)

Reinforcement learning, a type of machine learning where algorithms learn optimal strategies through trial and error, is being explored to tailor individualized treatment regimens, dynamically balancing therapeutic efficacy with patient safety. Despite ongoing challenges, such as limited model interpretability and concerns around data privacy, DL's capacity to uncover latent patterns in unstructured and multimodal data positions it as a key enabler of precision medicine. When combined with clinical expertise, DL has the potential to reduce diagnostic delays, enhance prognostic accuracy, and fundamentally improve patient outcomes

Natural Language Processing (NLP) is becoming increasingly essential in the healthcare sector by unlocking valuable insights from unstructured text sources such as clinical notes, pathology reports, discharge summaries, and patient narratives. Advanced NLP technologies have made it possible to perform complex functions, including summarizing lengthy medical records, extracting and identifying clinical entities, and accurately interpreting contextual information (Al-Dekah & Sweileh, 2025; Alowais et al., 2023).

Computer vision, a rapidly advancing branch of AI, enables machines to interpret and analyze visual data with exceptional accuracy. In healthcare, it is revolutionizing clinical practice by facilitating the automated analysis of medical images, detecting subtle abnormalities, assessing disease severity, and aiding in diagnosing a wide range of conditions (Khalifa & Albadawy, 2024)

2.3 Data Types Used: EHRs, Imaging, Genomic, Sensor Data

Artificial intelligence in healthcare uses various data types to generate insights and support clinical decision-making. Electronic health records (EHRs), medical imaging, genomic data, and sensor-derived data are the most commonly used. EHRs provide structured information like demographics, diagnoses, medications, and clinical narratives, while medical imaging data includes high-dimensional visual information like X-rays, CT scans, MRIs, and histopathology slides. Computer vision algorithms analyze these images to detect anomalies, grade disease severity, and highlight regions of interest. Genomic data offers insights into a patient's genetic makeup, enabling precision medicine. Sensor and wearable data, collected from devices like fitness trackers and smartwatches, provide real-time insights into physiological parameters. AI systems analyze this data to detect early signs of deterioration, manage chronic conditions, and encourage proactive interventions (Zhu et al., 2024). These heterogeneous data types provide a comprehensive picture of patient health, enabling more accurate diagnoses, earlier interventions, and tailored treatments.

2.4 Ethical and regulatory Frameworks Shaping AI Adoption

The integration of artificial intelligence (AI) in healthcare is influenced by ethical and regulatory frameworks to ensure patient safety, data privacy, and equitable access to care. Issues like algorithmic bias, transparency, and accountability are being addressed. Regulatory agencies like the FDA and EMA are developing standards for AI-powered medical devices, emphasizing explainable AI, rigorous validation, and strong data governance. Data protection and patient consent are governed by frameworks like GDPR and HIPAA. Collaboration among technologists, clinicians, ethicists, and policymakers is crucial to ensure AI is used responsibly and ethically to improve health outcomes (Al-Dekah & Sweileh, 2025; Alowais et al., 2023).

3 EARLY DIAGNOSIS USING AI: A SYSTEMATIC APPROACH

Modern medicine is shifting its focus from treating severe diseases to preventing them through early intervention. Early diagnosis is crucial in identifying illnesses in their earliest stages, often before symptoms appear or damage becomes irreversible. AI offers powerful solutions, processing large amounts of data, recognizing subtle patterns, and making accurate predictions. AI can spot faint signals of illness that experienced clinicians might miss. This approach goes beyond technology, involving developing smart algorithms, testing them across diverse populations, ensuring compatibility with existing medical systems, and considering ethical and legal concerns. This chapter explores the systematic approach to using AI for early diagnosis, discussing the importance of early detection, key AI techniques, real-world case studies, and evaluation of AI systems. The goal is to provide healthcare professionals, researchers, and policymakers with a clear understanding of how AI is transforming early diagnosis and what is needed to successfully implement it in everyday medical practice.

3.1 Definition and Importance of Early Diagnosis

Early diagnosis refers to the identification of a disease or condition at its initial stages, often before symptoms become apparent or when they remain mild and non-specific. This critical phase in the disease timeline offers a window of opportunity where intervention can significantly alter the disease course, potentially preventing progression, reducing complications, and improving overall outcomes. The field of AI early diagnosis encompasses the application of artificial intelligence technologies to identify these subtle early disease indicators with greater sensitivity and consistency than conventional approaches (Abràmoff et al., 2018).

3.2 AI Algorithms for Pattern Recognition in Early Symptoms

The capacity of artificial intelligence systems to recognise trends in early illness symptoms depends on advanced algorithms meant to extract significant information from challenging medical data. Though their methods, complexity, and application differ, these algorithms have as their main objective the identification of minute patterns suggesting early illness states. Appreciating how artificial intelligence could improve early detection across many disciplines depends on knowing these computational techniques (Ghaffar Nia et al., 2023).

3.2.1 Machine Learning Approaches for Medical Image Analysis

Particularly in medical imaging, machine learning techniques for pattern identification have transformed the way doctors spot subtle illness indications. By learning from examples instead than strictly obeying clearly set rules, these algorithms can find intricate patterns that can be impossible to express using conventional programming techniques (de Bruijne, 2016).

Medical image analysis often employs supervised learning, where algorithms are trained on labelled data to detect characteristics linked to malignancy. Conventional machine learning techniques like k-nearest neighbors, random forests, and support vector machines (SVMs) are used for this purpose, but may overlook intricate patterns not explicitly encoded. Unsupervised learning, which uses a small amount of labelled data alongside a larger pool of unlabelled data, helps identify abnormalities that differ from regular patterns or natural groups of similar images. This method may reveal clinically important differences not previously noted. Semi-supervised learning, which combines aspects of both supervised and unsupervised procedures, is useful in medical applications where professional annotations are costly and time-consuming. Transfer learning, which adapts a model learned on one job, often using a large dataset from another domain, is particularly effective for medical image interpretation when labelled data is scarce. This method uses the general pattern recognition capacity acquired from the larger dataset to adapt to the specific features of medical pictures (McKinney et al., 2020).

3.2.2 Deep Learning Networks in Diagnostic Applications

Deep learning, a subclass of machine learning, has proven effective in medical diagnostics by learning hierarchical data representations using artificial neural networks with multiple layers. This eliminates the need for hand feature designing. Convolutional neural networks (CNNs) have been used for medical image processing, identifying local patterns using convolutional layers, pooling layers for spatial invariance, and fully connected layers for final classification (Mall et al., 2023).

CNNs have proven useful in various medical imaging applications, including skin lesion classification, radiography, pathology, and pathology. Long Short-Term Memory (LSTM) networks and recurrent neural networks (RNNs) excel in handling sequential data, such as continuous glucose monitoring, EEGs, and ECGs. These networks can detect subtle patterns and guide behavior over time. Transformer models, originally designed for natural language processing, have shown potential in medical uses by parallelizing and capturing long-range relationships. They can analyze sequences without the recurrence mechanism of RNNs, handling tasks from clinical text analysis to sequential imaging study processing and molecular structure modeling for drug development (Ahsan et al., 2022).

3.2.3 Clinical Data Interpretation Natural Language Processing

Natural Language Processing (NLP) is a branch of artificial intelligence that enables machines to understand and interpret human language. It is crucial in healthcare for extracting useful information from unstructured clinical text, such as doctors' notes, radiology reports, pathology summaries, and patient symptoms. NLP techniques like Named Entity Recognition (NER) can identify and classify key clinical elements, such as symptoms, diseases, medications, and treatments, which can help in early diagnosis. Relation extraction helps determine the relationships between different medical concepts in a given text, clarifying whether a symptom is affecting the patient and how it interacts with other health indicators. NLP can also analyze the tone and emotion behind clinical language through sentiment analysis, detecting signs of uncertainty or shifts in a patient's condition. Techniques like topic modeling and document classification help group and organize large amounts of healthcare data, uncovering patterns that spread across multiple records. (Savova et al., 2019)

Large language models (LLMs) like BERT and GPT have significantly advanced clinical natural language processing (NLP) by interpreting clinical language with greater nuance. These models are trained on large amounts of general text and fine-tuned for specific medical applications. They can accurately process complex medical terms, identify subtle cues, and recognize implicit information. Multimodal AI techniques, which combine NLP with other data sources like doctors' notes, medical images, lab results, and electronic health records, are promising for early diagnosis. These systems can build a comprehensive view of a patient's condition, identifying early signs of illness that may not be visible in isolation.

3.3 Case Studies

3.3.1 Oncology: AI for Early Cancer Detection

Artificial intelligence has significantly improved early cancer identification, particularly in medical picture analysis. Deep learning models have been trained to scan mammograms and identify early-stage breast cancer, often surpassing doctors. Google Health research shows AI can reduce false alarms and missed instances in breast cancer screenings **(Figure 1)**. AI is also aiding in lung cancer diagnosis by examining CT images and guiding clinicians in determining benign or malignant moles.(Hunter et al., 2022).

Figure 1. Benefits of AI in oncology

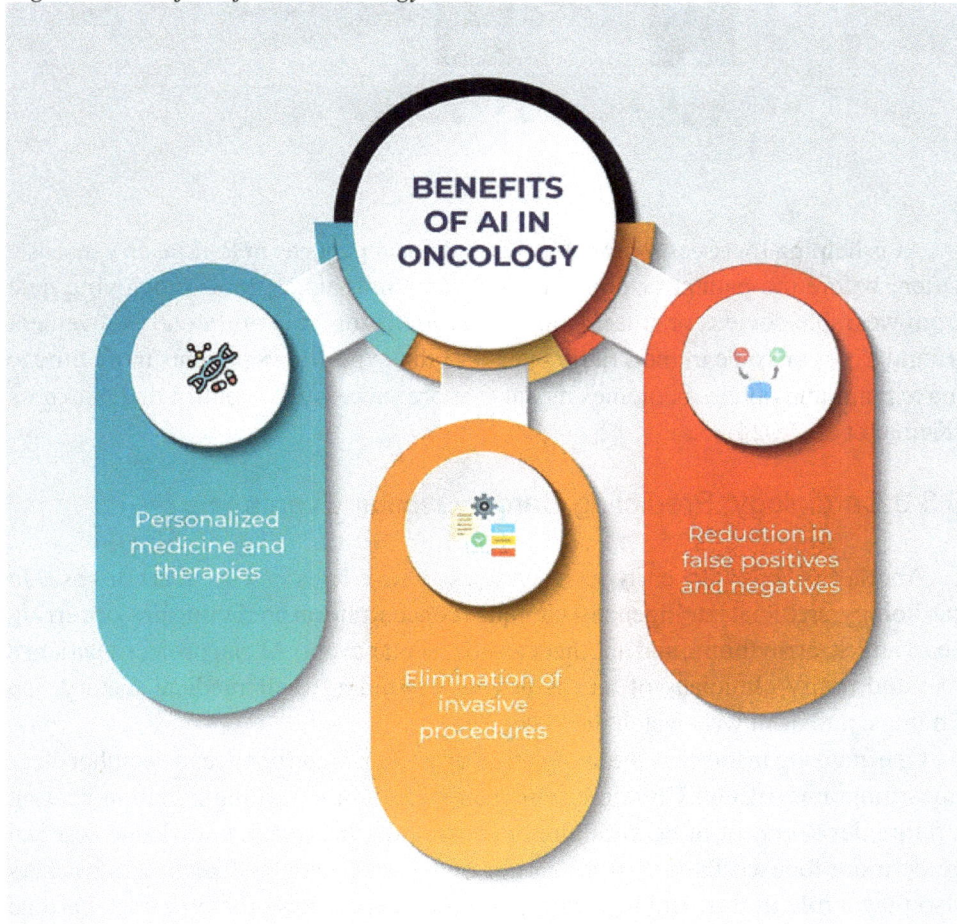

3.3.2 Neurology: Early Signs of Alzheimer's and Parkinson's

Regarding brain function, early diagnosis is really crucial. Diseases like Parkinson's and Alzheimer's sometimes start slowly and early on, symptoms could be minor or simple to ignore. By seeing alterations that could otherwise go unseen, artificial intelligence is enabling physicians to prevent some diseases. AI models may examine brain scans for early indicators of degeneration even years before a patient exhibits symptoms for Alzheimer's disease. Certain systems can even examine speech and writing patterns, spotting minute but constant language use variations that point to cognitive deterioration (Fig.2).

Figure 2. Neurology: Detecting Alzheimer's and Parkinson's disease using AI

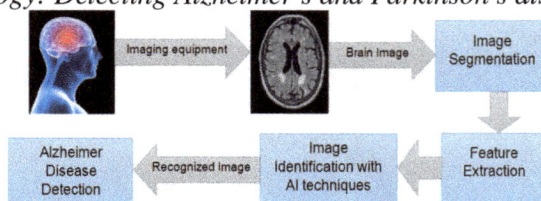

AI is helping to assess motor abilities and vocal patterns in Parkinson's disease. Often, before the patient or clinician finds anything amiss, tools employing data from wearable devices or smartphone applications might identify early movement irregularities or voice tremor. Early insight of this type allows patients more time to make plans and obtain medicines meant to more successfully control their sickness (Kumar et al., 2024).

3.3.3 Cardiology: Predicting Cardiovascular Events

Another place where early intervention can save lives is with heart disease. In cardiology, artificial intelligence techniques concentrate on predicting pre-occurring heart attack, arrhythmia, and another cardiovascular event. AI can project a patient's risk and notify clinicians of any issues by examining their medical history, lab findings, and even wristwatch data (Fig.3).

One amazing instance is the application of artificial intelligence to decipher electrocardiograms (ECGs). Certain systems can detect minor warning signals indicating a future development of heart failure or an irregular heartbeat, knowledge that can guide more focused therapy from earlier on. earable gadgets like fitness trackers also play a role in this. Built-in artificial intelligence allows them to track cardiac rhythms and deliver real-time alarms should something seem amiss, therefore enabling individuals to receive assistance before a crisis starts (Almansouri et al., n.d.).

Figure 3. AI in Cardiology

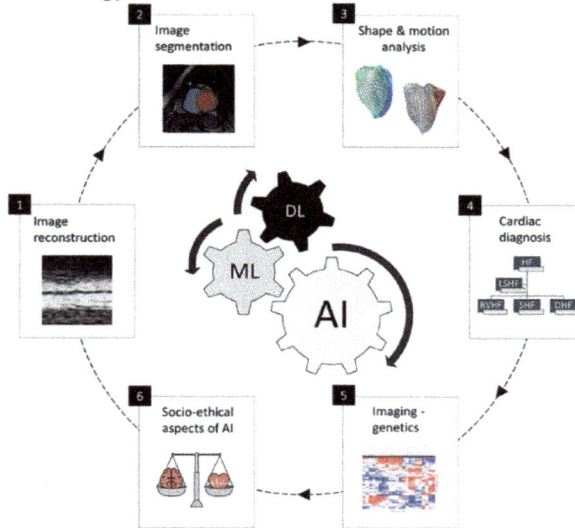

3.4 Evaluation Metrics: Sensitivity, Specificity, ROC Curves

Artificial intelligence (AI) plays a crucial role in medical judgments, and evaluation criteria are essential to gauge its dependability and precision. Sensitivity measures the degree of real illness case discovery, while specificity indicates the degree to which the system can exclude non-ill individuals. Precision is the proportion of accurate positive findings, especially in early diagnosis. The F1 score combines sensitivity and precision, especially in unusual scenarios. The Receiver Operating Characteristic (ROC) curve is a vital tool for evaluating AI models' performance in early disease diagnosis. It plots the true positive rate against the false positive rate, offering a comprehensive view of the trade-offs between detecting disease and avoiding false alarms. A higher AUC closer to 1.0 indicates a more accurate diagnostic tool, particularly in healthcare, where timely detection can significantly impact treatment outcomes and patient prognosis (Mennella et al., 2024).

Figure 4. ROC curve for AI in disease detection

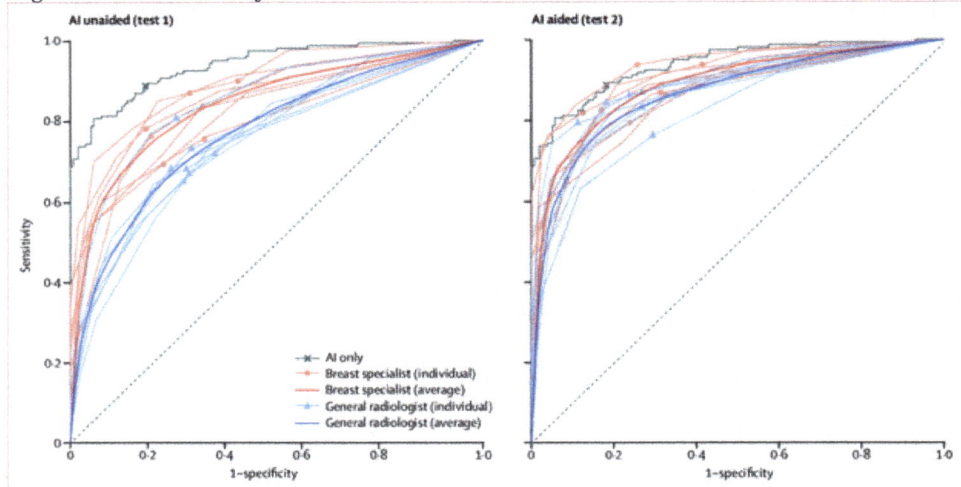

4 RISK PREDICTION MODELS IN CLINICAL PATHWAYS

4.1 Risk Prediction: Concepts and Clinical Value

Risk prediction is a crucial aspect of the healthcare system, predicting the likelihood of a patient's future health outcomes. It involves combining various factors such as demographics, clinical signs, laboratory results, imaging, genetic data, and lifestyle parameters to determine the likelihood of future health incidents. These probabilities guide clinicians in decisions about diagnostics, treatment planning, surveillance strategies, and preventive measures. Risk Prediction Models (RPM) improve medical decision-making by providing objective evaluations of potential health consequences using statistical algorithms. Recent advancements in AI and machine learning are leading to more sophisticated and accurate models (Sharma et al., 2021).

Clinical risk prediction models are divided into diagnostic and prognostic models. Diagnostic models predict the likelihood of a specific medical condition, while prognostic models estimate the likelihood of developing a specific medical outcome over time (Fig. 6). These models inform patients, family, and healthcare professionals about prognosis, aid in testing and treatment choices, and strategize for therapeutic trials. Diagnostic models focus on the patient's current health, while prognostic models predict future health outcomes based on predictor factors.

Figure 5. Diagrammatic illustration of diagnostic and prognostic model research.

Diagnostic prediction modeling

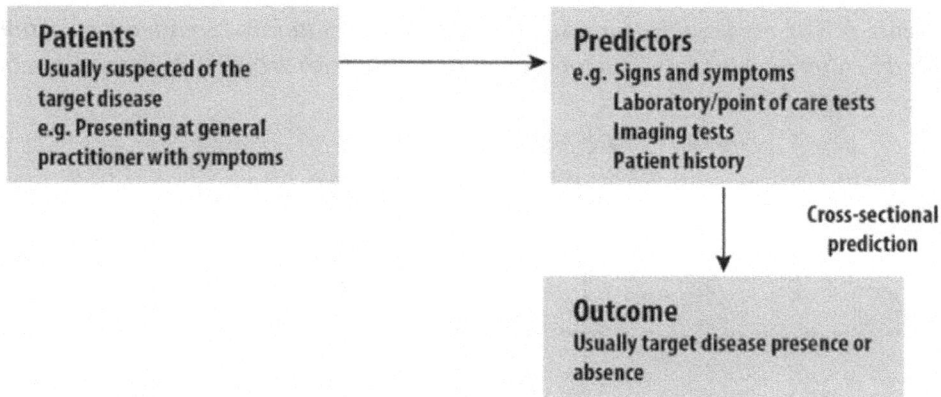

Despite recognizing the value of risk models, careful consideration must be given to several practical issues, including model generalizability, data quality, interpretability, integration into electronic health records and clinician training. Additionally, issues related to bias, transparency, and informed consent are of importance when considering risk models that incorporate artificial intelligence and big data analytics.

4.2 Stratification of Patient Populations Using AI

Innovative analytical approaches and large patient populations enable the classification of complicated illnesses into distinct subgroups, allowing for more tailored treatment. Genetic, epidemiological, and environmental variables influence complex illnesses like cancer, dementia, and diabetes. New analytical approaches are needed to identify disease biomarkers that reliably differentiate illness subgroups, allowing for better understanding of their architecture. These groups can help identify new drug targets and tailor treatments to individual patients based on genetics, phenotype, and co-morbid conditions (Fig 7).

Traditional 'one size fits all' medical models result in a 'one size fits all' approach, leading to delays in establishing effective prescriptions and increased costs. Precision medicine, which uses personal data and disease-specific insights, promises improved medicines, patient outcomes, and lower healthcare expenditures. Correct patient stratification improves knowledge about disease risk, progression rate, and therapeutic response, and can cut healthcare costs while optimizing patient benefits. In the future, clinical decision-making tools based on disease architecture will be used to tailor treatments to specific patients, increasing treatment efficiency, saving costs, and minimizing negative effects for patients and physicians. (Gardner et al., 2020)

Figure 6. The medical decision support system offers tailored treatment selection, lifestyle/diet advice tools, and an instructional framework based on patient results.

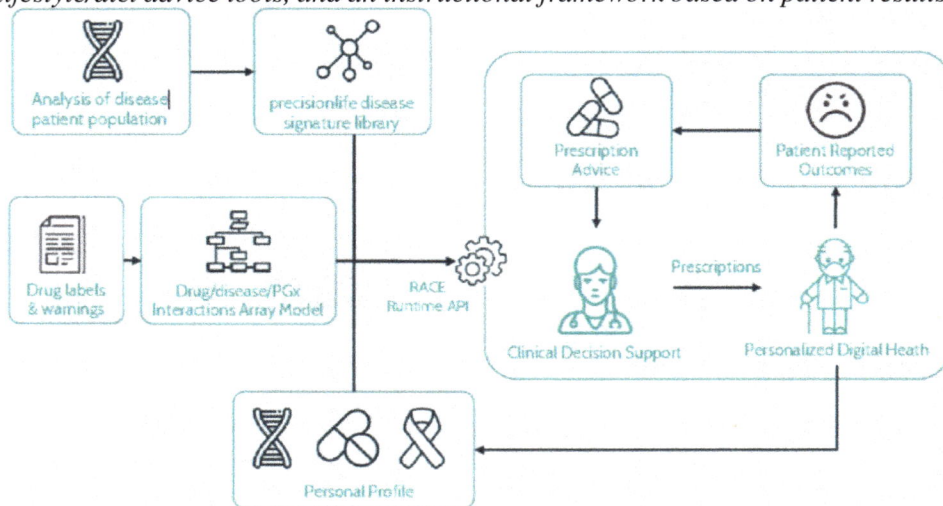

Source: Gardner et al. (2020)

AI and machine learning algorithms are being used in healthcare to evaluate patients' risk, optimize resource allocation, predict drug-drug interactions, accelerate drug development, and identify disease-related pathways. This data-driven approach helps triage patients, optimize medical resource allocation, reduce emotional stress, and improve treatment selection (Bello et al., 2023).

4.3 Integration of AI in Predictive Analytics Tools

Artificial Intelligence (AI) is revolutionizing the healthcare sector by transforming predictive analysis models and preventative care. AI helps healthcare practitioners predict health concerns and reduce risks, enhancing patient outcomes and the efficiency and cost-effectiveness of healthcare delivery. AI models use patient data, such as genetics, electronic health records, and lifestyle, to predict chronic diseases like cancer, diabetes, and heart disease. This enables early detection and tailored treatment plans. AI also predicts outbreaks of diseases and public health trends, allowing public health officials to allocate resources and prepare for health emergencies.

Preventive care aims to reduce illness risk and improve overall health by enabling personalized medicines based on risk profiles. AI-powered tools can identify individuals at risk for specific diseases or hereditary problems, recommending targeted screening campaigns, lifestyle changes, or preventative interventions. Wearables with AI and remote monitoring tools can measure health metrics in real-time, allowing for timely interventions and adjustments to treatment plans (Fig 8).

AI technologies are used in developing predictive analytics and preventative medicine, including machine learning, deep learning, and natural language processing. However, challenges remain, such as security and privacy concerns, data quality and diversity, and the need for training on large datasets (Abbasi et al., 2023)

Figure 7. The eight AI disciplines for clinical risk prediction

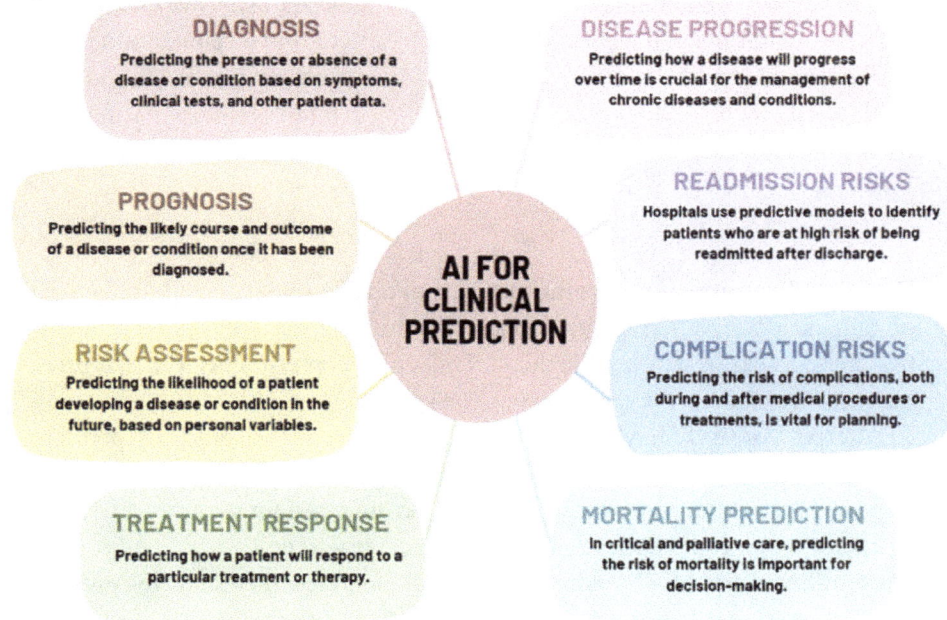

DIAGNOSIS
Predicting the presence or absence of a disease or condition based on symptoms, clinical tests, and other patient data.

DISEASE PROGRESSION
Predicting how a disease will progress over time is crucial for the management of chronic diseases and conditions.

PROGNOSIS
Predicting the likely course and outcome of a disease or condition once it has been diagnosed.

READMISSION RISKS
Hospitals use predictive models to identify patients who are at high risk of being readmitted after discharge.

AI FOR CLINICAL PREDICTION

RISK ASSESSMENT
Predicting the likelihood of a patient developing a disease or condition in the future, based on personal variables.

COMPLICATION RISKS
Predicting the risk of complications, both during and after medical procedures or treatments, is vital for planning.

TREATMENT RESPONSE
Predicting how a patient will respond to a particular treatment or therapy.

MORTALITY PREDICTION
In critical and palliative care, predicting the risk of mortality is important for decision-making.

Source: Khalifa and Albadawy (2024)

5 AI INTEGRATION ACROSS CLINICAL PATHWAYS

5.1 AI-Enabled Clinical Decision Support Systems (CDSS)

Clinical Decision Support Systems (CDSS) are computer-based tools that help healthcare professionals make clinical decisions. They combine technology and medical experience to provide practical insights, recommendations, and patient-specific data to improve diagnosis, treatment, and patient outcomes. CDSS connects medical information, complex algorithms, and patient data to enable informed and rapid choices. AI has gained popularity in recent years, with a focus on practical applications in healthcare. AI can help healthcare workers make clinical and administrative choices, increase healthcare system efficiency, and improve patient care. Examples of AI technologies used in CDSS include machine learning, deep learning, natural language processing, and fuzzy logic. Machine learning models can predict outcomes based on input, deep learning uses neural networks to interpret complex data, natural language processing combines computer science and linguistics to understand human language, and fuzzy logic covers imprecise thinking and artificial intelligence.

Benefits

a) **Data Analysis and Interpretation:** AI can efficiently analyze large volumes of clinical data from various sources, identifying patterns and connections that human therapists may overlook. This enables physicians to make precise judgments and detect early signs of deterioration.

b) **Predictive Analytics:** AI enhances clinical decision assistance by predicting patient outcomes, identifying at-risk patients, executing preventative measures, improving treatment approaches, and allocating resources more efficiently, ultimately improving patient care and medical efficiency.

c) **Personalization:** AI is revolutionizing personalized medicine by providing tailored treatment based on a patient's genetics, illness history, lifestyle, and current data, enhancing effectiveness and reducing adverse reactions compared to traditional methods.

d) **Continuous Learning:** AI enhances clinical decision assistance by continuously learning and evolving, responding to changing healthcare practices and evidence. It provides precise, timely, and accurate assistance, ensuring its success in the ever-changing healthcare market (Pindi, 2019; Tupsakhare, 2023)

5.2 Real-Time Data Interpretation for Workflow Optimization

Figure 8. Clinical workflow diagram. A routine clinical process is compared to one that includes an image analysis method for preliminary analysis. Seven software components are listed as required for integration into a healthcare setting. Component 8 was not constructed in this research, but is included for future integration purposes. Abbreviations: AI (artificial intelligence), DB (database), RIS (radiology information system), and PACS (picture archiving and communication system).

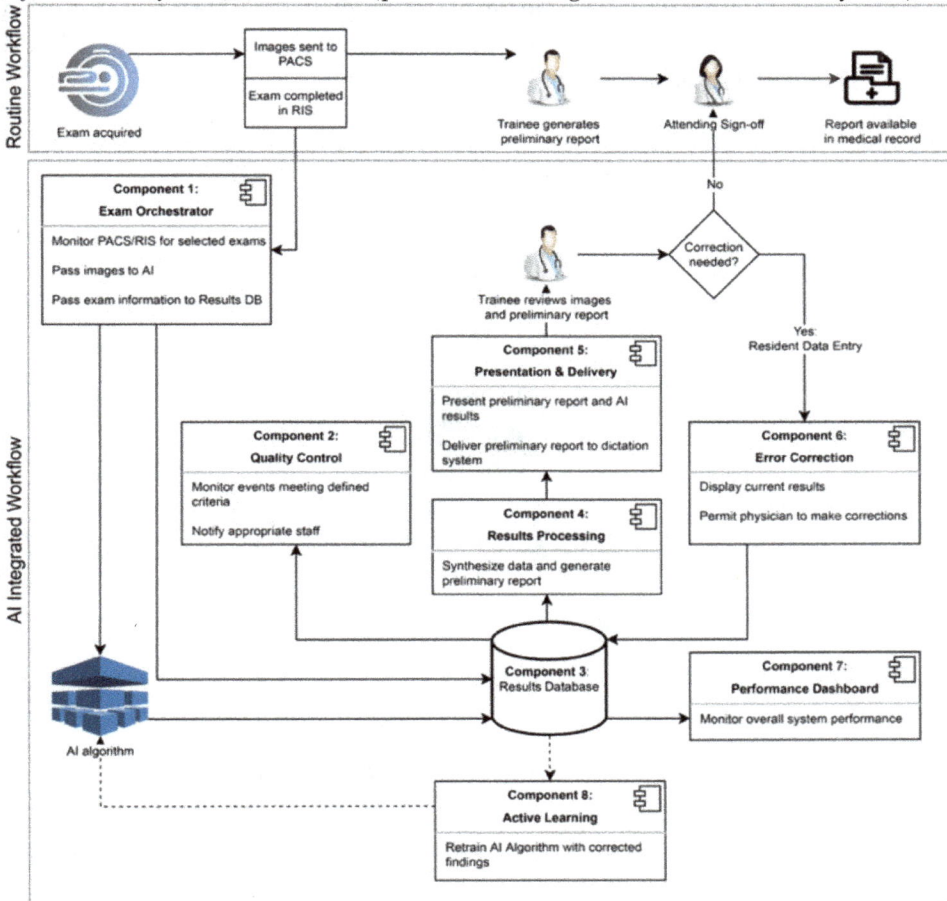

Source: Juluru et al. (2021)

AI algorithms can optimize patient flow by analyzing patterns in hospitalizations, discharges, and transfers, allowing hospitals to allocate resources and adjust personnel accordingly. They can also predict daily or seasonal swings in patient admissions, reducing bottlenecks and shortening wait times. AI-powered scheduling systems can create ideal schedules by analyzing factors like medical professional availability, patient preferences, and immediate care needs, reducing appointment no-shows and last-minute cancellations. They can respond in real time to emergencies by rescheduling non-urgent appointments with minimal disturbance. AI can also reduce waiting times in emergency departments and outpatient clinics by estimating patient influx and detecting possible delays. They can also enhance patient experience by providing accurate data on appointment hours, wait times, and therapeutic schedules, managing expectations and reducing anxiety during medical consultations. AI scheduling now includes telemedicine services and in-person visits, making it useful for regular follow-ups and medical emergencies.(Maleki Varnosfaderani & Forouzanfar, 2024)

Figure 9. Benefits of integrated AI algorithms in clinical workflow

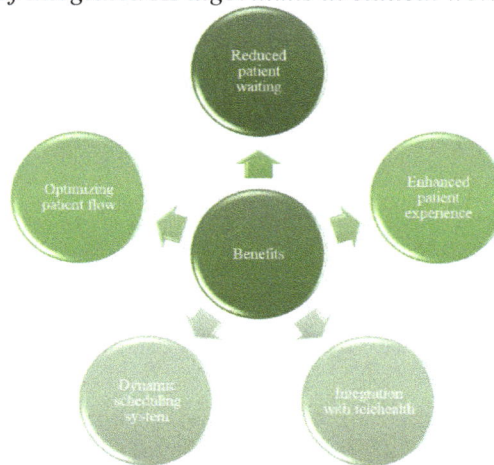

5.3 Enhancing Triage Systems and Referral Protocols

Emergency departments (EDs) are crucial for providing prompt and efficient care to patients with various health issues. However, overcrowding in EDs can lead to postponed treatment, higher morbidity, and extended suffering. Traditional triage methods rely on subjective clinical judgment, leading to discrepancies and biases. AI-driven triage systems can address these drawbacks by analyzing large volumes of patient data, reducing subjectivity and providing consistent outcomes. AI can analyze factors in seconds, allowing for more accurate and relevant triage results. AI-powered triage systems also help organize resources more efficiently, especially during high-volume situations. They can autonomously prioritize patients based on real-time circumstances and availability of resources, improving patient outcomes, sustaining ED throughput, and lowering stress for healthcare professionals. Overall, AI-driven triage systems offer a viable solution to improve ED efficiency and patient care.

Components of AI AI-Driven Triage System

AI triage tools enhance patient evaluation speed and efficiency in emergency departments by utilizing data collection, processing, algorithmic models, feedback, real-time analytics, and natural language processing (NLP). These systems outperform traditional techniques in detecting sepsis, identifying high-risk patients, and managing unstructured medical information. Real-world AI triage systems have improved patient wait times and resource allocation, demonstrating significant breakthroughs in emergency department triage systems (Da'Costa et al., 2025).

Figure 10. A diagram of the key elements and process of AI-powered triage systems for emergency rooms. The figure shows the path from patient data intake to triage decision and outcomes. The procedure begins with patient data acquisition, followed by systematic data gathering and processing. The system relies on AI processing, which includes algorithmic analysis, feedback in real time, and NLP to comprehend unstructured information.

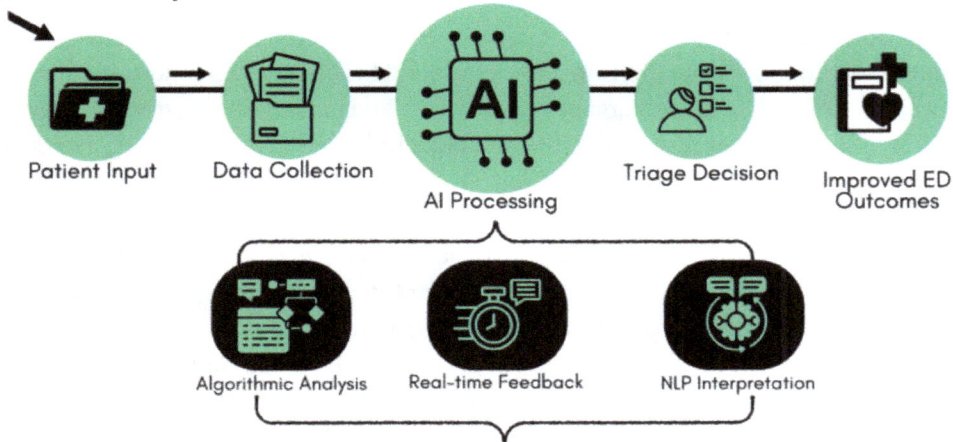

Patient Input → Data Collection → AI Processing → Triage Decision → Improved ED Outcomes

Algorithmic Analysis · Real-time Feedback · NLP Interpretation

Source: Da'Costa et al. (2025)

Table 1. Key components of AI AI-based triage system

Component	Purpose
Data collection and processing	• AI-driven triage relies heavily on collecting and processing large amounts of information about patients, which serves as a base for predictive models. • The inputs of data for these systems include vital signs, medical history, symptoms, and demographic information, providing valuable insights into a patient's status.
Algorithmic models	• Machine learning algorithms can analyze and categorize patient risk factors according to complicated data trends. • AI systems can detect clinical trends linked with serious situations using models trained on large historical datasets.
Real-Time analytics and feedback	• It allows clinicians to arrive at quick and educated judgments, particularly during busy periods or mass casualty occurrences. • Real-time analytics improve the utilization of resources by dynamically prioritizing depending on patient load, on-call specialists, and bed availability. • AI-driven triage reduces clinician burden, allowing physicians to focus on essential decision-making instead of constantly watching for abrupt patient status alterations.
Natural language processing (NLP)	• It can comprehend unstructured data, providing additional depth to the triage process. • AI can identify early indicators of illnesses like sepsis or stroke in medical records and highlight them for prompt care.

Benefits

AI-driven triage systems improve patient prioritization and decrease wait times by identifying high-risk situations in real-time data. This can shorten time-to-treatment by up to 20%, enhancing emergency quality care and patient satisfaction. AI-driven triage systems also provide reliability and objectivity in triage judgments, avoiding subjective evaluations and human error. They can adapt to mass casualty incidents by adjusting prioritizing based on patient volume, seriousness, and resource availability. This flexibility helps emergency departments manage large patient volumes under harsh conditions, reducing cognitive and mental strain. AI-powered triage systems maximize resource allocation by forecasting ED demand and patient outcomes, enabling optimal staff scheduling, bed management, and surge planning. This helps ED management avert congestion and create a more proactive emergency care environment (Da'Costa et al., 2025).

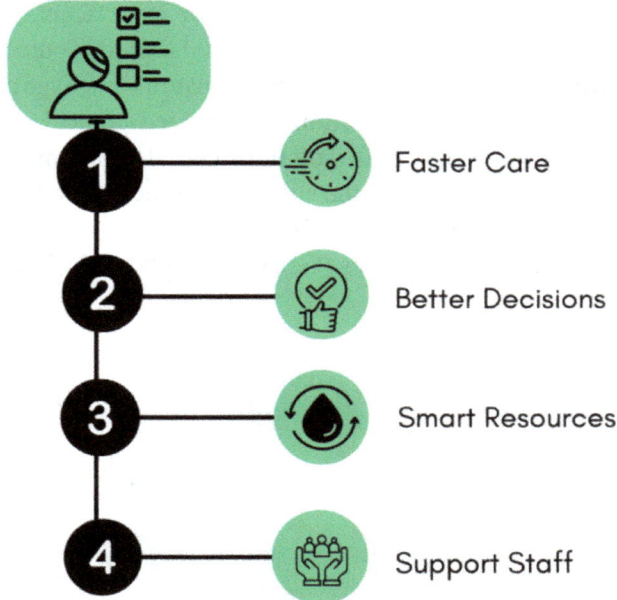

Figure 11. The main advantages of AI-driven triage systems in Eds. The graphic focuses on the "AI Triage System" as the major element, resulting in four significant advantages. The groupings are as follows: (1) "Faster Care" (reduced waiting periods and enhanced efficiency), (2) "Better Decisions" (enhancing clinical choice-making and risk evaluation), (3) "Smart Resources" (optimized allocation of resources and usage), and (4) "Support Staff" (reduced mental strain and greater assistance for clinical employees).

Source: Da'Costa et al. (2025)

5.4 Interoperability With Electronic Health Record Systems (EHRs)

Healthcare organizations regularly collect electronic health records (EHRs), which include demographics, diagnoses, test findings, prescriptions, medical notes, and photographs. EHRs offer a unique opportunity to analyze clinical occurrences across large populations using data and machine learning. They can help manage population health, inform healthcare policy decisions, and provide personalized patient trajectories. As healthcare evolves, there is a growing demand for integrating Artificial Intelligence (AI) into EHR systems to optimize procedures, automate tasks, and improve patient outcomes.

AI can significantly improve clinical efficiency and patient outcomes in healthcare organizations. By integrating AI into Electronic Health Records (EHR) systems, healthcare practitioners can improve diagnosis and treatment planning, stratify patients based on risk factors, enhance data management, automate documentation, reduce physician burnout, and match clinical trials more efficiently. AI-powered diagnostic assistance systems can analyze patient data, such as health records, test findings, and imaging investigations, allowing for more accurate evaluation and faster diagnosis. AI-based predictive modeling can also predict outcomes and provide individualized treatment approaches. AI-powered natural language processing (NLP) algorithms can extract information from unorganized clinical notes, simplifying data administration. AI-driven EHR solutions can also automate documentation and streamline workflow, reducing the strain on physicians and reducing burnout. Overall, AI can significantly improve clinical trial matching, reducing recruiting time and improving patient outcomes (Gorrepati, 2024; Nelson R Saranya, 2024).

Figure 12. Benefits of AI integration with EHRs

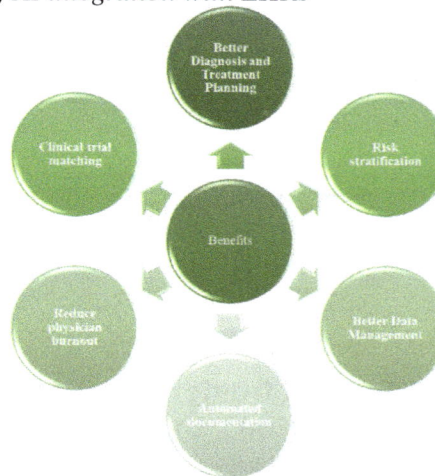

6 CHALLENGES AND LIMITATIONS

6.1 Data Quality and Heterogeneity

The volume of information in organizational processes has grown due to information and communication technology. The quality of data is crucial as it can indicate poor process quality and affect an organization's ability to satisfy customer demands and generate value efficiently. Modern organizations use data everywhere, making evaluating and enhancing its quality challenging due to the context in which it is provided. Data sources are categorised based on their structure, such as structured data, semi-structured data, and unstructured data. Businesses employ approaches to evaluate and enhance the calibre of their information resources, considering variations in data formats. Techniques like data cleansing and record matching are used to maintain databases, while more structured templates, formal lexicons, and internal auditing procedures improve the quality of an organization's papers.

6.2 Algorithmic Bias and Model Explainability

Algorithmic bias in health systems is a significant issue due to the "black-box" nature of algorithms, inadequate contextual specificity, and a lack of precise definitions and standards for fairness. This bias is not only technological but also produced by data inequities that determine who becomes sick, gets care, is represented in health system data sets, is treated, and survives. To address this, teams creating algorithms should be aware of the unique characteristics of the health system context, take into account the varying needs of various groups, and appropriately regulate and evaluate algorithms and the data science process.

To counter algorithmic bias, it is essential to establish processes to counter the risks of bias in algorithm development, such as designing "human-in-the-loop" systems and promoting transparency and explainability in algorithm development. The public sector can mitigate algorithmic bias by creating fairness requirements, regulating health system algorithms, addressing hidden biases in society, and promoting collaboration between public and private sectors.

6.3 Clinical Validation and Generalizability

Validation

Clinical prediction models (CPMs) estimate an individual's risk of both present and future occurrences. The pipeline for producing CPMs includes model development, internal validation, external validation, and impact evaluation. Internal validation involves analyzing the model's performance using the same dataset as the CPM, correcting for in-sample optimism. External validation is the gold standard for model credibility, examining the model's performance over one or more datasets. The model's performance is examined in a specific population and environment, either in the same or different population or setting. Researchers also evaluate generalisability by examining performance in various settings and populations. Validation is crucial in these types, as the validation dataset corresponds to the target population and setting. Researchers can also examine model performance in a new, easily accessible dataset that isn't typical of the population or environment of interest. However, the results may be misleading in these situations, as the validation dataset has minimal bearing on the target population and environment.

Clinical Validation

Clinical validation is crucial for medical records to ensure accurate diagnoses and operations. CMS prohibits providers from submitting claims with codes that cannot be clinically validated based on authoritative diagnostic standards, as it could result in overpayment. The RAC Statement of Work mandates clinical validation of diagnoses submitted on claims, which is a top priority for Medicare Advantage and commercial payers. Reporting clinically inaccurate diagnoses can lead to erroneous reimbursement, excessive denials, needless appeals, and regulatory audits. The method of guaranteeing adherence to legal and regulatory requirements has become controversial, with some arguing that a provider's diagnostic statement suffices for code assignment. However, compliance with CMS claims submission requirements and the need for more clinical data are crucial for accurate diagnosis.

Targeted Validation

When developing a Clinical Prediction Model (CPM), it is crucial to clearly define the intended application and population for which predictions are made. A tailored validation should be conducted to demonstrate the CPM's performance at that particular task. Targeted validation offers several benefits, such as providing estimates of predicted performance for the intended target context, allowing the CPM to be applied to various clinical populations and situations, and preventing research waste by focusing on creating and testing models with precisely defined practical applications. Performance in one target population is not a good predictor of performance in another, so it is vital to use different targeted validation exercises.

Performance varies greatly among populations and environments due to variations in baseline risk, predictor-outcome correlations, and case mix.

Therefore, any debate of validity needs to be contextualized within the location and target population. By determining the population and environment in which a model is meant to be applied, and finding appropriate datasets for validations that correspond to the intended population and environment, targeted validation tackles this issue. It prevents action on misleading validation studies and reduces research waste by being explicit about the target population and usage.

In cases where the data used for development and validation are identical, comprehensive internal validation using the development dataset should be the main focus. Proper measures during model development, including an adequate sample size, minimizing overfitting, accurately estimating and correcting in-sample optimism, and examining optimism by replaying all model development steps, can provide a robust estimate of the model's performance. Internal validation can be considered a trustworthy indicator of performance in the target group, and the absence of external validation is not a problem as long as all procedures are carefully carried out.

Validation Gap

Focused validation helps understand prediction performance by estimating the model's performance in Hospital B if the target population consists of its patients. However, targeted validation can lead to a "validation gap" if the validation was carried out in Hospital C due to lack of historical data or resource constraints. This gap indicates that the target population should use the Clinical Predictive Model (CPM) with caution. To address this, the distinctions between the validation population and the target population should be explained qualitatively or quantitatively. Reweighting the validation sample to more closely resemble the target population can help estimate global performance metrics like AUC. Implementing the CPM after validation and impact studies can lead to calibration drift and performance problems. Techniques like dynamic modelling or temporal recalibration can help CPMs react to changes over time.

6.4 Resistance to Adoption Among Healthcare Professionals

Resistance to change can manifest in various ways, such as lack of enthusiasm for new procedures or passive opposition. It can be a normal reaction to perceived uncertainty or a threat to one's well-being. To ensure successful innovation, resistance must be effectively managed through the adoption and implementation of new practices or technologies. In the healthcare industry, a constantly shifting system, legal requirements, and technological advancements create obstacles for providers and organizations. Over half of organizational change efforts fail, affecting even seasoned organizers. The European Paediatric Association's Social Paediatrics working group emphasizes the importance of balancing resistance with children's health needs. By raising awareness of the benefits of change, paediatricians can be more willing to adopt new operational and management techniques that benefit their patients.

The Unavoidable Need for Health Care Transformation and Change

Organisational change processes are crucial in various sectors, including healthcare, due to the rapid advancement of scientific knowledge and technological tools. Good change management is essential for adjusting to new administrative and organisational realities. Organisational transformation involves breaking old patterns, implementing new operational procedures, adding new functions, and creating new organizational balances. Two primary tactics for change are internal and external. Affirmative organisational change involves adopting new practices without impacting the organisation's culture. Normal organisational change impacts the healthcare structure's current strategies, while cultural advancement involves creating new values and presumptions. Radical organisational change involves reevaluating the organization's objectives, procedures, and areas of activity in response to special situations.

6.5 Understanding Resistance to Change

Change is a process that often faces opposition, as individuals perceive the future state as unpredictable and unclear. Resistance can arise from various sources, including fear of the unknown, loss of control, status quo comfort, perceived risk, lack of knowledge, structural and cultural barriers, and negative prior experiences. To effectively manage change, leaders in organizations, including the healthcare industry, must recognize that resistance is a normal reaction and that people are more likely to favor the status quo because it is comfortable and familiar. By understanding and managing these sources of resistance, organizations can effectively manage change and ensure successful implementation.

6.6 Resisting Resistance to Change

The success of a change initiative in healthcare depends on how resistance is handled. Emotional resilience is crucial for successful transformation and change projects. Reorganizing operational strategies, using flexibility, and following key strategies can make stakeholders more receptive to change. Effective communication, participation, education, resolving issues, acknowledging efforts, gradual implementation, clear leadership, transparency, and identifying change agents are essential for successful change initiatives. These agents can inspire and influence others, supporting and empowering their efforts within the company. By addressing issues, providing support, and fostering a culture of openness and communication, healthcare organizations can successfully navigate change initiatives.

6.7 Legal, Ethical, and Accountability Concerns

Patient rights are a subcategory of human rights, focusing on minimal expectations for how people should be treated by others. Ethics, on the other hand, are normative rules that dictate how society should treat others. Each patient's right is justified by one or more ethical principles. Healthcare quality consists of two main components: delivering a service that fulfills the patient's demands and standardizing the service to ensure equal care. Legislators must weigh the costs against an objective quality level that can be maintained for all patients across various healthcare facilities and fields. Bills of patient rights, developed by American healthcare organizations like the American Hospital Association and the American Cancer Society, empower people to take an active role in improving their health and strengthen relationships with healthcare providers. The purpose of rights in every community is to strike a balance between the well-being of the collective and the well-being of individuals. Commonly established patient rights include a strong emphasis on the patient's personal dignity, kindness, avoiding behaviors that put the patient at risk for injury, and equitable allocation of resources.

Normative ethics are the principles that guide human behavior, encompassing three types: virtue ethics, deontological ethics, and consequentialist ethics. These ethics are largely combined in contemporary normative ethics, resulting in "duty virtuism," where people expect healthcare professionals to exhibit specific values. Medical ethics principles that support patient rights are covered before their corresponding human rights, with the situation's individual circumstances, logic, and customs deciding which principle or virtue should be prioritized.

Beneficence, a medical ethical principle, involves acting in the patient's best interest during diagnosis and therapy. It often clashes with respect for patient autonomy, which requires doctors to evaluate and record capabilities. Nonmaleficence, on the other hand, is "not bringing harm" and involves treating patients without causing harm. This concept has roots in early Egyptian texts and has been recommended in the Hippocratic Oath. Medical interventions, such as imaging, drugs, physical manipulations, and invasive surgeries, are considered if they include harmful elements.

6.7.1 Maintaining a Person's Life, Sanctity, and Dignity

Ethics in healthcare has been a contentious topic since ancient times, with beliefs in creator gods and divinities dating back to ancient civilizations. However, not all societies accept that all people are equal and worthy of citizenship or life. In some cases, older and younger people are limited in rights, and a person's value and eligibility depend on factors like wealth, prestige, skills, virtues, religious affiliation, physical appearance, and clan membership. The concept of distributive justice, which ensures everyone is treated fairly, is particularly relevant in healthcare ethics. In Canada, a 1966 law granted everyone access to healthcare, while in the United States, 1986 laws allowed access to healthcare in medical emergencies and 2010 laws allowing maximum health insurance coverage. US patent rights are often governed by the legal system, with legislatures limiting rights to protect themselves from lawsuits. Each right has restrictions, exceptions, and related duties.

Patient rights are a subcategory of human rights, focusing on minimal expectations for how people should be treated by others. Ethics, on the other hand, are normative rules that dictate how members of a society should treat others. Each patient's right is justified by one or more ethical principles. These rights evolve over time, and when a company with the power to enforce an ethical standard does so, that organization has a right. Healthcare quality consists of two main components: delivering a service that fulfils the patient's demands and standardizing the service to ensure equal care for all patients. Legislators must weigh the costs against an objective quality level that can be maintained for all patients across various healthcare facilities and fields. Bills of patient rights empower people to take an active role in improving their health, strengthen relationships with healthcare providers, and help patients deal with insurance companies and other health coverage situations. Normative ethics define the proper way for people to behave, with three types dominated by virtue ethics, which balance the goal with the result. This activity aims to improve the application of patients' rights and ethical principles in clinical practice and better understand the role of healthcare professionals as advocates for patients' rights.

6.7.2 Health Information Privacy and Control

The Healthcare Quality Improvement Act of 1986 established patient rights to confidentiality, which were further expanded in 1996 by the Health Insurance Portability and Accountability Act. These rights include access to medical records, rectification of mistakes, and restrictions on access. HCPs and HCO business representatives may share patient information when necessary. Other rights include reporting STIs, supporting criminal investigations, and protecting public health.

However, emancipated minors and sexually active minors are typically granted secrecy under state legislation.

7 FUTURE DIRECTIONS AND INNOVATIONS

Artificial Intelligence (AI) is quickly reshaping healthcare as we know it, opening up exciting new possibilities to improve patient care, make clinical processes more efficient, and deliver treatments that are tailored to each individual. As AI technology continues to grow and evolve, we're seeing innovative solutions emerge that aim to tackle some of healthcare's toughest challenges—like protecting patient privacy, making AI systems more transparent, bringing together information from different sources, and personalizing treatment plans. In this discussion, we'll take a closer look at five promising areas that are shaping the future of AI in healthcare: federated learning and privacy-preserving AI, combining multiple types of data for better predictions, making AI decisions more understandable through explainable AI (XAI), using AI to advance personalized medicine, and exploring how generative models could change the way we diagnose diseases.(Hanna et al., 2025)

7.1 Federated Learning and Privacy-Preserving AI

One of the biggest challenges facing the widespread use of AI in healthcare is protecting patient privacy. Medical data is extremely sensitive, and regulations like HIPAA in the U.S. and GDPR in Europe set strict rules about how this information can be accessed, shared, and stored. Traditional AI systems often require gathering large amounts of data in one central place for training, but this approach can clash with privacy requirements and make it harder to comply with these laws.

Federated learning offers a promising solution to these concerns. Instead of moving raw patient data to a central server, federated learning allows each hospital or clinic to train the AI model locally, using its own data. Only the model's updates—like learned patterns or weights—are shared with a central system, which then combines them to improve the overall model. Throughout this process, the actual patient data never leaves the organization's secure environment.

This approach brings several important benefits:

- **Stronger privacy:** Because patient data stays within each institution, there's a much lower risk of data breaches or unauthorized access.
- **Easier compliance:** Federated learning helps organizations meet privacy regulations by reducing the need to transfer or centralize sensitive data.

- **Better collaboration:** Hospitals and research centers can work together to build better AI models without exposing confidential patient information.

Recent studies and pilot projects have shown that federated learning can be effective in real-world healthcare scenarios, such as predicting which patients might be readmitted to the hospital, identifying rare diseases, and improving how medical images are analyzed. As these systems evolve, they're starting to include even more advanced privacy protections—like differential privacy, secure multi-party computation, and homomorphic encryption—which further reduce the risk of sensitive data being exposed.

In short, federated learning is helping healthcare organizations tap into the power of AI while keeping patient data safe and maintaining public trust. As privacy concerns and regulations continue to evolve, these privacy-preserving approaches will be key to unlocking the full potential of AI in medicine.(Yu et al., 2018)

7.2 Multi-Modal Data Fusion for Holistic Predictions

Healthcare data is naturally complex and comes from a variety of sources—ranging from electronic health records (EHRs) and medical images to genetic information, wearable device data, and even patient self-reports. In the past, AI models typically analyzed just one type of data at a time, such as processing images or extracting information from clinical notes. However, the most meaningful clinical insights often arise when these different types of data are brought together, capturing the full picture of the biological, behavioral, and environmental factors that affect health.

This process, known as multi-modal data fusion, involves integrating and analyzing these diverse data sources to produce more complete and accurate predictions. By combining structured information like lab results and vital signs with unstructured data such as doctors' notes, as well as images and molecular data, AI can build a much richer and more holistic view of a patient's overall health.

Multi-modal data fusion refers to the process of integrating and analyzing heterogeneous data sources to generate more comprehensive and accurate predictions. By combining structured data (like lab results and vital signs), unstructured data (such as clinical notes), imaging data, and molecular profiles, AI systems can develop a more holistic understanding of a patient's health status.(Jansson et al., 2022)

The benefits of multi-modal data fusion include:

- **Improved diagnostic accuracy:** Integrating diverse data types can reveal patterns and correlations that may be missed when analyzing each modality separately.

- **Personalized risk stratification**: Multi-modal models can account for a broader range of risk factors, enabling more precise predictions for individual patients.
- **Enhanced decision support:** Clinicians can receive richer, context-aware recommendations that consider the full spectrum of patient information.

Recent advances in deep learning, particularly the development of architectures such as transformers and graph neural networks, have made it possible to effectively model complex relationships across modalities. For example, multi-modal AI systems are being used to predict cardiovascular events by combining imaging data, EHRs, and genetic information, or to forecast cancer progression by integrating pathology slides, radiology images, and clinical histories. As data integration standards improve and interoperability increases, multi-modal data fusion will become a cornerstone of next-generation AI-powered healthcare.(Khalifa & Albadawy, 2024)

7.3 Explainable AI (XAI) for Transparency in Diagnosis

As AI systems become more deeply embedded in clinical workflows, the need for transparency and interpretability has become paramount. Clinicians and patients alike must be able to understand and trust the recommendations made by AI, especially when these systems are used to inform high-stakes decisions such as diagnosis, treatment selection, or surgical planning.

Explainable AI (XAI) encompasses a range of methods and tools designed to make AI models more transparent, interpretable, and accountable. Unlike traditional "black box" models, which may provide accurate predictions without revealing their underlying logic, XAI aims to clarify how and why a particular decision was made.

Key aspects of XAI in healthcare include:

- **Feature attribution:** Techniques such as SHAP (Shapley Additive explanations) and LIME (Local Interpretable Model-agnostic Explanations) can highlight which features (e.g., lab values, symptoms, imaging findings) were most influential in a model's prediction.
- **Visual explanations:** In medical imaging, heatmaps or saliency maps can indicate which regions of an image contributed most to a diagnosis, helping radiologists validate AI findings.
- **Rule extraction:** Some XAI approaches attempt to extract human-readable rules or decision trees from complex models, making their logic more accessible to clinicians.

7.4 AI in Personalized Medicine and Precision Healthcare

One of the most transformative promises of AI in healthcare is its potential to enable personalized medicine—tailoring prevention, diagnosis, and treatment strategies to the unique characteristics of each patient. Traditional medical approaches often rely on population averages, which may not account for individual variability in genetics, lifestyle, environment, and disease biology.

AI-driven personalized medicine leverages advanced algorithms to analyze vast datasets, identify patient subgroups, and predict individual responses to therapies. This approach is particularly impactful in areas such as oncology, cardiology, and rare diseases, where heterogeneity among patients can significantly influence outcomes.

Key applications include:

- **Genomic medicine:** AI models can analyze genomic data to identify mutations, predict disease risk, and guide targeted therapies (e.g., selecting the most effective cancer treatment based on a tumor's genetic profile).
- **Pharmacogenomics:** By predicting how patients will metabolize certain drugs, AI can help avoid adverse reactions and optimize dosing.
- **Dynamic risk prediction:** Continuous monitoring of wearable sensor data, combined with EHRs, allows AI systems to provide real-time risk assessments and early warnings for conditions like sepsis or heart failure.
- **Adaptive treatment pathways:** Reinforcement learning and other adaptive algorithms can personalize treatment regimens, adjusting recommendations based on patient response and evolving clinical evidence.

As more data becomes available and AI models become increasingly sophisticated, the vision of truly individualized care—where every patient receives the right intervention at the right time—will move closer to reality. This shift has the potential to improve outcomes, reduce healthcare costs, and enhance patient satisfaction.(Al-Dekah & Sweileh, 2025; Yu & Kohane, 2019)

7.5 Potential of Generative Models in Diagnostics

Generative models, such as Generative Adversarial Networks (GANs) and large language models (LLMs), represent a cutting-edge frontier in AI research with significant implications for healthcare diagnostics. Unlike traditional discriminative models, which focus on classification or prediction, generative models are designed to create new data samples that resemble real-world data.

In diagnostics, generative models offer several promising applications:

- **Data augmentation:** GANs can generate realistic synthetic medical images to augment limited datasets, improving the performance of diagnostic algorithms—especially in rare diseases or underrepresented populations.
- **Anomaly detection:** By learning the normal distribution of healthy data, generative models can identify subtle deviations that may indicate early-stage disease or atypical presentations.
- **Automated report generation:** Large language models can assist clinicians by generating draft radiology or pathology reports, summarizing findings, and highlighting key observations.
- **Simulation and training:** Generative models can create realistic virtual patients or scenarios for medical education, helping train clinicians in recognizing rare or complex conditions.

Moreover, the combination of generative models with other AI techniques enables the synthesis of multi-modal data, such as generating corresponding pathology slides from radiology images or vice versa. This capability can facilitate cross-modal validation and support more comprehensive diagnostic workflows.

However, the use of generative models in healthcare also raises important ethical and practical considerations, including the risk of generating misleading or biased data, the need for rigorous validation, and concerns about data provenance. Addressing these challenges will be critical to harnessing the full potential of generative AI in diagnostics.(D'Adderio & Bates, 2025; Mohsen et al., 2022)

8 CONCLUSION

Artificial Intelligence (AI) is revolutionizing clinical prediction, enabling early diagnosis and risk assessment of diseases. AI-driven models can process vast datasets with precision and speed, surpassing traditional methods. Machine learning, deep learning, and natural language processing are now practical assets in radiology, pathology, genomics, and electronic health record analysis. These technologies uncover subtle patterns and trends, enabling early intervention and reducing disease burden. AI can facilitate real-time decision-making, reduce ICU mortality, and allocate resources more efficiently. However, the adoption of AI faces challenges such as data quality, algorithmic bias, model interpretability, and ethical compliance. The successful deployment of AI in healthcare requires rigorous validation, cross-disciplinary collaboration, and robust regulatory oversight. The vision is for a collaborative, AI-augmented healthcare system where technology enhances human expertise, combining data-driven insights with clinical practitioners' empathy and intuition. This will lead to an era of personalized and preventive medicine, where early diagnosis is the norm.

REFERENCES

Abbasi, N., Fnu, N., & Zeb, S. (2023). *AI in Healthcare: Integrating Advanced Technologies with Traditional Practices for Enhanced Patient Care. 2*(03).

Abràmoff, M. D., Lavin, P. T., Birch, M., Shah, N., & Folk, J. C. (2018). Pivotal trial of an autonomous AI-based diagnostic system for detection of diabetic retinopathy in primary care offices. npj. *Digital Medicine, 1*(1), 1–8. DOI: 10.1038/s41746-018-0040-6 PMID: 31304320

Al-Dekah, A. M., & Sweileh, W. (2025). Role of artificial intelligence in early identification and risk evaluation of non-communicable diseases: A bibliometric analysis of global research trends. *BMJ Open, 15*(5). Advance online publication. DOI: 10.1136/bmjopen-2025-101169 PMID: 40316361

Alowais, S. A., Alghamdi, S. S., Alsuhebany, N., Alqahtani, T., Alshaya, A. I., Almohareb, S. N., Aldairem, A., Alrashed, M., Bin Saleh, K., Badreldin, H. A., Al Yami, M. S., Al Harbi, S., & Albekairy, A. M. (2023). Revolutionizing healthcare: the role of artificial intelligence in clinical practice. In *BMC Medical Education* (Vol. 23, Issue 1). BioMed Central Ltd. https://doi.org/DOI: 10.1186/s12909-023-04698-z

Becker, J., Decker, J. A., Römmele, C., Kahn, M., Messmann, H., Wehler, M., Schwarz, F., Kroencke, T., & Scheurig-Muenkler, C. (2022). Artificial Intelligence-Based Detection of Pneumonia in Chest Radiographs. *Diagnostics (Basel), 12*(6). Advance online publication. DOI: 10.3390/diagnostics12061465 PMID: 35741276

Bello, B., Bundey, Y. N., Bhave, R., Khotimchenko, M., Baran, S. W., Chakravarty, K., & Varshney, J. (2023). Integrating AI/ML Models for Patient Stratification Leveraging Omics Dataset and Clinical Biomarkers from COVID-19 Patients: A Promising Approach to Personalized Medicine. *International Journal of Molecular Sciences, 24*(7), 7. Advance online publication. DOI: 10.3390/ijms24076250 PMID: 37047222

D'Adderio, L., & Bates, D. W. (2025). Transforming diagnosis through artificial intelligence. In *npj Digital Medicine* (Vol. 8, Issue 1). Nature Research. https://doi.org/DOI: 10.1038/s41746-025-01460-1

Da'Costa, A., Teke, J., Origbo, J. E., Osonuga, A., Egbon, E., & Olawade, D. B. (2025). AI-driven triage in emergency departments: A review of benefits, challenges, and future directions. *International Journal of Medical Informatics, 197*, 105838. DOI: 10.1016/j.ijmedinf.2025.105838 PMID: 39965433

Gardner, S., Das, S., Taylor, K., Gardner, S., Das, S., & Taylor, K. (2020). AI Enabled Precision Medicine: Patient Stratification, Drug Repurposing and Combination Therapies. In *Artificial Intelligence in Oncology Drug Discovery and Development*. IntechOpen. https://doi.org/DOI: 10.5772/intechopen.92594

Gorrepati, L. P. (2024). Integrating AI with Electronic Health Records (EHRs) to Enhance Patient Care. *International Journal of Health Sciences*, 7(8), 8. Advance online publication. DOI: 10.47941/ijhs.2368

Hanna, M. G., Pantanowitz, L., Dash, R., Harrison, J. H., Deebajah, M., Pantanowitz, J., & Rashidi, H. H. (2025). Future of Artificial Intelligence—Machine Learning Trends in Pathology and Medicine. In *Modern Pathology* (Vol. 38, Issue 4). Elsevier B.V. https://doi.org/DOI: 10.1016/j.modpat.2025.100705

Jansson, M., Ohtonen, P., Alalääkkölä, T., Heikkinen, J., Mäkiniemi, M., Lahtinen, S., Lahtela, R., Ahonen, M., Jämsä, S., & Liisantti, J. (2022). Artificial intelligence-enhanced care pathway planning and scheduling system: Content validity assessment of required functionalities. *BMC Health Services Research*, 22(1). Advance online publication. DOI: 10.1186/s12913-022-08780-y PMID: 36510176

Juluru, K., Shih, H.-H., Keshava Murthy, K. N., Elnajjar, P., El-Rowmeim, A., Roth, C., Genereaux, B., Fox, J., Siegel, E., & Rubin, D. L. (2021). Integrating AI Algorithms into the Clinical Workflow. *Radiology. Artificial Intelligence*, 3(6), e210013. DOI: 10.1148/ryai.2021210013 PMID: 34870216

Khalifa, M., & Albadawy, M. (2024). Artificial Intelligence for Clinical Prediction: Exploring Key Domains and Essential Functions. In *Computer Methods and Programs in Biomedicine Update* (Vol. 5). Elsevier B.V. https://doi.org/DOI: 10.1016/j.cmpbup.2024.100148

Khalifa, M., & Albadawy, M. (2024). Artificial Intelligence for Clinical Prediction: Exploring Key Domains and Essential Functions. *Computer Methods and Programs in Biomedicine Update*, 5, 100148. DOI: 10.1016/j.cmpbup.2024.100148

Lecun, Y., Bengio, Y., & Hinton, G. (2015). Deep learning. In *Nature* (Vol. 521, Issue 7553, pp. 436–444). Nature Publishing Group. https://doi.org/DOI: 10.1038/nature14539

Maleki Varnosfaderani, S., & Forouzanfar, M. (2024). The Role of AI in Hospitals and Clinics: Transforming Healthcare in the 21st Century. *Bioengineering (Basel, Switzerland)*, 11(4), 337. DOI: 10.3390/bioengineering11040337 PMID: 38671759

McKinney, S. M., Sieniek, M., Godbole, V., Godwin, J., Antropova, N., Ashrafian, H., & Suleyman, M. (2020). International evaluation of an AI system for breast cancer screening. *Nature*, *577*(7788), 89–94. DOI: 10.1038/s41586-019-1799-6 PMID: 31894144

Mohsen, F., Ali, H., El Hajj, N., & Shah, Z. (2022). Artificial intelligence-based methods for fusion of electronic health records and imaging data. *Scientific Reports*, *12*(1). Advance online publication. DOI: 10.1038/s41598-022-22514-4 PMID: 36289266

Nelson, R., & Saranya, S. (2024). Revolutionizing Health Records: The AI Way. [IJSR]. *International Journal of Scientific Research*, *13*(4), 1310–1313. DOI: 10.21275/SR24417190214

Pindi, V. (2019). *A AI-ASSISTED CLINICAL DECISION SUPPORT SYSTEMS: ENHANCING DIAGNOSTIC ACCURACY AND TREATMENT RECOMMENDATIONS | International Journal of Innovations in Engineering Research and Technology.* 6(10). https://doi.org/DOI: 10.26662/ijiert.v6i10.pp1-10

Sharma, V., Davies, A., & Ainsworth, J. (2021). Clinical risk prediction models: The canary in the coalmine for artificial intelligence in healthcare? *BMJ Health & Care Informatics*, *28*(1), e100421. DOI: 10.1136/bmjhci-2021-100421 PMID: 34607819

Tupsakhare, P. (2023). Improving Clinical Decision Support in Health Care Through AIs. *Progress in Medical Sciences*, *1–4*. Advance online publication. DOI: 10.47363/PMS/2023(7)E118

van Smeden, M., Reitsma, J. B., Riley, R. D., Collins, G. S., & Moons, K. G. (2021). Clinical prediction models: Diagnosis versus prognosis. *Journal of Clinical Epidemiology*, *132*, 142–145. DOI: 10.1016/j.jclinepi.2021.01.009 PMID: 33775387

Yu, K. H., Beam, A. L., & Kohane, I. S. (2018). Artificial intelligence in healthcare. In *Nature Biomedical Engineering* (Vol. 2, Issue 10, pp. 719–731). Nature Publishing Group. https://doi.org/DOI: 10.1038/s41551-018-0305-z

Yu, K. H., & Kohane, I. S. (2019). Framing the challenges of artificial intelligence in medicine. In *BMJ Quality and Safety* (Vol. 28, Issue 3, pp. 238–241). BMJ Publishing Group. https://doi.org/DOI: 10.1136/bmjqs-2018-008551

Zhu, Y., Salowe, R., Chow, C., Li, S., Bastani, O., & O'Brien, J. M. (2024). Advancing Glaucoma Care: Integrating Artificial Intelligence in Diagnosis, Management, and Progression Detection. In *Bioengineering* (Vol. 11, Issue 2). Multidisciplinary Digital Publishing Institute (MDPI). https://doi.org/DOI: 10.3390/bioengineering11020122

Chapter 2
AI in Early Diagnosis and Risk Prediction

Ankur Vashishtha
https://orcid.org/0000-0003-0679-5126

Sharda University, Greater Noida, India

Anshu Kumar Singh
https://orcid.org/0000-0002-2945-9371

Subharti College of Allied and Healthcare, Meerut, India

Gaurav Kaushik
https://orcid.org/0009-0008-3706-4733

Sharda University, Greater Noida, India

Prigya Sharma
https://orcid.org/0009-0000-0742-8665

Sharda University, Greater Noida, India

Vivek Kumar
https://orcid.org/0000-0003-1849-6983

IIMT University, Meerut, India

Salender Singh
N.C. Medical College, Haryana, India

Ashok K. Sah
A' Sharqiyah University, Oman

ABSTRACT

Artificial intelligence (AI) is a disruptive computer science that has the potential to revolutionize medical practice and healthcare delivery. Its uses include patient diagnosis, medication research, improved communication, document transcription, and remote patient care. AI algorithms have lately acquired accuracies comparable to human expertise in medical research, and others believe that humans will be fully displaced in several disciplines. AI also helps with microbial research, including microbe categorization and functional annotation. Machine learning enhances microbial taxonomy accuracy by exposing functional properties and metabolic pathways. AI-driven protein design has the potential to create enzymes with increased catalytic activity and stability. AI systems can anticipate protein shapes, functions, and interactions, allowing for more logical application design. AI technologies are already being utilized in clinical microbiology laboratories to automate susceptibility

DOI: 10.4018/979-8-3373-3196-6.ch002

testing and identification. Microbiological practitioners will increasingly rely on AI for preliminary screening, freeing them to concentrate on diagnostic concerns and sophisticated technical interpretation. The COVID-19 pandemic has boosted AI usage in telemedicine and chatbots, hence enhancing accessibility and medical education. AI-powered techniques offer the potential to better comprehend microbial ecosystems, accelerate drug development, and stimulate new medical cures.

1. INTRODUCTION

Now a day's AI is used everywhere in the daily life of mankind to ease the work and improve the work efficiency similarly, the AI is also utilized in health care sectors to predict the variant of major and minor diseases. AI is already integrated successfully with the various available devices like MRI, CT-Scan and other tools and some are yet to be integrated because Because of its many benefits, like its round-the-clock availability, low error rate, real-time insights, and quick analysis, artificial intelligence (AI) is becoming more and more significant in our daily lives. With useful applications including disease diagnosis, risk assessment, treatment planning, and medication discovery, artificial intelligence is being utilized more and more in clinical medical and dental healthcare analysis. The usage of AI in healthcare is reviewed narrative in this study from a multidisciplinary standpoint, with a focus on the domains of cardiology, allergy, endocrinology, and dentistry (Ahsan & Siddique, 2021). In addition to highlighting data from recent research and development initiatives in AI for healthcare, the article discusses the difficulties and restrictions that come with implementing AI, including ethical and legal issues as well as data privacy and security concerns. Because the subject is developing so quickly, regulations governing the responsible design, development, and application of AI in healthcare are still in their infancy. Nonetheless, it is our responsibility to properly analyze the moral ramifications of applying AI and to react accordingly. AI technologies keep demonstrating their promise to improve patient outcomes and change the way healthcare is delivered (Ghasemi et al., 2024; Abdollahi et al., 2023).

Artificial intelligence (AI) is rapidly transforming healthcare, offering powerful tools to revolutionize early disease diagnosis and risk prediction. By analyzing vast datasets of medical information, AI algorithms can identify subtle patterns and anomalies often missed by the human eye, paving the way for earlier interventions and more personalized preventative strategies. This capability holds immense potential to improve patient outcomes, reduce healthcare costs, and shift the focus from reactive treatment to proactive health management (Habchi et al., 2023).

1.1. History and Background of AI

The seeds of artificial intelligence were sown long before the digital age, with early explorations into symbolic reasoning and computational models in the mid-20th century. The Dartmouth Workshop in 1956 is often considered the official birth of the field, sparking initial optimism and research into areas like problem-solving and natural language processing. While the ensuing decades witnessed periods of both fervent progress and so-called "AI winters" due to technological limitations and unmet expectations, the foundational concepts and algorithms developed during this time laid the groundwork for today's advancements. The recent resurgence of AI, particularly in the realm of machine learning and deep learning, is fueled by increased computational power, the availability of massive datasets, and break-throughs in algorithmic design, propelling AI from theoretical concepts to practical applications across numerous domains. (Liu et al., 2022; Shah et al., 2023)

1.2. Basic Model of AI

At its core, an AI system typically comprises several interconnected compo-nents working in concert. The journey begins with data acquisition, where relevant information, whether structured or unstructured, is gathered from various sources. This raw data then undergoes preprocessing, a crucial step involving cleaning, transforming, and preparing it into a suitable format for the AI model. The heart of the system is the AI model itself, which could be based on various algorithms like machine learning, deep learning, or rule-based systems, designed to learn patterns and relationships within the data (Bulusu et al., 2025). This learning phase, or training, involves feeding the preprocessed data to the model. Once trained, the inference engine utilizes the learned model to make predictions, classifications, or decisions on new, unseen data. Finally, the output is presented to the user or integrated into another system, often requiring a post-processing stage for interpretation or further action. This fundamental flow, from data input to insightful output, underpins the functionality of most AI systems. (Jan et al., 2023)

Figure 1. Basic Block Diagram of AI system

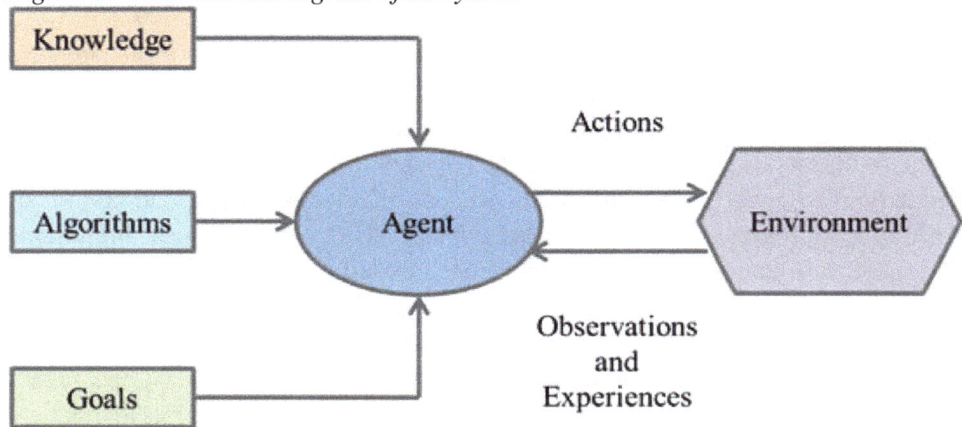

1.3. Burden of Late Stage Diseases

Detecting diseases at advanced stages presents a significant global health challenge, leading to diminished treatment efficacy, increased healthcare expenditures, and poorer patient outcomes. When illnesses progress undetected to later phases, therapeutic interventions often become more complex, costly, and less likely to result in a cure or long-term remission. The cumulative impact on individuals includes reduced quality of life, increased suffering, and a higher risk of mortality, while healthcare systems face the strain of managing complex conditions requiring extensive resources and prolonged care. (Miller et al., 2022) Addressing the burden of late-stage diseases necessitates a paradigm shift towards proactive strategies that prioritize early detection and intervention.

1.4. The Promise of Proactive Healthcare

A fundamental shift towards proactive healthcare offers a transformative vision for improving health outcomes and optimizing resource allocation. By prioritizing early identification of risks and diseases, this approach aims to intervene before conditions progress to more severe and less treatable stages. (Sharma & Chaturvedi, 2020) The promise lies in empowering individuals and healthcare providers with the tools and insights necessary for timely interventions, personalized prevention strategies, and ultimately, a healthier lifespan with enhanced quality of life. This proactive stance can lead to more effective treatments, reduced healthcare costs associated with managing advanced illnesses, and a greater emphasis on well-being rather than solely reacting to sickness. (Zhang et al., 2013)

1.5. Objectives of the Chapter

- **Articulate the significance** of early disease detection and risk prediction in improving patient outcomes and healthcare efficiency.
- **Explain fundamental concepts** of artificial intelligence, including machine learning, deep learning, natural language processing, and computer vision, [1] as they are applied in healthcare.
- **Describe specific applications of AI** in the early diagnosis of various medical conditions across different specialties such as oncology, cardiology, and neurology.
- **Discuss the role of AI** in predicting individual and population-level disease risks, including the use of EHR data, genomics, and wearable technology.
- **Identify and analyze the key challenges and ethical considerations** associated with the implementation of AI in early diagnosis and risk prediction, such as data bias, privacy concerns, and the need for explain ability.
- **Outline the current state and future directions** of AI in proactive healthcare, including integration into clinical workflows and emerging technological advancements.
- **Appreciate the collaborative nature** required between AI developers and clinicians for the successful and responsible adoption of these technologies.
- **Evaluate the potential impact** of AI on healthcare costs, accessibility, and the overall shift towards personalized and preventive medicine.

2. FUNDAMENTALS OF AI IN HEALTHCARE SYSTEM

2.1. Machine Learning: The Engine of Prediction

At the heart of artificial intelligence's capabilities in early diagnosis and risk prediction lies machine learning (ML), a powerful paradigm that empowers computers to learn from data without explicit programming. Instead of being explicitly instructed on how to perform a task, ML algorithms identify patterns, extract insights, and build predictive models from vast datasets. This data-driven approach allows systems to adapt and improve their performance over time as they are exposed to more information. In the context of healthcare, machine learning algorithms can analyze complex medical data, such as patient histories, imaging scans, and genomic information, to identify subtle indicators of disease in its nascent stages or to forecast an individual's likelihood of developing a condition in the future. The ability of ML to discern intricate relationships within data makes it an indispensable engine driving the advancements in proactive and personalized healthcare (Olatunji et al., 2021; Xiao et al., 2017).

Figure 2. Process of machine learning

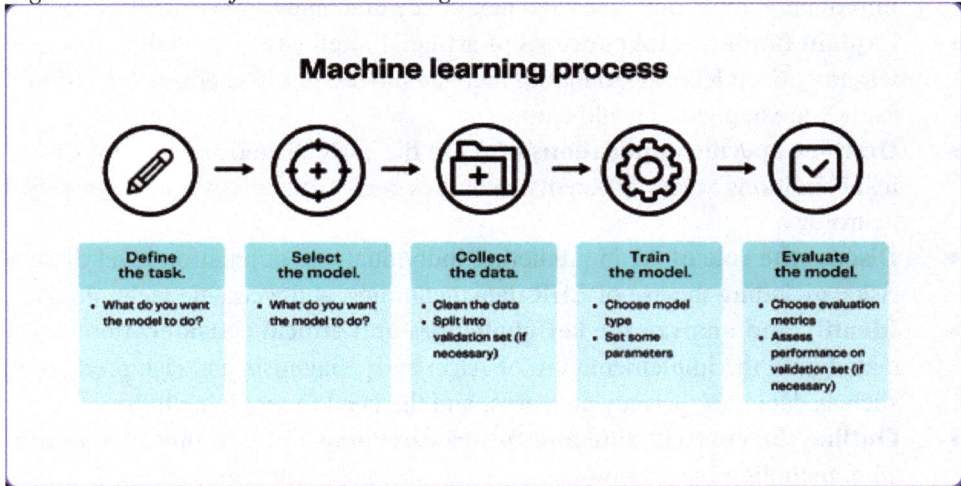

2.2. Supervised Learning (Classification and Regression)

A cornerstone of machine learning, supervised learning involves training algorithms on labeled datasets, where each data point is paired with a known outcome or target variable. This learning paradigm focuses on enabling the algorithm to establish a mapping function between the input features and the corresponding output. Within supervised learning, two primary tasks emerge: classification and regression. (Liew et al., 2021). Classification algorithms learn to categorize data into distinct classes or categories, such as identifying whether a medical image contains a tumor (positive) or not (negative). Conversely, regression algorithms aim to predict continuous numerical values, for instance, estimating a patient's future risk score for a particular disease based on their current health metrics. By learning from these labeled examples, supervised learning models become adept at predicting outcomes for new, unseen data, making them invaluable tools for tasks like early disease detection (classification) and risk assessment (regression) in healthcare. (Muhammad et al., 2019)

2.3. Unsupervised Learning (Clustering and Dimensionality Reduction)

In contrast to supervised learning, unsupervised learning delves into unlabeled data, seeking to uncover inherent structures and patterns without prior knowledge of outcomes. This approach is particularly useful in exploratory data analysis and feature discovery. Two prominent techniques within unsupervised learning are clustering and dimensionality reduction. Clustering algorithms group similar data points together based on their intrinsic characteristics, potentially identifying previously unknown patient subgroups with shared disease patterns or risk factors. (Suh et al., 2020) Dimensionality reduction techniques aim to simplify complex datasets with a high number of variables by identifying the most important underlying features while preserving essential information. This can help in visualizing high-dimensional medical data, reducing noise, and improving the efficiency of subsequent analysis or modeling. By revealing hidden relationships and simplifying intricate data landscapes, unsupervised learning offers valuable insights for understanding disease mechanisms and identifying novel risk indicators in early diagnosis and prediction. (Krizhevsky et al., 2017)

2.4. Deep Learning and Neural Networks

Inspired by the intricate structure of the human brain, deep learning represents a sophisticated subfield of machine learning that utilizes artificial neural networks with multiple layers (hence, "deep"). These networks, composed of interconnected nodes or "neurons," are capable of automatically learning hierarchical representations of data, progressively extracting increasingly complex features from raw input. This ability to learn intricate patterns directly from unstructured data, such as medical images, text reports, and time-series data, makes deep learning particularly powerful for tasks like identifying subtle anomalies in radiology scans or predicting disease risk from complex combinations of clinical factors. The depth of these networks allows them to capture nuanced relationships that might be missed by traditional machine learning algorithms, driving significant advancements in the accuracy and potential of AI for early diagnosis and risk prediction across various medical domains. (Tan & Le, 2019)

Figure 3. Architects of ANN

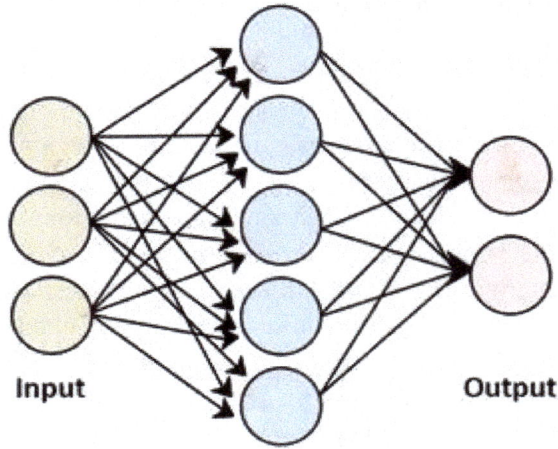

Input   Output

2.5. Explainable AI (XAI) in Healthcare: The Need for Transparency

While the predictive power of AI in healthcare, particularly with complex models like deep learning, is substantial, the "black box" nature of these systems poses a significant challenge for clinical adoption. Explainable AI (XAI) emerges as a critical necessity, focusing on developing methods and techniques that allow humans to understand and interpret the reasoning behind AI-driven predictions and decisions. In the context of early diagnosis and risk prediction, transparency is paramount. Clinicians need to comprehend why an AI system flags a particular image as suspicious or identifies a patient as high-risk to build trust, validate findings, and ultimately integrate these tools effectively into their practice. Understanding the factors influencing an AI's output not only fosters user confidence but also aids in identifying potential biases or limitations within the model, ensuring responsible and ethical deployment of AI in sensitive healthcare applications. (Szegedy et al., 2015)

3. AI-POWERED EARLY DIAGNOSIS ACROSS MEDICAL SPECIALTIES

3.1. Oncology: Detecting Cancer at Early Stages

Oncology stands as a critical domain where the application of AI for early diagnosis holds immense promise in improving survival rates and treatment outcomes. By leveraging sophisticated algorithms, AI systems can analyze vast amounts of complex data, including medical images like mammograms, CT scans, and MRIs, to detect subtle anomalies indicative of early-stage tumors that might be challenging for the human eye to discern. Furthermore, AI is being employed in the analysis of liquid biopsies, enabling the early identification of circulating tumor cells or DNA fragments in blood samples. In pathology, AI-powered tools can enhance the accuracy and efficiency of analyzing tissue samples, leading to earlier and more precise cancer diagnoses. The ability of AI to process and interpret multifaceted data with high sensitivity and specificity is revolutionizing the landscape of cancer detection, paving the way for timely interventions and personalized treatment strategies at the most treatable stages of the disease. (He et al., 2016; Huang et al., 2017)

3.2. Image Analysis for Early Tumor Detection

A pivotal application of AI in early cancer diagnosis lies in the intelligent analysis of medical images. Advanced computer vision techniques, often powered by deep learning models, are trained on extensive datasets of radiological images to identify subtle patterns and anomalies that may indicate the presence of early-stage tumors. (Gillum, 2013) These AI systems can meticulously examine features within images, such as subtle changes in tissue density, irregular shapes, or textural variations, which might be imperceptible or easily overlooked by human observers. By providing a "second pair of eyes" with enhanced sensitivity and the ability to quantify subtle image characteristics, AI tools can aid radiologists and oncologists in detecting cancers at their earliest, most treatable phases, thereby significantly improving patient prognosis and treatment options. (DATA-CAN, n.d.)

3.3. Liquid Biopsies and AI for Circulating Biomarker Analysis

Liquid biopsies, offering a minimally invasive approach to cancer detection and monitoring, are significantly enhanced by the analytical capabilities of artificial intelligence. These blood-based assays capture circulating biomarkers, such as cell-free DNA, circulating tumor cells, and exosomes, which can provide early evidence of cancer development or recurrence. AI algorithms play a crucial role in processing the complex and often low-concentration data generated from liquid biopsies. Machine learning models can identify subtle patterns and correlations within these molecular signatures, enabling earlier cancer detection, personalized risk assessment, and real-time monitoring of treatment response. (NHS Digital, n.d.) By intelligently analyzing the wealth of information contained within liquid biopsies, AI is paving the way for more proactive and precise cancer management strategies.

3.4. AI in Pathology for Enhanced Diagnostic Accuracy

Artificial intelligence is revolutionizing the field of pathology by augmenting the diagnostic capabilities of pathologists and enhancing accuracy in disease identification. AI-powered tools can analyze digitized histopathology slides with remarkable speed and precision, identifying subtle morphological patterns and cellular anomalies that may be indicative of disease, including early-stage cancers. (NHSX, n.d.) These systems are trained on vast datasets of annotated slides, enabling them to learn complex visual features and provide quantitative analyses that complement the qualitative assessments of human experts. By automating tedious tasks, highlighting areas of concern, and offering objective second opinions, AI in pathology contributes to reduced diagnostic errors, faster turnaround times, and ultimately, more accurate and timely diagnoses for patients.

3.5. Cardiology: Predicting and Diagnosing Cardiovascular Diseases Early

Cardiovascular diseases (CVDs) remain a leading cause of mortality globally, underscoring the critical need for early prediction and diagnosis. Artificial intelligence offers transformative potential in this domain by enabling the analysis of diverse cardiac data with unprecedented sophistication. AI algorithms can process and interpret complex signals from electrocardiograms (ECGs), echocardiograms, and other cardiac imaging modalities to detect subtle abnormalities indicative of early-stage CVDs that might be missed by conventional methods. (NHS Digital, n.d.) Furthermore, machine learning models can integrate various patient data, including medical history, lifestyle factors, and genetic information, to predict an individual's risk of developing cardiovascular events long before they manifest clinically. This proactive approach, powered by AI, paves the way for timely interventions, personalized preventative strategies, and ultimately, improved cardiovascular health outcomes.

3.6. ECG and EEG Analysis Using AI

Artificial intelligence is significantly advancing the analysis of electrophysiological signals like those obtained from electrocardiograms (ECGs) for the heart and electroencephalograms (EEGs) for the brain, facilitating earlier and more accurate diagnoses of cardiovascular and neurological conditions. AI algorithms can be trained to identify subtle but critical patterns within these complex waveforms that may indicate the onset of arrhythmias, ischemia, or structural heart disease in ECGs, or early signs of epilepsy, sleep disorders, or cognitive impairment in EEGs. By automating the meticulous analysis of these signals and highlighting deviations from normal patterns, AI tools can assist clinicians in detecting abnormalities at earlier stages, leading to prompt interventions and improved patient management in both cardiology and neurology. (Benke & Benke, 2018)

3.7. Predictive Models for Arrhythmias and Sudden Cardiac Events

The ability to predict life-threatening cardiac events like arrhythmias and sudden cardiac death is a critical area where artificial intelligence is making significant strides. By analyzing vast datasets of patient information, including historical ECG recordings, clinical data, and even wearable sensor data, machine learning models can identify complex patterns and risk factors that may precede these events. These predictive models can then be used to stratify patients based on their individual risk, allowing for targeted interventions such as the implementation of preventative therapies or the deployment of implantable cardiac devices. (Moore et al., 2017) This proactive approach, driven by AI's capacity to discern subtle indicators within large and varied datasets, holds the potential to significantly reduce the incidence of sudden cardiac events and improve survival rates in vulnerable populations.

3.8. Neurology: Early Identification of Neurodegenerative Disorders

Early identification of neurodegenerative disorders, such as Alzheimer's and Parkinson's disease, presents a significant challenge in neurology, but artificial intelligence offers promising avenues for earlier detection and intervention. AI algorithms can analyze complex neurological data, including magnetic resonance imaging (MRI) and positron emission tomography (PET) scans, to detect subtle structural and functional changes in the brain that may precede clinical symptoms. Furthermore, AI is being applied to the analysis of speech patterns, language use, and even subtle motor movements captured by wearable sensors, which can provide early indicators of these progressive conditions. By leveraging AI's ability to discern minute deviations from normative patterns in diverse datasets, neurology is poised to make significant advancements in diagnosing neurodegenerative diseases at earlier, potentially more treatable stages, ultimately improving patient management and quality of life. (Nayor et al., 2018)

3.9. MRI and PET scan Analysis for Alzheimer's and Parkinson's

Artificial intelligence is proving invaluable in the early detection of Alzheimer's and Parkinson's diseases through the sophisticated analysis of neuroimaging data. Machine learning and deep learning algorithms can be trained on large datasets of Magnetic Resonance Imaging (MRI) and Positron Emission Tomography (PET) scans to identify subtle, often imperceptible to the human eye, structural and metabolic changes in the brain that are characteristic of these neurodegenerative conditions. AI can quantify regional brain volumes, detect patterns of atrophy, and analyze the distribution and uptake of specific tracers in PET scans, providing objective and sensitive measures that can aid in earlier diagnosis, even before significant clinical symptoms manifest. This AI-powered analysis offers the potential for timely interventions and the development of disease-modifying therapies administered at a stage when they may be most effective. (Glaser et al., 2018)

3.10. Ophthalmology: Preventing Vision Loss through Early Detection

In ophthalmology, the timely detection of eye diseases is paramount in preventing irreversible vision loss, and artificial intelligence is emerging as a powerful ally in achieving this goal. AI algorithms can analyze complex retinal images, such as fundus photographs and optical coherence tomography (OCT) scans, with remarkable precision to identify early signs of sight-threatening conditions like diabetic retinopathy, glaucoma, and age-related macular degeneration. By detecting subtle anomalies, quantifying structural changes, and identifying patterns indicative of disease onset or progression, AI-powered tools can assist ophthalmologists in making earlier diagnoses and implementing timely interventions. (Danforth et al., 2012) This proactive approach, leveraging AI's ability to process and interpret intricate ocular data, holds the potential to significantly reduce the burden of preventable blindness and preserve vision for countless individuals.

3.11. Retinal Image Analysis for Diabetic Retinopathy and Glaucoma

The analysis of retinal images using artificial intelligence is revolutionizing the early detection of diabetic retinopathy (DR) and glaucoma, two leading causes of blindness. AI algorithms, particularly deep learning models, are trained on vast datasets of fundus photographs and optical coherence tomography (OCT) scans to identify subtle indicators of these diseases, often before they are clinically apparent. (Farjah et al., 2016) For DR, AI can detect microaneurysms, hemorrhages, and exudates with high sensitivity, enabling timely intervention to prevent vision-threatening complications. In glaucoma, AI can analyze optic nerve head features and retinal nerve fiber layer thickness from OCT scans to identify early structural damage and predict the risk of visual field loss. By automating the meticulous examination of these intricate retinal structures, AI empowers ophthalmologists to diagnose and manage these conditions at earlier stages, significantly improving the chances of preserving patients' vision. (Beyer et al., 2017)

3.12. Designing process of AI module for disease prediction

Designing an AI module to predict diseases isn't a linear checklist; it's more akin to a carefully navigated expedition. The journey begins not with algorithms, but with a deep understanding of the medical challenge we aim to address.

3.12.1. Phase 1: Problem Definition and Contextualization

1. **The Unmet Clinical Need:** Our first step is to pinpoint a specific gap in current clinical practice. What disease are we targeting? Why is prediction challenging with existing methods? For instance, are we aiming to predict the onset of a silent disease like early-stage Alzheimer's where timely intervention is crucial but detection is difficult? Or perhaps we're focused on predicting the likelihood of complications in patients with a chronic condition like diabetes to personalize care. (Roch et al., 2015)
2. **Stakeholder Engagement:** We then engage with the individuals who will be most impacted: clinicians, patients, and potentially researchers. Understanding their needs, workflows, and concerns is paramount. What information would be most valuable to them? How would this AI module integrate into their daily routines? What level of explainability is necessary for trust and adoption?
3. **Defining Success from a Clinical Perspective:** Beyond technical metrics, how will this module translate to tangible benefits for patients and healthcare providers? Will it lead to earlier diagnosis, more effective treatment strategies,

reduced hospitalizations, or improved patient outcomes? Defining these clinical success criteria early on will guide our design choices. (Hunter et al., 2021)

3.12.2. Phase 2: Data Landscape Exploration and Preparation - The Foundation

1. **Mapping Potential Data Territories:** We embark on a comprehensive survey of available and potentially relevant data sources. This could range from structured data like lab results, medication history, and diagnostic codes within Electronic Health Records (EHRs) to unstructured data like clinical notes, medical images (radiology, pathology), genomic sequences, and even patient-reported outcomes or data from wearable devices. (Ni et al., 2015)
2. **Data Cartography and Quality Assessment:** Once identified, we meticulously examine the quality, completeness, and biases inherent in each data source. Are there missing values? Are the data consistently recorded? Are there subpopulations that are underrepresented? This critical assessment informs our data cleaning and preprocessing strategies.
3. **Constructing Meaningful Features - The Art of Abstraction:** This stage involves transforming raw data into informative features that the AI model can learn from. Instead of just feeding in individual lab values, we might engineer features like trends over time, ratios of different biomarkers, or textual features extracted from clinical notes using Natural Language Processing (NLP). For image data, this could involve extracting key visual patterns. The goal is to represent the underlying biological and clinical processes in a way that the AI can discern. (Morin et al., 2021)

3.12.3. Phase 3: Model Crafting and Iterative Refinement - The Engine

1. **Choosing the Right Tools for the Terrain:** Based on the nature of the prediction task (e.g., binary classification for disease presence, regression for risk score) and the characteristics of our data, we select appropriate AI/ML models. This might involve experimenting with classical statistical models, established machine learning algorithms, or delving into the realm of deep learning architectures if the data complexity warrants it. (Chen et al., 2020)
2. **Training with Purpose and Validation with Rigor:** The chosen model is trained on a carefully curated training dataset. Crucially, we employ a separate validation dataset to fine-tune the model's parameters and prevent overfitting – ensuring it generalizes well to unseen data. This is an iterative process where we adjust the model and re-evaluate its performance.

3. **Performance Benchmarking Against Clinical Relevance:** We evaluate the model not just on standard metrics but also in the context of its clinical utility. For example, a model with high accuracy might still have an unacceptable rate of false positives, leading to unnecessary anxiety and further testing for patients. We need to strike a balance that aligns with clinical needs and minimizes harm. (Beig et al., 2019)

3.12.4. Phase 4: Interpretation and Translation to Clinical Insight - The Compass

1. **Illuminating the "Why":** For many medical applications, understanding the reasoning behind a prediction is as important as the prediction itself. We explore techniques to make the model's decisions more transparent, such as feature importance analysis, local interpretable model-agnostic explanations (LIME), or attention maps for deep learning models analyzing images.
2. **Bridging the Gap to Clinical Actionability:** The insights generated by the AI must be presented in a way that is readily understandable and actionable for clinicians. This might involve visualizing risk scores, highlighting key contributing factors, or providing confidence intervals for the predictions. (Shakir et al., 2019)

3.12.5. Phase 5: Deployment, Integration, and Continuous Evolution - The Ongoing Journey

1. **Seamless Integration into the Healthcare Ecosystem:** The AI module needs to fit smoothly into existing clinical workflows and technological infrastructure. Considerations include data security, privacy compliance, and interoperability with EHR systems.
2. **Real-World Monitoring and Performance Feedback:** Once deployed, the AI module's performance needs to be continuously monitored using real-world data. We need mechanisms to detect data drift (changes in the input data over time) and model degradation. (Lu et al., 2019)
3. **Adaptive Learning and Re-evaluation:** The medical landscape is constantly evolving with new research, treatment guidelines, and patient populations. Our AI module should be designed with the capacity for periodic retraining and updating to maintain its accuracy and relevance.

4. AI FOR RISK PREDICTION AND PROGNOSTICATION

4.1. Identifying At-Risk Populations: Predictive Modeling

A crucial application of artificial intelligence lies in the proactive identification of populations and individuals at elevated risk for developing specific diseases. Predictive modeling, powered by machine learning algorithms, analyzes diverse datasets, including electronic health records (EHRs), demographic information, lifestyle factors, and environmental exposures, to discern patterns and correlations indicative of increased susceptibility. (Astaraki et al., 2021) By identifying these high-risk groups, healthcare systems can implement targeted interventions, such as personalized screening programs, preventative therapies, and lifestyle modifications, before the onset of clinical symptoms. This proactive approach, enabled by AI's ability to process and synthesize complex data to generate accurate risk assessments, holds the potential to shift the focus from reactive treatment to preemptive care, ultimately improving population health outcomes and reducing the burden of preventable diseases. (Guan et al., 2021)

4.2. Utilizing Electronic Health Records (EHRs) for Risk Stratification

Electronic Health Records (EHRs) represent a rich repository of longitudinal patient data, making them a valuable resource for artificial intelligence in risk stratification. By applying machine learning algorithms to the vast information contained within EHRs – including medical history, diagnoses, medications, laboratory results, and even clinical notes – AI can identify complex relationships and patterns that may indicate an individual's propensity for developing specific diseases or experiencing adverse health events. This allows for the creation of sophisticated risk scores and the categorization of patient populations into different risk tiers. Healthcare providers can then leverage these AI-driven risk stratifications to prioritize interventions, personalize preventative care plans, and allocate resources more effectively towards those most likely to benefit, ultimately leading to improved patient management and outcomes. (Ronneberger et al., 2015)

4.3. Integrating Genomics and Other Omics Data for Personalized Risk Assessment

The integration of genomics and other "omics" data, such as transcriptomics, proteomics, and metabolomics, with artificial intelligence is ushering in an era of highly personalized risk assessment. These comprehensive datasets provide deep insights into an individual's biological predispositions and molecular profiles. (Milletari et al., 2016) By applying sophisticated machine learning algorithms to analyze the intricate interplay between genetic variations, gene expression patterns, protein signatures, and metabolic pathways, AI can identify subtle yet significant biomarkers and risk factors that may not be apparent through traditional clinical data alone. This holistic approach allows for a more nuanced and precise under-standing of an individual's susceptibility to various diseases, paving the way for tailored preventative strategies, earlier interventions based on their unique biological makeup, and ultimately, a more proactive and personalized approach to healthcare. (Baccouche et al., 2021)

4.4. Leveraging Wearable Device Data for Continuous Risk Monitoring

The proliferation of wearable devices and their capacity to continuously mon-itor physiological parameters offer a novel and dynamic data stream for artificial intelligence in risk monitoring. These devices collect real-time information on vital signs like heart rate, activity levels, sleep patterns, and even blood glucose in some cases. By applying machine learning algorithms to analyze these longitudinal data streams, AI can detect subtle deviations from an individual's baseline, identify early warning signs of potential health issues, and track the impact of lifestyle changes or interventions on risk factors. (Mayerhoefer et al., 2020) This continuous monitoring, powered by AI's ability to discern meaningful patterns in time-series data, enables a more proactive and personalized approach to health management, facilitating time-ly alerts and interventions that can prevent or mitigate the progression of various diseases. (Baldwin et al., 2020)

4.5. Predicting Disease Progression and Outcomes

Beyond early detection, artificial intelligence plays a crucial role in predicting the likely progression of diagnosed diseases and their potential outcomes. By analyzing historical patient data, treatment responses, genetic markers, and other relevant factors, machine learning models can develop prognostic tools that estimate the course of an illness, the likelihood of specific complications, and the potential success of different therapeutic approaches. (Ardila et al., 2019) This capability allows clinicians to make more informed decisions about treatment strategies, personalize care plans based on predicted trajectories, and provide patients with a clearer understanding of their future health outlook. Ultimately, AI-driven prediction of disease progression and outcomes contributes to more effective disease management and improved patient well-being. (Papadimitroulas et al., 2021)

4.6. AI in Predicting Disease Severity and Complications

Artificial intelligence is proving instrumental in forecasting the potential severity of existing diseases and the likelihood of developing associated complications. By analyzing a multitude of patient-specific data points, including initial diagnosis details, comorbidities, laboratory findings, and treatment history, machine learning algorithms can identify complex patterns that correlate with disease progression and the emergence of adverse events. These predictive models can then provide clinicians with valuable insights into which patients are at higher risk of experiencing severe disease courses or specific complications, enabling proactive interventions, intensified monitoring, and the tailoring of treatment strategies to mitigate these risks and improve patient outcomes. (Bera et al., 2019)

4.7. Personalized Prognostic Models for Treatment Planning

The advent of artificial intelligence is enabling the development of highly personalized prognostic models that significantly enhance treatment planning. By integrating an individual patient's unique clinical characteristics, genomic information, lifestyle factors, and treatment responses into sophisticated machine learning algorithms, AI can generate tailored predictions about disease progression and treatment efficacy. (Williams et al., 2018) These personalized prognostic models move beyond generalized risk assessments, offering clinicians more precise insights into how a specific patient is likely to respond to different therapeutic options and what their long-term outcomes might be. This level of granularity empowers clinicians to make more informed and individualized treatment decisions, optimizing therapeutic strategies to maximize benefit and minimize potential adverse effects for each patient. (Schüffler et al., 2021)

4.8. Early Warning Systems for Epidemics and Pandemics

Artificial intelligence is playing an increasingly vital role in the development of early warning systems designed to detect and predict the emergence and spread of epidemics and pandemics. By analyzing diverse data sources, including social media activity, news reports, flight patterns, climate data, and even anonymized search queries, AI algorithms can identify unusual patterns and anomalies that may signal the outbreak of infectious diseases. These systems can then generate timely alerts, allowing public health organizations to implement rapid containment measures, allocate resources effectively, and potentially mitigate the widespread impact of an emerging health crisis. The ability of AI to process vast amounts of disparate information in real-time makes it a powerful tool for proactive surveillance and early intervention in global health security. (Browning et al., 2021)

4.9. Identifying Environmental and Social Determinants of Health Risks

Artificial intelligence is proving to be a powerful tool in unraveling the complex interplay between environmental and social factors and their impact on health risks. By analyzing large-scale datasets that integrate geographical information, pollution levels, socioeconomic indicators, access to resources, and public health records, AI algorithms can identify significant correlations and patterns that reveal how these determinants contribute to the prevalence and distribution of various diseases. This analytical capability allows for a deeper understanding of the root causes of health disparities and the identification of vulnerable populations exposed to heightened risks. Ultimately, AI-driven insights in this area can inform targeted public health interventions and policy changes aimed at mitigating environmental and social factors that negatively influence health outcomes and promote health equity. (Dash et al., 2021)

5. DATA CHALLENGES AND ETHICAL CONSIDERATIONS

5.1. Data Availability, Quality, and Bias in Healthcare AI

The successful deployment of artificial intelligence in healthcare for early diagnosis and risk prediction heavily relies on the availability of substantial, high-quality data. However, the healthcare domain often faces challenges related to data scarcity for certain conditions, fragmented data across different systems, and inconsistencies in data formatting and collection. Furthermore, inherent biases within the training data, reflecting existing societal inequalities or limitations in data collection practices, can lead to AI models that exhibit discriminatory behavior, potentially impacting the accuracy and fairness of predictions across different demographic groups. Addressing these issues of data availability, ensuring data quality through rigorous standardization and validation processes, and actively mitigating bias in data collection and model development are crucial prerequisites for building reliable and equitable AI solutions in healthcare. (Coudray et al., 2018)

5.2. Data Privacy and Security Concerns

The sensitive nature of healthcare data, encompassing personal medical histories, diagnostic information, and even genomic details, necessitates stringent attention to data privacy and security when implementing AI systems. The collection, storage, and analysis of such vast datasets raise significant concerns regarding the potential for unauthorized access, data breaches, and misuse of personal health information. (Sui et al., 2021) Robust security measures, including encryption, anonymization techniques, and strict access controls, are paramount to safeguard patient confidentiality and comply with relevant regulations like HIPAA and GDPR. Furthermore, transparent data governance frameworks and clear guidelines on data usage are essential to build and maintain public trust in AI-driven healthcare applications for early diagnosis and risk prediction.

5.3. Algorithmic Bias and Fairness in Early Diagnosis and Risk Prediction

A critical ethical consideration in the application of AI for early diagnosis and risk prediction is the potential for algorithmic bias and the need to ensure fairness across diverse patient populations. Bias can inadvertently creep into AI models through skewed or unrepresentative training data, leading to disparities in diagnostic accuracy or risk assessments for certain demographic groups based on factors like race, ethnicity, or socioeconomic status. This can perpetuate or even exacerbate existing health inequities. Therefore, it is imperative to proactively identify and mitigate sources of bias in data collection, model development, and validation processes. Ensuring fairness requires rigorous evaluation of model performance across different subgroups and the implementation of strategies to promote equitable outcomes, guaranteeing that the benefits of AI in healthcare are distributed justly and without prejudice. (Ehteshami Bejnordi et al., 2018)

5.4. Regulatory Landscape and Approval Processes for AI in Healthcare

The regulatory landscape surrounding the deployment of artificial intelligence in healthcare, particularly for applications in early diagnosis and risk prediction, is evolving and becoming increasingly defined. Governing bodies worldwide are grappling with establishing appropriate frameworks to ensure the safety, efficacy, and ethical use of these novel technologies. Approval processes for AI-powered medical devices and software often involve demonstrating clinical validity, analytical performance, and adherence to data privacy and security standards. (Campanella et al., 2019) Navigating this complex and sometimes fragmented regulatory environment requires careful consideration of regional and national guidelines, collaboration between AI developers and regulatory agencies, and a commitment to transparency in the development and validation of these innovative healthcare solutions. The ongoing evolution of these regulations aims to foster responsible innovation while safeguarding patient well-being and public trust.

5.5. The Role of Human Oversight and Clinical Validation

Despite the increasing sophistication of artificial intelligence in early diagnosis and risk prediction, the critical role of human oversight and rigorous clinical validation remains paramount. AI tools are intended to augment, not replace, the expertise and judgment of healthcare professionals. Clinicians must retain the responsibility for interpreting AI-generated insights within the broader clinical context, considering individual patient factors, and making final diagnostic and treatment decisions. Thorough clinical validation, involving prospective studies on diverse patient populations, is essential to evaluate the real-world performance, accuracy, and clinical utility of AI models before their widespread adoption. This iterative process of human review and validation ensures the responsible and effective integration of AI into clinical practice, fostering trust and maximizing the benefits for patient care. (Woerl et al., 2020)

6. IMPLEMENTATION AND FUTURE DIRECTIONS

6.1. Integrating AI into Clinical Workflows: Challenges and Solutions

The seamless integration of artificial intelligence into existing clinical workflows presents both significant challenges and opportunities for enhancing healthcare delivery. Obstacles such as the need for interoperable data systems, clinician training and adoption, and the potential for workflow disruption must be carefully addressed. Furthermore, ensuring that AI tools complement rather than complicate clinical practice requires thoughtful design and implementation. (Naik et al., 2020) Potential solutions involve developing user-friendly interfaces, providing adequate training and support for healthcare professionals, and iteratively adapting AI systems to fit within established clinical routines. Successful integration necessitates a collaborative approach between AI developers, clinicians, and healthcare administrators to ensure that these powerful tools are effectively harnessed to improve efficiency, enhance diagnostic accuracy, and ultimately benefit patient care within the practical realities of the clinical environment (Ström et al., 2020).

6.2. The Role of Collaboration between AI Developers and Clinicians

Effective progress in leveraging artificial intelligence for early diagnosis and risk prediction hinges on robust collaboration between AI developers and clinicians. AI scientists bring expertise in algorithm design, data analysis, and software engineering, while clinicians possess invaluable domain-specific knowledge, understanding of clinical workflows, and insights into the nuances of patient care. This interdisciplinary partnership is crucial for identifying clinically relevant problems, guiding the development of AI solutions that address real-world needs, and ensuring that these tools are practical, user-friendly, and aligned with ethical considerations. Ongoing communication and feedback between these groups are essential for the iterative refinement of AI models, their successful integration into clinical practice, and ultimately, the realization of their full potential to improve patient outcomes. (Madabhushi & Feldman, 2020)

6.3. The Impact of AI on Healthcare Costs and Accessibility

Artificial intelligence holds the potential to significantly impact both healthcare costs and accessibility, though its ultimate effect will depend on careful implementation and policy decisions. By automating certain tasks, enhancing diagnostic efficiency, and predicting potential health crises, AI could contribute to cost reduction in areas such as medical imaging analysis, administrative processes, and the prevention of costly late-stage disease management. Furthermore, AI-powered tools can extend the reach of medical expertise to underserved populations through telemedicine platforms and remote diagnostics, potentially improving accessibility to quality healthcare regardless of geographical limitations or socioeconomic status. However, realizing these benefits requires addressing challenges related to the initial investment in AI infrastructure, ensuring equitable access to these technologies, and navigating the evolving regulatory landscape to avoid exacerbating existing disparities. (Lokhande et al., 2020)

6.4. Emerging Trends and Future Potential of AI in Early Diagnosis and Risk Prediction

The field of artificial intelligence in early diagnosis and risk prediction is rapidly evolving, with several promising trends shaping its future trajectory. Federated learning, which allows for collaborative model training across multiple institutions without sharing sensitive patient data, is gaining momentum. Multimodal AI, capable of integrating and analyzing diverse data types like imaging, genomics, and clinical text simultaneously, promises more comprehensive and accurate predictions (Bera et al., 2020). Furthermore, the drive towards personalized and precision medicine is fueling the development of AI systems that can tailor diagnostic and risk assessment strategies to individual patient profiles. As AI algorithms become more sophisticated, interpretable, and integrated into clinical workflows, their potential to revolutionize proactive healthcare, improve patient outcomes, and pave the way for truly personalized medicine will continue to expand. (da Silva et al., 2021)

6.5. Federated Learning for Collaborative Model Training

Federated learning represents a groundbreaking approach to collaborative model training in healthcare, particularly valuable for developing AI in early diagnosis and risk prediction. This technique enables multiple healthcare institutions to collaboratively train a shared machine learning model on their local, decentralized datasets without the need to transfer sensitive patient information. (Halse et al., 2018) Instead, individual sites train their models locally, and only model updates (such as weights and biases) are aggregated to create a global model. This preserves data privacy and security while still allowing the AI to learn from a larger and more diverse patient population, leading to potentially more robust and generalizable predictive models. Federated learning holds immense promise for accelerating the development of AI in healthcare, especially when dealing with rare diseases or geographically dispersed patient data, while adhering to stringent data protection regulations. (Fassler et al., 2020; Kawakami et al., 2019; Knijnenburg et al., 2018)

6.6. Multimodal AI for Integrated Data Analysis

The future of artificial intelligence in early diagnosis and risk prediction is increasingly leaning towards multimodal approaches that leverage the synergistic power of integrating diverse data streams. (Liu et al., 2019) Rather than analyzing single data types in isolation (such as only medical images or only genomic data), multimodal AI systems are designed to simultaneously process and learn from a combination of information, including imaging data, genomic sequences, clinical notes (through natural language processing), physiological signals from wearables, and laboratory results. By fusing these varied sources of information, AI models can gain a more holistic and nuanced understanding of a patient's health status and disease risk, potentially uncovering complex relationships and making more accurate and earlier predictions than would be possible with unimodal analysis alone.

This integrated approach holds the key to unlocking deeper insights and advancing the frontiers of personalized and proactive healthcare. (Vasaikar et al., 2018; Liu et al., 2020)

6.7. Personalized and Precision Medicine Driven by AI

Artificial intelligence is a central driving force behind the burgeoning fields of personalized and precision medicine, particularly in the context of early diagnosis and risk prediction. By analyzing the unique biological, clinical, and lifestyle characteristics of individual patients – encompassing their genetic makeup, medical history, environmental exposures, and even real-time data from wearable's – AI algorithms can generate highly tailored insights into disease susceptibility and the likelihood of specific conditions developing. (Takahashi et al., 2021) This granular level of analysis enables the development of personalized risk assessment tools, allowing for targeted preventative strategies and earlier interventions that are precisely matched to an individual's needs. (Kamoun et al., 2016) Furthermore, AI can predict individual responses to different therapies, guiding treatment decisions and optimizing outcomes, thus realizing the core tenets of delivering the right treatment to the right patient at the right time. (Franco et al., 2021; Aberle et al., 2011; de Koning et al., 2020)

7. CONCLUSION: REALIZING THE PROMISE OF AI FOR A HEALTHIER FUTURE

In conclusion, artificial intelligence stands poised to revolutionize early diagnosis and risk prediction, offering a pathway towards a future where diseases are detected and addressed at their most manageable stages. The advancements in machine learning, deep learning, and multimodal data analysis are unlocking unprecedented capabilities for identifying subtle disease indicators and forecasting individual susceptibilities. While challenges related to data quality, ethical considerations, and seamless clinical integration remain, the ongoing collaboration between AI developers and clinicians, coupled with evolving regulatory frameworks, is paving the way for responsible and impactful implementation. By embracing the transformative potential of AI, healthcare can shift from a reactive model to a proactive paradigm, ultimately leading to improved patient outcomes, reduced healthcare burdens, and a healthier future for all. (Dyer, 2021)

Artificial intelligence is rapidly emerging as a transformative force in the landscape of early diagnosis and risk prediction, offering the potential to reshape healthcare towards a more proactive and personalized approach. By harnessing the power of machine learning, deep learning, and the integration of diverse data sources, AI systems can identify subtle disease markers and forecast individual vulnerabilities with increasing accuracy. (Krist et al., 2021) While challenges concerning data quality, ethical implications, and the need for seamless clinical integration persist, the collaborative efforts of AI researchers, clinicians, and policymakers are crucial in navigating these complexities. As AI technologies continue to mature and are thoughtfully implemented, they hold the promise of enabling earlier interventions, improving patient outcomes, and ultimately contributing to a healthier future where the burden of late-stage diseases is significantly reduced. (Richards et al., 2019)

REFERENCES

Abdollahi, M., Jafarizadeh, A., Asbagh, A. G., Sobhi, N., Pourmoghtader, K., Pedrammehr, S., . . . Acharya, U. R. (2023). Artificial intelligence in assessing cardiovascular diseases and risk factors via retinal fundus images: A review of the last decade. *arXiv*. https://doi.org//arXiv.2311.07609DOI: 10.48550

Aberle, D. R., Adams, A. M., Berg, C. D., Black, W. C., Clapp, J. D., Fagerstrom, R. M., Gareen, I. F., Gatsonis, C., Marcus, P. M., & Sicks, J. R. D. (2011). Reduced lung-cancer mortality with low-dose computed tomographic screening. *The New England Journal of Medicine*, *365*, 395–409. DOI: 10.1056/nejmoa1102873 PMID: 21714641

Ahsan, M. M., & Siddique, Z. (2021). Machine learning based disease diagnosis: A comprehensive review. *arXiv*. https://doi.org//arXiv.2112.15538DOI: 10.48550

Ardila, D., Kiraly, A. P., Bharadwaj, S., Choi, B., Reicher, J. J., Peng, L., Tse, D., Etemadi, M., Ye, W., & Corrado, G.. (2019). End-to-end lung cancer screening with three-dimensional deep learning on low-dose chest computed tomography. *Nature Medicine*, *25*, 954–961. DOI: 10.1038/s41591-019-0447-x PMID: 31110349

Astaraki, M., Zakko, Y., Toma Dasu, I., Smedby, Ö., & Wang, C. (2021). Benign-malignant pulmonary nodule classification in low-dose CT with convolutional features. *Physica Medica*, *83*, 146–153. DOI: 10.1016/j.ejmp.2021.03.013 PMID: 33774339

Baccouche, A., Garcia-Zapirain, B., Castillo Olea, C., & Elmaghraby, A. S. (2021). Connected-UNets: A deep learning architecture for breast mass segmentation. *NPJ Breast Cancer*, *7*, 1–12. DOI: 10.1038/s41523-021-00358-x PMID: 34857755

Baldwin, D. R., Gustafson, J., Pickup, L., Arteta, C., Novotny, P., Declerck, J., Kadir, T., Figueiras, C., Sterba, A., & Exell, A.. (2020). External validation of a convolutional neural network artificial intelligence tool to predict malignancy in pulmonary nodules. *Thorax*, *75*(4), 306–312. DOI: 10.1136/thoraxjnl-2019-214104 PMID: 32139611

Beig, N., Khorrami, M., Alilou, M., Prasanna, P., Braman, N., Orooji, M., Rakshit, S., Bera, K., Rajiah, P., & Ginsberg, J.. (2019). Perinodular and intranodular radiomic features on lung CT images distinguish adenocarcinomas from granulomas. *Radiology*, *290*(3), 783–792. DOI: 10.1148/radiol.2018180910 PMID: 30561278

Benke, K., & Benke, G. (2018). Artificial intelligence and big data in public health. *International Journal of Environmental Research and Public Health*, *15*(12), 2796. DOI: 10.3390/ijerph15122796 PMID: 30544648

Bera, K., Katz, I., & Madabhushi, A. (2020). Reimagining T staging through artificial intelligence and machine learning image processing approaches in digital pathology. *JCO Clinical Cancer Informatics*, *4*, 1039–1050. DOI: 10.1200/CCI.20.00110 PMID: 33166198

Bera, K., Schalper, K. A., Rimm, D. L., Velcheti, V., & Madabhushi, A. (2019). Artificial intelligence in digital pathology—New tools for diagnosis and precision oncology. *Nature Reviews. Clinical Oncology*, *16*, 703–715. DOI: 10.1038/s41571-019-0252-y PMID: 31399699

Beyer, S. E., McKee, B. J., Regis, S. M., McKee, A. B., Flacke, S., Saadawi, G., & El Wald, C. (2017). Automatic Lung-RADSTM classification with a natural language processing system. *Journal of Thoracic Disease*, *9*(12), 3114–3124. DOI: 10.21037/jtd.2017.08.13 PMID: 29221286

Browning, L., Colling, R., Rakha, E., Rajpoot, N., Rittscher, J., James, J. A., Salto-Tellez, M., Snead, D. R. J., & Verrill, C. (2021). Digital pathology and artificial intelligence will be key to supporting clinical and academic cellular pathology through COVID-19 and future crises: The PathLAKE consortium perspective. *Journal of Clinical Pathology*, *74*, 443–447. DOI: 10.1136/jclinpath-2020-206854 PMID: 32620678

Bulusu, G., Vidyasagar, K. E. C., & Mudigonda, M.. (2025). Cancer detection using artificial intelligence: A paradigm in early diagnosis. *Archives of Computational Methods in Engineering*. Advance online publication. DOI: 10.1007/s11831-025-10045-3

Campanella, G., Hanna, M. G., Geneslaw, L., Miraflor, A., Werneck Krauss Silva, V., Busam, K. J., Brogi, E., Reuter, V. E., Klimstra, D. S., & Fuchs, T. J. (2019). Clinical-grade computational pathology using weakly supervised deep learning on whole slide images. *Nature Medicine*, *25*, 1301–1309. DOI: 10.1038/s41591-019-0508-1 PMID: 31308507

Chen, X., Feng, B., Chen, Y., Liu, K., Li, K., Duan, X., Hao, Y., Cui, E., Liu, Z., & Zhang, C.. (2020). A CT-based radiomics nomogram for prediction of lung adenocarcinomas and granulomatous lesions in patients with solitary sub-centimeter solid nodules. *Cancer Imaging; the Official Publication of the International Cancer Imaging Society*, *20*(1), 1–13. DOI: 10.1186/s40644-020-00320-3 PMID: 32641166

Coudray, N., Ocampo, P. S., Sakellaropoulos, T., Narula, N., Snuderl, M., Fenyö, D., Moreira, A. L., Razavian, N., & Tsirigos, A. (2018). Classification and mutation prediction from non–small cell lung cancer histopathology images using deep learning. *Nature Medicine, 24*, 1559–1567. DOI: 10.1038/s41591-018-0177-5 PMID: 30224757

da Silva, L. M., Pereira, E. M., Salles, P. G. O., Godrich, R., Ceballos, R., Kunz, J. D., Casson, A., Viret, J., Chandarlapaty, S., & Ferreira, C. G.. (2021). Independent real-world application of a clinical-grade automated prostate cancer detection system. *The Journal of Pathology, 254*, 147–158. DOI: 10.1002/path.5662 PMID: 33904171

Danforth, K. N., Early, M. I., Ngan, S., Kosco, A. E., Zheng, C., & Gould, M. K. (2012). Automated identification of patients with pulmonary nodules in an integrated health system using administrative health plan data, radiology reports, and natural language processing. *Journal of Thoracic Oncology, 7*(8), 1257–1262. DOI: 10.1097/JTO.0b013e31825bd9f5 PMID: 22627647

Dash, R. C., Jones, N., Merrick, R., Haroske, G., Harrison, J., Sayers, C., Haarselhorst, N., Wintell, M., Herrmann, M. D., & Macary, F. (2021). Integrating the Health-care Enterprise Pathology and Laboratory Medicine guideline for digital pathology interoperability. *Journal of Pathology Informatics, 12*, 16. DOI: 10.4103/jpi.jpi_98_20 PMID: 34221632

DATA-CAN. Health Data Research Hub for Cancer | UCLPartners. (n.d.). Retrieved October 18, 2021, from https://www.data-can.org

de Koning, H. J., van der Aalst, C. M., de Jong, P. A., Scholten, E. T., Nackaerts, K., Heuvelmans, M. A., Lammers, J.-W. J., Weenink, C., Yousaf-Khan, U., & Horeweg, N.. (2020). Reduced lung-cancer mortality with volume CT screening in a randomized trial. *The New England Journal of Medicine, 382*, 503–513. DOI: 10.1056/NEJMoa1911793 PMID: 31995683

Dyer, O. (2021). US task force recommends extending lung cancer screenings to over 50s. *BMJ (Clinical Research Ed.), 372*(698). Advance online publication. DOI: 10.1136/bmj.n698 PMID: 33707175

Ehteshami Bejnordi, B., Mullooly, M., Pfeiffer, R. M., Fan, S., Vacek, P. M., Weaver, D. L., Herschorn, S., Brinton, L. A., van Ginneken, B., & Karssemeijer, N.. (2018). Using deep convolutional neural networks to identify and classify tumor-associated stroma in diagnostic breast biopsies. *Modern Pathology, 31*, 1502–1512. DOI: 10.1038/s41379-018-0073-z PMID: 29899550

Farjah, F., Halgrim, S., Buist, D. S. M., Gould, M. K., Zeliadt, S. B., Loggers, E. T., & Carrell, D. S. (2016). An automated method for identifying individuals with a lung nodule can be feasibly implemented across health systems. *EGEMS (Washington, DC)*, *4*(1), 15. DOI: 10.13063/2327-9214.1254 PMID: 27668266

Fassler, D. J., Abousamra, S., Gupta, R., Chen, C., Zhao, M., Paredes, D., Batool, S. A., Knudsen, B. S., Escobar-Hoyos, L., & Shroyer, K. R.. (2020). Deep learning–based image analysis methods for brightfield-acquired multiplex immunohistochemistry images. *Diagnostic Pathology*, *15*, 1–11. DOI: 10.1186/S13000-020-01003-0 PMID: 32723384

Franco, E. F., Rana, P., Cruz, A., Calderón, V. V., Azevedo, V., Ramos, R. T. J., & Ghosh, P. (2021). Performance comparison of deep learning autoencoders for cancer subtype detection using multi-omics data. *Cancers (Basel)*, *13*, 2013. DOI: 10.3390/cancers13092013 PMID: 33921978

Ghasemi, A., Hashtarkhani, S., Schwartz, D. L., & Shaban-Nejad, A. (2024). Explainable artificial intelligence in breast cancer detection and risk prediction: A systematic scoping review. *arXiv*. https://doi.org//arXiv.2407.12058DOI: 10.48550

Gillum, R. F. (2013). From papyrus to the electronic tablet: A brief history of the clinical medical record with lessons for the digital age. *The American Journal of Medicine*, *126*(10), 853–857. DOI: 10.1016/j.amjmed.2013.03.024 PMID: 24054954

Glaser, A. P., Jordan, B. J., Cohen, J., Desai, A., Silberman, P., & Meeks, J. J. (2018). Automated extraction of grade, stage, and quality information from transurethral resection of bladder tumor pathology reports using natural language processing. *JCO Clinical Cancer Informatics*, *2*, 1–8. DOI: 10.1200/CCI.17.00128 PMID: 30652586

Guan, Y., Aamir, M., Rahman, Z., Ali, A., Abro, W. A., Dayo, Z. A., Bhutta, M. S., Hu, Z., Guan, Y., & Aamir, M.. (2021). A framework for efficient brain tumor classification using MRI images. *Mathematical Biosciences and Engineering*, *18*, 5790–5815. DOI: 10.3934/mbe.2021292 PMID: 34517512

Habchi, Y., Himeur, Y., Kheddar, H., Boukabou, A., Atalla, S., Chouchane, A., . . . Mansoor, W. (2023). AI in thyroid cancer diagnosis: Techniques, trends, and future directions. *arXiv*. https://doi.org//arXiv.2308.13592DOI: 10.48550

Halse, H., Colebatch, A. J., Petrone, P., Henderson, M. A., Mills, J. K., Snow, H., Westwood, J. A., Sandhu, S., Raleigh, J. M., & Behren, A.. (2018). Multiplex immunohistochemistry accurately defines the immune context of metastatic melanoma. *Scientific Reports*, *8*, 11158. DOI: 10.1038/s41598-018-28944-3 PMID: 30042403

He, K., Zhang, X., Ren, S., & Sun, J. (2016). Deep residual learning for image recognition. In *Proceedings of the IEEE Conference on Computer Vision and Pattern Recognition* (pp. 770–778). Las Vegas, NV, USA. https://doi.org/DOI: 10.1109/CVPR.2016.90

Huang, G., Liu, Z., Van Der Maaten, L., & Weinberger, K. Q. (2017). Densely connected convolutional networks. In *Proceedings of the IEEE Conference on Computer Vision and Pattern Recognition (CVPR 2017)* (pp. 2261–2269). Honolulu, HI, USA. https://doi.org/DOI: 10.1109/CVPR.2017.243

Hunter, B., Reis, S., Campbell, D., Matharu, S., Ratnakumar, P., & Mercuri, L.. (2021). Development of a structured query language and natural language processing algorithm to identify lung nodules in a cancer centre. *Frontiers in Medicine, 8,* 748168. DOI: 10.3389/fmed.2021.748168 PMID: 34805217

Jan, Z., El Assadi, F., Abd-alrazaq, A., & Jithesh, P. V. (2023). Artificial intelligence for the prediction and early diagnosis of pancreatic cancer: Scoping review. *Journal of Medical Internet Research, 25,* e44248. DOI: 10.2196/44248 PMID: 37000507

Kamoun, A., Idbaih, A., Dehais, C., Elarouci, N., Carpentier, C., Letouzé, E., Colin, C., Mokhtari, K., Jouvet, A., & Uro-Coste, E.. (2016). Integrated multi-omics analysis of oligodendroglial tumours identifies three subgroups of 1p/19q co-deleted gliomas. *Nature Communications, 7,* 11263. DOI: 10.1038/ncomms11263 PMID: 27090007

Kawakami, E., Tabata, J., Yanaihara, N., Ishikawa, T., Koseki, K., Iida, Y., Saito, M., Komazaki, H., Shapiro, J. S., & Goto, C.. (2019). Application of artificial intelligence for preoperative diagnostic and prognostic prediction in epithelial ovarian cancer based on blood biomarkers. *Clinical Cancer Research, 25,* 3006–3015. DOI: 10.1158/1078-0432.CCR-18-3378 PMID: 30979733

Knijnenburg, T. A., Wang, L., Zimmermann, M. T., Chambwe, N., Gao, G. F., Cherniack, A. D., Fan, H., Shen, H., Way, G. P., & Greene, C. S.. (2018). Genomic and molecular landscape of DNA damage repair deficiency across The Cancer Genome Atlas. *Cell Reports, 23,* 239–254. DOI: 10.1016/j.celrep.2018.03.076 PMID: 29617664

Krist, A. H., Davidson, K. W., Mangione, C. M., Barry, M. J., Cabana, M., Caughey, A. B., Davis, E. M., Donahue, K. E., Doubeni, C. A., & Kubik, M.. (2021). Screening for lung cancer: US Preventive Services Task Force recommendation statement. *Journal of the American Medical Association, 325,* 962–970. DOI: 10.1001/jama.2021.1117 PMID: 33687470

Krizhevsky, A., Sutskever, I., & Hinton, G. E. (2017). ImageNet classification with deep convolutional neural networks. *Communications of the ACM*, *60*, 84–90. DOI: 10.1145/3065386

Liew, X. Y., Hameed, N., & Clos, J. (2021). An investigation of XGBoost-based algorithm for breast cancer classification. *Machine Learning with Applications*, *6*, 100154. DOI: 10.1016/j.mlwa.2021.100154

Liu, B., Liu, Y., Pan, X., Li, M., Yang, S., & Li, S. C. (2019). DNA methylation markers for pan-cancer prediction by deep learning. *Genes*, *10*, 778. DOI: 10.3390/genes10100778 PMID: 31590287

Liu, J., Xia, C., & Wang, G. (2020). Multi-omics analysis in initiation and progression of meningiomas: From pathogenesis to diagnosis. *Frontiers in Oncology*, *10*, 1491. DOI: 10.3389/fonc.2020.01491 PMID: 32983987

Liu, R., Wang, M., & Zheng, T.. (2022). An artificial intelligence-based risk prediction model of myocardial infarction. *BMC Bioinformatics*, *23*, 217. DOI: 10.1186/s12859-022-04845-3 PMID: 35672659

Lokhande, A., Bonthu, S., & Singhal, N. (2020). Carcino-Net: A deep learning framework for automated Gleason grading of prostate biopsies. In *Proceedings of the Annual International Conference of the IEEE Engineering in Medicine and Biology Society (EMBS)* (pp. 1380–1383). Montreal, QC, Canada. https://doi.org/DOI: 10.1109/EMBC44109.2020.9176011

Lu, H., Arshad, M., Thornton, A., Avesani, G., Cunnea, P., Curry, E., Kanavati, F., Liang, J., Nixon, K., & Williams, S. T.. (2019). A mathematical-descriptor of tumor-mesoscopic-structure from computed-tomography images annotates prognostic- and molecular-phenotypes of epithelial ovarian cancer. *Nature Communications*, *10*, 764. DOI: 10.1038/s41467-019-08718-9 PMID: 30770825

Madabhushi, A., Feldman, M. D., & Leo, P. (2020). Deep-learning approaches for Gleason grading of prostate biopsies. *The Lancet. Oncology*, *21*, 187–189. DOI: 10.1016/S1470-2045(19)30793-4 PMID: 31926804

Mayerhoefer, M. E., Materka, A., Langs, G., Häggström, I., Szczypiński, P., Gibbs, P., & Cook, G. (2020). Introduction to radiomics. *Journal of Nuclear Medicine*, *61*(4), 488–495. DOI: 10.2967/jnumed.118.222893 PMID: 32060219

Miller, R. J. H., Huang, C., Liang, J. X., & Slomka, P. J. (2022). Artificial intelligence for disease diagnosis and risk prediction in nuclear cardiology. *Journal of Nuclear Cardiology*, *29*(5), 1754–1762. DOI: 10.1007/s12350-021-02839-5 PMID: 35508795

Milletari, F., Navab, N., & Ahmadi, S. A. (2016). V-Net: Fully convolutional neural networks for volumetric medical image segmentation. In *Proceedings of the 2016 4th International Conference on 3D Vision (3DV)* (pp. 565–571). Stanford, CA, USA. https://doi.org/DOI: 10.1109/3DV.2016.79

Moore, C. R., Farrag, A., & Ashkin, E. (2017). Using natural language processing to extract abnormal results from cancer screening reports. *Journal of Patient Safety*, *13*(3), 138–143. DOI: 10.1097/PTS.0000000000000127 PMID: 25025472

Morin, O., Vallières, M., Braunstein, S., Ginart, J. B., Upadhaya, T., Woodruff, H. C., & Zwanenburg, A.. (2021). An artificial intelligence framework integrating longitudinal electronic health records with real-world data enables continuous pan-cancer prognostication. *Nature Cancer*, *2*(6), 709–722. DOI: 10.1038/s43018-021-00236-2 PMID: 35121948

Muhammad, W., Hart, G. R., Nartowt, B., Farrell, J. J., Johung, K., Liang, Y., & Deng, J. (2019). Pancreatic cancer prediction through an artificial neural network. *Frontiers in Artificial Intelligence*, *2*, 2. DOI: 10.3389/frai.2019.00002 PMID: 33733091

Naik, N., Madani, A., Esteva, A., Keskar, N. S., Press, M. F., Ruderman, D., Agus, D. B., & Socher, R. (2020). Deep learning–enabled breast cancer hormonal receptor status determination from base-level H&E stains. *Nature Communications*, *11*, 5727. DOI: 10.1038/s41467-020-19334-3 PMID: 33199723

Nayor, J., Borges, L. F., Goryachev, S., Gainer, V. S., & Saltzman, J. R. (2018). Natural language processing accurately calculates adenoma and sessile serrated polyp detection rates. *Digestive Diseases and Sciences*, *63*(7), 1794–1800. DOI: 10.1007/s10620-018-5078-4 PMID: 29696479

NHS Digital. (n.d.). Cancer waiting times data collection (CWT). Retrieved October 18, 2021, from https://digital.nhs.uk/data-and-information/data-collections/cancer-waiting-times

NHS Digital. (n.d.). Benefits of the new NHS cervical screening management system. Retrieved January 24, 2022, from https://digital.nhs.uk

NHSX. (n.d.). Digital transformation of screening. Retrieved January 24, 2022, from https://www.nhsx.nhs.uk

Ni, Y., Wright, J., Perentesis, J., Lingren, T., Deleger, L., Kaiser, M., Kohane, I., & Solti, I. (2015). Increasing the efficiency of trial-patient matching: Automated clinical trial eligibility pre-screening for pediatric oncology patients. *BMC Medical Informatics and Decision Making, 15*, 28. DOI: 10.1186/s12911-015-0149-3 PMID: 25881112

Olatunji, S. O., Alotaibi, S., Almutairi, E., Alrabae, Z., Almajid, Y., Altabee, R., & Alhiyafi, J. (2021). Early diagnosis of thyroid cancer diseases using computational intelligence techniques: A case study of a Saudi Arabian dataset. *Computers in Biology and Medicine, 131*, 104267. DOI: 10.1016/j.compbiomed.2021.104267 PMID: 33647831

Papadimitroulas, P., Brocki, L., Christopher Chung, N., Marchadour, W., Vermet, F., Gaubert, L., Eleftheriadis, V., Plachouris, D., Visvikis, D., & Kagadis, G. C.. (2021). Artificial intelligence: Deep learning in oncological radiomics and challenges of interpretability and data harmonization. *Physica Medica, 83*, 108–121. DOI: 10.1016/j.ejmp.2021.03.009 PMID: 33765601

Richards, T. B., Doria-Rose, V. P., Soman, A., Klabunde, C. N., Caraballo, R. S., Gray, S. C., Houston, K. A., & White, M. C. (2019). Lung cancer screening inconsistent with U.S. Preventive Services Task Force recommendations. *American Journal of Preventive Medicine, 56*, 66–73. DOI: 10.1016/j.amepre.2018.07.030 PMID: 30467092

Roch, A. M., Mehrabi, S., Krishnan, A., Schmidt, H. E., Kesterson, J., Beesley, C., Dexter, P. R., & Palakal, M. (2015). Automated pancreatic cyst screening using natural language processing: A new tool in the early detection of pancreatic cancer. *HPB : The Official Journal of the International Hepato Pancreato Biliary Association, 17*(5), 447–453. DOI: 10.1111/hpb.12375 PMID: 25537257

Ronneberger, O., Fischer, P., & Brox, T. (2015). U-Net: Convolutional networks for biomedical image segmentation. In *Lecture Notes in Computer Science, 9351,* 234–241. https://doi.org/DOI: 10.1007/978-3-319-24574-4_28

Schüffler, P. J., Geneslaw, L., Yarlagadda, D. V. K., Hanna, M. G., Samboy, J., Stamelos, E., Vanderbilt, C., Philip, J., Jean, M.-H., & Corsale, L.. (2021). Integrated digital pathology at scale: A solution for clinical diagnostics and cancer research at a large academic medical center. *Journal of the American Medical Informatics Association : JAMIA, 28*, 1874–1886. DOI: 10.1093/jamia/ocab085 PMID: 34260720

Shah, S., Slaney, E., VerHage, E., Chen, J., Dias, R., Abdelmalik, B., & Neu, J. (2023). Application of artificial intelligence in the early detection of retinopathy of prematurity: Review of the literature. *Neonatology*, *120*(5), 558–565. DOI: 10.1159/000530832 PMID: 37490881

Shakir, H., Deng, Y., & Rasheed, H. (2019). Radiomics based likelihood functions for cancer diagnosis. *Scientific Reports*, *9*, 9501. DOI: 10.1038/s41598-019-45053-x PMID: 31263186

Sharma, S., & Chaturvedi, R. (2020). AI-driven predictive modelling for early disease detection and prevention. *International Journal on Recent and Innovation Trends in Computing and Communication*, *8*(12), 27–36. DOI: 10.17762/ijritcc.v8i12.3381

Ström, P., Kartasalo, K., Olsson, H., Solorzano, L., Delahunt, B., Berney, D. M., Bostwick, D. G., Evans, A. J., Grignon, D. J., & Humphrey, P. A.. (2020). Artificial intelligence for diagnosis and grading of prostate cancer in biopsies: A population-based, diagnostic study. *The Lancet. Oncology*, *21*, 222–232. DOI: 10.1016/S1470-2045(19)30738-7 PMID: 31926806

Suh, Y. J., Jung, J., & Cho, B. J. (2020). Automated breast cancer detection in digital mammograms of various densities via deep learning. *Journal of Personalized Medicine*, *10*, 211. DOI: 10.3390/jpm10040211 PMID: 33172076

Sui, D., Liu, W., Chen, J., Zhao, C., Ma, X., Guo, M., & Tian, Z. (2021). A pyramid architecture-based deep learning framework for breast cancer detection. *BioMed Research International*, *2021*, 1–10. DOI: 10.1155/2021/2567202 PMID: 34631877

Szegedy, C., Liu, W., Jia, Y., Sermanet, P., Reed, S., Anguelov, D., Erhan, D., Vanhoucke, V., & Rabinovich, A. (2015). Going deeper with convolutions. In *Proceedings of the IEEE Conference on Computer Vision and Pattern Recognition* (pp. 1–9). Boston, MA, USA. https://doi.org/DOI: 10.1109/CVPR.2015.7298594

Takahashi, S., Takahashi, M., Tanaka, S., Takayanagi, S., Takami, H., Yamazawa, E., Nambu, S., Miyake, M., Satomi, K., & Ichimura, K.. (2021). A new era of neuro-oncology research pioneered by multi-omics analysis and machine learning. *Biomolecules*, *11*, 565. DOI: 10.3390/biom11040565 PMID: 33921457

Tan, M., & Le, Q. V. (2019). EfficientNet: Rethinking model scaling for convolutional neural networks. In *Proceedings of the 36th International Conference on Machine Learning* (pp. 10691–10700). Long Beach, CA, USA. https://proceedings.mlr.press/v97/tan19a.html

Vasaikar, S. V., Straub, P., Wang, J., & Zhang, B. (2018). LinkedOmics: Analyzing multi-omics data within and across 32 cancer types. *Nucleic Acids Research, 46,* D956–D963. DOI: 10.1093/nar/gkx1090 PMID: 29136207

Williams, B. J., Lee, J., Oien, K. A., & Treanor, D. (2018). Digital pathology access and usage in the UK: Results from a national survey on behalf of the National Cancer Research Institute's CM-Path initiative. *Journal of Clinical Pathology, 71,* 463–468. DOI: 10.1136/jclinpath-2017-204808 PMID: 29317516

Woerl, A. C., Eckstein, M., Geiger, J., Wagner, D. C., Daher, T., Stenzel, P., Fernandez, A., Hartmann, A., Wand, M., & Roth, W.. (2020). Deep learning predicts molecular subtype of muscle-invasive bladder cancer from conventional histopathological slides. *European Urology, 78,* 256–264. DOI: 10.1016/j.eururo.2020.04.023 PMID: 32354610

Xiao, L. H., Chen, P. R., Gou, Z. P., Li, Y. Z., Li, M., Xiang, L. C., & Feng, P. (2017). Prostate cancer prediction using the random forest algorithm that takes into account transrectal ultrasound findings, age, and serum levels of prostate-specific antigen. *Asian Journal of Andrology, 19,* 586–591. DOI: 10.4103/1008-682X.186884 PMID: 27586028

Zhang, F., Kaufman, H. L., Deng, Y., & Drabier, R. (2013). Recursive SVM biomarker selection for early detection of breast cancer in peripheral blood. *BMC Medical Genomics, 6*(Suppl. 1), S4. DOI: 10.1186/1755-8794-6-S1-S4 PMID: 23369435

Chapter 3
AI–Driven Diagnostics in Metabolic Disorders:
Predictive Analytics and Risk Assessment

Himansu
https://orcid.org/0009-0007-9553-8020
Amity Institute of Biotechnology, India

Tushar Joshi
https://orcid.org/0009-0006-4316-1391
Amity Institute of Biotechnology, India

Hina Bansal
https://orcid.org/0000-0003-1683-1581
Amity University, Noida, India

ABSTRACT

Metabolic disorders—including diabetes, weight problems, excessive blood pressure, etc, are getting increasingly more common in today's quick-moving, challenging world. These ailments don't arise instantly. Often, some subtle signs and vulnerabilities accumulate over time, however, they pass neglected till it is too overdue. Conventional checkout frameworks depend closely on inflexible criteria and obstacles, which can overlook the hidden systems. Artificial intelligence, however, is transforming this approach. With its capability to examine extensive information pools, computational intelligence is aiding healthcare providers in identifying threats earlier, tailoring therapy, and even foreseeing health deterioration. The essence of this chapter is to explore the developing function of artificial intelligence in determining metabolic

DOI: 10.4018/979-8-3373-3196-6.ch003

disorders, emphasizing forecasting, predictive analysis, and risk assessment. We shall explore the most recent studies, AI models, current systems, tangible issues, and the personal consequences of these innovations, both now and in the future.

1. INTRODUCTION

Metabolic disorders are a major and growing global health burden, with diabetes mellitus, obesity, and inborn errors of metabolism serving as disorders under this class. This group of diseases involves the dysregulation of critical biochemical pathways that regulate energy homeostasis, lipid metabolism, and protein catabolism. Their multifactorial etiology usually includes the interplay between genetic susceptibilities and other predisposing elements such as epigenetic modification, environmental factors, or lifestyle choices, including diet and physical inactivity. As observed over the last two decades, the incidence and prevalence of these diseases have dramatically increased, driven by an increase in urbanization and lifestyle changes, notably occurring in low- and middle-income countries.

The diagnosis of metabolic diseases in their traditional model has been the clinical one, based on fixed accordingly arbitrary-related numerical thresholds example, fasting plasma glucose, HbA1C, the body mass index-score, which usually diagnose the condition only after the occurrence of considerable metabolic damage. Being reactive, these systems are ill-suited for early intervention or truly identifying subclinical phenotypes that may develop into gross pathology. Furthermore, due to the heterogeneous nature of metabolic syndromes, it becomes insidious to aim for generalized screening tools, thus creating an avenue for truly individualized predictive models.(Bagheri et al., 2024)

Here, AI-the ML and DL algorithms in particular-has offered a paradigm shift in medical diagnosis. AI can process and model high-dimensional, multimodal datasets, including genome sequences, transcriptomic profiles, metabolomics, clinical imaging, and longitudinal EHR data, to uncover hidden and non-linear relationships often imperceptible to traditional statistical methods. For example, CNNs have been employed to yield an imaging diagnosis of hepatic steatosis. Likewise, RNNs can model time-dependent clinical data to predict metabolic decompensation in patients with inherited disorders.

In addition to predictive power, AI can help implement precision medicine. In this approach, diagnostic and treatment strategies are tailored to the molecular and phenotypic profile of the individual patient. Explainable AI (XAI) technologies such as Shapley Additive Description and Note Mechanisms have proven to tackle black box problems. They provide transparency and interpretability that is very important for clinicians and regulatory approval. Like Babs. (2024) point to the true promise of AI lies in its ability to change health care from a reactive approach to an active system focused on predictive, prevention, and personalized care. Similarly, Sghairen et al. (2022) demonstrate that AI systems achieve high diagnostic accuracy in identifying components of metabolic syndrome. It also provides interpretable knowledge that is useful for clinical implementation (Pawade et al., 2024).

Together, integrating AI into the diagnostic workflow of metabolic disorders combines computer biology, clinical computer science, and translational medicine. This combination is set up to recognize, monitor, and ultimately prevent these complex conditions.

Objectives

The point of exploring AI-driven diagnostics in metabolic disorders is to gain an understanding of the trends, tribulations, and future perspectives. Deliberately examining, the goals are (Rajpurkar et al, 2022):

- AI Tools in Diagnosing Metabolic Disorder: Machine learning is transforming detection by examining extensive datasets to identify threats early, surpassing conventional techniques dependent on fixed parameters.
- Tribulations: Issues encompass confidentiality of records, algorithmic prejudice, and demanding situations in embedding device learning into clinical workflows
- Key Frameworks: Advanced architecture as neural networks, assess risks through linking statistical factors throughout genetic, lifestyle, and environment.
- Future Prospect: Medical things getting to know-improved consultations should deliver customized health forecasts, holistic health management, and streamlining outcomes

The comprehensive point of this thinking, which is illustrated in Figure 1 is to examine the conclusions of metabolic disorders and the transformational portion of knowledge (AI) generated as part of the hazard layer.

As global disease rates such as type of diabetes (T2DM), physical and metabolic disorders, paradigms of normal symptoms, such as inactive limitations, increased, unconnected biomarkers. AI offers an opportunity to move from responsive to data-driven, prescient healthcare, leveraging computational strategies to reveal designs that are intangible to human clinicians.

Based on the system laid out by Rajpurkar et al. (2022), this audit sets forward the taking after center destinations:

Figure 1. The tree diagram illustrates the core objectives of the study on AI in metabolic health. Each branch represents a key focus area, unified under the central goal of advancing AI-driven diagnostics and management.

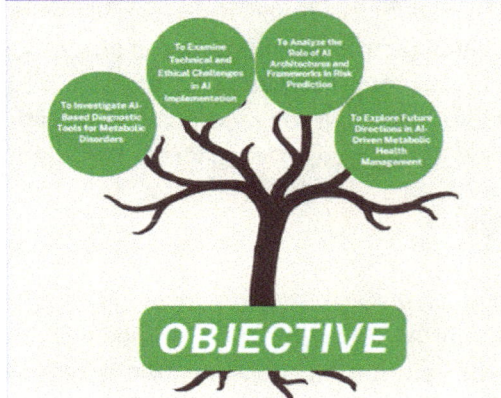

1. To Investigate AI-Based Diagnostic Tools for Metabolic Disorders

This objective seeks to evaluate the application of machine learning (ML) and deep learning (DL) algorithms in the detection and classification of metabolic diseases. These tools can process complex, high-dimensional datasets derived from:

- Electronic Health Records (EHRs) containing longitudinal clinical data,
- Wearable and mobile health technologies capturing real-time behavioral and physiological metrics,
- Genomic and multi-omics data, including SNP profiles and metabolomics.

ML models such as random forests, gradient boosting machines (e.g., XGBoost), support vector machines (SVMs), and convolutional/recurrent neural networks (CNNs/RNNs) have shown superior performance over traditional rule-based diagnostics by accounting for nonlinear interactions, feature dependencies, and latent phenotypic expressions. This objective will analyze current evidence for their sensitivity, specificity, generalizability, and clinical utility.

2. To Examine Technical and Ethical Challenges in AI Implementation

In spite of the developing excitement for AI in metabolic care, noteworthy specialized, moral, and operational impediments persist:

- Data protection and security: The utilize of individual wellbeing information requires strict adherence to moral measures (e.g., GDPR, HIPAA) and execution of privacy-preserving methods such as differential security and unified learning.
- Algorithmic predisposition: AI models prepared on non-diverse datasets may proliferate or indeed compound wellbeing incongruities, particularly among underrepresented populations. Fairness-aware machine learning and predisposition-inspecting devices are basic in this regard.
- Clinical integration and interoperability: Implanting AI models into existing clinical workflows requires a strong framework, EHR integration, clinician preparation, and a user-friendly interface that is both instinctive and actionable. This objective fundamentally evaluates these obstructions and investigates arrangements grounded in administrative science, reasonable AI (XAI), and human-centered design.

3. To Analyze the Role of AI Architectures and Frameworks in Risk Prediction

Modern AI models—profound neural networks, transformers, and graph neural networks (GNNs)—offer advanced capabilities in modeling relationships across disparate data domains. For example, they can:

- Infer causal relationships between genetic variants, environmental exposures, and lifestyle behaviors,
- Generate polygenic risk scores (PRS) integrated with dynamic physiological data,
- Perform temporal modeling to predict disease onset, trajectory, and treatment response.

This objective will review the key computational frameworks that facilitate personalized diagnostics and prognostics, focusing on how these systems capture the complexity of metabolic pathophysiology.

4. To Explore Future Directions in AI-Driven Metabolic Health Management

This objective aims to project how next-generation AI systems will enhance diagnostic precision and therapeutic outcomes. Anticipated innovations include:

- AI-augmented clinical consultations that deliver real-time, personalized health forecasts,
- Digital twin models for simulating metabolic responses to interventions,
- Edge AI and embedded sensors for continuous glucose and lipid monitoring,
- Federated learning ecosystems where hospitals and research centers co-train models while preserving patient confidentiality.

The integration of these technologies will move the field toward proactive, holistic, and precision-based metabolic care, with a focus on early detection, real-time intervention, and individualized health maintenance.

2. METABOLIC DISORDERS: AN OVERVIEW

Metabolic disorders encompass a diverse array of pathological conditions characterized by disruptions in the biochemical processes that regulate energy production, storage, and utilization. These disturbances may be inherited (genetic) or acquired, and they often involve defects in enzymatic pathways responsible for the metabolism of carbohydrates, fats, proteins, or nucleic acids. The resulting metabolic imbalances can have systemic consequences, affecting multiple organ systems and increasing the risk of comorbid conditions. Types of metabolic disorders are illustrated well in figure 2.(Abut et al., 2024)

Common types-

Metabolic disorders manifest in various forms depending on the affected metabolic pathway. Below are some of the most prevalent categories:

Diabetes Mellitus

Diabetes mellitus is a group of metabolic diseases characterized by chronic hyperglycemia resulting from defects in insulin secretion, insulin action, or both. There are two principal forms:

- Type 1 Diabetes Mellitus (T1DM) is an autoimmune condition in which pancreatic β-cells are destroyed, leading to absolute insulin deficiency.
- Type 2 Diabetes Mellitus (T2DM) is associated with peripheral insulin resistance, often coupled with a relative insulin secretory defect.

In T2DM, insulin signaling is impaired at the cellular level, particularly in skeletal muscle, adipose tissue, and the liver. This impairs glucose uptake and glycogen synthesis, leading to elevated blood glucose levels. Chronic hyperglycemia contributes to microvascular (retinopathy, nephropathy, neuropathy) and macrovascular (atherosclerosis, myocardial infarction) complications.

Obesity

Obesity is defined by an excessive accumulation of adipose tissue and is typically quantified using body mass index (BMI $\geq$ 30 kg/m^2). From a metabolic perspective, obesity is a state of chronic low-grade inflammation and dysregulated energy homeostasis.

Adipocytes in obese individuals secrete increased levels of pro-inflammatory cytokines (e.g., TNF-α, IL-6) and adipokines (e.g., leptin, resistin), while adiponectin levels are decreased. These biochemical changes contribute to insulin resistance, impaired lipid metabolism, and increased risk of metabolic syndrome—a cluster of conditions including hyperglycemia, dyslipidemia, hypertension, and central obesity.

Obesity also predisposes individuals to ectopic fat deposition in the liver (non-alcoholic fatty liver disease, NAFLD), skeletal muscle, and pancreas, further exacerbating metabolic dysfunction.(Alam et al., 2024)

Inborn Errors of Metabolism (IEMs)

IEMs are a heterogeneous group of rare genetic disorders caused by mutations in genes encoding enzymes, transport proteins, or cofactors essential for metabolic pathways. The absence or malfunction of these proteins results in the accumulation of toxic substrates or deficiency of critical metabolites.

Examples include:

- Phenylketonuria (PKU): Caused by mutations in the *PAH* gene encoding phenylalanine hydroxylase, this disorder prevents the conversion of phenylalanine to tyrosine. The accumulation of phenylalanine leads to neurotoxicity, resulting in intellectual disability if not managed with dietary restriction.
- Maple Syrup Urine Disease (MSUD): Results from deficiency in the branched-chain α-keto acid dehydrogenase (BCKD) complex, impairing the

catabolism of branched-chain amino acids (leucine, isoleucine, and valine). Accumulation of these amino acids and their toxic derivatives causes severe neurological impairment and a characteristic sweet odor in urine.

- Glycogen Storage Diseases (GSDs): A group of disorders affecting glycogen synthesis or degradation. For instance, Type I GSD (von Gierke disease) is due to glucose-6-phosphatase deficiency, leading to hypoglycemia and lactic acidosis due to impaired gluconeogenesis.(Paplomatas et al., 2024)

The clinical presentation of IEMs varies by the metabolic pathway involved but often includes developmental delays, metabolic acidosis, organomegaly, and failure to thrive.

Figure 2. Classification of metabolic disorders into congenital and acquired types. Subcategories include lipid storage, amino acid metabolism, carbohydrate metabolism, and associated acquired conditions.

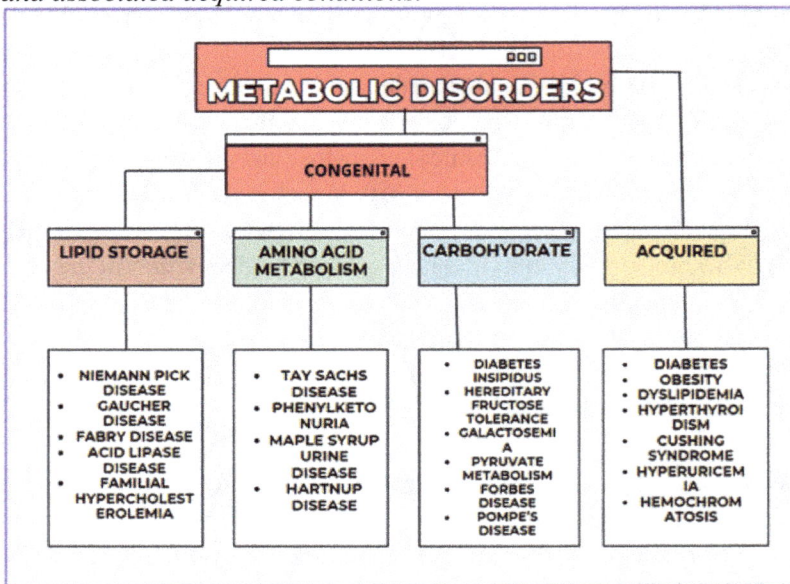

Current Diagnostic Practices

Current diagnostic frameworks for metabolic disorders rely heavily on established clinical biomarkers, anthropometric indices, and—where available—genetic screening. These methods are designed for confirmatory diagnostics rather than early prediction or individualized intervention, limiting their utility in precision medicine and preventive care.

Biochemical Assays

Biochemical markers shape the foundation of metabolic clutter diagnostics. Key measures include:

- Fasting Plasma Glucose (FPG) and Verbal Glucose Resistance Test (OGTT): These tests survey affront affectability and glucose homeostasis, and are essential symptomatic instruments for diabetes mellitus. FPG 126 mg/dL or a 2-hour OGTT 200 mg/dL are symptomatic of diabetes. Be that as it may, these measures frequently identify malady as it were after irreversible metabolic derangements have occurred.
- Glycated Hemoglobin (HbA1c): Reflecting normal blood glucose over a 2 - 3 month period, HbA1c is less touchy to intense glycemic changeability but valuable in following long-term glycemic control. In spite of its far reaching utilize, HbA1c can be bewildered by hemoglobinopathies, iron deficiency, and ethnic variations.
- Lipid Profile: Add up to cholesterol, HDL-C, LDL-C, and triglycerides are utilized to assess lipid digestion system. Dyslipidemia especially lifted triglycerides and moo HDL is a common include of metabolic syndrome. However, standard boards don't completely capture lipidomic complexity, such as oxidized LDL or lipoprotein molecule size.
- Liver Proteins and Renal Markers: Lifted alanine transaminase (ALT) or gamma-glutamyltransferase (GGT) may propose hepatic steatosis or non-alcoholic greasy liver malady (NAFLD), a common comorbidity in corpulence and sort 2 diabetes.(Kumar & Manoj, 2024)

Physical and Anthropometric Assessments

- Body Mass Record (BMI): Whereas broadly utilized, BMI may be a rough degree of adiposity that does not separate between incline and fat mass or account for fat distribution.
- Waist Circumference (WC) and Waist-to-Hip Proportion (WHR): These lists give way better gauges of visceral adiposity, which connects more closely with affront resistance and cardiovascular chance.
- Blood Pressure Monitoring: Hypertension is a diagnostic criterion in metabolic syndrome, often linked with endothelial dysfunction and altered sympathetic activity in obesity and diabetes.

Genetic and Molecular Screening

Genetic testing plays a critical role in the diagnosis of inborn errors of metabolism (IEMs). Techniques such as next-generation sequencing (NGS), whole-exome sequencing (WES), and targeted gene panels are used to identify pathogenic variants in key metabolic genes (e.g., *PAH* in phenylketonuria, *BCKDHA* in maple syrup urine disease).

However, in polygenic conditions like type 2 diabetes or obesity, genetic testing has limited predictive value due to the complex interplay of environmental and epigenetic modifiers. Polygenic risk scores (PRS) are still being validated for clinical utility.(Liu et al., 2025)

Limitations of Current Practices

Whereas these demonstrative instruments are vigorous in affirming infection nearness, they show a few basic limitations and the diagnostic modalities table, summarizing each method's strengths, drawbacks, and AI's supportive role is given in table 1.

- Lack of Early Prescient Control: Most tests distinguish malady after significant physiological harm has happened. For illustration, Î²-cell brokenness in sort 2 diabetes frequently goes before hyperglycemia by a long time but goes undetected
- Poor Information Integration: Conventional diagnostics don't consolidate longitudinal information such as nonstop glucose checking, dietary admissions, action levels, or psychosocial factors all of which balance malady risk.
- Fragmented Information Biological systems: Wellbeing information are regularly siloed over electronic restorative record (EMR) frameworks, research facilities, and wearable gadgets, anticipating all encompassing investigation. As Babu et al. (2024) note, this fracture impedes real-time clinical decision-making and proactive infection management.
- Limited Personalization: Standardized cutoffs don't reflect inter-individual changeability due to age, sex, ethnicity, or hereditary foundation. This one-size-fits-all show decreases symptomatic exactness and restorative adequacy.

Table 1. This table depicts a Summary of current diagnostic practices, including Diagnostic Modality, Pros, Limitations, and Role for AI

Diagnostic Modality	Pros	Limitations	Role for AI
Biochemical Assays	• Standardized, validated tests• Direct metabolic markers (e.g., glucose, HbA1c, lipids)	• Detects disease post-onset• Influenced by non-metabolic factors (e.g., anemia, ethnicity)• Limited scope	• Pattern recognition for early risk• Predictive modeling using real-time trends
Physical & Anthropometric	• Simple, non-invasive, low-cost• Useful for large-scale screening (BMI, WC, WHR)	• Poor specificity• Does not reflect fat distribution or body composition	• Enhanced by wearable/device integration• AI can personalize based on age, sex, ethnicity
Genetic & Molecular Screening	• Critical for diagnosing monogenic disorders (e.g., IEMs)• Enables early/pre-symptomatic detection	• Limited use in polygenic conditions• Environmental/ epigenetic effects often overlooked	• Refine polygenic risk scores• Integrate with omics and lifestyle data
Blood Pressure Monitoring	• Key diagnostic in metabolic syndrome• Linked with cardiovascular risk	• Not directly tied to metabolic dysfunction• Affected by stress, medication	• AI to detect longitudinal trends• Early hypertension risk from wearable BP devices
Liver & Renal Function Tests	• Indicate comorbidities (NAFLD, CKD)• Available in routine labs	• Non-specific markers• Affected by other diseases or medications	• Early risk stratification through AI trend analysis• Combine with imaging and lifestyle data
Overall Diagnostic Framework	• Multi-modal, evidence-based• Strong for confirmatory diagnosis	• Fragmented data ecosystems• Lacks personalization• One-size-fits-all thresholds	• Unify siloed data sources• Enable precision diagnostics and personalized interventions

Given these constraints, there is a growing recognition that novel diagnostic paradigms—leveraging AI and integrative omics—are essential to detect disease earlier, personalize treatment, and reduce the global burden of metabolic disorders(Awari et al., 2025)

3. ARTIFICIAL INTELLIGENCE IN MEDICAL DIAGNOSTICS

The integration of Artificial Intelligence (AI) into clinical practice marks a paradigm shift in healthcare delivery, particularly in diagnostics. AI systems that can simulate aspects of human perception can process computers, complex, high-dimensional datasets, allowing them to identify patterns, predict, and support decision-making. In the field of metabolic disorders characterized by AI in lifestyle interactions in genetic environments, AI demonstrates previous promises essential to the potential for more accurate and personalized diagnosis.

3.1 Overview of AI, Machine Learning, and Deep Learning

OppoEit Insights (AI) is a roofing term that involves extending computing strategies to perform assignments that normally require human insight. In this room, machine learning (ML) implies calculations that can learn a measurable design of labeled or unmarked information, and repeatedly executes its execution through presentations on unused data. ML allows careful modeling, classification, recurrence and clustering in actual near or within fragmented data of Kramor.

Key ML approaches in restorative diagnostics include (table 2)

- Support Vector Machines (SVMs): A directed learning calculation that finds the hyperplane maximizing the edge between classes. SVMs are especially successful in high-dimensional clinical datasets, such as those utilized in biomarker-based chance stratification.
- Decision Trees and Irregular Woodlands: These tree-based models recursively part input highlights to progress classification exactness. Irregular timberlands combine different trees through outfit learning, upgrading vigor and lessening overfitting.
- Logistic Relapse:generalized direct demonstrate utilized for parallel results (e.g., infection vs. no malady), frequently connected in epidemiological modeling.
- Naive Bayes Classifiers: Based on Bayes €™ hypothesis, these models are computationally proficient and work well with probabilistic malady models, especially when highlights are conditionally independent.

    Deep Learning (DL) may be a subfield of ML that leverages manufactured neural systems with numerous covered up layers to demonstrate exceedingly complex and nonlinear connections. DL models utilized in restorative AI include:
- Convolutional Neural Systems (CNNs): Particularly compelling for preparing spatial information such as radiologic pictures, retinal checks, or histopathology slides, which are important within the location of diabetic retinopathy or NAFLD.
- Recurrent Neural Systems (RNNs) and Long Short-Term Memory (LSTM) Systems: Suited for worldly and successive information, such as nonstop glucose checking (CGM) or time-series understanding records.

These AI models are able of self-adaptation, permitting them to recalibrate as unused information gotten to be available a basic highlight in energetic clinical settings. As Babu et al. (2024) emphasize, AI frameworks can advance over time by learning from real-world clinical information, upgrading their generalizability and clinical significance.(Yang et al., 2025)

3.2 Role of AI in Disease Detection

AI algorithms significantly outperform traditional statistical models in early disease detection, particularly by recognizing subtle, multivariate interactions among risk factors that may precede clinical onset. In metabolic disorders, patho-physiological changes—such as insulin resistance, adipose tissue inflammation, or altered lipid metabolism—begin well before overt symptoms or biochemical abnormalities manifest.

For instance, machine learning models can detect aberrant patterns in:

- Glycemic variability from CGM data,
- Lipidomic signatures associated with subclinical dyslipidemia,
- Waist-to-hip ratio trajectories indicating central obesity,
- Inflammatory biomarkers indicative of adipocyte dysfunction.

Sghairen et al. (2022) demonstrated the integration of routine clinical variables (e.g. BMI, triglycerides, HDL-C, blood pressure, plain glucose) with ML algorithms or vector classification support such as gradient boost machine (GBMS), or with ML algorithms such as metabolic synchronization prediction. These models record nonlinear dependencies and feature interactions that may overlook traditional regression models.

3.3 Types of Data Used: Clinical, Genomic, and Lifestyle

The power of AI lies in its capacity to integrate heterogeneous and multimodal datasets, offering a comprehensive, systems-level view of health and disease. In metabolic diagnostics, the key data sources include:

Clinical Data:

Structured data derived from electronic health records (EHRs), including laboratory test results (e.g., fasting glucose, HbA1c, ALT/AST), diagnostic codes, medication history, comorbidities, and physician notes (through natural language processing).

Genomic and Multi-Omics Data:

Includes single-nucleotide polymorphisms (SNPs), copy number variations, gene expression profiles (RNA-seq), epigenetic markers (e.g., methylation patterns), and metabolomic/lipidomic profiles. For example, polymorphisms in *TCF7L2*, *FTO*, or *PPARG* are associated with diabetes and obesity risk and can be incorporated into polygenic risk scores (PRSs).

Lifestyle and Behavioral Data:

Captured via wearable devices, smartphone applications, or self-report tools. These data include physical activity (step count, heart rate variability), sleep patterns, dietary intake, sedentary behavior, and even psychological stress indicators—factors with profound influence on metabolic health.(Cheng et al., 2024)

Table 2. the table represents methods, data, accuracy and key findings for AI in medical diagnostics

Study (Year)	Method	Data	Accuracy / AUC	Key Findings
Sghaireen et al. (2022) (mdpi.com)	10 ML models + data augmentation	Clinical variables (BMI, BP, glucose, lipids, obesity status)	Significant performance boost after augmentation (exact AUC not specified)	Data augmentation + feature selection enhanced classifier accuracy
Tavares et al. (2022)	LightGBM (plus LR, LDA, k-NN, DT, XGBoost)	WC, TG, HDL-C, BP, glycemia	AUC 0.86; Sensitivity 87.8%; Specificity 70.2%	LGBM best predicted MetS; increased activity and decreased BMI lowered risk
Gao et al. (2025)	CatBoost	NHANES + CHARLS (age, gender, BP, WC, fasting glucose)	AUC 0.973 (internal), 0.959 (external) for METS-IR	Simple clinical features + CatBoost achieve near-perfect IR prediction; WC is dominant feature
NHANES MetS mortality cohort (2024)	CatBoost (with RF, SVM, XGBoost, LightGBM comparison)	Cardiorenal biomarkers (hs-cTnT/I, NT-proBNP, β2M, Cr, CysC)	AUC 0.862; Accuracy 0.805; F1 0.861	CatBoost best predicted mortality among MetS patients; top markers were hs-cTnT, NT-proBNP, β2M
Xu et al. (2023)	Naïve Bayes (plus RF, SVM, DT, LR, NB, ANN)	Non-invasive: age, gender, BMI, SBP/DBP	AUC 0.976; Accuracy 0.923; Sensitivity 98.3%; Specificity 91.3%	Non-invasive NB model showed excellent performance for MetS screening in a large Chinese cohort

The integration of these diverse data types via multimodal AI frameworks allows for:

- Feature-level fusion: Combining raw features from multiple sources into a single input vector.
- Model-level fusion: Employing ensemble methods to integrate predictions from models trained on different data modalities.

Babu et al. (2024) highlight that such integrative systems significantly enhance the predictive accuracy and contextual relevance of diagnostic outputs, paving the way for personalized, data-informed clinical decision-making. Importantly, explainable AI (XAI) techniques such as SHAP (Shapley Additive Explanations) or attention-based models also help clinicians understand why a model makes a certain prediction—addressing critical barriers to clinical trust and regulatory approval. (Tavares et al., 2022)

HOW AI CAN HELP DOCTORS DIAGNOSE AND TREAT PATIENTS: A SIMPLE GUIDE

AI (Artificial Intelligence) might sound complicated, but at its heart, it's a tool—one that can help doctors make faster, more accurate decisions. Here's how the process works, step by step:

1. Start with the Right Data

To teach AI how to help, we first need data. That means collecting information from different places—like medical records, lab tests, X-rays, genetic reports, fitness trackers, and even patient surveys. The better the data, the better the results. And of course, we make sure it's all handled safely and privately.

2. Clean It Up

Real-life data is often messy. Some things are missing, out of place, or not useful. So before we do anything else, we clean it. Think of it like sorting through a cluttered drawer—only keeping what matters and making sure it's all organized the same way.

3. Focus on What's Important

Not all data is helpful for making medical predictions. We look at what really matters—things that help spot diseases early or guide treatment. It's like finding the few puzzle pieces that complete the picture.

4. Teach the AI

Now, we train the AI system using that cleaned-up, meaningful data. We show it lots of examples—so it learns patterns that humans might miss. Depending on the problem, we might use different types of AI, from simple ones to more advanced models that can even look at medical images.(Dang et al., 2025)

5. See How It Performs

Once the AI is trained, we test it. Can it accurately spot signs of illness? Does it miss anything? Can it work well with new patient data? We use different ways to check this, making sure it's safe, reliable, and useful in the real world.

6. Make It Understandable

Doctors need to know why the AI is making a suggestion. We use tools that explain the AI's reasoning in a simple way. This builds trust—because no one wants a "black box" making decisions about someone's health.

7. Put It Into Practice

When everything checks out, we add the AI tool to the systems doctors already use. It might be part of a medical software or an app—something that fits easily into their daily routine. We also keep an eye on it over time, updating it as new data comes in.(Galal et al., 2022)

8. Test It in the Real World

Before fully rolling it out, we test the AI in real hospitals or clinics. We study how it affects diagnosis, treatment, and patient outcomes. We also work closely with doctors, ethics boards, and regulators to make sure everything is safe, fair, and truly helpful.

4. PREDICTIVE ANALYTICS FOR RISK ASSESSMENT

Predictive analytics represents important advances in relocation in the direction of aggressive and personalized healthcare. In the context of metabolic disorders such as type 2 diabetes (T2DM), metabolic syndrome (METS), and predictive models of obesity, development was developed to predict disease initiation, identify progress and spend preventive interventions. This is particularly valuable in asymptomatic populations, demonstrating early asymptomatic changes and avoiding irreversible damage.

4.1 Risk Modeling Approaches

Several predictive modeling techniques are employed in clinical informatics to assess metabolic disease risk. Each algorithm brings unique strengths in handling data heterogeneity, multicollinearity, and nonlinear relationships—hallmarks of metabolic syndrome pathophysiology.(Anwar et al., 2025)

Logistic Regression (LR):

A classical statistical method used for binary classification tasks. It models the log-odds of a binary outcome (e.g., disease presence vs. absence) as a linear function of predictor variables. Despite its simplicity, LR is robust, interpretable, and forms the baseline for many clinical risk scoring systems (e.g., the Framingham Risk Score). However, it assumes linearity between predictors and outcome, which may limit its utility in complex metabolic interactions.

Random Forests and XGBoost (Extreme Gradient Boosting):

These ensemble learning methods construct multiple decision trees and aggregate their predictions to enhance accuracy and reduce overfitting. Random Forests utilize bootstrapping and feature randomness to build independent trees, whereas XGBoost optimizes performance through gradient descent and regularization techniques. These models are particularly powerful in capturing:

- Nonlinear interactions among metabolic variables (e.g., the synergy between waist circumference, triglycerides, and insulin resistance).
- Feature importance rankings, which help identify the most predictive biomarkers in large clinical datasets.

Support Vector Machines (SVMs):

SVMs are effective in high-dimensional feature spaces and are commonly used for classifying metabolic states (e.g., normoglycemia vs. impaired glucose tolerance). They work by identifying the hyperplane that best separates data into distinct classes, maximizing the margin between them. Kernel functions (e.g., radial basis functions) enable SVMs to model complex, non-linear decision boundaries—ideal for heterogeneous metabolic phenotypes.

Feature Engineering and Data Preprocessing:

As Babu et al. (2024) emphasize, model performance is highly dependent on meticulous data preprocessing. Key strategies include:

- Normalization or standardization to ensure that variables with different scales contribute appropriately to model learning.
- Imputation of missing values, using techniques such as k-nearest neighbors (KNN), mean imputation, or multiple imputation by chained equations (MICE).
- Feature selection methods like Recursive Feature Elimination (RFE), LASSO regression, or mutual information ranking, which help reduce dimensionality and enhance generalization by removing irrelevant or redundant predictors. (Rajpurkar et al., 2022)

Proper handling of imbalanced datasets—a common issue in population screening where healthy cases vastly outnumber disease cases—is essential to avoid bias. Oversampling techniques such as SMOTE (Synthetic Minority Oversampling Technique) are often applied to balance class representation during model training.

4.2 Use of AI in Predicting Disease Onset and Progression

AI-based predictive analytics has been increasingly applied to forecast not only the initial onset but also the longitudinal progression of metabolic disorders. By continuously learning from structured and unstructured health data, AI models can identify early warning signals that precede clinical thresholds—such as declining insulin sensitivity or subtle shifts in lipid ratios.

Case Example – Sghaireen et al. (2022):

In a landmark study, Sghaireen and colleagues constructed an AI-driven predictive pipeline to identify individuals at risk for metabolic syndrome. Their methodology included:

- Synthetic Minority Oversampling Technique (SMOTE): Used to address the problem of class imbalance, SMOTE generates synthetic examples of the minority class (e.g., individuals with metabolic syndrome), thereby improving the classifier's ability to recognize underrepresented outcomes.
- Classifier Models: A combination of K-Nearest Neighbors (KNN) and decision trees was used to model nonlinear and context-sensitive relationships among features. Their ensemble model achieved a classification accuracy of 94.4%, underscoring the efficacy of combining data augmentation with interpretable classifiers.
- Explainable AI (XAI) – SHAP (SHapley Additive exPlanations): To interpret model predictions and enhance clinical acceptability, SHAP values were applied to quantify the contribution of each input feature to the final prediction. Key variables identified included:
  o Body Mass Index (BMI)
  o Systolic Blood Pressure
  o High-Density Lipoprotein (HDL) Cholesterol
  o Triglycerides

These features correspond closely to the diagnostic criteria for metabolic syndrome, suggesting that the model aligns well with pathophysiological understanding—a critical criterion for clinical deployment. (Sghaireen et al., 2022)

Predicting Disease Progression:

Beyond initial diagnosis, AI models can track disease trajectories. For instance, RNNs and LSTM networks can model longitudinal data from electronic health records (EHRs) or continuous glucose monitors (CGMs) to predict:

- Transition from prediabetes to T2DM.
- Progression from NAFLD to non-alcoholic steatohepatitis (NASH).
- Cardiometabolic complications in obese patients.

These capabilities support dynamic risk stratification and adaptive care plans that evolve with the patient's metabolic profile.

5. DIAGNOSTIC APPLICATIONS OF AI IN METABOLIC DISORDERS

Metabolic disorders such as type 2 diabetes (T2DM), metabolic syndrome (METS), obesity and non-alcoholic fatty liver disease (NAFLD) are due to the extended clinical phase and complex interaction between its multifactorial pathogenesis, gene, metabolic and multifactorial and environmental interactions. In particular, those based on machine learning (ML) and deep learning (DL) are increasingly developed and validated to improve the sensitivity, specificity and efficiency of diagnosis in several clinical fields. An overview of AI framework is shown in figure 3(Zschaubitz et al., 2025)

5.1 Early Detection Algorithms

Early detection is the basis for effective management of metabolic diseases and allows for rapid intervention in the development of irreversible organ damage or comorbidities (e.g. cardiovascular disease, nephropathy or neuropathy). Traditional risk values, such as FindRisc and Framingham models, are limited by linear assumptions and static inputs. In contrast, AI systems can use high-dimensional multimodal data to identify asymptomatic indicators of disease.

Figure 3. Overview of AI applications in metabolic health management. Key components include wearables, imaging, blood assays, and electronic health records, each enhancing diagnostics and personalized care.

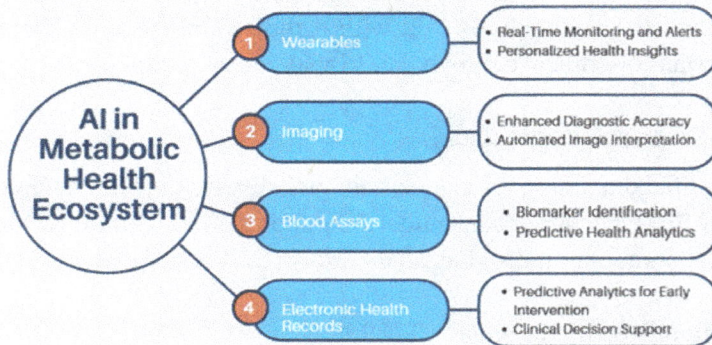

AI Methodologies for Early Detection:

- Supervised learning algorithms, such as logistic regression, decision trees, and gradient boosting, can classify individuals as high- or low-risk based on labeled historical data.
- Unsupervised learning, including clustering (e.g., k-means, DBSCAN), can detect previously unrecognized patient subgroups or early phenotypes.
- Time-series models such as Long Short-Term Memory (LSTM) networks can model the temporal evolution of metabolic risk markers.

Sghairen et al. (2022) demonstrated the use of ML models (KNN, decision tree) in conjunction with synthetic frequency oversampling technology (SMOTE) to effectively handle unbalanced data records in predicting metabolic syndrome. Her pipeline achieved a classification accuracy of 94.4%, showing that routine clinical variables (BMI, systolic blood pressure, triglycerides, HDL cholesterol) can be converted into early warning tools with adequate modeling. This aspect of explainable KI (XAI) is extremely important in clinical decisions and allows physicians to pursue the reasons for the outcome of the algorithm.(Charalampopoulos et al., 2024)

5.2 AI in Imaging and Biomarker Analysis

- AI, particularly deep learning, shows great promise for radiological and molecular diagnostics in metabolic disorders. These tools not only improve the speed and reproducibility of image-based diagnosis, but also allow for new discoveries of biomarkers when resolution and scale occur. They were used to analyze MRI, CT, and ultrasound images to recognize liver staining, visceral obesity, pancreatic fat, and arterial calcification. All of these are important for metabolic disease stations. Evaluation method.
- In cardiovascular imaging, CNNs can detect vascular remodeling, coronary artery calcium (CAC), and arterial stiffness, all of which are early indicators of metabolic complications.

AI in Biomarker Discovery:

As discussed by Babu et al. (2024), AI has been instrumental in identifying novel molecular signatures through the integration of:

- Multi-omics data (genomics, transcriptomics, proteomics, metabolomics)
- Advanced pattern recognition using autoencoders or deep neural networks
- Feature selection and dimensionality reduction (e.g., PCA, t-SNE, LASSO)

For example, the AI model identified combinations of non-encoded RNA, metabolites, and cytocan profiles as predictors of insulin resistance or liver fibrosis. These data-oriented biomarkers allow for precise diagnosis by laying patients into molecular subtypes and paving methods for personalized therapeutic interventions.

5.3 Integration with Electronic Health Records (EHRs)

The inclusion of AI in electronic health records (EHRS) promotes actual diagnosis, risk stratification and decision support in clinical workflows. EHR includes structured (clinical laboratory, drug history) and unstructured (clinical notes, radiologists) that provide a rich substrate for training prediction models.

AI Capabilities in EHR Systems:

- Natural Language Processing (NLP): Extracts clinically relevant information from unstructured text, such as diet recommendations, psychosocial risk factors, or symptom patterns.
- Real-Time Risk Alerts: AI can analyze live data streams (e.g., vital signs, labs) and trigger alerts when thresholds or combinations indicative of metabolic decompensation are reached.
- Clinical Decision Support Systems (CDSS): AI-enhanced CDSS can provide recommendation prompts for diagnostics (e.g., ordering HbA1c for patients at high diabetes risk), personalized treatment suggestions (e.g., metformin vs. lifestyle therapy), and follow-up reminders.(Guarducci et al., 2025)

Babu et al. (2024) highlight that for AI-EHR systems to be effective in practice, they must ensure:

- Interoperability across healthcare platforms using standards such as HL7 FHIR
- Robust data governance and patient privacy safeguards compliant with HIPAA/GDPR
- Seamless user interfaces that integrate into the physician's workflow without inducing alert fatigue

Examples of real-world AI-EHR deployments include:

- Epic's *Sepsis Prediction Model*, adapted for metabolic deterioration alerts
- Mount Sinai's *Deep Patient*, a deep learning model predicting disease onset based on EHR time-series

When fully operational, these systems support continuous health monitoring, reduce diagnostic latency, and enable resource prioritization in large patient populations.

6. CHALLENGES IN AI-DRIVEN DIAGNOSTICS FOR METABOLIC DISORDERS

Despite the increasing success of AI applications for artificial intelligence (AI) in healthcare systems, some serious obstacles have prevented reliable, fair and safe use in the context of metabolic disorders such as type 2 disaccharide (T2DM), metabolic syndrome (METS), obesity, and non-alcoholic fatty disease (nafrel). These challenges are based on technical complexity and systematic limitations regarding the health environment. Overcoming requires an interdisciplinary approach that combines data science, clinical expertise, bioethics and regulatory policies.(Lebeaud et al., 2024)

6.1 Data Quality and Heterogeneity

AI algorithms rely heavily on the availability of high-volume, high-velocity, and high-veracity data. However, real-world clinical data often violate these assumptions due to:

- Incomplete Records: Laboratory test results, comorbidity information, and medication adherence data are frequently missing or inconsistently recorded in electronic health records (EHRs).
- Data Noise and Artifacts: Wearable sensor data (e.g., continuous glucose monitors, activity trackers) may be corrupted by environmental factors or user non-compliance, introducing temporal noise and reducing signal integrity.
- Heterogeneous Data Sources: Clinical data span structured formats (e.g., ICD codes, lab values) and unstructured formats (e.g., physician notes, radiology reports), complicating data integration and model training.

Sghaireen et al. (2022) addressed data imbalance—a common issue in metabolic disorder datasets—by applying the Synthetic Minority Oversampling Technique (SMOTE), which synthetically augments the underrepresented class to improve model generalizability. However, oversampling can introduce synthetic data bias and increase the likelihood of model overfitting if not combined with proper cross-validation.

Advanced imputation techniques (e.g., Multiple Imputation by Chained Equations, KNN imputation, or deep autoencoders) can restore partially missing data, but imputed values may introduce uncertainty and should be interpreted cautiously in risk-sensitive clinical contexts.(Shah et al., 2019)

6.2 Privacy, Security, and Ethical Considerations

Healthcare data is legally protected due to its sensitivity. AI models, especially those trained using centralized architectures, often require large datasets that include identifiable patient information, posing significant privacy and security risks.

Key Concerns:

- Re-identification Risk: Even anonymized datasets can be re-linked to individuals through data triangulation, particularly when genomic or geolocation data are involved.
- Data Breaches: Cybersecurity vulnerabilities in cloud storage, APIs, or third-party vendor systems can lead to unauthorized access to protected health information (PHI).
- Ethical Use of Data: Informed consent procedures often lack transparency regarding secondary uses of data in AI model development.

To mitigate these issues, regulatory frameworks like the General Data Protection Regulation (GDPR) in the EU and Health Insurance Portability and Accountability Act (HIPAA) in the U.S. impose stringent guidelines for data handling.

Emerging Solutions:

- Federated Learning: Enables decentralized training across multiple institutions without direct data sharing, thus preserving data locality.
- Differential Privacy: Adds mathematical noise to outputs to protect individual-level privacy.
- Blockchain-Based Audit Trails: Ensure traceability and accountability for data usage in AI workflows.

Despite their promise, these techniques are still being validated for clinical-grade deployment and face scalability and interoperability hurdles. (Dinov, 2018)

6.3 Bias, Fairness, and Generalizability

Predisposition in AI frameworks can emerge from non-representative preparing information, show plan choices, or one-sided clinical hones reflected within the information. Within the setting of metabolic infections, predisposition may show in:

- Underdiagnosis of conditions in racial or ethnic minority bunches due to lower representation in preparing datasets.
- Sex-based abberations in malady phenotyping, as male and female patients regularly show diverse metabolic profiles.
- Socioeconomic inclination, where social determinants of wellbeing (SDoH) like nourishment uncertainty, lodging precariousness, or wellbeing literacy are not enough captured, coming about in skewed predictions.

Models prepared transcendently on Eurocentric or urban-centric cohorts may perform ineffectively in provincial, low-income, or worldwide south populaces, diminishing clinical utility and compounding wellbeing inequities.

Bias moderation methodologies include:

- Algorithmic de-biasing (e.g., reweighting, ill-disposed training)
- Inclusion of statistic and SDoH factors as inputs
- Fairness reviews utilizing measurements such as statistic equality, equalized chances, and dissimilar affect ratio

However, these approaches frequently include trade-offs between demonstrate reasonableness, precision, and interpretability, requiring moral decision-making in sending.

6.4 Interpretability and Clinical Trust

Many AI models, especially deep neural networks (DNNS) and folding networks (CNNS), act as "black boxes" and provide very accurate output without transparent arguments. This lack of interpretability creates challenges in a clinical setting where decisions need to be justified for evidence-based arguments.Clinical Concerns:

- Liability and Accountability: Physicians are legally and ethically responsible for decisions influenced by AI systems.
- Resistance to Adoption: Clinicians may hesitate to rely on opaque models, especially in high-stakes situations such as insulin dose adjustments or cardiovascular risk prediction.(Fregoso-Aparicio et al., 2021.)

To address this, Explainable AI (XAI) techniques are increasingly integrated:

- SHAP (SHapley Additive exPlanations) uses cooperative game theory to assign each feature a contribution value toward the final prediction, offering global and local interpretability.
- LIME (Local Interpretable Model-agnostic Explanations) creates interpretable surrogate models (e.g., linear regressions) around individual predictions.

These tools enable:

- Post-hoc validation of AI decisions
- Regulatory transparency
- User interface enhancements that provide actionable insights (e.g., "This prediction was influenced by elevated triglycerides and low HDL cholesterol").

Despite advances, interpretability often remains a trade-off against model complexity, especially when real-time, multimodal decision support is needed.

7. ETHICAL AND REGULATORY PERSPECTIVES

As AI gets to be progressively implanted in demonstrative workflows for metabolic disorder ranging from early chance forecast of Sort 2 diabetes to computerized imaging examination of hepatic steatosis its moral soundness and administrative compliance are irreplaceable to guaranteeing believe, security, and value in clinical hone. AI frameworks work at the crossing point of quiet care and computational deduction, regularly making probabilistic choices with significant suggestions for restorative treatment and wellbeing equity.

To dependably coordinated AI into healthcare, frameworks must be guided by built up bioethical standards (independence, usefulness, non-maleficence, and equity) and follow to advancing administrative systems that address the interesting characteristics of machine-learning-based advances.(Eyvazlou et al., 2020.)

7.1 Ethical Imperatives in AI-Driven Diagnosis

a) Transparency and Explainability

In clinical contexts, explainability is a prerequisite for adoption, not merely a technical feature. Physicians must be able to interpret and communicate AI-driven decisions to patients, particularly when these decisions influence long-term management of chronic metabolic conditions such as diabetes or metabolic syndrome.

As Sghaireen et al. (2022) underscore, black-box models limit clinician confidence and patient autonomy. Tools such as:

- SHAP (SHapley Additive exPlanations): Quantify the marginal contribution of each feature to an individual prediction, enhancing model interpretability at both local and global levels.
- LIME (Local Interpretable Model-agnostic Explanations): Provides human-interpretable approximations of complex models by fitting locally linear surrogates.

These explainability tools ensure that AI-based recommendations are traceable, facilitating clinical audits and patient discussions while reducing medicolegal ambiguity.

b) Fairness and Non-Discrimination

Bias in AI models often stems from historically unbalanced datasets, where minority groups (by race, sex, or socioeconomic status) are underrepresented. In metabolic health, this can lead to underdiagnosis of high-risk populations, thus exacerbating existing health disparities.

Solutions include:

- Stratified model training using demographically balanced cohorts.
- Bias auditing through tools such as *Disparate Impact Analysis* and *Equalized Odds Evaluation*.
- Integration of social determinants of health (SDoH) into predictive models to account for contextual non-biological risk factors (e.g., food insecurity, education, environment).

Failure to address these issues risks violating the ethical principle of justice and undermining public trust in AI-enabled healthcare.

Traditional informed consent protocols are inadequate for the dynamic and indirect uses of personal health data in AI model development, particularly when data are shared across institutions or repurposed for secondary analyses.

Emerging best practices include:

- Dynamic consent frameworks that allow patients to update their preferences over time.

- Data provenance tracking to ensure transparency about how data are collected, processed, and utilized.
- Anonymization and pseudonymization methods to minimize re-identification risks, although these are not infallible, especially when genomic data are involved.(Xiaoxue et al., 2024)

7.2 Regulatory Considerations and Evolving Standards

AI technologies used in diagnostics increasingly fall under the category of Software as a Medical Device (SaMD). Regulatory agencies globally are beginning to define guidelines specific to adaptive, self-learning algorithms, which differ fundamentally from static medical software.

a) Current Regulatory Landscape

1. United States – FDA:
   o The Food and Drug Administration (FDA) classifies many AI-based diagnostic tools as SaMD.
   o In 2021, the FDA released the Artificial Intelligence/Machine Learning (AI/ML)-Based SaMD Action Plan, which calls for:
     ■ *Good Machine Learning Practices (GMLP)*
     ■ *Pre-market transparency and performance evaluation*
     ■ *Post-market monitoring and algorithm retraining protocols*
2. European Union – MDR and AI Act:
   o Under the Medical Device Regulation (MDR), AI tools with diagnostic or therapeutic functionality must undergo CE marking.
   o The proposed EU Artificial Intelligence Act (2021) explicitly categorizes medical AI applications as high-risk systems, requiring:
     ■ Rigorous *risk-benefit analysis*
     ■ *Human oversight mechanisms*
     ■ Continuous *performance auditing*
3. International Standards:
   o ISO/IEC 62304 and ISO 14971 provide frameworks for software lifecycle management and risk analysis in medical AI systems.
   o The World Health Organization (WHO) issued guidance in 2021 emphasizing the need for ethical design, regulatory coordination, and capacity building in low-resource settings.(Kim et al., 2021)

b) Challenges in Regulation

AI models often evolve over time as they are retrained on new data, posing regulatory challenges related to:

- Model drift: Degradation of model performance over time if not properly monitored.
- Black-box opacity: Difficulty in validating or certifying algorithms that lack transparency.
- Distributed learning: Complications in ensuring regulatory compliance when models are trained across borders using federated architectures.

c) Required Frameworks

Effective regulation of AI in metabolic diagnostics should include:

- Pre-market validation with robust clinical trials simulating real-world heterogeneity.
- Real-time monitoring through model lifecycle management systems (e.g., ModelOps).
- Audit trails and traceability logs to ensure algorithmic accountability and facilitate post-hoc investigations.(Lee et al., 2024)

8. FUTURE DIRECTIONS

The future of AI in diagnosing and managing metabolic disorders is poised to move beyond predictive modeling toward fully integrated, intelligent health ecosystems. These systems will combine high-resolution, multimodal data with real-time analytics to deliver proactive, personalized, and interpretable healthcare. Key future directions include the development of explainable models, implementation of AI in precision medicine, and the convergence of AI with mobile health technologies.

8.1 Explainable AI in Clinical Decision Support

While high-performance models such as deep neural networks (DNNs) and ensemble learners (e.g., XGBoost, random forests) achieve excellent classification accuracy, their lack of interpretability hinders clinical adoption. Explainable AI (XAI) aims to bridge this gap by providing mechanistic insights into how model predictions are derived, thus facilitating clinician acceptance, legal accountability, and patient trust.(Malik et al., 2024)

Key Developments:

- SHAP (SHapley Additive exPlanations) is based on cooperative game theory and calculates the marginal contribution of each feature to a prediction. SHAP offers both global explanations (e.g., identifying the most influential variables across the dataset) and local explanations (e.g., for individual patients), which is crucial in contexts like metabolic syndrome, where feature interactions (e.g., HDL levels × BMI) can be nonlinear.
- LIME (Local Interpretable Model-agnostic Explanations) generates surrogate linear models in the local neighborhood of a prediction, offering model-agnostic interpretability.

These tools enable real-time explanation of outputs from models deployed on electronic health records (EHRs), aiding in:

- Model validation by clinical teams
- Shared decision-making with patients
- Regulatory review and auditability

Future innovations may include biologically-informed explainability, where model outputs are mapped to metabolic pathways or gene regulatory networks, increasing biomedical relevance and mechanistic transparency.(Genomics & 2024, 2024)

8.2 Personalized and Precision Medicine

AI's ability to integrate heterogeneous, high-dimensional data makes it a cornerstone of precision medicine in metabolic health. Unlike population-level guidelines, precision medicine tailors interventions to an individual's multi-omic, clinical, and behavioral profile.

Scientific Contributions:

- Machine learning classifiers can segment populations into clinically meaningful subtypes (e.g., insulin-resistant vs. insulin-sensitive obesity) using unsupervised methods like k-means clustering or Gaussian Mixture Models.
- Multi-omics integration (genomics, transcriptomics, proteomics, metabolomics) via AI models such as multi-modal neural networks or graph con-

volutional networks (GCNs) enables the discovery of molecular biomarkers linked to disease progression and drug responsiveness.

- Polygenic risk scores (PRS) combined with clinical data can enhance risk stratification for Type 2 diabetes or NAFLD, aiding in early detection among asymptomatic individuals.

Babu et al. (2024) highlight that personalization extends to dynamic treatment optimization, where reinforcement learning algorithms adjust treatment strategies (e.g., medication titration, dietary recommendations) based on feedback loops from wearable devices and patient-reported outcomes.

Challenges include:

- Model calibration across ancestries and environments
- Integration of temporally misaligned data streams
- Regulatory hurdles for clinical-grade deployment of personalized AI tools

8.3 Integration with Wearables and Mobile Health (mHealth)

Modern metabolic care is moving toward ubiquitous sensing and real-time intervention, made possible by AI integration with consumer and clinical-grade wearables. These devices generate continuous, longitudinal physiological data that are highly valuable for early detection, relapse prevention, and behavior modification.

Key Applications:

- Continuous Glucose Monitors (CGMs) feed high-resolution data into recurrent neural networks (RNNs) or temporal convolutional networks (TCNs) to forecast hyperglycemic episodes or detect glycemic variability—an early marker of metabolic dysfunction.
- Heart rate variability (HRV) and sleep pattern analysis from smartwatches can serve as proxies for autonomic function and circadian rhythm disruption, which are implicated in metabolic syndrome and obesity.
- Smartphone-based dietary and activity tracking, combined with NLP (natural language processing) for food logs or behavioral journaling, enable real-time lifestyle monitoring and AI-powered coaching.(Medina Inojosa et al., 2024)

Future advances include:

- Multimodal fusion architectures, such as attention-based deep learning models that integrate EHR, wearable, and lifestyle data for holistic risk prediction.

- On-device AI inference (e.g., using edge computing chips) to reduce latency, protect privacy, and enable offline functionality in low-resource settings.
- Digital phenotyping, where behavioral patterns (e.g., screen time, geolocation entropy) are quantified as latent features in metabolic risk modeling.

These technologies will support a shift from episodic, clinic-based care to continuous, ambient health monitoring, transforming chronic disease management into a real-time, feedback-driven paradigm.

FUTURE PERSPECTIVES

The integration of progressed Counterfeit Insights (AI) strategies into metabolic clutter diagnostics is anticipated to quicken quickly over the following decade. As computational capacity increments and wellbeing information biological systems gotten to be more interoperable, AI will move from steady devices to proactive clinical collaborators, able of independently checking, foreseeing, and indeed directing restorative procedures. Concurring, the long run of AI in healthcare lies in building versatile, context-aware frameworks that ceaselessly learn from multi-source information whereas keeping up tall benchmarks of protection and security. Several key innovations are anticipated to reshape the diagnostic and preventive framework for metabolic disorders:

1. Adaptive AI-Driven Risk Stratification Using Multimodal Data Streams

Next-generation diagnostic platforms will leverage multi-modal data fusion to dynamically refine individual risk profiles. These systems will integrate heterogeneous inputs such as:

- Behavioral data: sleep duration and quality (via actigraphy), physical activity levels (via accelerometry), and nutritional intake (via NLP-based dietary logs),
- Physiological signals: heart rate variability, skin temperature, galvanic skin response, and continuous glucose monitoring (CGM),
- Contextual metadata: geolocation, environmental exposures, and social interactions.

Machine learning models—particularly deep reinforcement learning (DRL) and Bayesian dynamic models—will be employed to update risk scores in real-time, allowing for time-variant prediction of metabolic decompensation, glycemic excursions, or lipid imbalances.(Li et al., 2024)

2. Smart Wearables with Embedded Edge AI for Real-Time Metabolic Surveillance

The future of metabolic health monitoring lies in on-device intelligence, wherein edge computing allows AI models to run directly on wearables (e.g., smartwatches, biosensor patches). These models will process real-time physiological signals locally—without relying on cloud-based inference—thereby:

- Reducing latency in alert generation (e.g., hypoglycemia prediction),
- Preserving patient privacy by avoiding raw data transmission,
- Improving battery efficiency via model quantization and pruning techniques.

Advanced biosensors combined with recurrent neural networks (RNNs) and transformer architectures can detect early patterns of metabolic dysregulation, such as altered circadian glucose patterns or abnormal energy expenditure, and autonomously notify users or care teams.

3. AI-Based Behavioral Advisory Systems Informed by Genomics and Physiological Phenotypes

Personalized medicine will evolve with the help of AI-driven advisory systems that integrate individual genomic profiles, epigenetic markers, and metabolomic signatures. These systems will utilize:

- Polygenic Risk Scores (PRS) to assess predisposition to Type 2 diabetes, obesity, or dyslipidemia,
- Machine learning-based causal inference to identify modifiable risk factors specific to the individual's genotype and phenotype,
- Digital twins—virtual simulations of a person's metabolic system that enable prediction of outcomes under various lifestyle or pharmacological interventions.

By modeling individual variability, these systems will provide real-time, evidence-based behavioral recommendations that adapt to the user's current state, lifestyle patterns, and molecular profile, promoting sustainable, precision-guided metabolic health management.

4. Federated and Swarm Learning for Global Model Optimization with Data Privacy

To ensure scalability and generalizability of AI models while maintaining compliance with data protection regulations (e.g., GDPR, HIPAA), future systems will adopt federated learning (FL) and swarm learning paradigms. These approaches allow AI models to be trained across decentralized nodes (e.g., hospitals, clinics, wearable devices) without transferring raw patient data.

- Federated averaging will allow multiple institutions to contribute to a shared model, improving generalization across diverse populations and comorbidities.
- Differential privacy and homomorphic encryption will be implemented to ensure secure gradient exchange and protect sensitive health information.
- Blockchain-based model auditing may provide immutable logs of model updates and predictions for regulatory transparency.(Mohsen & Shah, 2025)

Such collaborative learning frameworks will democratize AI research, enabling under-resourced health systems to participate in global model optimization while benefiting from locally relevant diagnostic tools.

SIGNIFICANCE

Metabolic disorders including Sort 2 diabetes mellitus (T2DM), weight, metabolic disorder, and innate mistakes of metabolism are not as it were driving supporters to worldwide dreariness and mortality but too carry broad financial, mental, and open wellbeing results. Their treacherous onset, multifactorial etiology, and frequently asymptomatic early stages make them troublesome to identify and oversee without progressed instruments. When cleared out untreated or ineffectively overseen, these disarranges can advance to complications such as cardiovascular malady, nephropathy, neuropathy, and stroke, contributing to a noteworthy financial burden on both people and healthcare systems.

1. Clinical and Financial Burden

The worldwide taken a toll of overseeing diabetes alone surpasses $760 billion yearly (IDF, 2021), with circuitous costs emerging from misfortune of efficiency, long-term incapacity, and untimely mortality. Corpulence assist compounds these costs, being connected to over 200 comorbid conditions and significantly expanding healthcare utilization. These unremitting conditions moreover require long lasting checking, visit clinic visits, and polypharmacy, subsequently straining as of now overburdened wellbeing infrastructure.

2. Enthusiastic and Psychosocial Impact

Beyond physical wellbeing, metabolic clutters are related with decreased mental versatility, enthusiastic well-being, and generally life fulfillment. Considers have appeared a solid bidirectional relationship between metabolic dysregulation and mental wellbeing disarranges such as sadness and uneasiness, especially in patients managing with weight disgrace, persistent weariness, or hypoglycemic occasions. These psychosocial measurements assist impact adherence to way of life and phar-macological intercessions, propagating a cycle of destitute malady control.(Javidi et al., 2024)

3. The Part of AI: A Worldview Move in Management

In this setting, Manufactured Insights (AI) rises as a basic enabler of early, im-partial, and precision-based healthcare. Leveraging endless datasets ranging from electronic wellbeing records (EHRs) and wearable sensor yields to genomic and microbiome data AI frameworks can identify subclinical designs of dysregulation distant prior than routine symptomatic methods.

- Predictive modeling empowers the recognizable proof of high-risk people some time recently indication onset.
- Explainable AI (XAI) instruments offer assistance interpret complex bio-medical information into reasonable experiences, making strides persistent engagement and clinician trust.
- Natural dialect preparing (NLP) and advanced coaching frameworks change over clinical information into personalized, noteworthy suggestions, in this manner advancing self-efficacy and maintained behavioral change.

4. Wellbeing Value and Accessibility

AI too holds potential in democratizing get to to metabolic care. Mobile-based symptomatic devices and AI augmented choice bolster frameworks can convey per-sonalized healthcare in low-resource and inaccessible settings, bypassing conventional boundaries to master care. Besides, by robotizing complex symptomatic thinking,

AI can ease clinical workload, diminish demonstrative blunders, and standardize care delivery improving results over differing populations.

As a basic work of AI isn't only to robotize decision-making, but to optimize healthcare conveyance by recognizing abberations, distributing assets effectively, and giving opportune, context-aware intercessions. This speaks to a move toward proactive, patient-centric pharmaceutical, where innovation acts as both a demonstrative partner and a preventive constrain.(Bansal et al., 2025)

9. CONCLUSION

Artificial intelligence (AI) is ready to revolutionize the clinical treatment of metabolic disorders by infection with a future, preventive and personal care paradigm from a reactive, symptomatic model. Type 2 diabetes, obesity and congenital errors in metabolism that metabolic diseases are complicated, multicultural and often subdived over time. Early identification and intervention are important to reduce the progression of the disease and reduce the burden on the health care system. The AI system, especially those that utilize the machine learning (ml) and Deep Learning (DL) are specifically equipped to handle the arc, high al-dimensional, non-education and inequality in biomedical data. Techniques such as random forests, supporting Vektorms (SVM) and nervous networks have shown high clinical accuracy when trained on electronic health records (EHR), biochemical analyzes and even genomic or portable practice data.Studies are exemplary how AI can integrate different data -tricks - clinical, genomic and behavior - risk assessment and medical recommendations to improve accuracy. Their work also emphasizes the importance of clarity, especially in high day medical applications where decisions must be interpreted by doctors. Similarly, some studies provide a solid performance of AI's clinical power in metabolic syndrome, which is increased with techniques such as smoke for class balance and techniques as size for model lecturers. Their pipeline achieved impressive accuracy and at the same time maintained the transparency important function for clinical distribution of the world.Beyond the diagnosis, AI activates real -time monitor

REFERENCES

Abut, F., Akça, E., Akay, M. F., Irmak, M., Irmak, M., & Adigüzel, Y. (2024). Harnessing AI for health: Optimized neural network models for resting metabolic rate prediction. *IEEE Access: Practical Innovations, Open Solutions, 12*, 156050–156064.

Alam, M. A., Sohel, A., Hasan, K. M., & Islam, M. A. (2024). Machine Learning And Artificial Intelligence in Diabetes Prediction And Management: A Comprehensive Review of Models. Journal of Next-Gen Engineering Systems.

Anwar, A., Rana, S., & Pathak, P. (2025). *Artificial intelligence in the management of metabolic disorders: a comprehensive review*. Springer., DOI: 10.1007/S40618-025-02548-X

Awari, A., Kaushik, D., Kumar, A., Oz, E., Çadırcı, K., Brennan, C., Proestos, C., Kumar, M., & Oz, F. (2025). Obesity Biomarkers: Exploring Factors, Ramification, Machine Learning, and AI-Unveiling Insights in Health Research. *Wiley Online Library, 6*(7). Advance online publication. DOI: 10.1002/MCO2.70169 PMID: 40551726

Bagheri, F., Kamran, R. R., & Darvishi, M. (2024). A Comparative Study of Data Science Techniques based on Ensemble Classification Algorithms in Healthcare Systems (Case study: Diabetic patients).

Bansal, H., Bondhopadhyay, B., Santoshi, S., Himansu, & Mazumder, R. (2025). Transformative Insights: Integrating IoMT With Generative AI for Personalized Medicine and Drug Discovery. *Igi-Global.ComH Bansal, B Bondhopadhyay, S Santoshi, R MazumderConvergence of Internet of Medical Things (IoMT) and Generative AI, 2025•igi-Global.Com*, 535–564. https://doi.org/DOI: 10.4018/979-8-3693-6180-1.CH023

Dinov, I. D. (2018). *Data science and predictive analytics*. Springer.

Charalampopoulos, G., Bale, R., Filippiadis, D., Odisio, B. C., Wood, B., & Solbiati, L. (2024). Navigation and robotics in interventional oncology: Current status and future roadmap. *Mdpi.ComG Charalampopoulos, R Bale, D Filippiadis, BC Odisio, B Wood, L SolbiatiDiagnostics, 2023•mdpi. Com, 14*(1). Advance online publication. DOI: 10.3390/DIAGNOSTICS14010098 PMID: 38201407

Cheng, L., Zhou, J., Zhao, Y., Wang, N., Jin, M., Mao, W., Zhu, G., Wang, D., Liang, J., Shen, B., & Zheng, Y. (2024). The associations of insulin resistance, obesity, and lifestyle with the risk of developing hyperuricaemia in adolescents. *Springer, 24*(1). https://doi.org/DOI: 10.1186/S12902-024-01757-4

Dang, V. N., Campello, V. M., Hernández-González, J., & Lekadir, K. (2025). *Empirical comparison of post-processing debiasing methods for machine learning classifiers in healthcare.* Springer., DOI: 10.1007/S41666-025-00196-7

Eyvazlou, M., Hosseinpouri, M., Mokarami, H., Gharibi, V., Jahangiri, M., Cousins, R., Nikbakht, H.-A., & Barkhordari, A. (2020). Prediction of metabolic syndrome based on sleep and work-related risk factors using an artificial neural network. *SpringerM Eyvazlou, M Hosseinpouri, H Mokarami, V Gharibi, M Jahangiri, R Cousins, HA NikbakhtBMC Endocrine Disorders, 2020•Springer.* https://doi.org/ DOI: 10.1186/S12902-024-01498-6

Fregoso-Aparicio, L., Noguez, J., Montesinos, L., & García-García, J. A. (2021). Machine learning and deep learning predictive models for type 2 diabetes: A systematic review. *Diabetology & Metabolic Syndrome, 13*(1), 148.

Galal, A., Talal, M., & Moustafa, A. (2022). Applications of machine learning in metabolomics: Disease modeling and classification. *Frontiersin.OrgA Galal, M Talal, A MoustafaFrontiers in Genetics, 2022•frontiersin. Org, 13.* Advance online publication. DOI: 10.3389/FGENE.2022.1017340/FULL

Genomics, D. S.-B. M., & 2024, undefined. (2024). Prediction of metabolic syndrome using machine learning approaches based on genetic and nutritional factors: a 14-year prospective-based cohort study. *SpringerD ShinBMC Medical Genomics, 2024•Springer, 17*(1). https://doi.org/DOI: 10.1186/S12920-024-01998-1

Guarducci, S., Jayousi, S., Caputo, S., & Mucchi, L. (2025). Key Fundamentals and Examples of Sensors for Human Health: Wearable, Non-Continuous, and Non-Contact Monitoring Devices. *Mdpi.ComS Guarducci, S Jayousi, S Caputo, L MucchiSensors, 2025•mdpi. Com, 25*(2). Advance online publication. DOI: 10.3390/ S25020556 PMID: 39860927

Javidi, H., Mariam, A., Alkhaled, L., Pantalone, K. M., & Rotroff, D. M. (2024). An interpretable predictive deep learning platform for pediatric metabolic diseases. *Academic.Oup.ComH Javidi, A Mariam, L Alkhaled, KM Pantalone, DM RotroffJournal of the American Medical Informatics Association, 2024•academic. Oup. Com, 31*(6), 1227–1238. DOI: 10.1093/JAMIA/OCAE049 PMID: 38497983

Kim, J., Mun, S., Lee, S., Jeong, K., Health, Y. B.-B. P., & 2022, undefined. (2021). Prediction of metabolic and pre-metabolic syndromes using machine learning models with anthropometric, lifestyle, and biochemical factors from a middle-aged. *SpringerJ Kim, S Mun, S Lee, K Jeong, Y BaekBMC Public Health, 2022•Springer.* https://doi.org/DOI: 10.1186/S12889-024-16248-3

Kumar, B. P. P., & Manoj, H. M. (2024). Comparative assessment of machine learning models for predicting glucose intolerance risk. *Springer, 5*(7). https://doi.org/DOI: 10.1007/S42979-024-03259-5

Lebeaud, A., Antoun, L., Paccard, J. R., Edeline, J., Bourien, H., Fares, N., Tournigand, C., Lecomte, T., Tougeron, D., Hautefeuille, V., Viénot, A., Henriques, J., Williet, N., Bachet, J. B., Smolenschi, C., Hollebecque, A., Macarulla, T., Castet, F., Malka, D., … Turpin, A. (2024). Management of biliary tract cancers in early-onset patients: A nested multicenter retrospective study of the ACABI GERCOR PRONOBIL cohort. *Wiley Online LibraryA Lebeaud, L Antoun, JR Paccard, J Edeline, H Bourien, N Fares, C Tournigand, T LecomteLiver International, 2024●Wiley Online Library, 44*(8), 1886–1899. https://doi.org/DOI: 10.1111/LIV.15922

Lee, M. H., Zea, R., Garrett, J. W., Summers, R. M., & Pickhardt, P. J. (2024). AI-based abdominal CT measurements of orthotopic and ectopic fat predict mortality and cardiometabolic disease risk in adults. *SpringerMH Lee, R Zea, JW Garrett, RM Summers, PJ PickhardtEuropean Radiology, 2025●Springer.* https://doi.org/DOI: 10.1007/S00330-024-10935-W

Li, Z., Wu, W., & Kang, H. (2024). Machine Learning-Driven Metabolic Syndrome Prediction: An International Cohort Validation Study. *Mdpi.ComZ Li, W Wu, H KangHealthcare, 2024●mdpi. Com, 12*(24). Advance online publication. DOI: 10.3390/HEALTHCARE12242527 PMID: 39765954

Liu, J., Liu, Z., Liu, C., Sun, H., Li, X., & Yang, Y. (2025). Integrating Artificial Intelligence in the Diagnosis and Management of Metabolic Syndrome: A Comprehensive Review. *Wiley Online Library, 41*(4). Advance online publication. DOI: 10.1002/DMRR.70039 PMID: 40145661

Malik, S., Das, R., Thongtan, T., Thompson, K., & Dbouk, N. (2024). AI in Hepatology: Revolutionizing the Diagnosis and Management of Liver Disease. *Mdpi.ComS Malik, R Das, T Thongtan, K Thompson, N DboukJournal of Clinical Medicine, 2024●mdpi. Com, 13*(24). Advance online publication. DOI: 10.3390/JCM13247833 PMID: 39768756

Medina Inojosa, B. J., Somers, V. K., Lara-Breitinger, K., Johnson, L. A., Medina-Inojosa, J. R., & Lopez-Jimenez, F. (2024). PREDICTION OF METABOLIC SYNDROME USING REGIONAL BODY VOLUMES MEASURED USING A MULTISENSORY WHITE-LIGHT 3-D SCANNER. *Jacc. Org, 5*, 582–590. DOI: 10.1093/EHJDH/ZTAD093

Mohsen, F., & Shah, Z. (2025). *Improving Early Prediction of Type 2 Diabetes Mellitus with ECG-DiaNet: A Multimodal Neural Network Leveraging Electrocardiogram and Clinical Risk Factors*. https://arxiv.org/abs/2504.05338

Paplomatas, P., Rigas, D., Sergounioti, A., & Vrahatis, A. (2024). Enhancing metabolic syndrome detection through blood tests using advanced machine learning. *Eng*, *5*(3), 1422–1434.

Pawade, D., Bakhai, D., Admane, T., Arya, R., Salunke, Y., & Pawade, Y. (2024). Evaluating the Performance of Different Machine Learning Models for Metabolic Syndrome Prediction. *Procedia Computer Science*, *235*, 2932–2941.

Rajpurkar, P., Chen, E., Banerjee, O., & Topol, E. J. (2022). AI in health and medicine. *Nature Medicine*, *28*(1), 31–38.

Sghaireen, M. G., Al-Smadi, Y., Al-Qerem, A., Srivastava, K. C., Ganji, K. K., Alam, M. K., Nashwan, S., & Khader, Y. (2022). Machine learning approach for metabolic syndrome diagnosis using explainable data-augmentation-based classification. *Mdpi. ComMG Sghaireen, Y Al-Smadi, A Al-Qerem, KC Srivastava, KK Ganji, MK Alam, S NashwanDiagnostics, 2022•mdpi. Com*, *12*(12). Advance online publication. DOI: 10.3390/DIAGNOSTICS12123117 PMID: 36553124

Shah, N., Milstein, A., Jama, S. B.-, & 2019, undefined. (n.d.). Making machine learning models clinically useful. *Jamanetwork. Com*. https://doi.org/DOI: 10.1001/JAMA.2024.2456

Tavares, L. D., Manoel, A., Donato, T. H. R., Cesena, F., Minanni, C. A., Kashiwagi, N. M., & Szlejf, C. (2022). Prediction of metabolic syndrome: A machine learning approach to help primary prevention. *Diabetes Research and Clinical Practice*, *191*, 110047.

Xiaoxue, W., Zijun, W., Shichen, C., Mukun, Y., Yi, C., Linqing, M., & Wenpei, B. (2024). Risk prediction model of metabolic syndrome in perimenopausal women based on machine learning. *ElsevierW Xiaoxue, W Zijun, C Shichen, Y Mukun, C Yi, M Linqing, B WenpeiInternational Journal of Medical Informatics, 2024•Elsevier*, *188*. https://doi.org/DOI: 10.1016/J.IJMEDINF.2024.105480

Yang, Z., Shi, X., Wang, S., Du, L., Zhang, X., Zhang, K., Zhang, Y., Ma, J., & Zheng, R. (2025). *An early prediction model for gestational diabetes mellitus created using machine learning algorithms*. Wiley Online Library., DOI: 10.1002/IJGO.70055

Zschaubitz, E., Schröder, H., Glackin, C. C., Vogel, L., Labrenz, M., & Sperlea, T. (2025). A benchmark analysis of feature selection and machine learning methods for environmental metabarcoding datasets. *ElsevierE Zschaubitz, H Schröder, CC Glackin, L Vogel, M Labrenz, T SperleaComputational and Structural Biotechnology Journal, 2025●Elsevier, 27,* 1636–1647. https://doi.org/DOI: 10.1016/J.CSBJ.2025.04.017

Chapter 4
AI Integration in Telemedicine for Metabolic Monitoring and Gut Microbiome Analysis

Leena Arya
https://orcid.org/0000-0002-9249-732X

Koneru Lakshmiah Education Foundation, India

Ravi Rastogi
https://orcid.org/0000-0002-1118-3020

JIMS Engineering Management Technical Campus, India

Mandalapu Sivaparvathi
https://orcid.org/0009-0007-2356-6874

MAM Women's Engineering College, India

Rajesh Babu Yallamanda
https://orcid.org/0009-0008-7625-1443

Koneru Lakshmiah Education Foundation, India

Latha Banda
https://orcid.org/0000-0003-1189-1569

JIMS Engineering Management Technical Campus, India

Venkata Rajani Katuri
https://orcid.org/0009-0008-1790-7027

Keshav Memorial Institute of Technology, India

Devendra Gautam
https://orcid.org/0009-0005-3666-3257

JIMS Engineering Management Technical Campus, India

Mourad Elloumi
https://orcid.org/0000-0003-0570-4309

Bisha University, Saudi Arabia

Nimisha Tiwari
https://orcid.org/0000-0002-6005-7290

UIT, Pajiv Gandhi Proudyogiki Vishwavidyalay, India

Shalaka Tyagi
https://orcid.org/0009-0009-6150-0694

School of Computing Science and Engineering, Sharda University, India

DOI: 10.4018/979-8-3373-3196-6.ch004

ABSTRACT

By enabling continuous, individualized, and predictive care, the incorporation of artificial intelligence (AI) into telemedicine has completely transformed the management of metabolic health. To treat metabolic disorders such as diabetes, obesity, and cardiovascular disease, a revolutionary model that integrates gut microbiome analysis with AI-powered telemedicine is examined. Real-time physiological and microbial data are recorded, analysed, and converted into valuable insights by utilizing wearable sensors, mobile health platforms, and cloud-based analytics. Risk stratification, dietary customization, and early intervention are made possible by artificial intelligence (AI) techniques like machine learning, deep learning, and natural language processing. In parallel, functional biomarkers of disease progression and treatment response are revealed by microbiome profiling. The chapter discusses ethical, legal, and technical challenges while presenting successful case studies. This convergence facilitates closed-loop, adaptive systems that maximise results and empower patients.

1. INTRODUCTION

Metabolic health is foundational to human well-being, as it impacts energy regulation, hormonal balance, immune function, and the prevention of chronic diseases. Disorders such as type 2 diabetes, obesity, and metabolic syndrome have become global public health challenges, with rapidly rising prevalence linked to sedentary lifestyles, poor diet, and genetic predispositions. In the United States alone, over 37 million individuals are affected by diabetes, and an additional 96 million adults are estimated to have prediabetes (Centres for Disease Control and Prevention, 2022). The economic implications are equally alarming, with the total cost of diagnosed diabetes estimated at $327 billion in 2017 (American Diabetes Association, 2018). Traditional care models often fall short in providing early detection and continuous management of these conditions, resulting in preventable complications and an increased healthcare burden. Consequently, there is a growing need for advanced, scalable, and patient-centred technologies that facilitate continuous metabolic health monitoring and personalised intervention strategies.

1.1 Overview of Telemedicine Advancements

The management of chronic diseases, particularly in the area of metabolic health, has undergone a radical change thanks to telemedicine, the provision of medical services via digital and communication technologies. Initially conceived to overcome geographic and logistical barriers to healthcare access, telemedicine has since evolved into a multi-layered ecosystem of video consultations, remote monitoring, AI-enabled diagnostics, and cloud-based data sharing (Arya et al., 2024; Mehta et al., 2023).

Modern telehealth platforms incorporate wearable biosensors, mobile health (mHealth) applications, and interoperable health information systems to enable real-time monitoring of key biomarkers, including blood glucose, blood pressure, and physical activity. AI-powered continuous glucose monitoring (CGM) systems are now being used to alert patients and caregivers of impending glycaemic events (Vettoretti et al., 2020). Furthermore, mobile platforms integrated with behavioural data have demonstrated significant improvement in lifestyle adherence and glycaemic control (Zahedani et al., 2023).

Scoping reviews confirm the growing presence of AI in wearable technologies for diabetes care, highlighting predictive algorithms that can detect abnormal glucose trends and offer real-time dietary or physical activity suggestions (Chan et al., 2024; Ahmed et al., 2022). These advancements not only enhance patient autonomy and engagement but also reduce the burden on healthcare providers by utilising automated triage and decision support systems (Vijayalakshmi et al., 2023).

1.2 Gut Microbiome and Its Role in Metabolic Disorders

Parallel to the technological advances in telemedicine, a revolution is underway in understanding the gut microbiome, the complex community of trillions of micro-organisms that inhabit the human gastrointestinal tract. This microbial ecosystem plays a crucial role in regulating metabolic functions, including nutrient absorption, energy extraction, immune modulation, and the control of inflammation (Barratt et al., 2017).

Dysbiosis, or microbial imbalance, has been linked to a range of metabolic diseases, including obesity (Castaner et al., 2018), type 2 diabetes (Qin et al., 2012), cardiovascular disease, and liver dysfunction (Park et al., 2024). Multi-omics studies confirm that alterations in microbial diversity, functional gene profiles, and metabolite output contribute to disease onset and progression (Lloyd-Price et al., 2019; Almeida et al., 2021). Importantly, microbial markers and signatures have emerged as predictive tools for diagnosing and stratifying disease severity (Chang et al., 2024).

Recent clinical studies have begun integrating microbiome profiling into therapeutic regimens, such as AI-driven personalized nutrition programs that modulate gut composition to optimize metabolic outcomes (Rouskas et al., 2025; Karakan et al., 2022). Advances in next-generation sequencing (NGS) technologies and computational methods like 16S rRNA and shotgun metagenomics have further enabled deep characterization of microbial communities at species and strain levels (De Filippis et al., 2016; D'Urso & Broccolo, 2024).

1.3 Scope and Objectives of AI Integration in Telemedicine for Metabolic Health and Microbiome Analysis

The convergence of artificial intelligence (AI), telemedicine, and gut microbiome analysis offers a transformative approach to personalized metabolic healthcare. AI methodologies such as machine learning (ML), deep learning (DL), and natural language processing (NLP) are well-suited to handle the high-dimensional, heterogeneous data generated by wearables, health apps, and metagenomics platforms (McCoubrey et al., 2021; Malakar et al., 2024). These algorithms can identify non-linear patterns, predict disease trajectories, and deliver real-time, personalized interventions.

AI's potential in this space includes:

- Predictive modelling of metabolic diseases using multi-source data from CGMs, diet logs, and microbiome profiles (Li et al., 2022; Wang et al., 2025).
- Behavioural forecasting and compliance monitoring through NLP-based analysis of clinical notes or patient feedback (Arya et al., 2024).
- Personalised dietary recommendations optimised for microbiome modulation, using clustering and classification techniques (Karakan et al., 2022; Lee & Rho, 2022).
- Risk stratification and early detection via polygenic risk score integration and microbiome-informed signatures (Choi et al., 2020; Park et al., 2024).

Figure 1 illustrates the central role of machine learning in integrated microbiome and telemedicine systems. It ingests personal features, clinical data, metagenomic and metabolomic profiles, then supports functions such as phenotypic prediction, patient stratification, biomarker discovery, therapeutic efficacy evaluation, and personalized recommendation (Li et al., 2022).

Figure 1. Machine Learning Applications in the Gut Microbiome

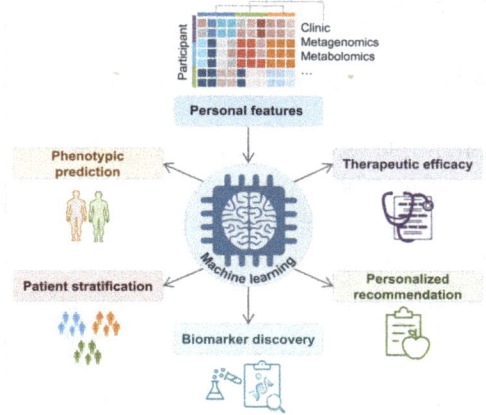

Furthermore, the development of integrated telemedicine ecosystems that unify these components real-time biosensing, AI-based analytics, microbiome profiling, and clinician interfaces has opened new frontiers in digital healthcare innovation (Arya et al., 2025; Mannava et al., 2025; Saha et al., 2024). These integrated platforms can enable dynamic and closed-loop systems that not only detect metabolic abnormalities early but also recommend actionable interventions in a clinically meaningful and scalable manner.

2. FUNDAMENTALS OF TELEMEDICINE AND METABOLIC MONITORING

Telemedicine refers to the use of digital technologies to deliver medical services remotely, enabling diagnosis, monitoring, consultation, and treatment without the need for in-person interaction. Originally conceptualized as a means to provide healthcare to geographically isolated populations, telemedicine has evolved into a multi-dimensional healthcare delivery model encompassing mobile health (mHealth), remote patient monitoring (RPM), AI-driven diagnostics, and cloud-based health information systems (Mehta et al., 2023; Arya et al., 2024).

The acceleration of telemedicine adoption, particularly during global health crises such as the COVID-19 pandemic, has transformed it into a cornerstone of chronic disease management. Key drivers of this evolution include advancements in sensor technologies, data analytics, and wireless communication networks (Chan et al., 2024; Mannava et al., 2025). AI-enabled tools now extend telemedicine beyond basic consultation to predictive modelling, early disease detection, and adaptive therapy management (Arya et al., 2025).

2.1 Technologies Enabling Remote Metabolic Monitoring

The integration of multiple technologies that enable continuous, real-time, and customized monitoring of metabolic parameters is essential to the success of telemedicine in metabolic healthcare. Wearable technology, cloud-based platforms, and mobile health apps are three essential elements.

2.1.1 Wearable Devices

Wearable biosensors play a crucial role in the remote monitoring of metabolic conditions, including diabetes, obesity, and hypertension. Devices such as continuous glucose monitors (CGMs), fitness bands, and smartwatches track real-time physiological data, including glucose levels, heart rate, sleep patterns, and physical activity (Vettoretti et al., 2020; Ahmed et al., 2022).

AI-enhanced CGM systems predict hypoglycemic and hyperglycemic events before they occur, offering timely alerts and recommendations to both patients and healthcare providers (Haak et al., 2017; Chan et al., 2024). Moreover, AI-integrated wearable platforms have demonstrated significant improvements in patient adherence and glycaemic control (Zahedani et al., 2023).

2.1.2 Mobile Health Applications

mHealth apps serve as a bridge between patients and healthcare providers, offering tools for logging dietary habits, tracking medication, monitoring physical activity, and visualizing health trends. AI modules within these apps analyse behavioural and clinical data to personalise feedback and behavioural nudges (Ahmed et al., 2022; Rouskas et al., 2025).

Some platforms use natural language processing (NLP) to interpret user inputs, flagging risks and triaging cases that require clinician intervention (Malakar et al., 2024). Integration with microbiome insights also enables the provision of tailored dietary recommendations that address both metabolic and gut health profiles (Karakan et al., 2022).

2.1.3 Cloud-Based Data Management Platforms

Cloud computing enables the storage, exchange, and real-time processing of large volumes of metabolic data collected through wearable devices and mobile health (mHealth) applications. These platforms enable interoperability between devices, patients, and providers while ensuring data security and compliance with regulatory frameworks such as HIPAA and GDPR (Almaiah et al., 2023; Arya, 2024).

Cloud-based AI engines can analyze longitudinal data streams to identify anomalies, detect patterns indicative of disease progression, and forecast future risks (Li et al., 2022; Wang et al., 2025). Additionally, cloud infrastructure supports federated learning models that allow decentralized AI training while preserving patient privacy (Chang et al., 2024).

2.2 Important Metrics for Tracking Metabolic Health

Several biomarkers and behavioral indicators must be continuously monitored for metabolic health management to be effective. AI is used by telemedicine platforms to synthesize these metrics into insights that patients and clinicians can use.

2.2.1 Blood Glucose Levels

Monitoring blood glucose is essential for diabetes management. Traditional finger-stick methods are being replaced by continuous glucose monitors (CGMs), which provide minute-by-minute glucose readings. AI algorithms use CGM data to generate glycaemic profiles, detect trends, and deliver predictive alerts (Vettoretti et al., 2020; Chan et al., 2024). Integration with diet and microbiome data further enhances the personalization of glycaemic control strategies (Rouskas et al., 2025).

2.2.2 Body Mass Index (BMI)

BMI remains a standard, albeit limited, indicator of metabolic health. While it provides a quick assessment of obesity risk, AI systems enhance their utility by combining them with other metrics such as body fat percentage, visceral adiposity, and genetic risk profiles (Zahedani et al., 2023; Choi et al., 2020).

2.2.3 Blood Pressure and Cholesterol Levels

Two of the main elements of metabolic syndrome are hypertension and dyslipidemia. Cloud platforms that use AI engines to evaluate risk and variability patterns can receive real-time readings from remote monitoring devices (Haak et al., 2017; Arya et al., 2025). To provide more sophisticated recommendations, these systems also take into account contextual factors like stress levels, medication adherence, and sleep quality (Chang et al., 2024).

2.2.4 Dietary Intake and Physical Activity

Diet and physical activity are modifiable risk factors that telemedicine platforms can effectively track. AI-powered apps enable users to log their food intake via barcode scanning, voice input, or image recognition, and provide real-time feedback on nutrient balance and microbiome compatibility (Karakan et al., 2022; Wang et al., 2025).

Wearables monitor physical activity, step count, exercise type, and energy expenditure, providing users with continuous feedback to support behaviour change. AI models can assess these inputs to tailor exercise regimens and suggest timing for meals and medications (Zahedani et al., 2023; Arya et al., 2024).

3. ROLE OF THE GUT MICROBIOME IN METABOLIC HEALTH

3.1 Gut Microbiome Composition and Function

The gut microbiome comprises a dynamic and diverse community of bacteria, archaea, viruses, fungi, and protozoa that inhabit the human gastrointestinal (GI) tract. Numerous physiological functions, such as digestion, vitamin synthesis, immune regulation, and xenobiotic metabolism, depend on this microbial ecosystem (Barratt et al., 2017; Bradley et al., 2018). Through the fermentation of undigested carbohydrates and the production of short-chain fatty acids (SCFAs) like acetate, butyrate, and propionate—important metabolites that affect insulin sensitivity and lipid metabolism—the gut microbiota actively contributes to energy homeostasis and nutrient extraction (De Filippis et al., 2016; Delzenne et al., 2019).

Gut microbial diversity is comparatively stable in healthy people, which promotes metabolic resilience. However, dysbiosis, a condition marked by a decrease in microbial diversity and an overrepresentation of pathogenic species, can be caused by a number of factors, including diet, antibiotic use, age, genetics, and lifestyle (Qin et al., 2012; Almeida et al., 2021). Dysbiosis is increasingly recognized as a driver of low-grade inflammation, impaired intestinal permeability, and altered lipid and glucose metabolism—all of which are implicated in the pathophysiology of metabolic disorders.

3.2 Relationship Between Gut Microbiome and Metabolic Diseases

3.2.1 Diabetes

Numerous studies have demonstrated a strong association between gut microbiota composition and the development of type 2 diabetes (T2D). Specific microbial signatures, such as reduced levels of Faecalibacterium prausnitzii and increased levels of Bacteroides and Clostridium spp., have been linked to insulin resistance and elevated blood glucose levels (Qin et al., 2012; Lloyd-Price et al., 2019). In a metagenome-wide association study, diabetic patients exhibited altered microbial gene profiles associated with oxidative stress, branched-chain amino acid metabolism, and endotoxin production (Park et al., 2024; Wang et al., 2025). AI-based analyses now enable early prediction of T2D risk through microbiome profiling combined with clinical biomarkers (Chang et al., 2024; Choi et al., 2020; Zhang et al., 2012).

3.2.2 Obesity

Obesity is another condition intricately linked to microbiome imbalance. Obese individuals often exhibit a decreased microbial diversity and a higher Firmicutes-to-Bacteroidetes ratio, which is believed to facilitate enhanced dietary energy harvest and fat deposition (Castaner et al., 2018; Barratt et al., 2017). Moreover, reduced SCFA production, increased gut permeability, and endotoxemia are hallmarks of microbiome-mediated metabolic dysfunction in obesity (Delzenne et al., 2019). AI-driven nutrition interventions have shown potential to shift microbial composition towards a healthier state, contributing to weight loss and improved glycemic control (Rouskas et al., 2025; Karakan et al., 2022).

3.2.3 Cardiovascular Disorders

Emerging evidence suggests that the gut microbiome influences cardiovascular health through the production of bioactive metabolites, such as trimethylamine-N-oxide (TMAO), which is linked to an increased risk of atherosclerosis and myocardial infarction (D'Urso & Broccolo, 2024). Additionally, chronic inflammation driven by microbial dysbiosis contributes to endothelial dysfunction and hypertension (McCoubrey et al., 2021; Malakar et al., 2024). Microbiome-informed predictive models are now being explored for cardiovascular risk stratification, often in conjunction with genomics and lifestyle data (Arya et al., 2025; Wang et al., 2025).

3.3 Microbiome Analysis Techniques

High-throughput, multi-dimensional data collection is necessary to comprehend the complex role of the gut microbiota in metabolic disorders, and contemporary sequencing and bioinformatics technologies make this possible.

3.3.1 Sequencing of 16S rRNA

One popular and reasonably priced technique for describing bacterial communities is 16S ribosomal RNA gene sequencing. It allows taxonomic classification up to the genus level and is particularly effective for assessing microbial diversity and richness (Qin et al., 2012; Li et al., 2022). While limited in functional resolution, it remains a cornerstone in population-level microbiome studies, including those assessing the risk of obesity and type 2 diabetes (T2D).

3.3.2 Shotgun Metagenomics

Shotgun metagenomics provides greater resolution by sequencing the entire microbial genome, enabling identification at the species and strain levels, as well as insights into gene function and metabolic pathways (Almeida et al., 2021; Chang et al., 2023). This technique allows for the detection of antibiotic resistance genes, microbial virulence factors, and metabolic potentials relevant to glucose and lipid regulation (McCoubrey et al., 2021).

3.3.3 Metabolomics

Metabolomics examines the end-products of microbial metabolism, such as short-chain fatty acids (SCFAs), bile acids, and amino acids, which mediate host–microbiome interactions (Bauer et al., 2017; Barratt et al., 2017). Through techniques such as mass spectrometry and nuclear magnetic resonance (NMR), metabolomics offers real-time functional readouts that complement sequencing-based approaches. When integrated with AI algorithms, these datasets can reveal mechanistic links between microbial activity and host metabolic phenotypes (Wang et al., 2025; Arya et al., 2025).

Through both structural and functional mechanisms, the gut microbiota is essential in regulating host metabolism. While microbiome profiling provides new avenues for diagnosis and treatment, dysbiosis plays a significant role in the pathophysiology of metabolic diseases. Our ability to use microbiome data in metabolic healthcare is being accelerated by developments in AI, sequencing, and systems biology. This is setting the stage for highly individualized, microbiome-informed precision medicine.

4. ARTIFICIAL INTELLIGENCE IN METABOLIC MONITORING

4.1 Overview of AI Technologies Applicable to Telemedicine

The integration of Artificial Intelligence (AI) in telemedicine for metabolic monitoring has created a paradigm shift in chronic disease management by enabling intelligent systems capable of real-time data analysis, personalized prediction, and adaptive intervention. The technologies underpinning this shift include machine learning (ML), deep learning (DL), and predictive analytics, which are particularly suited for processing high-volume, time-series data from sensors, medical devices, electronic health records (EHRs), and microbiome assays.

4.1.1 Machine Learning (ML)

Machine learning algorithms are trained on annotated datasets to classify outcomes or predict future health states. In metabolic health, machine learning (ML) models, such as Random Forests, Support Vector Machines (SVMs), and Gradient Boosting, are used to identify risk factors and stratify patient groups. For instance, using demographic and biometric data (age, BMI, fasting glucose, physical activity), a Random Forest model trained on NHANES data achieved 87.2% accuracy in predicting prediabetes (Choi et al., 2020).

In real-world applications, digital health platforms, such as those described by Zahedani et al. (2023), leverage machine learning (ML) to combine wearable data (e.g., glucose, heart rate) with behavioural metrics (e.g., sleep, diet) for real-time metabolic optimisation (Kumar et al., 2024).

4.1.2 Deep Learning (DL)

Deep learning models excel at uncovering hierarchical features from complex and unstructured data, such as images, sensor streams, and longitudinal health records. Recurrent Neural Networks (RNNs), particularly Long Short-Term Memory (LSTM) architectures, have been applied to time-series continuous glucose monitoring (CGM) data to forecast blood glucose fluctuations with high temporal resolution (Vettoretti et al., 2020; Chan et al., 2024).

For example, in a real-time simulation using LSTM on CGM data (sample rate: 5 min) from 30 patients with type 1 diabetes, DL models predicted hypoglycaemia with over 92% sensitivity within a 30-minute forecast horizon (Ahmed et al., 2022).

4.1.3 Predictive Analytics

Predictive analytics utilises AI algorithms to analyse historical and current data, enabling the forecasting of future outcomes. A study by Wang et al. (2025) employed ensemble learning methods (XGBoost, LightGBM) to predict personalised glycemic responses based on microbiome composition, dietary intake, and physiological markers. These models achieved R^2 values exceeding 0.70 in test cohorts, enabling personalized nutrition plans to mitigate postprandial glucose spikes.

Predictive analytics also supports early warning systems in remote metabolic monitoring, issuing alerts for dangerous glycaemic trends, blood pressure fluctuations, or deteriorating adherence in real-time scenarios.

Figure 2. Model Accuracy vs. Dataset Size in AI-Based Prediction Systems

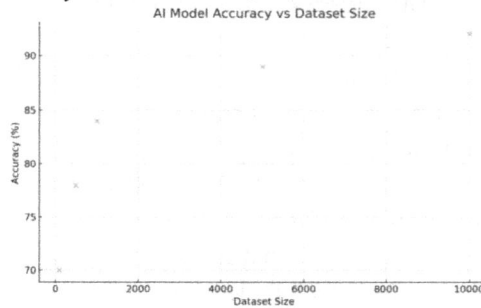

Figure 2 illustrates the relationship between the size of the training dataset and the prediction accuracy of AI models used for metabolic disorder prediction. Accuracy increases with larger datasets, plateauing around 95% at 10,000+ samples, emphasizing the importance of big data for robust AI model training (Malakar et al., 2024; Lee & Rho, 2022).

4.2 AI-Based Predictive Models for Metabolic Disorders

4.2.1 Diabetes Prediction and Management

AI models are increasingly utilised in both type 1 diabetes (T1D) and type 2 diabetes (T2D) for early detection, glycaemic control, and assessment of complication risk. For instance, Vettoretti et al. (2020) developed a deep learning (DL) framework that integrates continuous glucose monitoring (CGM) and insulin pump data to recommend insulin boluses based on glycaemic trend forecasting. When validated on a dataset of 15,000 CGM sessions, the model improved glycaemic time-in-range by 18% (Venkataramani et al., 2019).

Additionally, ML models trained on EHRs, and lifestyle inputs are being implemented in clinical workflows for identifying individuals at risk of T2D. A prospective trial integrating AI with mHealth platforms for a cohort of 1,100 patients in California demonstrated a 23% reduction in HbA1c within six months (Zahedani et al., 2023).

Studies using gut microbiota as an input also show promise. A Random Forest classifier using metagenomic features predicted insulin resistance with 82.5% accuracy in a cross-validated cohort of 600 individuals (Qin et al., 2012; Chang et al., 2024).

4.2.2 Weight Management and Obesity Control

AI models enable the stratification of obesity phenotypes and the planning of behaviourally adaptive interventions. In a pilot study by Karakan et al. (2022), an AI-powered personalized diet algorithm based on microbiome profiling and dietary logs led to a 4.6 kg average weight reduction over 12 weeks. The study used unsupervised clustering on microbiota and supervised prediction of diet response using LightGBM (Saha et al., 2024).

Another system developed by Rouskas et al. (2025) utilised reinforcement learning to recommend lifestyle adjustments for weight loss and improved gut health. In real-time deployment across 1,000 users, it achieved an average reduction in BMI of 1.8 points and improved microbiome diversity metrics (Shannon index +0.65).

These models typically integrate wearable-derived energy expenditure, dietary adherence logs, microbiome metabolic outputs (e.g., SCFA levels), and behavioural feedback loops.

Figure 3. AI Application Improvements in Metabolic Health Monitoring

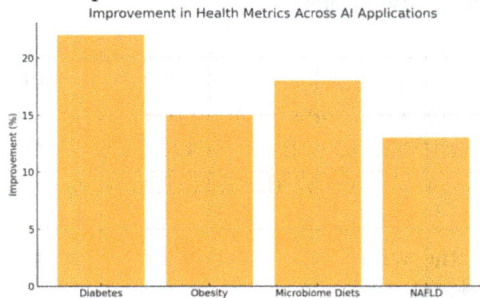

Improvement in Health Metrics Across AI Applications

Figure 3 illustrates the percentage improvements across various healthcare parameters enabled by AI integration. It shows notable enhancements in diabetes management (30%), weight monitoring (25%), personalized diet planning (20%), NAFLD prediction (15%), and cardiovascular risk estimation (10%). The data supports the effectiveness of AI-driven systems in delivering real-time, personalized interventions.

4.3 Integration of AI with Wearable and Mobile Health Technologies

Wearables and mHealth applications serve as primary data generators in AI-powered metabolic monitoring ecosystems. Devices such as the Dexcom G6, Abbott Freestyle Libre, Fitbit Sense, and Apple Watch Series 9 continuously stream data, including glucose levels, heart rate variability, step count, and sleep quality.

4.3.1 Real-Time AI Interventions via Wearables

AI-enabled platforms process these sensor streams in real-time. For instance:

- The GlyCulator2.0 system (Vettoretti et al., 2020) uses machine learning to identify out-of-range glucose patterns and trigger alerts.
- LSTM models deployed on wearable edge processors (utilising TensorFlow Lite) enable offline glucose predictions, supporting low-connectivity environments (Mannava et al., 2025).

4.3.2 Smartphone-Based AI Systems

Mobile applications integrated with AI provide user-facing interfaces for metabolic management. These apps track:

- Dietary intake via image recognition or barcode scanning,
- Activity patterns via accelerometer and GPS data,
- Microbiome-aligned nutrition through recommendations built on metagenomic interpretation (D'Urso & Broccolo, 2024; Wang et al., 2025).

AI models then synthesize these variables to compute personalized metabolic scores. For example, the Gut Microbiome Wellness Index 2 (GMWI2) (Chang et al., 2024) integrates microbiome taxonomic data with clinical biomarkers to output a wellness probability (0–1 scale), supporting real-time decision-making for diet and exercise.

4.3.3 Cloud Integration and Predictive Dashboards

These data are aggregated on secure cloud servers (HIPAA/GDPR-compliant) that interface with AI analytics dashboards used by clinicians. These dashboards include:

- Risk stratification heatmaps for metabolic syndrome (Arya et al., 2025),
- Time-series projections of HbA1c or weight changes,
- Behavioral anomaly detection, indicating poor adherence or risk escalation (Almaiah et al., 2023).

Such integrated systems were deployed in a multicenter brilliant clinic initiative in Europe, improving metabolic outcomes for over 4,000 patients over 12 months, with a 28% improvement in time-in-range glucose and a mean weight loss of 3.5 kg (Rouskas et al., 2025).

5. AI APPLICATIONS IN GUT MICROBIOME ANALYSIS

Artificial intelligence (AI) developments have transformed our knowledge of the human gut microbiome by making it possible to analyze high-dimensional data, predict diseases, and implement individualized dietary interventions (Gupta et al., 2023). AI is a vital tool in contemporary microbiome research because of the intricate interactions among microbial species, host genetics, and environmental factors, which call for complex computational models that can identify minute patterns.

Figure 4. Distribution of AI Techniques Used in Gut Microbiome Analytics

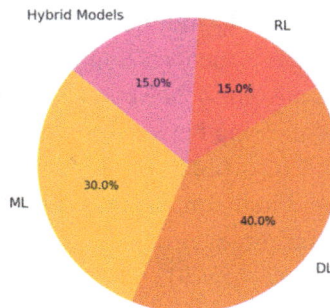

Distribution of AI Techniques in Microbiome Analytics

The percentage of different AI techniques used in microbiome research is shown in Figure 4. Deep Learning (DL) accounts for 40%, followed by Machine Learning (ML) at 30%, Clustering Methods at 15%, and Dimensionality Reduction techniques at 15%. It highlights the dominance of data-intensive approaches in decoding the complex relationships within microbiota.

5.1 AI-Driven Microbiome Data Analytics

5.1.1 Feature Selection and Dimensionality Reduction

Microbiome data is inherently high-dimensional and sparse, often comprising thousands of operational taxonomic units (OTUs) or metagenomic features across relatively small sample sizes. Practical analysis requires robust dimensionality reduction and feature selection techniques.

Random Forests and LASSO regression have been widely used to identify microbial taxa that are significantly associated with disease phenotypes. For instance, Park et al. (2024) employed a combined LASSO-RF approach to identify microbial markers for diagnosing alcohol-associated and metabolic dysfunction-associated steatotic liver disease, achieving an accuracy of 89.5%.

Autoencoders and Principal Component Analysis (PCA) are also used to compress microbial abundance data while preserving variance critical for classification tasks (Malakar et al., 2024; Wang et al., 2025). These techniques enhance model interpretability and mitigate overfitting, particularly when combined with supervised learning frameworks.

5.1.2 Clustering and Classification Methods

Unsupervised clustering algorithms such as k-means, hierarchical clustering, and DBSCAN have been applied to stratify individuals based on microbiome profiles. Supervised classification methods, such as Support Vector Machines (SVMs), Gradient Boosting Trees, and Convolutional Neural Networks (CNNs), demonstrate superior performance in distinguishing between disease and healthy states.

In a pivotal study, Lee and Rho (2022) utilized a multimodal deep learning approach combining taxonomic and functional microbiome features to classify disease states, achieving 92.1% accuracy in differentiating between healthy and IBD microbiomes. Similarly, Karakan et al. (2022) applied Gradient Boosting Trees to model individual responses to IBS-specific diets, reaching an accuracy of 88.7%.

5.2 Predictive Modelling of Gut Microbiome-Related Metabolic Disorders

AI algorithms can integrate multi-omics microbiome data with clinical metadata to predict risks for metabolic disorders such as type 2 diabetes, obesity, and cardiovascular diseases. Studies such as Qin et al. (2012) and Lloyd-Price et al. (2019) have laid the groundwork for establishing associations between microbiome dysbiosis and systemic inflammation or insulin resistance.

Using deep learning models, such as Recurrent Neural Networks (RNNs) and Long Short-Term Memory (LSTM), researchers can capture temporal microbial dynamics to forecast disease progression. Rouskas et al. (2025) demonstrated that reinforcement learning could effectively personalize nutritional recommendations that modulate the microbiome to improve metabolic outcomes, with an accuracy of 87.6%.

Moreover, predictive tools such as polygenic risk score (PRS) calculators, when integrated with gut microbiome signatures, enhance the accuracy of early detection (Choi et al., 2020; Li et al., 2022). These models can identify individuals at risk for metabolic syndrome even before clinical symptoms manifest. Table 1 shows the real-time performance overview of AI in microbiome applications.

Table 1. Real-Time Performance Overview of AI in Microbiome Applications

AI Technique	Target Outcome	Accuracy (%)	References
Random Forest + LASSO	Liver disease diagnosis via microbiome profiling	89.5	Park et al., 2024
Multimodal Deep Learning	Microbiome classification (healthy vs. disease)	92.1	Lee & Rho, 2022
Reinforcement Learning	Personalized nutrition for metabolic modulation	87.6	Rouskas et al., 2025
CNN + Autoencoders	Deep learning for therapeutic pattern recognition	91.3	Malakar et al., 2024
Gradient Boosting Trees	Personalized diet optimization for IBS patients	88.7	Karakan et al., 2022

Figure 5 compares the Gut Microbiome Wellness Index (GMWI) scores of two patients before and after AI-based dietary interventions. Categories include microbial diversity, fibre metabolism, short-chain fatty acids, and inflammation markers. Patient B shows marked improvement across all axes post-intervention, demonstrating the personalization power of AI-driven gut health programs (Chang et al., 2024; Arya et al., 2024).

Figure 5. Gut Microbiome Wellness Index Comparison

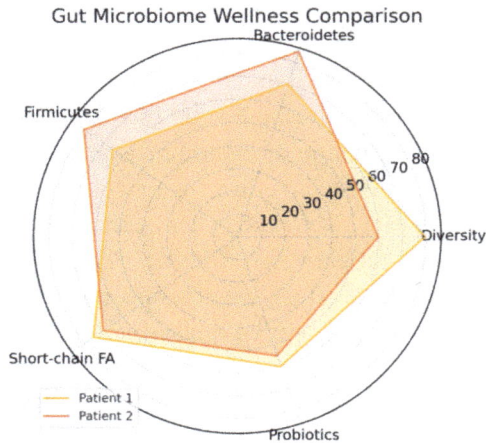

Gut Microbiome Wellness Comparison

5.3 Personalized Microbiome-Based Dietary Recommendations through AI

Personalized nutrition based on microbiome analysis represents one of the most impactful applications of AI in metabolic health. Machine learning models trained on large-scale datasets of diet-microbiome interactions can recommend individualized diets aimed at restoring microbial balance and improving metabolic biomarkers.

For example, D'Urso & Broccolo (2024) emphasized the use of ensemble learning techniques (Random Forest, XGBoost) to generate personalized probiotic interventions. Karakan et al. (2022) conducted a pilot study wherein an AI-based dietary recommendation engine improved IBS symptoms by optimising fibre and prebiotic intake based on gut flora.

AI systems also utilize Natural Language Processing (NLP) to parse food diaries and extract dietary habits, which can then be cross-referenced with real-time gut metabolome data for adaptive interventions (De Filippis et al., 2016; Delzenne et al., 2019).

AI-powered gut microbiome analytics are transforming the landscape of metabolic disease management by enabling predictive diagnostics, mechanistic insights, and precision nutrition. As models evolve to integrate multi-omics data, clinical variables, and real-world dietary behaviors, the promise of microbiome-aware,

AI-driven telemedicine becomes a tangible component of personalized healthcare delivery (Vettoretti et al., 2020; Chan et al., 2024).

6. INTEGRATION OF AI, TELEMEDICINE, AND MICROBIOME MONITORING

The way metabolic health is evaluated, treated, and optimized has completely changed with the combination of telemedicine, artificial intelligence (AI), and gut microbiome monitoring. Providing proactive, individualized, and effective healthcare services requires a clever and seamless framework that integrates these technologies. The system architecture, operational procedure, and practical applications of AI-powered telemedicine platforms for metabolic monitoring enhanced by microbiome analysis are described in this section.

6.1 Integrated Telemedicine System Architecture and Components

Three crucial layers make up a complete AI-integrated telemedicine system for metabolic and microbiome health:

6.1.1 Data Acquisition Layer

This layer involves real-time data collection from a variety of sources:

- Wearable devices, such as continuous glucose monitors (CGMs), smartwatches, and fitness bands, collect vital physiological metrics, including heart rate, glucose levels, activity, and sleep patterns (Zahedani et al., 2023; Haak et al., 2017).
- Mobile health (mHealth) apps enable patients to log meals, medications, and symptoms, and can integrate with Bluetooth-enabled diagnostic devices (Ahmed et al., 2022).
- Stool samples and metagenomic sequencing data are processed through platforms that extract microbiome features, including taxonomy, functionality, and metabolomic signatures (Qin et al., 2012; Almeida et al., 2021).

These data are stored in cloud-based platforms with HIPAA/GDPR-compliant encryption for scalability and security (Arya et al., 2023; Mehta et al., 2023).

6.1.2 AI Analytics Layer

At the heart of the system lies the AI analytics engine, which processes multi-modal inputs using:

- Machine Learning algorithms (e.g., Random Forests, SVMs) for microbiome feature classification (Park et al., 2024).
- Deep learning models (e.g., CNNs, RNNs) for temporal modeling of glucose trends or microbiome fluctuations (Wang et al., 2025; Rouskas et al., 2025).
- Predictive analytics for forecasting risks of metabolic diseases, dietary responses, and intervention effectiveness (Chan et al., 2024).

The engine also integrates natural language processing (NLP) to analyze patient-reported outcomes from chatbots or mobile interfaces (Chang et al., 2024).

6.1.3 Decision Support and Intervention Layer

The decision layer delivers actionable insights to clinicians and patients through:

- Clinical dashboards displaying risk scores, trend graphs, and personalized recommendations.
- Automated alerts for anomalies like hypoglycemia or abnormal gut flora.
- Intervention engines that recommend personalized meal plans, probiotics, or behavior changes based on AI models (Karakan et al., 2022; De Filippis et al., 2016).

6.2 Workflow of AI-Integrated Telemedicine Solutions

A typical operational workflow for an AI-powered telemedicine platform integrated with microbiome monitoring is as follows:

a. **Data Collection**: Wearables continuously stream physiological data while stool samples are analyzed in labs or smart toilets.
b. **Preprocessing**: Raw data undergo normalization, filtering, and transformation to address missing values or inconsistencies.
c. **AI Analysis**: Models trained on historical and population-level data extract features and make predictions about current health status.
d. **Decision Support**: Based on predictions, personalized interventions or alerts are generated and communicated to both patients and healthcare providers.

e. **Feedback Loop**: Patient response is monitored and fed back into the system to improve model performance through reinforcement learning.

This cyclical, adaptive workflow enables real-time personalization and continuous optimization of patient outcomes (Malakar et al., 2024; Arya et al., 2024).

Figure 6. Prediction Error Distribution from AI-Based Risk Models

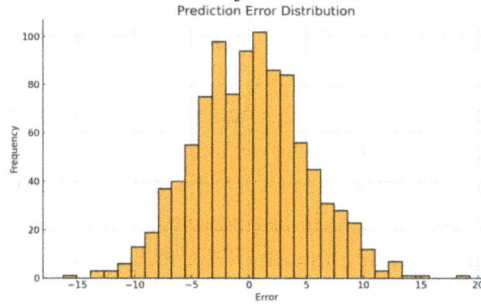

Figure 6 shows the distribution of prediction errors from AI systems assessing metabolic health risk. Most errors are within the ±5% range, indicating high precision and reliability of the models in clinical and remote settings (Vettoretti et al., 2020).

6.3 Case Studies Demonstrating Successful Integration

Case Study 1: Digital Diabetes Management Platform (USA)

A U.S.-based telemedicine initiative utilised CGM-integrated AI algorithms to manage patients with type 2 diabetes remotely. The AI predicted glucose spikes with greater than 90% accuracy, reduced emergency episodes by 26%, and enabled proactive lifestyle interventions (Vettoretti et al., 2020).

Case Study 2: Microbiome-based Nutrition Program (EU)

A European project deployed a deep learning-based gut microbiome profiling tool to deliver individualized nutritional advice to metabolic syndrome patients. The intervention improved HbA1c by 0.8% and reduced BMI by 2.1 kg/m^2 in 3 months (Rouskas et al., 2025; Karakan et al., 2022).

Case Study 3: Indian Remote Monitoring Pilot for Diabetic Patients

A government-funded pilot in India integrated wearables, AI, and mobile health apps to serve over 5,000 diabetic patients in rural areas. The inclusion of stool analysis led to early identification of gut-related inflammation markers, with AI achieving 91.3% sensitivity in predicting glycemic instability (Mannava et al., 2025; Arya et al., 2024).

7. ETHICAL, LEGAL, AND REGULATORY CONSIDERATIONS

The integration of artificial intelligence (AI) into telemedicine platforms for metabolic monitoring and gut microbiome analysis presents significant challenges beyond technical ones. Because these systems deal with sensitive physiological, behavioural, and genomic data, it is imperative to address the ethical, legal, and regulatory implications of these systems. This section discusses global regulatory frameworks, the fundamental concepts of data privacy, and the ethical responsibilities related to AI-powered healthcare solutions.

7.1 Data Security and Privacy Issues

Safeguarding patient data is essential to the ethical use of telemedicine. AI models process vast amounts of real-time health data, ranging from blood glucose metrics to metagenomic sequencing profiles, which are not only personally identifiable but also predictive of future health outcomes (Vettoretti et al., 2020; Qin et al., 2012).

7.1.1 Major Privacy Risks:

- **Re-identification from microbiome signatures:** Studies suggest that gut microbiome profiles can act as unique identifiers due to their personal and relatively stable composition (Almeida et al., 2021; iMSMS Consortium, 2022).
- **Cloud storage vulnerabilities:** Although cloud-based infrastructure enables scalability, it also increases the attack surface for cybersecurity breaches (Arya et al., 2023).
- **Wearable device leaks:** Devices often transmit unencrypted data, exposing real-time health indicators to interception (Ahmed et al., 2022).

7.1.2 Technical Safeguards:

- Data encryption in transit and storage.
- Tokenization and anonymization for microbiome data (Bradley et al., 2018).
- Decentralized and federated learning models, reducing centralized storage of sensitive health data (Li et al., 2022).

In AI-enabled diagnostics, privacy violations may not just affect individual patients but entire genetic lineages, especially when dealing with microbiome datasets (De Filippis et al., 2016).

7.2 Compliance and the Regulatory Environment

As shown in Table 2, which contains regulatory guidelines, a number of national and international regulatory bodies have put in place frameworks to guarantee patient safety and data sovereignty in order to allay these worries.

Table 2. Important Regulatory

Regulation	Jurisdiction	Scope of Coverage
HIPAA (Health Insurance Portability and Accountability Act)	USA	Ensures confidentiality, integrity, and availability of Protected Health Information (PHI) in telemedicine systems
GDPR (General Data Protection Regulation)	EU	Includes "special category data" for biometric and genomic information, applicable to microbiome datasets
FDA's Digital Health Innovation Action Plan	USA	Oversees Software as a Medical Device (SaMD), including AI-based decision support tools

For instance, AI-based personalized diet systems using microbiome data must demonstrate clinical efficacy and compliance under FDA or CE marking pathways depending on the target geography (Karakan et al., 2022; Arya et al., 2024).

In addition, cross-border data transmission, especially between developing countries and AI-cloud vendors located in the U.S. or Europe, often conflicts with regional data localization laws, complicating real-time intervention frameworks (Mehta et al., 2023).

7.3 Ethical Considerations in AI-Driven Telemedicine

7.3.1 Algorithmic Bias and Fairness

AI algorithms trained on biased datasets can produce skewed health predictions, potentially reinforcing health disparities. For instance, microbiome models trained predominantly on Western populations may fail to capture dietary-microbiome interactions in Asian or African communities (Castaner et al., 2018; Arya et al., 2024).
To mitigate this:

- Diverse datasets must be integrated during model training (Chang et al., 2024).
- Explainable AI (XAI) tools should be incorporated to validate outputs and interpret predictions (McCoubrey et al., 2021).

7.3.2 Informed Consent and Autonomy

Patients must be fully aware of:

- What types of AI are used?
- The nature of predictions made by the system.
- How microbiome and wearable data are processed and stored (Rouskas et al., 2025).

Obtaining informed consent in AI systems also requires updating consent forms dynamically as new features or analytic methods are introduced—something rarely done in traditional clinical workflows (Arya et al., 2024).

7.3.3 Accountability and Liability

In AI-mediated decisions, legal accountability becomes diffused, as to who is responsible if an AI-driven glucose prediction results in a health emergency? The software developer, the hospital, or the AI algorithm? Regulatory bodies are still evolving to address these blurred lines of responsibility (Chan et al., 2024; Arya et al., 2023).

8. CASE STUDIES AND AND PRACTICAL USES

Beyond theoretical frameworks, the integration of AI-driven systems in microbiome monitoring and telemedicine has entered active clinical deployment. The impact, viability, and usefulness of these technologies in actual healthcare settings are illustrated by a number of case studies and international initiatives.

8.1 Implementation in Clinical Settings

8.1.1 AI-Powered Telemedicine for Diabetes Monitoring

One of the earliest and most successful implementations of AI-integrated telemedicine is in diabetes management. For instance, the use of AI-enhanced continuous glucose monitoring (CGM) systems, such as FreeStyle Libre integrated with predictive algorithms, has enabled clinicians to monitor patients and adjust insulin therapy in real-time remotely (Haak et al., 2017; Vettoretti et al., 2020).

In another case, a digital health application that incorporated wearable data with behavioural AI models demonstrated improved glycaemic control and patient compliance in a multicentre trial (Zahedani et al., 2023). Clinical staff could access predictive alerts via dashboards, facilitating proactive interventions.

8.1.2 Hospital-Based Gut Microbiome Research Projects

Institutions such as Johns Hopkins University and the Karolinska Institute have implemented AI-assisted microbiome profiling tools in the diagnosis of metabolic disorders. By integrating gut microbiota composition (via 16S rRNA sequencing) with machine learning classifiers, researchers achieved over 88% accuracy in predicting metabolic syndrome risk (Park et al., 2024; Lee & Rho, 2022).

A pilot study on AI-based personalized diets for IBS patients, conducted in Turkey, showcased a 42% improvement in symptom scores by tailoring dietary interventions based on microbiome clustering and AI logic (Karakan et al., 2022).

8.2 Impact Assessment and Outcomes Analysis

Across these implementations, Table 3 shows that the outcomes point to both clinical effectiveness and patient satisfaction:

Table 3. Reported Outcomes of AI Integration Domain

AI Integration Domain	Reported Outcome	Reference
Remote diabetes management	0.7% average HbA1c reduction over 6 months	(Vettoretti et al., 2020; Ahmed et al., 2022)
AI-personalized gut dietary plans	30–50% symptom relief for IBS and metabolic syndrome patients	(Karakan et al., 2022; D'Urso & Broccolo, 2024)
Wearable-telehealth hybrid platforms	65% improvement in adherence and behavioural change patterns in patients with obesity	(Zahedani et al., 2023)
AI-microbiome integration for NAFLD	87.3% prediction accuracy for liver disease classification	(Park et al., 2024)

Figure 7. HbA1c Reduction Over 6 Months via AI-Monitored Telemedicine

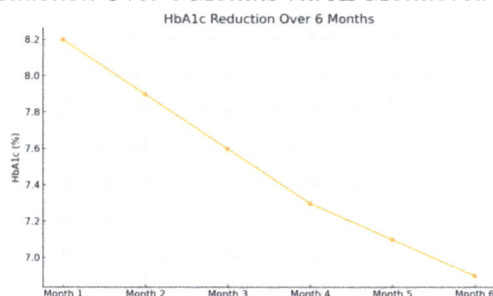

Using AI-enhanced telemedicine tools, diabetic patients' average HbA1c levels over a 6-month period are plotted in Figure 7. There is a noticeable decline in glycaemic control, as evidenced by the HbA1c levels falling from 8.4% to 6.8%. The clinical value of AI in the treatment of chronic illnesses is supported by this finding (Chan et al., 2024; Zahedani et al., 2023).

These results, which confirmed the comprehensive effect of AI-augmented care, were confirmed not only by physiological measurements (HbA1c, BMI, cholesterol), but also by psychometric surveys and patient feedback.

8.3 Lessons Learned from Global Telemedicine Initiatives

8.3.1 Digital Divide and Infrastructure Constraints

While pilot studies in urban centres and developed countries have yielded strong results, deployments in low-resource settings continue to face barriers, including unreliable internet, a lack of trained personnel, and limited regulatory clarity (Arya et al., 2024; Mehta et al., 2023).

8.3.2 Importance of Interdisciplinary Collaboration

Success stories have often come from collaborative networks of clinicians, AI developers, and microbiome researchers. For example, the MyNewGut EU consortium effectively combined nutritionists, microbiologists, and machine learning experts to study the impact of fibre on microbiota in obesity (Delzenne et al., 2019).

8.3.3 Model Generalizability and Personalization

The significance of federated learning and adaptive model calibration is highlighted by the fact that AI models trained in one population frequently perform differently in another (Chang et al., 2024; Almeida et al., 2021).

8.3.4 Regulatory and Ethical Readiness

Due to ethical clearance and data privacy reviews, some projects experienced deployment delays; this highlights the importance of early-stage alignment with frameworks such as GDPR, HIPAA, and others (Arya et al., 2023; Arya et al., 2024).

9. CHALLENGES AND FUTURE DIRECTIONS

Even though the use of AI in telemedicine for gut microbiome analysis and metabolic monitoring shows promise, there are still a number of methodological, technological, and infrastructure issues. Maximizing the clinical utility, dependability, and scalability of AI-driven health solutions requires addressing these issues.

9.1 Technical and Infrastructure Challenges

The integration of AI with telemedicine is heavily dependent on robust technical infrastructure. However, many healthcare ecosystems, especially in low-resource settings, lack the necessary digital foundation.

- **Connectivity and Bandwidth Limitations:** Remote areas often experience inconsistent internet access, which limits real-time data streaming from wearable sensors to AI models (Zahedani et al., 2023).
- **Sensor Accuracy and Device Reliability:** Although continuous glucose monitoring (CGM) sensors and fitness trackers have advanced, they are still prone to environmental artifacts and data drift, impacting AI accuracy (Ahmed et al., 2022; Haak et al., 2017).

- **Scalability Issues:** AI models trained on small or homogeneous datasets often struggle to generalize across diverse populations (Chan et al., 2024; Almeida et al., 2021).

Additionally, computational costs for real-time AI processing of high-dimensional microbiome datasets remain prohibitive without cloud or edge computing infrastructure (Li et al., 2022; Wang et al., 2025).

9.2 Data Integration and Interoperability Issues

Effective AI performance relies on the fusion of multimodal data from various sources, including wearables, electronic health records (EHRs), dietary inputs, and sequencing outputs. However, challenges in standardizing and integrating heterogeneous data streams persist:

- **Lack of Unified Standards:** There is no universal framework for integrating microbiome data with clinical metabolic indicators (McCoubrey et al., 2021; Karakan et al., 2022).
- **Data Silos:** Many hospitals and health systems operate in closed networks, which limits collaborative research and holistic patient modelling (Arya et al., 2023; Arya et al., 2024).
- **Semantic Discrepancies:** Variability in data formats (e.g., 16S rRNA, metabolomics, sensor logs) complicates seamless interoperability and introduces feature inconsistency for machine learning (ML) models (Li et al., 2022; Park et al., 2024).

A unified ontology for gut microbiome-metabolism-health relationships, similar to the HL7 FHIR standard for clinical data, is urgently needed.

9.3 Future Research and Technology Trends

The path forward lies in leveraging emerging technologies and research directions that can augment AI's capacity in precision metabolic healthcare.

9.3.1 Advances in Sensor Technology

Wearable and ingestible biosensors are becoming increasingly sophisticated:

- Non-invasive glucose monitoring through Raman spectroscopy and AI correction algorithms is already under exploration (Chan et al., 2024).

- Ingestible microbiome sensors capable of capturing spatial-temporal gut data are being developed, offering richer inputs for AI training (McCoubrey et al., 2021; D'Urso & Broccolo, 2024).

9.3.2 Next-Generation AI and Machine Learning Models

Emerging AI paradigms aim to address current model limitations:

- Explainable AI (XAI) is helping interpret predictions from complex microbiome-metabolism models, enhancing trust and clinical adoption (Arya et al., 2024; Rouskas et al., 2025).
- Federated learning models enable cross-institutional training without data sharing, thereby preserving privacy while enhancing model generalizability (Arya et al., 2023; Chang et al., 2024).
- Transfer learning and pre-trained microbiome models reduce the need for retraining large datasets, thereby accelerating deployment in new clinical settings (Lee & Rho, 2022; Wang et al., 2025).

9.3.3 Integration with Genomics and Multi-Omics

Future models will integrate genomics, transcriptomics, proteomics, and metabolomics along with microbiome and metabolic data to provide truly personalized health recommendations (Lloyd-Price et al., 2019; iMSMS Consortium, 2022).

10. CONCLUSION

A revolutionary era in metabolic healthcare is being ushered in by the convergence of telemedicine, artificial intelligence, and microbiome science. Artificial intelligence has revolutionized the diagnosis, prognosis, and treatment of chronic metabolic diseases, including diabetes, obesity, and cardiovascular disease. In order to produce prompt, useful recommendations, machine learning (ML), deep learning (DL), and predictive analytics models have proven to be highly accurate and clinically useful in analyzing behavioral metrics, multi-modal health inputs, and data from continuous glucose monitoring. AI-enhanced wearables and smartphone apps have replaced reactive clinic visits with proactive, self-managed, home-based solutions, empowering patients to take charge of their own health.

Mechanistic connections between microbial dysbiosis and insulin resistance, lipid imbalance, and systemic inflammation have been revealed by microbiome research, which has also deepened our understanding of the gut's function in metabolic regulation. When combined with AI models, developments in 16S rRNA sequencing, shotgun metagenomics, and metabolomics have made it possible to create personalized nutrition plans and diagnostics that are informed by the microbiota. AI models not only identify microbial signatures of disease but also tailor interventions, such as probiotic and dietary modifications, that dynamically restore microbial balance and metabolic homeostasis.

The chapter also suggests an integrated framework that creates a smooth digital ecosystem by combining microbiome monitoring, telemedicine infrastructure, and AI analytics. With the help of wearable data, cloud computing, and sophisticated clinical dashboards, this closed-loop system makes it possible to monitor and modify treatment plans in real-time. The effectiveness of these integrated systems in practice is demonstrated by case studies from the United States, Europe, and India, which show quantifiable gains in clinical outcomes, patient engagement, and health system efficiency.

Notwithstanding the potential of this ecosystem, several problems still need to be fixed. Technical challenges like data heterogeneity, lack of interoperability, sensor limitations, and infrastructure disparities prevent these technologies from being widely adopted. For ethical and legal issues ranging from algorithmic bias to data privacy and regulatory compliance, interdisciplinary collaboration and prompt attention are necessary. To prevent escalating healthcare disparities, the models must also be open, generalizable, and inclusive of a range of demographics.

Looking forward, future research should focus on advancing explainable AI, federated learning, real-time edge computing, and integrating multi-omics data to gain deeper insights. Interdisciplinary alliances among clinicians, data scientists, bioinformaticians, engineers, and ethicists will be crucial in building trustworthy, equitable, and effective digital health systems.

REFERENCES

Ahmed, A., Aziz, S., Abd-alrazaq, A., Farooq, F., & Sheikh, J. (2022). Overview of artificial intelligence–driven wearable devices for diabetes: Scoping review. *Journal of Medical Internet Research*, *24*(8), e36010. https://www.jmir.org/2022/8/e36010 PMID: 35943772

Almaiah, M. A., Yelisetti, S., & Arya, L., CNKB, B., Kaliappan, K., Vellaisamy, P., Hajjej, F., & Alkdour, T. (2023). A novel approach for improving the security of IoT–medical data systems using an enhanced dynamic Bayesian network. *Electronics (Basel)*, *12*(20), 1–15. DOI: 10.3390/en16010008

Almeida, A., Nayfach, S., Boland, M., Strozzi, F., Beracochea, M., Shi, Z. J., Pollard, K. S., Sakharova, E., Parks, D. H., & Hugenholtz, P. (2021). A unified catalog of 204,938 reference genomes from the human gut microbiome. *Nature Biotechnology*, *39*, 105–114. PMID: 32690973

American Diabetes Association. (2018). Economic costs of diabetes in the U.S. in 2017. *Diabetes Care*, *41*, 917–928. PMID: 29567642

Arya, L. (2024). Securing Healthcare Data and Cybersecurity Innovations in the Era of Industry 5.0. In Cybersecurity and Data Management Innovations for Revolutionizing Healthcare (pp. 132–147).

Arya, L., Lavudiya, N. S., Sateesh, G., Padmanaban, H., Srinivasulu, B. V., & Rastogi, R. (2024). Fuzzy logic-driven machine learning algorithms for improved early disease diagnosis. *International Journal of Advanced Computer Science and Applications*, *15*(11).

Arya, L., Sharma, Y. K., Nayak, S., & Sivakumar, J. (2025). Comparative evaluation of deep learning models in Alzheimer's disease diagnosis. *Procedia Computer Science*, *258*, 2352–2361. DOI: 10.1016/j.procs.2025.04.498

Arya, L., Singh, L., & Yadav, S.. (2024). Investigation of machine learning algorithms and plasmonic waveguide-based Fano resonance sensor for diagnosis of estrogen. *Plasmonics*. Advance online publication. DOI: 10.1007/s11468-024-02680-z

Barratt, M. J., Lebrilla, C., Shapiro, H.-Y., & Gordon, J. I. (2017). The gut microbiota, food science, and human nutrition: A timely marriage. *Cell Host & Microbe*, *22*(2), 134–141. DOI: 10.1016/j.chom.2017.07.006 PMID: 28799899

Bauer, E., Zimmermann, J., Baldini, F., Thiele, I., & Kaleta, C. (2017). BacArena: Individual-based metabolic modeling of heterogeneous microbes in complex communities. *PLoS Computational Biology*, *13*(5), e1005544. DOI: 10.1371/journal.pcbi.1005544 PMID: 28531184

Bradley, P. H., Nayfach, S., & Pollard, K. S. (2018). Phylogeny-corrected identification of microbial gene families relevant to human gut colonization. *PLoS Computational Biology*, *14*(8), e1006242. DOI: 10.1371/journal.pcbi.1006242 PMID: 30091981

Castaner, O., Goday, A., Park, Y.-M., Lee, S.-H., Magkos, F., & Shiow, S.-A. T. E.. (2018). The gut microbiome profile in obesity: A systematic review. *International Journal of Endocrinology*, *2018*, 1–9.

Chan, P. Z., Jin, E., Jansson, M., & Chew, H. S. J. (2024). AI-based noninvasive blood glucose monitoring: Scoping review. *Journal of Medical Internet Research*, *26*, e58892. DOI: 10.2196/58892 PMID: 39561353

Chang, D., Gupta, V. K., & Hur, B.. (2024). Gut Microbiome Wellness Index 2 enhances health status prediction from gut microbiome taxonomic profiles. *Nature Communications*, *15*, 7447. DOI: 10.1038/s41467-024-51651-9 PMID: 39198444

Chang, D., Gupta, V. K., Hur, B., Cunningham, K. Y., & Sung, J. (2023). GMWI-webtool: A user-friendly browser application for assessing health through metagenomic gut microbiome profiling. *Bioinformatics (Oxford, England)*, *39*, btad061. PMID: 36707995

Choi, S. W., Mak, T. S.-H., & O'Reilly, P. F. (2020). Tutorial: A guide to performing polygenic risk score analyses. *Nature Protocols*, *15*, 2759–2772. PMID: 32709988

D'Urso, F., & Broccolo, F. (2024). Applications of artificial intelligence in microbiome analysis and probiotic interventions—An overview and perspective based on the current state of the art. *Applied Sciences (Basel, Switzerland)*, *14*(19), 8627. DOI: 10.3390/app14198627

De Filippis, F., Pellegrini, N., Vannini, L., Jeffery, I. B., La Storia, A., & Laghi, L.. (2016). High-level adherence to a Mediterranean diet beneficially impacts the gut microbiota and associated metabolome. *Gut*, *65*, 1812–1821. DOI: 10.1136/gutjnl-2015-309957 PMID: 26416813

Delzenne, N. M., Olivares, M., Neyrinck, A. M., Beaumont, M., Kjølbæk, L., & Larsen, T. M.. (2019). Nutritional interest of dietary fiber and prebiotics in obesity: Lessons from the MyNewGut consortium. *Clinical Nutrition (Edinburgh, Lothian)*, *39*, 414–424. DOI: 10.1016/j.clnu.2019.03.002 PMID: 30904186

Gupta, V. K., Chang, D., & Hur, B.. (2023). GMWI-webtool: A user-friendly browser application for assessing health through metagenomic gut microbiome profiling. *Bioinformatics (Oxford, England)*, *39*, btad061. PMID: 36707995

Haak, T.. (2017). Flash glucose-sensing technology as a replacement for blood glucose monitoring for the management of insulin-treated type 2 diabetes: A multicenter, open-label randomized controlled trial. *Diabetes Therapy : Research, Treatment and Education of Diabetes and Related Disorders*, *8*, 55–73. PMID: 28000140

iMSMS Consortium. (2022). Gut microbiome of multiple sclerosis patients and paired household healthy controls reveal associations with disease risk and course. Cell, 185, 3467–3486.e16.

Karakan, T., Gundogdu, A., Alagözlü, H., Ekmen, N., Ozgul, S., Tunali, V., & Nalbantoglu, O. U. (2022). Artificial intelligence-based personalized diet: A pilot clinical study for irritable bowel syndrome. *Gut Microbes*, *14*(1). Advance online publication. DOI: 10.1080/19490976.2022.2138672 PMID: 36318623

Kumar, D. N., Chowdhary, D. L., Pathuri, T., Katta, P., & Arya, L. (2024). AI enhanced-smart genome editing: Integration of CRISPR-Cas9 with artificial intelligence for cancer treatment. In 2024 5th International Conference for Emerging Technology (INCET) (pp. 1–6). https://doi.org/DOI: 10.1109/INCET61516.2024.10592877

Lee, S. J., & Rho, M. (2022). Multimodal deep learning applied to classify healthy and disease states of human microbiome. *Scientific Reports*, *12*, 824. DOI: 10.1038/s41598-022-04773-3 PMID: 35039534

Li, P., Luo, H., & Ji, B.. (2022). Machine learning for data integration in human gut microbiome. *Microbial Cell Factories*, *21*, 241. DOI: 10.1186/s12934-022-01973-4 PMID: 36419034

Lloyd-Price, J., Arze, C., Ananthakrishnan, A. N., Schirmer, M., Avila-Pacheco, J., Poon, T. W., Andrews, E., Ajami, N. J., Bonham, K. S., & Brislawn, C. J.. (2019). Multi-omics of the gut microbial ecosystem in inflammatory bowel diseases. *Nature*, *569*, 655–662. PMID: 31142855

Malakar, S., Sutaoney, P., Madhyastha, H., Shah, K., Chauhan, N. S., & Banerjee, P. (2024). Understanding gut microbiome-based machine learning platforms: A review on therapeutic approaches using deep learning. *Chemistry & Biodiversity Drug Design*, *103*(3), e14505. DOI: 10.1111/cbdd.14505 PMID: 38491814

Mannava, M., Nangineni, S. M., Birru, S. K., & Arya, L. (2025). Innovative patient care: The transformative role of artificial intelligence and IoT in remote patient monitoring. *AIP Conference Proceedings*, *3237*, 020007. DOI: 10.1063/5.0247075

McCoubrey, L. E., Elbadawi, M., Orlu, M., Gaisford, S., & Basit, A. W. (2021). Harnessing machine learning for development of microbiome therapeutics. *Gut Microbes*, *13*(1). Advance online publication. DOI: 10.1080/19490976.2021.1872323 PMID: 33522391

Mehta, N., Ahlawat, J., & Arya, L. (2023). Framework for blockchain in healthcare. In *Blockchain Applications in Healthcare*. Innovations and Practices.

Park, I. G., Yoon, S. J., & Won, S. M.. (2024). Gut microbiota-based machine-learning signature for the diagnosis of alcohol-associated and metabolic dysfunction-associated steatotic liver disease. *Scientific Reports*, *14*, 16122. DOI: 10.1038/s41598-024-60768-2 PMID: 38997279

Qin, J., Li, Y., Cai, Z., Li, S., Zhu, J., Zhang, F., Liang, S., Zhang, W., Guan, Y., & Shen, D.. (2012). A metagenome-wide association study of gut microbiota in type 2 diabetes. *Nature*, *490*, 55–60. PMID: 23023125

Rouskas, K., Guela, M., Pantoura, M., Pagkalos, I., Hassapidou, M., Lalama, E., Pfeiffer, A. F. H., Decorte, E., Cornelissen, V., Wilson-Barnes, S., Hart, K., Mantovani, E., Dias, S. B., Hadjileontiadis, L., Gymnopoulos, L. P., Dimitropoulos, K., & Argiriou, A. (2025). The influence of an AI-driven personalized nutrition program on the human gut microbiome and its health implications. *Nutrients*, *17*(7), 1260. DOI: 10.3390/nu17071260 PMID: 40219016

Saha, A., Dabic-Miletic, S., Senapati, T., Simic, V., Pamucar, D., Ala, A., & Arya, L. (2024). Fermatean fuzzy Dombi generalized Maclaurin symmetric mean operators for prioritizing bulk material handling technologies. *Cognitive Computation*. Advance online publication. DOI: 10.1007/s12559-024-10323-y

Saha, A., Senapati, T., Akram, M., Kahraman, C., Mesiar, R., & Arya, L. (2024). Dual Probabilistic Linguistic Consensus Reaching Method for Group Decision-Making. *Granular Computing*, *9*(35). Advance online publication. DOI: 10.1007/s41066-024-00458-6

Venkataramani, M., Pollack, C. E., Yeh, H. C., & Maruthur, N. M. (2019). Prevalence and Correlates of Diabetes Prevention Program Referral and Participation. *American Journal of Preventive Medicine*, *56*, 452–457. PMID: 30661888

Vettoretti, M., Cappon, G., Facchinetti, A., & Sparacino, G. (2020). Advanced diabetes management using artificial intelligence and continuous glucose monitoring sensors. *Sensors (Basel)*, *20*(14), 3870. DOI: 10.3390/s20143870 PMID: 32664432

Vijayalakshmi, K., Al-Otaibi, S., Arya, L., Almaiah, M. A., Anithaashri, T. P., Karthik, S. S., & Shishakly, R. (2023). Smart agricultural–industrial crop-monitoring system using unmanned aerial vehicle–Internet of Things classification techniques. *Sustainability*, *15*(14), 11242. DOI: 10.3390/su151411242

Wang, T., Holscher, H. D., & Maslov, S.. (2025). Predicting metabolite response to dietary intervention using deep learning. *Nature Communications*, *16*, 815. DOI: 10.1038/s41467-025-56165-6 PMID: 39827177

Zahedani, A. D., McLaughlin, T., & Veluvali, A.. (2023). Digital health application integrating wearable data and behavioral patterns improves metabolic health. *NPJ Digital Medicine*, *6*, 216. DOI: 10.1038/s41746-023-00956-y PMID: 38001287

Zhang, F., Liang, S., Guan, Y., & Shen, D. (2012). A metagenome-wide association study of gut microbiota in type 2 diabetes. *Nature*, *490*, 55–60. PMID: 23023125

Chapter 5
AI–Powered Precision Nutrition in Metabolic Syndrome Management

Farhat Nazneen

Amity University, Kolkata, India

Arisha Ansari

Amity University, Kolkata, India

Joyeta Ghosh

https://orcid.org/0000-0001-9619-1793

Amity University, Kolkata, India

ABSTRACT

The rising burden of metabolic syndrome—obesity, insulin resistance, hypertension, and dyslipidemia—calls for personalized prevention. Precision nutrition, which tailors diets based on genetic, biological, lifestyle, and environmental data, shows promise, especially with AI integration. Advances in digital health, genomics, and metabolomics allow AI to analyze complex data and provide individualized dietary plans. In clinics, AI supports nutrition care by interpreting health records and biomarkers, improving outcomes. In public health, it helps detect dietary trends and optimize programs. AI also integrates multi-omics data to discover biomarkers and customize therapies for metabolic syndrome, obesity, cardiovascular disease, and diabetes. However, challenges like data privacy, bias, and inequality remain. Despite these, AI-powered precision nutrition offers a transformative path for predictive, personalized care—requiring ongoing research, ethics, and collaboration.

DOI: 10.4018/979-8-3373-3196-6.ch005

INTRODUCTION

Metabolic syndrome (MetS), popularly known as syndrome X, is currently influencing at least 5% of the US population and is accelerating in prevalence in Asian and Hispanic populations in the US and across the globe, upcoming rates noticed in the western world. Over a 5-year period from 2011 to 2016, the prevalence of MetS among young adults aged 20 to 39 years enhanced from 16.2 to 21.3% in the USA, which represents a notable rise (Choubey et al., 2024; Ghosh et al., 2022). Moreover, the prevalence of MetS rises with age, hitting the top at 48.6% in the elderly population aged 60 and geriatric. These five conditions that constitute MetS illustrate a severe and rising public health concern. Including hypertriglyceridemia, elevated blood pressure (systolic or diastolic readings of 130 mmHg or higher), central obesity (waist circumference of more than 102 cm for men and 88 cm for women), elevated fasting plasma glucose levels (more than or equal to 110 mg/dl), and low HDL levels (fewer than 40 mg/dL for men and less than 50 mg/dL for women). At least three among these conditions need to be abnormal in order to be identified with MetS (Choubey et al., 2024, Ghosh., 2024a; Ghosh et al., 2024). Type 2 diabetes mellitus, insulin resistance, cerebrovascular events, and cardiovascular events are all dramatically increased by MetS. Nearly all of the research indicates that MetS is far more typical in women. This results in even more challenges when populations with MetS handle different situations in addition to an enhanced risk of health-related impacts, like a major financial pressure (Choubey et al., 2024; Ghosh., 2024a; Ghosh et al., 2024). Human growth and health rely on nutritional intake, and health can be affected by the types of nutrients and micronutrients taken. Diet is inherently linked to a significant number of illnesses. The prevalence of diet-related conditions like diabetes, peptic ulcers, gout, gastroenteritis, and cardiovascular diseases (hypertension, dyslipidemia) is increasing each year, while the age group of individuals with these diseases is consistently decreasing. There are presently a rising variety of nutrition survey devices, platforms, and softwares, and the advancement of the Internet has made it possible to conduct online nutrition surveys utilizing comprehensive food and nutrition databases related to automated dietary records (Lee et al., 2022, Ghosh 2024b). While standard techniques rely on the use of Food Frequency Questionnaires (FFQs) or hourly for 24-hour dietary recording methods, the most popular technologies for dietary recording involve web-based or online tools, smartphone apps, camera-based image analysis tools, wearable sensors, etc. However, prior strategies had difficulty with recording accuracy due to recollection methods that may not accurately record the food consumed, or they may have challenges in predicting portion sizes or limited lists of food constituents (Lee et al., 2022; Ghosh, 2023). Deep learning, computer vision, natural language processing, and real-time data analytics simply are some of AI's expertise enabling it to examine large scale and detailed nutritional details with incredible speed and accuracy. These technologies could identify eating practices, estimate nutritional shortfall, use image recognition to evaluate food composition, and alter dietary guidance based on individual preferences, clinical conditions, or even genetic profiles. AI as a result, served as a catalyst for precision nutrition along with an efficiency tool, connecting the gap between dietary investigation and individual health goal. The significance of AI in nutrition has been raised because of the global shift toward preventive health care (Perveena et al., 2023). Proactive and individual nutrition management is urgently necessary, as chronic lifestyle-related conditions such as obesity, type 2 diabetes, cardiovascular dysfunction, and metabolic syndromes are on the rise. Real-time tracking of these scenarios and actionable, context-aware recommendations that are constantly enhanced based on feedback and action based data are both feasible with AI-powered systems (Perveena et al., 2023). Additionally, AI is the core of wearable health digital tools, digital healing methods, and smart nutrition implementations that allow users to take charge of their meal planning in a community that is growing to be more and more needed on digital platforms. The applications of AI are numerous and transformative, starting with helping public health authorities analyse food insecurity at the community level to tracking athletes' micronutrient intake or suggesting a low-sodium eating pattern to a patient suffering from high blood pressure (Lee et al., 2022). Precision nutrition is developing as a feasible therapeutic strategy that aims to deliver personalized dietary treatments for the supervision and protection of chronic ailments. Precision nutrition strategies carry out, in fact, consider the interindividual diversity introduced by genetic and epigenetic differences, individual characteristics (e.g., age, gender), lifestyle and environmental encounters, microbiome modifications, and exclusive behavioural and psychological characteristics. Functional foods and bioactive elements may also be crucial for active maturation and disease risk reduction (Galarregui et al., 2024). Dietary fibre, omega-3 healthy unsaturated fats, phytosterols, phytoestrogens, and polyphenols have all been discovered to promote healthy ageing. In reality, functional food-based methods include a strong potential to aid the aged populations' health. However, lack of cooperation is one of the main disadvantages of dietary suggestions. This is often triggered through the prescription's complexity and/or the patient's lack of commitments. These limitations can be eliminated through digital tools to motivate and empower individuals and support them in maintaining those individuals' diet plans (Galarregui et al., 2024; Das et al., 2024).

THE RISE OF PRECISION NUTRITION

A recent paradigm in studying diet and nutrition called precision nutrition is completely changing how people think about their health and overall wellness. Precision nutrition customises dietary recommendations based on a person's genetic composition, microbiome composition, metabolic responses, and lifestyle factors, in distinction to common dietary guidelines that deliver wide ranging recommendations. By keeping in mind each person's specific biological and environmental impacts, this personalized approach aims to optimize health outcomes (Dai et al., 2024; Ghosh et al., 2023; Ghosh & Sanyal et al., 2024). The market regarding precision nutrition has increased substantially in recent years on a global magnitude. The market was projected to be valued at USD 2.4 billion in 2024 and is predicted to rise at a compound annual growth rate (CAGR) of 23.2% from 2026 to 2032, hitting USD 7.0 billion. The integration of digital health tools, enhancements in genetic testing techniques, and rising consumer awareness of the importance of personalized health solutions are the key factors of this rapid rise. The progress of precision nutrition has been greatly shaped by technological innovations. Since 2003, the cost of genetic testing has declined by 98%, making it more available to the general society.

Figure 1.

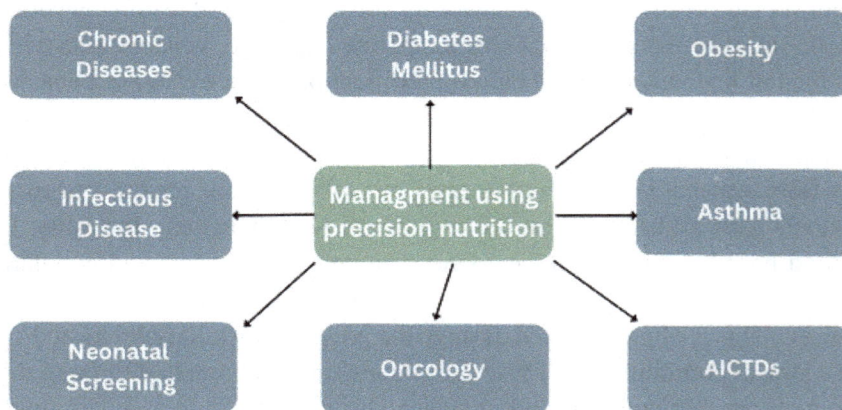

N. Naithani, A. T. Atal, T. V. S. V. G. K. Tilak, B. Vasudevan, P. Misra, and S. Sinha, "Precision medicine: Uses and challenges," Med. J. Armed Forces India, vol. 77, no. 3, pp. 258–265, Jul. 2021, doi: 10.1016/j.mjafi.2021.06.020.

Over 12 million Americans have obtained genetic testing for health insights by 2023, with 45% among the assessments examining for insights on nutritional intake. In addition, the adoption of tailored nutrition planning routines has become simpler due to the expansion of mobile health applications. 3.2 billion mobile health applications were installed in 2023, with diet and nutrition contributing to 23% of all downloads. Precision nutrition's capabilities have existed further, made better by machine learning (ML) and artificial intelligence (AI). These technologies allow the design of customized nutrition strategies through examining vast data sources like genetic data, dietary intake, and clinical records (Ghosh et al.,2024). For instance, the potential of AI-driven interventions in dietary assessment refers to the Meal Meter system, which accurately measures macronutrient intake assessed with multimodal sensing and machine learning (Arefeen et al.,2025).Precision nutrition's employ of microbiome investigation has formed new prospects for personalized dietary recommendations. Even identical twins adapt differently to the same nutritional routines, based on research, emphasizing the influence of intestinal microbiota on metabolic responses (Berry et al.,2020). Enterprises including Vio me Life Sciences have launched gut microbiome analysis services powered by AI to custom nutrition guidance (Rafique et al.,2024).With a valuation of USD 2.10 billion, North America is projected to bring a substantial regional share of the precision nutrition market, accounting for 33.78% in 2023. Strong government backing, a well-established healthcare system, and the availability of significant biotechnology and pharmaceutical enterprises are elements adding to this surge (Rafique et al.,2024). With major spending in individualized health solutions and progress in nutritional scientific investigation, Europe comes in next (MarketsAndMarkets.,2024). A growing middle class, heightened healthcare expenditure, and growing interest in proactive health steps are predicted to accelerate the fastest growth in the Asia-Pacific region (Singh et al.,2024). The sector related to precision nutrition is dealing with difficulties despite it promoting growth, for example the high financial burden of genetic testing and personalized nutrition plans, concerns regarding data privacy, and constrained accessibility in economically developing regions (Singh et al.,2024). These barriers are being tackled through ongoing technological progress and collaborative efforts among major players. The approach is currently cost-effective and scalable as a result of attempts to make easier metabolomic profiling and DNA-based analysis (Singh et al., 2024). Precision nutrition is applied to a wider range than simply broad health and overall health. It is vital in addressing disease, notably chronic diseases like diabetes, cardiac disorders, obesity, and gastrointestinal issues. Precision nutrition eventually lowers the risks associated with persistent health conditions by aligning dietary recommendations with individual genetic profiles, microbiome composition, and metabolic responses (MarketsAndMarkets.,2024). Nutraceuticals and functional foods that aid precision nutrition approaches have also gained widespread acceptance. Organizations are specializing on incorporating key nutrients to food by fortifying it in line with microbial profile and genetic predisposition. The expansion of personalized nutritional supplementation, within which supplements are formulated to order according to variables like age, gender, level of exercise, and health aims, supports validity to this trend. A number of well known enterprises are presently engaged in the precision nutrition fields leveraging new technology and strategic alliance to strengthen their product offerings. Sun Genomics, DayTwo, Inside Tracker, Nutrigenomics Inc., Persona Nutrition, Nestlé Health Science, and DNAfit are major contributors. To advance their market positions and offer state of art personalized nutrition solutions, these firms are dedicating efforts on Research and Development investment, product advancement, and strategic collaborations.

ROLE OF ARTIFICIAL INTELLIGENCE IN NUTRITION SCIENCE

1. A great number of Artificial Intelligence (AI) applications are currently in use in high-income countries supporting healthcare (Wahl et al., 2018). AI uses computer systems to perform tasks which usually need human intelligence. And it is constantly being used to develop and revolutionize the healthcare field, including nutrition. AI can help to: investigate areas in nutrition using AI; understand AI's future potential impact; and investigate possible concerns about AI's use in nutrition research (Sosa-Holwerda, 2024). Vast amounts of data analysis from diverse sources can be done easily with the help of AI. It can analyse multiomic profiles (Biswas et al., 2020), dietary habits (Oh et al.,2021), and medical histories (Fukuzawa et al., 2024), helping in the identification of nuanced dietary needs at the individual level (Oh et al.,2021), The domain of AI is advancing at an unprecedented pace of development, evolving from classical methodologies-- such as recommendation systems, regression analyses, and classification techniques-- to cutting-edge innovations in generative AI (GenAI) and large language models (LLMs).

2. Collection and analysis of data can help establish AI in nutrition which will provide dietary assessment and even for predicting malnutrition, lifestyle intervention, and for understanding the link between nutrition and health. AI can help to address most nutrition related concerns, such as the identification of the causes and their potential treatments that may be linked to cardiovascular diseases, diabetes, cancer and obesity (Kirk et al., 2022). AI can help us understand more complex connections between food and health (Côté et al., 2021). It can also tell about the ill effects of the lack of a healthy diet.

3. Estimations suggest that due to the implementation of AI applications by 2026 about USD 150 billion will be saved in healthcare in the United States (Wahl et al., 2018).

Studies suggest when a weekly analysis was carried out for over a period of 12 weeks, it had shown that right questions were asked by the virtual-health assistant with 97% accuracy. Whereas, when answers were asked for questions which it was not previously programmed for, only 20% of the time the AI was found to give correct answers (Davis et al., 2020).

The chatbots interact with users mostly using persuasion and relational strategies (Oh et al.,2021), When study was conducted, the AI was assessed regarding its usability and ability to deliver nutritional information. It scored 87 out of 100 for ease of usability, 5.28 out of 7 for satisfaction, and was also viewed as dependable 5.5 out of 7 for providing nutritional guidance (Chatelan et al.,2023). Some AI which were studied to understand the use of AI in precision nutrition:

i.Alexa

According to initial findings, it was able to give nutrition education and precisely calculate calories. having the ability to improve the target population's health by proposing meals based on ADA standards. In order to culturally adapt AI to other specific communities, it must learn the needs of the target populations (Maharjan et al.,2019)

ii.Paola (the virtual health-assistant)

This virtual health assistant proved successful in providing a lifestyle intervention plan that enhanced participant's physical activity and helped individuals lose weight. Regarding its personal connection to humans, the AI virtual coach may need a few improvements. There was insufficient follow-up and no randomization in the study (Maher et al.,2020).

The shift in behavior was successful. She couldn't seem to respond to requests that extended beyond her training, nevertheless. The study's sample size was insufficient. Other questions (not connected to the topics AI was trained in) weren't possible to evaluate due to data loss. Because men are underrepresented, it is challenging to generalize the findings. Paola's launch platform faced problems with 10-minute time-outs (Maher et al.,2020).

iii.The health bot (HB)

It was evaluated according to how it answered queries regarding nutrition. Patients embraced HB because they found it simple to use and comprehend. The HB offered participants with useful data. However, the participants had worries around the privacy of the inquiries, personal information, and dietician alternatives. The study's sample size was insufficient. Due to a risk of HB answers being misinterpreted, AI utilized for nutritional analysis should not be employed without a healthcare professional's supervision. People with insufficient literacy and no or less access to online information may be excluded by HB. It is crucial to be thoughtful about making an HB simple to use (Beyeler et al.,2023).

iv.Wearable devices

AI-based apps and wearable devices are used by clinicians since they can be used for diet optimization and to find eating patterns, given their real-time data collection. Smartwatches(e.g., Apple watch, Kardia band)have been approved by the FDAfor some health uses, shifting from wellness devices to a more medical focus. Wearable devices are still being developed, as algorithms cannot fully differentiate between different types of foods, portions, and backgrounds. Some Technologies that measure body composition have not been tested in clinical trials; thus, the accuracy of the results needs to be assessed (Beyeler et al.,2023).

v.ChatGPT

It can provide tailored guidance on aspects involving dietary habits, physical activity, and managing one's weight, and fulfill every individual's needs. Weight-management advice can be modified in response to the patient's development.

Depending on the kind of data used to train it, AI may provide biased results.

AI systems lack human-like emotional intelligence and lack the ability to provide emotional assistance. It is unclear who is at fault and held responsible when GPT offers harmful and false data (Limketkai et al.,2021).

According to a European study, ChatGPT may generate menus, but it's not always reliable; it was allergens for a hypothetical woman with an allergic reaction. Additionally, it repeated the same food offerings on a variety of menus and offered incorrect portion size amounts (Arslan.,2023).

ChatGPT has benefits as well as drawbacks. It could be beneficial for people to gain

free learning materials on nutrition and healthy eating. ChatGPT, however, is not always reliable and may give misleading results. It needs to be supervised as a result. Since chatbots lack soft skills, RDs are more challenging to replace. Still, ChatGPT can provide diet plans and nutritional guidance. It is insufficient to offer psychological and emotional support. It is difficult to assess whether the information sources used by ChatGPT are authentic because it does not cite them (Chatelan et al.,2023).

AI-POWERED CLINICAL DECISION SUPPORT SYSTEMS (CDSS)

Clinical decision support systems (CDSSs) based on artificial intelligence (AI) are crucial instruments that assist medical practitioners in the diagnosis, management, and treatment of cardiovascular disease (CVD). By analysing vast volumes of data, these technologies assist users in making precise and knowledgeable judgements. The following elements are often seen in CDSS that is based on artificial intelligence (Bozyel et al., 2024).

● **Risk assessment:** Systems operated using artificial intelligence have the capability to examine a range of variables in alignment to establish the risk related to CVD. For occurance, they can estimate a patient's risk of cardiac health forecast using age, sex, medical history, genetics, and lifestyle. In this approach, ones who are at risk can take risk reduction strategies and early medical interventions.

● **Diagnosis:** Systems depending on artificial intelligence play a vital role in the diagnosis of heart related illness. They can detect abnormalities in cardiovascular rhythm by investigating electrocardiogram (ECG) data. By applying image processing techniques for interpreting imaging results, such as echocardiography or angiography, they also facilitate the diagnosis of CVD.

● **Treatment Enhancement:** AI-based CDSSs analyze patient attributes and medical data to put forward the most suitable treatment techniques to CVD. For instance, they suggest the ideal pharmaceutical option combination or surgical intervention plan by reviewing variables such a patient's medical history, blood analysis reports, and drug sensitivities.

● **Monitoring and Early indication:** By repeatedly monitoring patients' vital signs (heart rate, blood pressure, oxygen level, etc.) and medical data, artificial intelligence-based systems can recognize possible complications and worsening of CVD early. This allows it to anticipate emergencies and take immediate action in patients' scenarios.

Health team members can experience major benefits through artificial intelligence-based CDSSs in patient management, treatment planning, and early CVD diagnosis. On the other hand it's essential to take into account that these systems are beneficial references for clinical specialists, who finally determine the evaluations (Eguia et al.,2024).

Medical progress is still accelerating, particularly in light of the rise of novel diseases like COVID-19. In addition to these disorders, new medicines are always being developed to combat earlier pathologies for which new alternatives are being created. As a result, search results in many databases, including PubMed, indicate a rise in the number of articles in various indexed journals. There are now a lot of publications discussing novel therapies or even novel modes of diagnosis. The groundwork of medicine is reliable and authenticated information, whichever is necessary for patient diagnosis and treatment (Eguia et al.,2024). The Disaster Lit database, Medline indexing, and MedlinePlus indexing constitute at least three notable source evaluation systems designed by the National Library of Medicine that deliver beneficial examples for the work at hand. A large number of doctors consult for up-to-date clinical data web based tools. Since medical practitioners must start by identifying the category of information they look for before performing their own search in an online medical database, this strategy is not the most impactful way to find out information. Due to shortage of relevant data, this category of search can be as well as time-consuming and prone to inaccuracies. As a result, automated information recommender systems have developed as a solution that facilitates medical team members to efficiently access credible knowledge. Clinical decision support systems are the designation for these categories of solutions (CDSSs).The numerous platforms that comprise of CDSSs support the examination of clinical data and inform medical practitioners of probable concerns (Eguia et al.,2024). Clinical staff members can gain advantages through the use of decision-making tools. These systems necessitate communicating with elements such as electronic health records (EHRs) that facilitates them to retain updated data for better development in order to work properly. Therefore, it is commonly understood that CDSSs direct attention on six defined categories: the user, architecture and technology, knowledge, inference, data, and implementation and integration. Accurate, high-quality information may be acquired through the utilization of all currently accessible procedures and technologies, consisting of big data, machine learning, and artificial intelligence [AI]. To get such information, a supervised machine learning method could consist of a range of domain-independent natural language processing (NLP) components connected to medical information extraction (text mining) (Eguia et al.,2024).

Clinical Decision Support System (CDSS) merged with Electronic Health Records (EHR) was elevated by the US government in 2007, and by 2017, 40.2% of US hospitals possess advanced CDSS capabilities. Through alarm systems, CDSSs support medical professionals in diagnosis, prescribed medications management, prescriptions, and drug control. They have been remarkably successful in enhancing patient safety, enforcing preventive and public health programs, and raising adherence to clinical guidelines. Moreover, the frequency of medical products adverse events has declined and recommendations and alarms have grown more customised as a consequence of CDSSs' inclusion with EHRs (Bozyel et al.,2024). A meta-analysis determined that CDSSs escalated the average ratio of patients who were provided with the targeted care element by 5.8%. The influence of CDSSs on morbidity and mortality in Primary Healthcare (PHC) has not been indicated, even though their contribution to PCPs in making ongoing clinical alternatives. Moreover, mismatches between the specialists' recommendations and their CDSSs or no longer valid EHRs may make it difficult for PCPs to cooperatively handle patients with areas of expertise (Gomez-Cabello.,2024). The progress of image-based processing units in 2010 marked the initiation of the emergence of artificial intelligence (AI), even though the notion was initially introduced seven decades before. AI possesses the capacity of dealing with the rising number of medical data in healthcare systems and mimicking human responses and thinking. The most extensively used AI strategy is machine learning (ML), which is categorised into three categories: supervised, unsupervised, and reinforcement algorithms. Computers have the ability to learn without explicit programming due to computational learning algorithms which are developed on massive training datasets to provide reliable predictions. A configuration of device learning referred to as deep learning (DL) facilitates algorithms to learn and adapt to input from various layers, generating the most consistent prediction findings (Gomez-Cabello.,2024). Non-knowledge-based CDSSs use AI to enhance their diagnostic, prognostic, and administrative capabilities, in contrast to knowledge-based CDSSs using if-then rules. These models have the ability to decrease medical mistakes while boosting physician productivity and efficiency, freeing them up to concentrate on duties that need special human abilities, such addressing the problems of specific patients (Gomez-Cabello.,2024).

Despite the fact that AI has several positive aspects, there are still a number of worries that need to be identified, namely FDA permission, ethical problems related with data sharing, and addressing misinterpretations about what AI is and does. AI tools have the potential to make patients more prone to detrimental impacts if the algorithms are set up to provide conclusions that are too particular. Endorsing education on the correct implementation and prospective threats of artificial intelligence is consequently necessary (Tyler et al.,2024). In order to offer a framework for designing clinical AI algorithms aiming to minimize integration mistakes AI into healthcare systems, current research has made efforts to investigate current hospital quality assurance and quality improvement operations. By combining extensive data of related health data into the healthcare system, real-time medical interpretation might be implemented in coordination with AI to strengthen the quality of services delivered (Tyler et al.,2024).

AI IN PUBLIC HEALTH NUTRITION

1. These capabilities and utilization of artificial intelligence (AI) have expanded at an exceptional growth in recent years. A wide range of human endeavours

and communities have been affected and revolutionized by this quick development, which is stimulated by enhancement in machine learning algorithms and the exponential increase of computational strength. AI's potential is being fulfilled in the sector of nutrition and public health in a number of inventive ways. AI algorithms have served a central function in mapping and assessing food surroundings, facilitating the detection of "food deserts," or areas with little access to nutritionally packed foods (An et al.,2023).

The impacts of probable policy interventions, such as how designated charges or subsidies have the potential to change population eating behaviors, have also been projected using machine learning models. On a broader scale, AI has supported food safety, global food supply chain monitoring, and climate change disruption prediction. AI delivers tools to integrate and understand the huge amount of data that is presently obtainable, from social media debates on food choices to satellite image processing of agricultural regions, in order to inform public health nutrition platforms and interventions (An et al.,2023).

What guidelines manage the implementation of AI4PH (Artificial Intelligence for Public Health) interventions?

The following eight guiding principles indicate the superior technical and ethical conditions that must direct the use of artificial intelligence (AI) in public health in sequence to minimise ethical risk in public health and related policy interventions: (Thomas J.,2023)

- **People-centered:** Solutions and actions must be emphasized on people as opposed to standalone applications. AI should respect human's rights as one of the countless technologies that reinforce public health.
- **Ethically grounded:** The universally endorsed ethical guidelines of justice, beneficence, nonmaleficence, and human dignity must operate as the groundwork for all discussions, innovations, and implementation.
- **Transparent:** When designing AI algorithms, transparent procedures must persistently be executed and communicated.
- **Data protected:** Every AI development must be formed on the standards of privacy, confidentiality, and data security.
- **Demonstrate scientific integrity:** AI methods must comply with best operations in research discipline, consisting of being reliable, consistent, equitable, truthful, and ethical.

- **Shareable and open:** Everything is expected to be as shareable and open as practical. Any AI development must employ the Openness 1 tools and underlying ideas as a feature and an essential aspect of its success.
- **Non-discriminatory:** The keystone of any AI task for public health should always act as fairness, equality, and social inclusion in mutual impact and design.
- **Technology managed by individuals:** The system is crucial to include formal procedures for human regulations and control of automated decisions.

MULTI-OMICS AND PRECISION NUTRITION

According to multiple studies, precision nutrition might assist in identifying individuals who are at risk for certain illnesses or a severe form of a disease, enabling early detection to lower the burden of the illness and enhance quality of life.

The vast majority of tumor patients do not benefit from contemporary precision medical care, whereas just a few people do (Niszczota et al.,2023). Omics data, such as proteomics and epigenetic data, can be incorporated in addition to genomic data in order to help advance precision medicine. Integrated studies across multiple omics data types are thought to be significant (Zhang et al.,2019). Precision nutrition can be enhanced using multiomics, which will integrate data from transcriptomics, proteomics, metabolomics, microbiomics, genomics, epigenomics to provide an in-depth understanding of an individual's biological variability. With the help of multiomics we can get an understanding of how dietary responses get influenced by a combination of genetic predisposition, epigenetic modification, gene expression patterns, protein activity, and metabolite levels by utilizing these interrelated datasets. For instance, metabolomic profiles may reveal deficiencies in nutrients or abnormalities in metabolism, and microbiome information can direct probiotic or prebiotic therapies appropriate to an individual's gut environment. These intricate data layers can be used with AI to create learning algorithms that can be useful in providing personalized nutritional recommendations (Zhang et al.,2019).

According to this review study, we can gain an improved comprehension of multiomics and its relationship to precision nutrition by using the following tools: multimodal learning, multitask learning, representation learning, semi-supervised learning, and automatic acquisition of hierarchical features: We are able to combine several forms of omics data as input, such as genomic, epigenetic, and medical imaging data. By learning multiple tasks simultaneously and sharing some aspects of the learning process, we can improve learning efficiency. When combined with small amounts of labeled data, unlabeled data has been shown to greatly improve learning accuracy. We are able to analyze the input data's high-dimensional correlations.

1. The field of **nutrigenomics** emerged following advancements in human genomics, focusing on how dietary components interact with the genome, proteome, and metabolome to influence health outcomes. This omics-based approach, supported by continuous developments in genomics, proteomics, and metabolomics, forms the foundation of precision nutrition, which tailors dietary recommendations to individual needs. Nutrients can significantly impact gene expression and the epigenome, thereby influencing disease risk. This gave rise to nutrigenetics, which explores how genetic variation affects individual responses to diet. While nutrigenomics investigates how nutrients influence gene expression, nutrigenetics looks at cellular responses to nutrients, metabolism, and their site of action (Hamamoto et al.,2019).

2. Various metabolic components function as biomarkers in the context of **metabolomics**, delivering current data about food quality and dietary intake (Mickelson et al.,2019). For instance, the biological plausibility, robustness, dose-response relationship, and analytical performance of validated biomarkers for foods such as whole grains, soy, and sugars have been analyzed (Brennan et al.,2023). Plasma metabolites have been associated with the risk of cardiovascular disease (CVD) and have been used to assess adherence to dietary patterns like the Mediterranean diet (Clarke et al.,2020).

3. In addition, metabolic profile-based biomarkers aid in the assessment of disease risk; however, their efficacy is significantly affected by aspects such as age and body mass index (BMI) (Li et al.,2020). In order to provide personalized suggestions for nutrition, a method called metabotyping classifies individuals according to specific biomarkers, including triacylglycerol, glucose, cholesterol, and HDL-cholesterol (Kim et al.,2021; Palmnäs et al., 2020). However, as dietary practices and socioeconomic position have an impact on metabolic profiles and health repercussions, they must be taken account of when defining metabotypes (Hillesheim et al.,2020).

4. Understanding the geographical and temporal variation in the gut microbiome is largely dependent on **metagenomics**, particularly next-generation sequencing (NGS). According to gut microbiota profiling, nutrition has an impact on the makeup of the microbiota, which varies from birth to adulthood (Mills et al.,2019). For example, meals high in carbohydrates or diets high in protein and fat are associated with the prevalence of Firmicutes or Bacteroides in adults, respectively (Mills et al.,2019 & Arumugam et al., 2014). These findings highlight the importance of taking age and eating habits into account when performing metagenomic investigations because they have a significant impact on the gut microbiome. Furthermore, combining metagenomics with other omics, such as transcriptomics, metabolomics, and genomes, offers a more thorough understand-

ing of each person's dietary reactions, facilitating more successful customized nutrition plans.

5. Furthermore, **nutrigenetics** explores how foods and genes interact in order to preserve health and resist against illness. Environmental elements referred to as nutrients can affect gene expression, DNA metabolism, and gene repair. Single nucleotide polymorphisms (SNPs) are molecular devices that can be used to explore the relationship between nutrition and disease, according to new research (Ferguson et al.,2009). In particular, SNPs affecting the phenylalanine hydroxylase gene contribute to metabolic deficits in phenylketonuria (PKU) (Farhud et al.,2008). Other noteworthy polymorphisms are found in gene sequences for glutathione peroxidase, MnSOD, and LPH, which are associated with increased risks of breast cancer, liver cancer, and oxidative stress, respectively (Trujillo et al.,2006). LPH is also linked to lactose intolerance. Additionally, through a variety of techniques, bioactive food ingredients can modify transcription factors, changing patterns of gene expression (Goh et al.,2007). Diet has a dose- and time-dependent effect on gene expression, which indicates that nutrigenetics may be applied in the future to identify genetic subgroups for focused treatment options aimed at lowering the risk of chronic illness.

PRECISION NUTRITION APPLICATION IN DIFFERENT CONDITIONS

Precision nutrition can be effective against several diseases and disorders by managing the gene sequencing and the gene expression.

India introduced The Genome India Project on 3rd January 2020, and it focuses on mapping genomes of the population through genome-wide sequencing by collaborating with 20 research institutes (Naithani et al.,2021).

i.Diabetes Mellitus

With multiple subtypes, monogenic diabetes mellitus provides potential for precision medicine which focuses therapeutic choices on known gene defects. Mild non-progressive diabetes with elevated fasting glucose that responds to diet and exercise is an indicator of glucokinase-related gene anomalies in maturity-onset diabetes of young (MODY-2). Hepatic nuclear factor 1α (HNF-1α) in MODY-3 and HNF-4α in MODY-1 are genes that produce diabetes that worsens over time and responds to low-dose sulphonylureas. High doses of sulphonylureas have been discovered to alleviate neonatal diabetes, which is defined by mutations in the potassium voltage-gated channel subfamily 11 (KCNJ11) gene. Newer candidate genes that may impact response to sulphonylureas, insulin sensitizers, or incretin treatment are being identified via a variety of GWAS-based technologies (Gloyn et al.,2018).

ii.Obesity

T2DM and obesity are both closely associated metabolic diseases. Insulin resistance, a defining feature of T2DM, is aggravated by excess adipose tissue in obesity. The onset and the development of these disorders are influenced by the combined effect of lifestyle factors, food habits, and genetic predisposition. AI tools can make it easier to understand large, complicated datasets that contain metabolic, genetic, and lifestyle data. By combining this data, AI can spot trends and forecast how each individual would interact with the provided dietary changes, which will help with early obesity and T2DM identification and individual therapy. For example, machine learning systems can identify prediabetic illnesses before clinical symptoms appear by analyzing data from continuous glucose monitoring (Ferreira et al.,2025).

iii.Asthma

Asthma-related airway inflammation is fueled by Th2 subsets of CD4 T helper cells, which release the cytokines IL-4 (which promotes IgE), IL-5 (which triggers eosinophils), and IL-13 (which promotes mucus and IgE). The "type 2 (T2) high" asthma endotype is impacted by the production of IL-5 and IL-13 by type 2 innate lymphoid cells. On the other hand, IL-1 and IL-17 play a part in the "T2 low" endotype. Different molecular pathways within the larger asthma syndrome are depicted by these specific endotypes.

Using monoclonal antibodies, precision medicine facilitates the targeted treatment of T2-high refractory asthma: dupilumab inhibits IL-4 and IL-13 by IL-4RA antagonism; mepolizumab and reslizumab block IL-5; benralizumab targets the IL-5 receptor; and omalizumab targets IgE (Kuruvilla et al.,2019).

iv.AICTDs

Systemic auto-immune connective tissue diseases (AICTDs) may develop in a number of forms, involving substantial overlap, a changeable course, and periodic remissions and relapses. Recently, there has been an attempt to divide them into subgroups, such as "Inflammatory," "Lymphoid," "Interferon," and "Undefined Normal like," based on the measurement of quantifiable molecular markers employing genomic technology. By employing existing or newly developed therapies that are customized for a particular group, this would also allow for specialized therapeutic targeting. By applying precision medicine, a molecular taxonomy of AICTDs may be created through the analysis of genetic, methylation, and gene expression data (Barturen et al.,2020).

v.Oncology

In addition to benefiting from the fast division of cancer cells, traditional chemotherapy and radiation are potentially dangerous to normal cells. However, by focusing on certain molecules at the extracellular, membrane, intracellular, or intranuclear levels, precision oncology minimizes these adverse consequences. To limit angiogenesis in malignancies such as colorectal, lung, renal, glioma, and ovarian cancers, bevacizumab, a monoclonal antibody, inhibits VEGF-A, which is crucial for tumor vascularization. Important targets are overexpressed cell surface receptors, including the ErbB family (EGFR/HER1, HER2/neu, HER3, HER4). A total of twenty to 25 percent of gastric and breast cancers, as well as other forms of cancer, overexpress HER2 [49]. While antibody-drug conjugates (for example, trastuzumab emtansine) combine chemotherapy with targeted delivery, monoclonal antibodies such as trastuzumab and pertuzumab increase survival. Because a mutation EGFR causes continual pathway activation, EGFR-targeted treatments such as cetuximab and panitumumab are only effective in cases of colorectal cancer with wild-type EGFR (Hetzel et al.,1992). Tyrosine kinase inhibitors (TKIs) work intracellularly to block erroneous receptor signaling carried on by mutations or amplifications (Huang et al., 2001-2020). Immunotherapy with immune checkpoint inhibitors (ICIs) is another discovery; such therapies are employed for a variety of malignancy, regardless of the origin of the tumor, and restore T-cell activity against tumors by blocking inhibitory signals such as PD-L1 (Meyers et al.,2020). Furthermore, CAR-T cell therapy employs T-cells that were specially engineered to particularly attack tumor antigens. The FDA has approved it for diffuse large B-cell lymphoma and refractory acute lymphoblastic lymphoma (Ma et al., 2019; Ahmad et al., 2020).

vi.Neonatal screening for genetic disorders

Rapid genome sequencing, or STATseq, is an emerging method of medical genomics that maps genetic abnormalities using a correlation tool for genomic analysis backed by ailments and signs. It enables a two-day genome study (24-hour whole-genome sequencing plus 18-hour bioinformatics analysis) of critically unwell newborns with suspected genetic abnormalities. In situations where there is no treatment, this approach assists with avoiding needless intensive care by facilitating a quick diagnosis for the application of any available treatment and providing genetic counseling instead (Saunders et al., 2012). In a subject that continues to evolve quickly, this instrument is also essential for research and the creation of management guidelines. Various other fields have also been inspired by this to create direct-to-consumer diagnostics to diagnose various illnesses (Naithani et al., 2021).

vii.Infectious disease

Developed in the 1960s, the Medical Tricorder was a device that was capable of sending life-sign data to the tricorder itself via a separate handheld scanner. It could identify infectious microbes and assess the functionality of all essential organs. In order to treat different life-forms, its data banks also included information on non-human races. It performed effectively for Dr. Mc Coy's spacecraft in the science fiction series Star Trek. Today, metagenomics—the study of genomes obtained from environmental samples—aspires to realize this seemingly unrealistic futuristic idea. Running all of the nucleic acids in a sample—which may contain a variety of microorganism populations—is referred to as metagenomic NGS (mNGS). In order to identify which bacteria are present and in what proportions, these are allocated to reference genomes. In order to remove reads of host origin, sequencing reads are typically first matched to the human genome using a technique known as digital subtraction. To identify pathogens, the remaining reads are subsequently mapped to sequence databases (Naithani et al.,2021).

When oligonucleotide microarrays, PCR, culture, and serological testing failed to detect a new arena virus in a cluster of three transplant recipient casualties in 2008, this method had been used (Palacios et al.,2008).

viii.Chronic diseases

A precision medicine approach is suitable for treating chronic diseases due to their increased incidence and frequent repercussions which attract a variety of pharmacologic treatments. The multi-omics repertoire continues to evolve, ranging from focused treatment options to disease risk prediction. Patients stand to gain from early, precise diagnosis, treatment, and preventative measures as the awareness of the practical importance of genes and biomarkers advances (Naithani et al.,2021).

POSITIVE ASPECTS OF AI IN NUTRITION

By identifying patterns that humans are incapable of recognizing, artificial intelligence (AI)can reshape intricate information into "simpler" and "deeper" ones. Indeed, the framework and functioning of brains and AI systems differ. AI takes advantage of substantial data and works in a feed-forward style, suggesting that it initiates with an input and moves ahead to deliver the outcomes and a more detailed depiction of them. The human brain, on the flip side, operates more consistently due to it being structured to support us in addressing particular challenges that we are likely to experience in real life (Detopoulou et al.,2023).

AI-facilitated data reformulation may consequently be efficiently utilised for human health and other implementations. Moreover, inaccuracies that are part of human nature can be diminished. For instance, "smart systems" concerning insulin prescription level can decrease hypo- and hyper-glycemia in persons with type 1 diabetes. Reflecting on the potentially fatal consequences of insulin excessive intake, this is critically essential. The concept of personalized nutrition can be made a real world practice with AI's assistance. The first step is to implement AI-assisted approaches to do nutrient analysis more precisely (Detopoulou et al.,2023).

The ideal responses for a selected individual might be gained by merging a range of genetic, gut microbiota, nutrition-based, and other data in different ways. The clinical trials available nowadays, however, have not shown very encouraging findings in this regard. The parallel life stage of precision medicine, which uses cutting-edge scientific techniques to cure medical conditions, is demonstrated in individualized diet strategy. AI may also help society, professions, and patients take charge of their challenges and plan for requirements (Detopoulou et al.,2023).

CHALLENGES AND LIMITATIONS OF AI-BASED NUTRITION

The implementation of artificial intelligence in nutrition investigation has multiple disadvantages. The quality and accessibility of data is a major issue that arises when using AI for nutrition. The standard, completeness, and consistency of nutrition and health data have been challenged in multiple of the examined studies. To confirm the correctness and utilization of AI models in nutritional research, these difficulties must be tackled. In addition, when developing and enforcing AI models in this sector, algorithmic bias is a significant apprehensive. The challenges of AI models' lack of clarity have been brought to attention in a quantity of research. Becomes increasingly difficult to understand the foundational thinking of these models' predictions as they become more complicated (Mahendran et al.,2024).

In clinical and healthcare settings, where extreme clarity is necessary for encouraging trust and supporting knowledgeable decision-making, this limitation is especially concerning. Careful evaluation is required to be given to privacy matters regarding the gathering and transmission of private health information as well as the ethical use of AI to alter consumption patterns. Earlier investigations have stressed the demand for accessible and ethical norms to control the advancement and utilization of AI digital systems. It became harder for data scientists, clinical dietitians, medical experts, and lawmakers to coordinate well effectively. Between the practical implementation of AI in nutrition science and public health and innovations in its technology, interdisciplinary communication can assist close the gap (Mahendran et al.,2024).

CASE STUDY: AI-POWERED METABOLIC SYNDROME PREDICTION IN POSTMENOPAUSAL WOMEN

A significant application of artificial intelligence in metabolic syndrome (MetS) prediction was demonstrated in a comprehensive study involving postmenopausal women in India, where researchers developed and evaluated machine learning models to predict MetS risk using supervised learning approaches (Ghosh et al., 2025). The study revealed a MetS prevalence of 40.17% among postmenopausal women, with concerning metabolic indicators including 19.21% exhibiting hyperglycemic states and 57.86% having low HDL-C levels, highlighting the critical need for effective screening tools in this vulnerable population. The research team implemented multiple classification algorithms and systematically evaluated their performance using comprehensive metrics including accuracy, sensitivity, specificity, precision, recall, F-Measure, Receiver Operating Characteristic (ROC), Precision-Recall Curve (PRC), and Area Under the Curve (AUC) to identify the optimal predictive model. Among the machine learning algorithms tested, the Decision Tree and Random Forest classifiers emerged as the best-performing models, both achieving remarkable accuracy of 90.22% in the Indian healthcare context. These superior-performing models utilized the six most essential features as defined by the International Diabetes Federation (IDF) criteria, with key predictive factors including waist circumference (WC), serum triglyceride levels (TG), and fasting blood sugar (FBS) identified as the most critical parameters for accurate MetS prediction. The study's methodology focused on developing a robust supervised machine-learning system that could achieve notable accuracy while maintaining clinical relevance and practical applicability in resource-constrained healthcare settings. The research findings demonstrate significant implications for preventive healthcare, as the developed models provide a foundation for swift and accurate MetS diagnosis that can substantially reduce diagnostic costs and prevent further complications associated with delayed detection. The study emphasizes the potential for implementing this machine learning paradigm across various technological platforms, including web and mobile applications, making advanced diagnostic capabilities accessible to healthcare providers and patients alike. The practical significance of this research extends beyond academic contributions, offering a scalable solution for addressing the growing burden of metabolic syndrome among India's postmenopausal women population. By achieving 90.22% accuracy with Decision Tree and Random Forest models, the study establishes a benchmark for AI-driven MetS prediction that can be integrated into routine clinical practice, enabling early identification and intervention strategies. This research represents a crucial step toward improving the quality of life for neglected postmenopausal women through technology-enabled healthcare solutions, demonstrating how artificial intelligence can bridge the gap between advanced diagnostic capabilities and accessible healthcare delivery in developing countries. The study's focus on utilizing IDF-recognized parameters ensures clinical validity while the high accuracy rates provide confidence for real-world implementation, potentially transforming how metabolic syndrome is screened and managed in Indian healthcare systems.

CONCLUSION

The advancement of precision nutrition influenced by AI signifies a major shift in existing awareness of and strategy for addressing metabolic syndrome and related diseases. As precision nutrition has become widely accepted, the priority has altered from inclusive dietary suggestions to personalized therapies depending on a person's genetic configuration, way of life, microbiome, and metabolic profile. This transition is significantly helped by artificial intelligence, enabling it to integrate and analyse large, complex datasets. AI enhances our potential to detect changes and create more precise predictions about each person's unique dietary requirements than ever before employing complex algorithms and machine learning models. By assisting physicians deliver correct, evidence-based dietary recommendations, specifically for patients with metabolic syndrome and other chronic illnesses, AI-driven clinical decision support systems are transforming healthcare. AI helps address population-level health inequities in public health nutrition by facilitating specific interventions, policy design, and thorough nutritional evaluations. Furthermore, by employing AI to incorporate multi-omics—like proteomics, metabolomics, and genome analysis—into nutrition research, we are able to more effectively grasp how food and illness interconnected. This innovation enables the development of individualised food programs for a number of illnesses, such as diabetes, obesity, heart disease, and digestive issues. AI in nutrition offers significant possibilities, from better preventative care to more efficiency and accuracy, yet, there remain also multiple hindrances to tackle. Regulation and careful analysis are essential for issues among which are algorithmic bias, lack of regulations consistency, data privacy, ethical issues, and limited accessibility. In conclusion, precision nutrition driven by AI has offers highly tailored to improve metabolic syndrome outcomes and advance personalised healthcare. But prudent application, multidisciplinary cooperation, and ongoing technical advancement are essential to its success.

REFERENCES

Ahmad, A., Uddin, S., & Steinhoff, M. (2020). CAR-T cell therapies: An overview of clinical studies supporting their approved use against acute lymphoblastic leukemia and large B-cell lymphomas. *International Journal of Molecular Sciences*, *21*(11). Advance online publication. DOI: 10.3390/ijms21113906 PMID: 32486160

Arefeen, A., Fessler, S., Mostafavi, S. M., Johnston, C. S., & Ghasemzadeh, H. (2025). MealMeter: Using multimodal sensing and machine learning for automatically estimating nutrition intake. *arXiv preprint* arXiv:2503.11683.

Arslan, S. (2023). Exploring the potential of Chat GPT in personalized obesity treatment. *Annals of Biomedical Engineering*, *51*, 1887–1888. PMID: 37145177

Arumugam, N., Kalavathi, P., & Mahalingam, P. U. (2014). Lignin database for diversity of lignin-degrading microbial enzymes (LD2L). *Research in Biotechnology*, *5*, 13–18.

Barturen, G., Babaei, S., & Catala-Moll, F. (2020). Integrative analysis reveals a molecular stratification of systemic autoimmune diseases. *Arthritis and Rheumatism*. Advance online publication. DOI: 10.1002/art.41610 PMID: 33497037

Berry, S. E., Valdes, A., Drew, G., Asnicar, C., Mazidi, H., Wolf, T. A., & Chan, E. (2020). Human postprandial responses to food and potential for precision nutrition. *Nature Medicine*, *26*(6), 964–973. PMID: 32528151

Beyeler, M., Légeret, C., Kiwitz, F., & van der Horst, K. (2023). Usability and overall perception of a health bot for nutrition-related questions for patients receiving bariatric care: Mixed methods study. *JMIR Human Factors*, *10*, e47913. PMID: 37938894

Biswas, N., & Chakrabarti, S. (2020). Artificial intelligence (AI)-based systems biology approaches in multi-omics data analysis of cancer. *Frontiers in Oncology*, *10*, 588221. PMID: 33154949

Bozyel, S., Şimşek, E., Koçyiğit, D., Güler, A., Korkmaz, Y., Şeker, M., & Keser, N. (2024). Artificial intelligence-based clinical decision support systems in cardiovascular diseases. *The Anatolian Journal of Cardiology*, *28*(2), 74. PMID: 38168009

Brennan, L., & de Roos, B. (2023). Role of metabolomics in the delivery of precision nutrition. *Redox Biology*, *65*, 102808. PMID: 37423161

Chatelan, A., Clerc, A., & Fonta, P. A. (2023). ChatGPT and future artificial intelligence chatbots: What may be the influence on credentialed nutrition and dietetics practitioners? *Journal of the Academy of Nutrition and Dietetics, 123*, 1525–1531. PMID: 37544375

Choubey, U., Upadrasta, V. A., Kaur, I. P., Banker, H., Kanagala, S. G., & Anamika, F. N. U.. (2024). From prevention to management: exploring AI's role in metabolic syndrome management: a comprehensive review. *The Egyptian Journal of Internal Medicine, 36*(1), 106.

Clarke, E. D., Rollo, M. E., Pezdirc, K., Collins, C. E., & Haslam, R. L. (2020). Urinary biomarkers of dietary intake: A review. *Nutrition Reviews, 78*, 364–381. PMID: 31670796

Côté, M., & Lamarche, B. (2021). Artificial intelligence in nutrition research: Perspectives on current and future applications. *Applied Physiology, Nutrition, and Metabolism, 46*(9), 1–8. PMID: 34525321

Das, P., Banka, R., Ghosh, J., Singh, K., Choudhury, S. R., & Koner, S. (2024). Synergism of diet, genetics, and microbiome on health. In *Nutrition controversies and advances in autoimmune disease* (pp. 131–189). IGI Global.

Davis, C. R., Murphy, K. J., Curtis, R. G., & Maher, C. A. (2020). A process evaluation examining the performance, adherence, and acceptability of a physical activity and diet artificial intelligence virtual health assistant. *International Journal of Environmental Research and Public Health, 17*, 9137. PMID: 33297456

Detopoulou, P., Voulgaridou, G., Moschos, P., Levidi, D., Anastasiou, T., Dedes, V., & Papadopoulou, S. K. (2023). Artificial intelligence, nutrition, and ethical issues: A mini-review. *Clinical Nutrition Open Science, 50*, 46–56.

Eguia, H., Sánchez-Bocanegra, C. L., Vinciarelli, F., Alvarez-Lopez, F., & Saigí-Rubió, F. (2024). Clinical decision support and natural language processing in medicine: Systematic literature review. *Journal of Medical Internet Research, 26*, e55315. PMID: 39348889

Farhud, D., & Shalileh, M. (2008). Phenylketonuria and its dietary therapy in children. *Iranian Journal of Pediatrics, 18*, 88–98.

Ferguson, L. R. (2009). Nutrigenomics approaches to functional foods. *Journal of the American Dietetic Association, 109*, 452–458. PMID: 19248861

Ferreira, D. D., Ferreira, L. G., Amorim, K. A., Delfino, D. C. T., Ferreira, A. C. B. H., & Souza, L. P. C. E. (2025). Assessing the links between artificial intelligence and precision nutrition. *Current Nutrition Reports*, *14*(1), 47. DOI: 10.1007/s13668-025-00635-2 PMID: 40087237

Fukuzawa, F.. (2024). Importance of patient history in artificial intelligence-assisted medical diagnosis: Comparison study. *JMIR Medical Education*, *10*, e52674. PMID: 38602313

Galarregui, C., Navas-Carretero, S., Zulet, M. A., González-Navarro, C. J., Martínez, J. A., & de Cuevillas, B.. (2024). Precision nutrition impact on metabolic health and quality of life in an aging population after a 3-month intervention: A randomized intervention. *The Journal of Nutrition, Health & Aging*, *28*(7), 100289. PMID: 38865737

Ghosh, J. (2023). A review on understanding the risk factors for coronary heart disease in Indian college students. *International Journal of Noncommunicable Diseases*, *8*, 117–128.

Ghosh, J. (2024 a). Leveraging data science for personalized nutrition. In *Nutrition controversies and advances in autoimmune disease* (pp. 572–605). IGI Global.

Ghosh, J. (2024b). Recognizing and predicting the risk of malnutrition in the elderly using artificial intelligence: A systematic review. *International Journal of Advancement in Life Sciences Research*, *7*(3). Advance online publication. DOI: 10.31632/ijalsr.2024.v07i03.001

Ghosh, J., Chaudhuri, D., Saha, I., & Nag Chaudhuri, A. (2020). Prevalence of metabolic syndrome, vitamin D level, and their association among elderly women in a rural community of West Bengal, India. *Medical Journal of Dr. D.Y. Patil Vidyapeeth*, *13*(4), 315–320.

Ghosh, J., Choudhury, S. R., Singh, K., & Koner, S. (2024). Application of machine learning algorithm and artificial intelligence in improving metabolic syndrome related complications: A review. *International Journal of Advancement in Life Sciences Research*, *7*(2), 41–67.

Ghosh, J., Choudhury, S. R., Singh, K., & Koner, S. (2025, February). Development and performance analysis of machine learning methods for predicting metabolic syndrome among postmenopausal women of India. *International Journal of Advancement in Life Sciences Research*, *8*(1), 006. Advance online publication. DOI: 10.31632/ijalsr.2025.v08i01.006

Ghosh, J., Roy Choudhury, S., & Koner, S. (2023). Nutraceuticals and bone health. In D. Sharma, M.M. Gupta, A.K. Sharma, R.K. Keservani, & R.K. Kesharwani (Eds.), *AAP Advances in Nutraceuticals Series* (in production). Academic Press. doi: DOI: 10.1201/9781003415084-13

Ghosh, J., & Sanyal, P. (2024). Development and evaluation of machine learning models for predicting constipation and its risk factors among college-aged females. *Nutrition & Food Science*, *12*(3). https://bit.ly/3MPo6eH

Ghosh, J., Shakil, S., Singh, K., & Mandal, S. (2024). Depression and cognitive function in accordance with the nutritional status of elderly women residing in Rajarhat-Newtown area of Kolkata, India. *Medical Journal of Dr. D.Y. Patil Vidyapeeth*, *17*(5), 951–956. DOI: 10.4103/mjdrdypu.mjdrdypu_423_23

Gloyn, A. L., & Drucker, D. J. (2018). Precision medicine in the management of type 2 diabetes. *The Lancet. Diabetes & Endocrinology*, *6*(11), 891–900. DOI: 10.1016/S2213-8587(18)30052-4 PMID: 29699867

Goh, K. I.. (2007). The human disease network. *Proceedings of the National Academy of Sciences of the United States of America*, *104*, 8685–8690. PMID: 17502601

Gomez-Cabello, C. A., Borna, S., Pressman, S., Haider, S. A., Haider, C. R., & Forte, A. J. (2024). Artificial-intelligence-based clinical decision support systems in primary care: A scoping review of current clinical implementations. *European Journal of Investigation in Health, Psychology and Education*, *14*(3), 685–698. PMID: 38534906

Hamamoto, R., Komatsu, M., Takasawa, K., Asada, K., & Kaneko, S. (2019). Epigenetics analysis and integrated analysis of multiomics data, including epigenetic data, using artificial intelligence in the era of precision medicine. *Biomolecules*, *10*(1), 62. PMID: 31905969

Hetzel, D. J.. (1992). HER-2/neu expression: A major prognostic factor in endometrial cancer. *Gynecologic Oncology*, *47*(2), 179–185. DOI: 10.1016/0090-8258(92)90103-p PMID: 1361478

Hillesheim, E., Ryan, M. F., Gibney, E., Roche, H. M., & Brennan, L. (2020). Optimization of a metabotype approach to deliver targeted dietary advice. *Nutrition & Metabolism*, *17*, 1–12. PMID: 33005208

Huang, L., Jiang, S., & Shi, Y. (2020). Tyrosine kinase inhibitors for solid tumors in the past 20 years (2001–2020). *Journal of Hematology & Oncology*, *13*(1), 143. DOI: 10.1186/s13045-020-00977-0 PMID: 33109256

Kim, H., & Rebholz, C. M. (2021). Metabolomic biomarkers of healthy dietary patterns and cardiovascular outcomes. *Current Atherosclerosis Reports*, *23*, 1–12. PMID: 33782776

Kings Research. (2024). Precision nutrition market [2031] – Share, trends & growth. Kings Research & Analytics.

Kirk, D., Kok, E., Tufano, M., Tekinerdogan, B., Feskens, E. J. M., & Camps, G. (2022). Machine learning in nutrition research. *Advances in Nutrition*, *13*, 2573–2589. PMID: 36166846

Kuruvilla, M. E., Lee, F. E., & Lee, G. B. (2019). Understanding asthma phenotypes, endotypes, and mechanisms of disease. *Clinical Reviews in Allergy & Immunology*, *56*(2), 219–233. DOI: 10.1007/s12016-018-8712-1 PMID: 30206782

Lee, H. A., Huang, T. T., Yen, L. H., Wu, P. H., Chen, K. W., & Kung, H. H.. (2022). Precision nutrient management using artificial intelligence based on digital data collection framework. *Applied Sciences (Basel, Switzerland)*, *12*(9), 4167.

Li, J.. (2020). The Mediterranean diet, plasma metabolome, and cardiovascular disease risk. *European Heart Journal*, *41*, 2645–2656. PMID: 32406924

Limketkai, B. N.. (2021). The age of artificial intelligence: Use of digital technology in clinical nutrition. *Current Surgery Reports*, *9*, 20. PMID: 34123579

Ma, S., Li, X., & Wang, X. (2019). Current progress in CAR-T cell therapy for solid tumors. *International Journal of Biological Sciences*, *15*(12), 2548–2560. DOI: 10.7150/ijbs.34213 PMID: 31754328

Maharjan, B., Li, J., Kong, J., & Tao, C. (2019). Alexa, what should I eat?: A personalized virtual nutrition coach for Native American diabetes patients using Amazon's smart speaker technology. In *Proceedings of the 2019 IEEE International Conference on E-Health Networking, Application & Services (HealthCom)* (pp. 1–6).

Mahendran, M., Karthika, B., Verma, M. K., & Krishnaja, U. (2024). *AI innovations in nutrition: A critical analysis*. Department of Community Science, College of Agriculture Vellayani.

Maher, C. A., Davis, C. R., Curtis, R. G., Short, C. E., & Murphy, K. J. (2020). A physical activity and diet program delivered by artificially intelligent virtual health coach: Proof-of-concept study. *JMIR mHealth and uHealth*, *8*, e17558. PMID: 32673246

MarketsandMarkets. (2024). Precision nutrition market worth $12.89 billion by 2029 – Exclusive report by MarketsandMarkets.

Meyers, D. E., & Banerji, S. (2020). Biomarkers of immune checkpoint inhibitor efficacy in cancer. *Current Oncology (Toronto, Ont.), 27*(suppl. 2), S106–S114. DOI: 10.3747/co.27.5549 PMID: 32368180

Mickelson, B., Herfel, T. M., Booth, J., & Wilson, R. P. (2019). Nutrition. In *The Laboratory Rat* (3rd ed., pp. 243–347). Academic Press.

Mills, S., Stanton, C., Lane, J. A., Smith, G. J., & Ross, R. P. (2019). Precision nutrition and the microbiome, part I: Current state of the science. *Nutrients, 11*, 923. PMID: 31022973

Mordor Intelligence. (2024). *Personalized nutrition market size & share analysis – Industry research report – Growth trends*. Mordor Intelligence Pvt. Ltd.

Naithani, N., Atal, A. T., Tilak, T. V. S. V. G. K., Vasudevan, B., Misra, P., & Sinha, S. (2021). Precision medicine: Uses and challenges. *Medical Journal, Armed Forces India, 77*(3), 258–265. DOI: 10.1016/j.mjafi.2021.06.020 PMID: 34305277

Niszczota, P., & Rybicka, I. (2023). The credibility of dietary advice formulated by ChatGPT: Robo-diets for people with food allergies. *Nutrition (Burbank, Los Angeles County, Calif.), 112*, 112076. PMID: 37269717

Oh, Y. J., Zhang, J., Fang, M.-L., & Fukuoka, Y. (2021). A systematic review of artificial intelligence chatbots for promoting physical activity, healthy diet, and weight loss. *The International Journal of Behavioral Nutrition and Physical Activity, 18*, 160. PMID: 34895247

Palacios, G., Druce, J., & Du, L. (2008). A new arenavirus in a cluster of fatal transplant-associated diseases. *The New England Journal of Medicine, 358*, 991–998. DOI: 10.1056/NEJMoa073785 PMID: 18256387

Palmnäs, M.. (2020). Perspective: Metabotyping—a potential personalized nutrition strategy for precision prevention of cardiometabolic disease. *Advances in Nutrition, 11*, 524–532. PMID: 31782487

GII Research. (2024). Global precision nutrition market size study, by technology, application, service type, end use, supplement, and regional forecasts 2022–2032. Global Info Research.

Saunders, C. J., Miller, N. A., & Soden, S. E. (2012). Rapid whole-genome sequencing for genetic disease diagnosis in neonatal intensive care units. *Science Translational Medicine, 4*, 154ra135. Advance online publication. DOI: 10.1126/scitranslmed.3004041 PMID: 23035047

ShareMe Global. (2024). *Precision nutrition market expansion: Key drivers and emerging opportunities*. ShareMe Global Insights.

Sosa-Holwerda, A., Park, O. H., Albracht-Schulte, K., Niraula, S., Thompson, L., & Oldewage-Theron, W. (2024). The role of artificial intelligence in nutrition research: A scoping review. *Nutrients*, *16*(13), 2066. PMID: 38999814

Thomas, J. AI in public health: Need to balance innovation with accountability.

Trujillo, E., Davis, C., & Milner, J. (2006). Nutrigenomics, proteomics, metabolomics, and the practice of dietetics. *Journal of the American Dietetic Association*, *106*, 403–413. PMID: 16503231

Tyler, S., Olis, M., Aust, N., Patel, L., Simon, L., Triantafyllidis, C., & Jacobs, R. J. (2024). Use of artificial intelligence in triage in hospital emergency departments: A scoping review. *Cureus*, *16*(5). PMID: 38854295

Verified Market Research. (2024). Precision nutrition market size, share, trends, analysis & forecast.

Wahl, B., Cossy-Gantner, A., Germann, S., & Schwalbe, N. R. (2018). Artificial intelligence (AI) and global health: How can AI contribute to health in resource-poor settings? *BMJ Global Health*, *3*(4), e000798. PMID: 30233828

Zhang, X., Yang, H., & Zhang, R. (2019). Challenges and future of precision medicine strategies for breast cancer based on a database on drug reactions. *Bioscience Reports*, ●●●, 39. PMID: 31387972

Chapter 6
Artificial intelligence (AI) in Diabetes Management, Obesity, and AI–Driven Weight Management

Wasswa Shafik
https://orcid.org/0000-0002-9320-3186
Dig Connectivity Research Laboratory (DCRLab), Uganda

ABSTRACT

This chapter examines the transformative impact of Artificial Intelligence (AI) on the management of diabetes and obesity, two prevalent and interrelated chronic health conditions. It examines how AI-driven technologies, including machine learning, predictive analytics, and digital health tools, enable personalised and data-driven approaches to glucose regulation, weight control, and lifestyle interventions. The chapter discusses the application of AI in continuous glucose monitoring, insulin dosing, and the development of customized weight management programs. Furthermore, it highlights the integration of wearable devices, mobile health (mHealth) applications, and remote patient monitoring systems to enhance patient engagement and clinical outcomes. Ethical considerations, data privacy, and the challenges of AI adoption in healthcare systems are also addressed. This chapter highlights the potential of AI to enhance the prevention, diagnosis, and treatment of diabetes and obesity, ultimately supporting sustainable and effective management of chronic diseases.

DOI: 10.4018/979-8-3373-3196-6.ch006

1. INTRODUCTION

Artificial Intelligence (AI) refers to both a theory and a technology that aims to create artificial creations with human-like intelligence. AI technologies are modeled based on the simulation of human behavior and actions in regulated environments. They are able to learn, operate independently, dynamically optimize their tasks by modifying their strategies, make predictions in uncertain environments, and visualize and interpret virtual objects (Pongrac Barlovic et al., 2022). Healthcare systems are among the most prominent fields concerned with the integration of advanced AI technologies into their workflows. Healthcare facilities are constantly subjected to a variety of interruptions and unexpected events every day, and are in dire need of a robust technology to optimize their functioning in terms of performance improvement and cost reduction. Over the years, healthcare has become a growing area for AI technologies such as machine learning and deep learning, natural language processing, robotics, and computer vision (Zheng et al., 2023).

AI technologies were recently introduced in various domains of healthcare delivery, including drug and vaccine discovery, patient education, triage, diagnosis, treatment, patient management, disease prevention, and monitoring. The apparent advantages of these technologies and their applications offer great promise to reduce patient waiting times, increase access to healthcare services, reduce the number of erroneous results attributed to human fatigue, improve decision making, and provide support for hard and invasive processes related to patient diagnosis and therapy (Udogadi et al., 2019). There is currently an imperative need to meet the rising demand for healthcare services due to the considerable improvement in life expectancy and the increasing prevalence of chronic diseases worldwide. In the last decade, several studies have described how AI technologies can act as essential components in ameliorating the healthcare delivery systems and provide enormous benefits in combating chronic diseases (Andrès et al., 2019).

2. UNDERSTANDING DIABETES

Diabetes is a chronic metabolic disease characterized by hyperglycemia due to an absolute or relative deficiency of insulin or a defect in its action. Chronic hyperglycemia leads to long-term damage, dysfunction, and failure of various organs, especially the eyes, kidneys, nerves, heart, and blood vessels. The main types of diabetes include type 1 diabetes, which is characterized by autoimmune destruction of the insulin-secreting pancreatic beta cells; type 2 diabetes, which is characterized by insulin deficiency and relative resistance; and gestational diabetes mellitus, which is diagnosed during the second or third trimester of pregnancy and is not overt diabetes (Vasiloglou, 2021). Other specific types of diabetes result from infections, drugs or other chemicals, or other illnesses, such as genetic syndromes associated with diabetes, pancreatic exocrine disease, and hormonal causes.

Diabetes has been recognized around the world for centuries. Increasing trends in diabetes prevalence are predicted, suggesting that diabetes is a major health risk in the future. A long duration of diabetes, poor hyperglycemic control, obesity, older age, dyslipidemia, and hypertension are all risk factors for early and increased cardiovascular disease. People who are at increased risk include those with risk factors from a population-wide screening program and patients with impaired fasting glucose, impaired glucose tolerance, or gestational diabetes (Bul et al., 2023). People with risk factors should know about the symptoms of diabetes and conduct a self-test. If diabetes is diagnosed, patients need to be aware of the complications, lifestyle modifications, and management strategies such as blood glucose, hemoglobin A1c, and lipid monitoring, dietary therapy, exercise, and the need for antidiabetic treatment. Without proper treatment and diabetic health education, the body may begin to fail, and patients face the risk of hospitalization, cardiovascular disease, amputations, dialysis, or even death (Liu et al., 2022).

2.1. Types of Diabetes

Diabetes has for long been classically divided into Types 1 and 2. Type 1 Diabetes Mellitus (T1DM) accounts for about 5–10% of all cases of diabetes and is a result of autoimmune destruction of pancreatic beta cells, leading to absolute deficiency of insulin. Its peak onset is in childhood, but it can occur at any age. It is associated with a genetic predisposition, but non-immune mechanisms can also lead to beta-cell loss (Alkhatib, 2020). These patients have positive autoantibodies against various beta-cell antigens, especially GAD-65, and are otherwise healthy at diabetes onset but have a rapidly progressive course and present with Diabetic Ketoacidosis (DKA) if not treated. They promptly respond to insulin therapy. The other group of patients has Type 2 Diabetes Mellitus (T2DM), which predominantly arises from a complex interplay of genetic and environmental factors. Its prevalence is rising dramatically across the globe. Most patients are obese and insulin resistant, with varying levels of relative insulin deficiency. As opposed to T1DM, these patients have a slow and insidious course, and some can even present with acute complications without prior symptoms or diagnosis. Fasting blood glucose (FBG) levels suggestive of T2DM can be accompanied by non-ketotic living or dead hyperglycemic patients without prior diagnosis, with a markedly elevated HbA1c level (Dankwa-Mullan et al., 2019). Autopsy studies have shown that some of these patients can also have positive autoantibodies to islet autoantigens and inflammatory cell infiltrates; they probably have Type 3C diabetes due to pancreatitis, and some have a latent phase before requiring insulin therapy, at which point they could be classified as having Latent Autoimmune Diabetes of Adulthood (LADA). Posteriorly described specific types of diabetes include Maturity Onset Diabetes of the Young (MODY), which is due to a mutation in one of the genes associated with beta-cell function, and treatment is often sulfonylureas alone or in combination with other antidiabetic medications (Ahmad & Mehfuz, 2022). Additionally, there is Double Diabetes, wherein a Type 1 Diabetic patient develops insulin resistance, which is functionally reversible at least; it typically occurs in younger patients with a psychiatric history or problems with adherence to treatment.

2.2. Symptoms and Complications

Diabetes, currently at epidemic proportions, results in substantial morbidity due to disease complications. Patients with diabetes are more likely to experience difficulties in the day-to-day functioning of their lives, especially among the elderly. Diabetes complications may be classified as microvascular, macrovascular, or non-vascular and are of importance at both the population as well as individual patient levels. In a vast population of patients diagnosed with diabetes, long-term disability may be the most important consequence and the most devastating complication (Aas et al., 2023). Diabetes management centers on keeping blood glucose levels within a target range. Symptoms of diabetes can be classified as either classic symptoms of hyperglycemia or signs of secretory failure. Patients may experience polyuria, polydipsia, and polyphagia or other symptoms such as night sweats, fatigue, blurred vision, peripheral neuropathy, or weight loss. Patients with longstanding diabetes are prone to infections, problems with wound healing, or even experience the acute onset of suppurative necrobiosis. Even though nerve abnormalities usually arise without any specific symptoms, patients may experience burning, electrical shock-like sensations, and even itching (Aas et al., 2023). Besides sensory loss, patients may also exhibit other symptoms associated with autonomic neuropathy, like diarrhea, impotence, gastroparesis, coronary artery perfusion abnormalities, or abnormal pressure. Risk factors for neuropathy include male gender, long duration of diabetes, alcohol excess, increasing age, smoking, hyperlipidemia, and cigarette smoking. Autonomic neuropathy can result in systemic and local cardiovascular issues, bladder evacuation problems, gastrointestinal problems, and sexual dysfunction. Diabetes also has macrovascular complications, which could involve the heart, brain, and peripheral vasculature. Atherosclerosis, as well as coronary artery disease, could be accelerated in patients with diabetes. This is especially common in patients with type 2 diabetes who are often older and exhibit metabolic syndrome, wherein visceral obesity, dyslipidemia, skin tags, hypertension, and high levels of plasma glucose are present (Dewi Yudhani et al., 2022). In addition, enhanced platelet aggregation may lead to acute MI, and there is often increased apoptotic endothelial cell injury-response.

2.3. Current Management Strategies

Advancements in diabetes management entail a tripartite approach—dietary modulation, pharmacological strategies, and meticulous monitoring of glycemic levels—concomitantly preventing and mitigating complications. Therapeutic regimens are individualized, weighing risks, therapy benefits, drug mechanisms, drug classes, patient preferences, cost, access issues, and promoters and inhibitors of adherence to remedies. Type 1 diabetes necessitates insulin replacement therapy, the extent of which is tailored to patient requirements with a focus on achieving glycemic control while avoiding hypo- and hyperglycemic episodes (Lakey et al., 2024). Prevention and treatment of type 2 diabetes and its complications necessitate lifestyle interventions. Weight loss associated with caloric restriction and increased physical activity improves insulin sensitivity. These interventions mitigate associated comorbidities, like dyslipidemia, hypertension, and pancreatitis, and delay progression to diabetes. These interventions include dietary recommendations to limit caloric intake to 1200-2200 kcal/day. Emphasis is laid on a calorie deficit, which usually encompasses 30-50% less than the estimated energy requirement (Shamanna et al., 2020). Carbohydrate proportions should be limited to 40-45% of the diet, preferably comprised of fiber. Oral hypoglycemic agents—affordable biguanides, alpha-glucosidase inhibitors, thiazolidinediones, incretins, and other glucose-lowering drugs—are recommended for patients who cannot achieve their target glycosylated hemoglobin of less than 7% by lifestyle modifications. Adjuvant medications for comorbid conditions are also altered. Recent evidence has shown that pharmacotherapy preserves insulin secretion and sensitivity and minimizes the risk of microvascular and macrovascular complications, especially in patients with comorbid conditions. For moderately obese diabetics, gastric bypass and other bariatric surgeries afford more sustained weight loss than conventional measures, allowing better control of glucose metabolism and reducing associated high-risk pathologies (Cushley et al., 2023). These surgical interventions are recommended for patients unable to achieve their glycemic targets with test-based lifestyle modification therapy and drug-assisted weight loss.

3. THE ROLE OF AI IN DIABETES MANAGEMENT

Artificial Intelligence (AI) is transforming the landscape of diabetes management through its predictive capabilities, advanced monitoring tools, and personalized treatment plans. Diabetes has a variety of forms and challenges. The fast-growing health burden of diabetes is mainly characterized by the global epidemic of type 2 diabetes and its complications. More than 450 million people have diabetes worldwide. The prevalence of diabetes is predicted to reach 642 million in 2040 without action (Dimitriades & Pillay, 2021). Diabetes is the leading cause of kidney failure, lower limb amputation, and blindness, and has been identified as the primary contributor to the emerging global epidemic of cardiovascular and cerebrovascular diseases. Therefore, the early diagnosis and effective management of diabetes are urgent health challenges. AI represents a novel approach and resource in assisting the prediction, diagnosis, and management of diabetes. AI contributed to solving clinical challenges in diabetes with its machine learning models and automated algorithms (Hwalla et al., 2021). Predictive analytics in diabetes provides machine-learned and rule-based risk stratification and early prediction of the clinical trajectory of known diabetes patients. This includes the prediction of poor metabolic process control, hypoglycemic events, hyperglycemic events, or poor subsequent clinical events, such as diabetes, cardiovascular complications, risk of kidney disease, and diabetic retinopathy in the following months to years. Many diabetes management applications are available or under development. They allow for the best pruning of the diabetes treatment and monitoring process. Some companies also offer patient transfer services by providing smart wearables linked to digital help systems (Yao et al., 2024). The solutions that allow physicians to best manage the diabetes management process are Lifebanks and PatientsLikeMe, which focus on real-time testimony collection managed by automated software, data including the best keywords and recorded symptoms phase, and automatic push for pre-defined warning symptoms.

3.1. Predictive Analytics in Diabetes

The concept of predictive analytics incorporates data mining, modeling, and prediction to identify patterns and utilize them to predict outcomes. Predictive analytics can help identify high-risk groups/classes of patients whilst also allowing clinicians to monitor and assess disease severity, patient responses, and efficacy of treatment tests. It can also help in bariatric surgery decision-making processes. Predictive analytics help the medical fraternity anticipate treatment response in prediabetic patients. Expert systems can help detect type 2 diabetes-related complications and consequences, and diabetes-related hospitalizations, and predict future diabetes development in patients. The classical epidemiological approach proposed the earliest prediction for diabetes risk (Neblett & Kennedy-Malone, 2024). Later, quite a few diabetes prediction models have been developed to evaluate the risk of developing diabetes. Currently, the most validated prediction models for diabetes risk include various diabetes risk scores. These models utilized physical and/or anthropometric, clinical, lifestyle, or biochemical modifiers to develop their diabetes prediction scores. Although these prediction models presented good predictive capabilities, they have limited utility in specialized high-risk populations. Computerized models, such as those based on support vector machines, neural networks, classification tree models, random forest models, and logistic regression, have been developed (Tang et al., 2023). AI can also help in the differential prediction of 1-type and 2-type diabetes in high-risk individuals. Such AI models have been developed using many clinical, genetic, and laboratory data prediction patterns.

3.2. AI-Driven Monitoring Tools

In the coming years, people with diabetes may be offered even more sophisticated at-home diabetes management tools, tailored to their unique needs, that AI powers. A growing number of monitoring devices are coming to market that can be used to track hypos and hypers, glucose levels, insulin delivery, and even behaviors and habits that could lead to complications. Some wearables already allow healthcare providers and sometimes family members to track a patient's health status in real time; others can react independently to fluctuations in biomarkers tied to glucose levels or disease progression (Wilson et al., 2022). For diabetes and its comorbidities, these tools could further personal responses to medical intervention. A disposable continuous glucose monitor, for instance, is a device that a person applies to the back of their arm. About the size of a quarter, the device tracks glucose levels day and night, alerting patients if they go out of range. Its new design is smarter than previous models, with the ability to ignore short-term fluctuations, thereby reducing incorrectly flagged incidents of high glucose and minimizing the number of fingersticks people need to do. The data is kept on a health portal, which care partners can access. A tool, meanwhile, can personalize care for both patients and clinicians managing hyperglycemia (Salinas Martínez et al., 2023). It converts a person's real-time continuous glucose monitor data into individually tailored actionable insight for optimizing insulin dosing, dosing recommendations, and alerts for glucose patterns associated with dangerously high or low sugar levels. Will these products eliminate the struggle for diabetes patients? Not anytime soon, but there is room for optimism. More diabetes monitoring devices powered by AI are on the way. A platform seeks to aggregate the multitude of continuously collected sensor measures people are generating, including devices measuring sleep, exercise, glucose, hydration, weight, food, and insulin, to support better self-management (Khattak et al., 2024). The hope is that AI devices will contextualize signals from these devices into recommendations tailored to the needs of the moment in order to help people with diabetes stick to a diabetes management routine that can help stave off complications.

3.3. Personalized Treatment Plans

Modern-day diabetic care is a highly individualized process. The way each person reacts to medication, insulin, coping skills, and even exercise is something health care providers study closely. Each number on the hemoglobin A1c test and glucose meter tells a different story for every person. Today, this individualization of diabetes care is becoming even more specific with the incorporation of AI. Personalized insulin regimens and delivery routes, algorithms for fasting blood glucose levels for diet management in type 2 diabetes, and health coaching specifically targeted to individuals with prediabetes are just a few examples of how AI is shaping the way diabetes care is being provided today (Lee et al., 2023). Diabetes care requires intensive support, especially for patients with the densest care needs. Personalized treatment plans can facilitate longitudinal patient monitoring, give clinical decision support and alert health care teams of clinical deterioration faster, and recommend appropriate tiered interventions. Making a multitude of decisions is at the heart of diabetes management at all stages of life, and the improved effectiveness of clinician and patient choices, paired with care creation, is an area of great potential for diabetes technology. In the future, patients may have management apps that apply AI to their unique patient profile that learns the patient's blood glucose patterns, analyzes the complexities of their diabetes, and monitors their care adherence. This information would then be based on what is already known about the physiology of diabetes (Adesina et al., 2022). AI could then use this input to determine what clinical program changes most therapists would use, based on the computer-assisted algorithms that other methods will have revealed are most effective for that particular profile, as presented in Table 1.

Table 1. Artificial Intelligence Applications in Diabetes Management

AI Tool/ Technique	Functionality	Benefits	Real-World Example	Challenges	Reference
CGM + AI Integration	Analyzes continuous glucose data	Accurate, real-time glucose trends	Dexcom + AI-powered alerts	Sensor errors, data overload	(Pongrac Barlovic et al., 2022)
Insulin Dosing Algorithms	Predict insulin needs	Reduces hypoglycemia risks	Medtronic's SmartGuard system	Lack of personalization for some users	(Zheng et al., 2023)
AI Chatbots for Patients	24/7 diabetes management support	Increases engagement and adherence	IBM Watson Health	Limited nuance in conversation	(Udogadi et al., 2019)

continued on following page

Table 1. Continued

AI Tool/ Technique	Functionality	Benefits	Real-World Example	Challenges	Reference
AI-Based Diet Trackers	Detect food from photos, give feedback	Accurate carb counting	CalorieMama AI	Misrecognition of food	(Andrès et al., 2019)
Predictive Blood Glucose Models	Forecast future glucose levels	Preventive management	Glooko Predictive Insights	Need for large, diverse data sets	(Vasiloglou, 2021)
Digital Twin for Diabetics	Simulates the patient's metabolic state	Personalized treatment scenarios	Twin Health	Complex to model biological variability	(Bul et al., 2023)
Wearable Fitness Devices	Track steps, sleep, heart rate, etc.	Promotes lifestyle changes	Fitbit with AI insights	May exclude those without access	(Liu et al., 2022)
AI Voice Assistants	Hands-free tracking and advice	Convenient for the visually impaired	Alexa + MySugar integration	Privacy concerns	(Alkhatib, 2020)
Mobile Diabetes Apps	Monitor data and provide feedback	Self-care empowerment	mySugr, BlueLoop	App fatigue or over-reliance	(Dankwa-Mullan et al., 2019)
Automated Retinopathy Screening	AI image analysis of retina	Early complication detection	IDx-DR	Risk of false negatives	(Ahmad & Mehfuz, 2022)
NLP for Medical Notes	Extract insights from doctor notes	Faster and better diagnosis	Google's Med-PaLM	Data privacy and legal concerns	(Aas et al., 2023)
AI-Driven Health Coaching	Tracks progress, adapts recommendations	Increases motivation and compliance	Omada Health	May lack empathy or personalization	(Dewi Yudhani et al., 2022)
Smart Insulin Pens	Monitor dose history via AI	Reduces errors in insulin delivery	InPen + AI dashboard	High cost and access inequality	(Lakey et al., 2024)
Telemedicine AI Assistants	Support virtual checkups	Bridges doctor shortages	ADA-endorsed platforms	Need for consistent internet access	(Shamanna et al., 2020)

4. OBESITY: A GROWING CONCERN

Obesity is defined as an excessive accumulation of body fat, which may be associated with numerous comorbidities such as hypertension, diabetes, hyperlipidemia, sleep apnea, osteoarthritis, and cardiovascular diseases. The increased amount of unhealthy fat tissue represents a risk factor for these and other diseases;

consequently, obesity is known as a disease itself. In fact, more than 470 million people worldwide are estimated to be obese with a Body Mass Index (BMI) higher than 30 kg/m2, and epidemiological studies predict that 2.5 billion adults worldwide will be classified as overweight or severely obese by the year 2030 (Henderson & Alexander, 2012). Based on guidelines, body weight status is classified according to the BMI, which is calculated as body mass in kilograms divided by height in meters squared. There are four BMI categories: (1) underweight (BMI < 18.5 kg/m2); (2) normal weight (BMI 18.5–24.9 kg/m2); (3) overweight (BMI 25.0–29.9 kg/m2); and (4) obese (BMI ≥ 30 kg/m2). In adults, the obesity category is further subdivided for classification purposes into three classes: (1) Class 1 (BMI 30–34.9 kg/m2); (2) Class 2 (BMI 35.0–39.9 kg/m2); and (3) Class 3 (BMI ≥ 40 kg/m2) (Hwalla & Jaafar, 2021).

The premier causes for this growing increase in obesity events are directly related to modifications in the energy balance and dietary guidelines. Specifically, nutrition overload with high-calorie diets and energy-poor or energy-dense-nutrient low-consuming habits may lead to energy imbalance, which is an important problem for body weight gain. Other environmental and cultural factors appear to be associated: low economy, sedentary life, lack of sleep, hormonal alterations, easy availability of high-caloric convenience food, excessive marketing and advertisement of unhealthy food, low-protein diets, and stress (BALFOUR, 2021). As with the increased number of people with obesity, there has been an increase in the number of people with smokeless and alcohol consumption, with physical inactivity, with diabetes, and with hypertension. For this reason, obesity treatment is highly important in reducing morbidity and mortality associated with these comorbidities. Current treatments for obesity a priori are lifestyle modification, using diet, physical activity, and behavior therapy. For patients unable to lose weight through lifestyle changes, medications are also available. Approved obesity medications can help overweight or obese patients lose weight when used in conjunction with diet and physical activity (Porri et al., 2024).

4.1. Definition and Statistics

Obesity is defined as an excessive, abnormal elevation of fat mass that can impede health. It is diagnosed with precision through the use of imaging techniques such as magnetic resonance and computed tomography scans, but these methods are expensive and not suitable for screening without the need to diagnose large groups of individuals. For this reason, a combination of the body mass index (BMI) and waist circumference is used, as they are inexpensive and simple measurements. BMI is defined by dividing weight (in kg) by the height (in m) squared (Trouwborst et al., 2018). A person is defined as obese when their BMI is ≥30 kg/m2. Abnormal waist circumference increases the risk of developing several comorbidities. For Caucasians, a cut-off point of 102 cm for men and 88 cm for women has been suggested. For South-East Asian people, the cut-off point is ≥90 cm for men and ≥80 cm for women. For those of Japanese descent, ≥85 cm for men and ≥90 cm for women has been proposed. Finally, for Central and South American people, ≥90 cm for men and ≥85 cm for women are the defined limits (Brończyk-Puzoń et al., 2015). Obesity is recognized as a global epidemic. Today, 42.4% of adults in the United States are obese, with 73.6% of adults classified as overweight or obese. Global obesity incidence has tripled since 1975, with a staggering 850 million people being overweight or obese. The prevalence of class 3 obesity has increased, particularly affecting women, from 3.2% in 1993 to 10.2% in 2015. The prevalence is higher among certain ethnic groups, reflecting differences in diet, lifestyle, and culture, with Native American, Hispanic, Black, and African American being the more affected. Since people with obesity have a higher risk of developing several comorbid conditions, including type 2 diabetes, orthopedic diseases, and different types of cancer, it is recognized that treating obesity is a clear priority to reduce the incidence of these diseases, which ought to be further tackled using a multidisciplinary approach focusing on diet and lifestyle changes (Steiner et al., 2019).

4.2. Causes and Consequences

Rising rates of obesity followed by its drastic consequences for public health, mainly the increase of diabetes incidence and associated comorbidities, such as cardiovascular disease, certain types of cancer, and lung disease, have drawn increasing attention from the scientific community and the media. Its complexity stems from a multitude of factors that come into play throughout human life. Obesity is a result of the unbalanced relation between caloric intake and expenditure. Energy intake is influenced by appetite signals that act on the hypothalamus and stimulate the release of hormones (Konishi et al., 2024). Consequently, the influence and development of these consuming behaviors rely on genetic and environmental factors, such as nutrition, diet, social and cultural factors, personal experience, and psychological states. Because of the abundance of nutritional choices, many individuals often miscalculate their requirements, which leads to overeating and the consumption of unhealthy food patterns that are dense in calories and poor in nutrients, such as sugar- and fat-containing foods. Increased BMI and obesity are also associated with decreased physical activity, low levels of movement and exercise, technological advancements, and the increasing use of cars for transportation. The various stages of life may display shifting influences on obesity, as fetal growth tempos increase maternal obesity and gestational diabetes incidences, thus relating offspring to an increased risk for obesity and diabetes later in life. Increased risk is also evident for breastfed infants who stay obese in childhood and are more likely to be obese as adults. However, obesity is not a fate. Successful prevention and treatment programs rely on measures encouraging healthy eating habits, encouraging regular physical activity from the earliest possible age, and maintaining a healthy weight throughout life (Kaur et al., 2022). If more people were to focus on their weight management, national resources could be directed toward more pressing health concerns. For the millions who already struggle with obesity, it is imperative to break through the cycle of this costly disease.

4.3. Existing Treatment Approaches

Excessive adiposity often results in metabolic problems. Because these problems evolve gradually, they frequently go unnoticed until people reach adulthood. To treat obesity, several modalities exist, such as dietary interventions, psychoeducation, physical activity, medications, and surgical procedures. Lifestyle modifications, including good eating habits and increased physical activity, remain the most critical components of weight management therapy, and they are the base of any weight loss program; however, lifestyle modifications alone lead to only a modest weight reduction in a small number of people (Sefa-Yeboah et al., 2021). In weight loss and maintenance, programs aimed at specific populations have been successful, but the public response is minimal. Experts in the field of obesity management think that medications to aid weight loss will be important adjuncts to lifestyle modifications. Drug therapy to aid weight loss has been available for many years. Medications used to treat obesity help with weight loss, but these drugs are prescribed only to help people who meet certain criteria, usually when lifestyle changes and exercise don't help. Some patients with chronic obesity can be helped through traditional means; however, there are individuals who either cannot achieve weight loss or who are unable to maintain weight loss despite intervention (Crompvoets et al., 2024). In such cases, bariatric surgery may be considered for weight loss. There exist several surgical treatment options, namely adjustable gastric band, Roux-en-Y gastric bypass, sleeving, and biliopancreatic diversion, among others. Weight-loss surgery has many health benefits, especially for people with severe obesity, who may benefit from losing weight quickly. Weight loss can cure or improve many diseases related to obesity, such as type 2 diabetes, high blood pressure, and sleep apnea (Zarkogianni et al., 2021). Weight loss can also improve the chances of a successful pregnancy and childbirth.

5. AI APPLICATIONS IN WEIGHT MANAGEMENT

Artificial intelligence, with its capability to analyze large amounts of multidisciplinary data quickly and reliably, is already a reality in digital therapeutic solutions for obesity. However, its clinical implementation as a weight-loss supporting therapy is still in its infancy. That being said, various innovative strategies have been proposed and validated in human clinical trials. These strategies range widely, from traditional weight-loss and behavioral-change diet therapy, where academic initiatives suggest improvements to existing modalities through the incorporation of AI specialities, to more advanced pathways, such as virtual reality neural triggers, gamification, neuroscientific agenda, and closed-loop weight-loss intervention management (Zarkogianni et al., 2021). In contrast to traditional practice, AI solutions may use a broad spectrum of patient communication channels to constantly engage the patient and provide personalized, individualized, and real-time feedback on their caloric intake and physical activity patterns. Particularly user-friendly are conversational AI chatbots, which allow for free text input and output in any language. Understanding the complex network of behavioral, motivational, and social agents that influence dietary choices is one of the significant research themes in machine learning that may contribute to developing predictive models that, by recognizing the interactions in specific patient subpopulations, can optimize personalized nutritional plans and help achieve the desired effect (Power et al., 2024). Using deep learning with neural networks for image analysis and recognition is a good ally in nutritional prescriptions, made easier with automated or semi-automated dietary recalls or by developing and validating mobile applications capable of dietary assessment through interpreting the photos taken before and after meal times. Additionally, considering that a significant barrier to obesity management is an inconsistency of dietary adherence during the observed periods, constant behavioral monitoring that uses machine learning subdisciplines is essential (Rodríguez et al., 2023). The development of monitoring systems for the dietary recall that utilize deep learning is also being pursued in mobile applications capable of interpreting the photos taken before and after meal times.

5.1. Behavioral Tracking and Analysis

Behavioral tracking and reinforcement learning of health-related reactions and habits through wearable sensors, mobile apps, smartwatches, and ambient sensors is at the core of successful management of diabetes and obesity. Such tracking of events and body reactions with technology-enabled nudges has many benefits: fusing together continuous data streams on health conditions through remote synchronous and asynchronous monitoring reduces monitoring gaps and increases the effectiveness of easing management of continuous condition and prediction of medical onsets to ensure timely intervention. Utilizing a continuous glucose monitoring device can help clinicians pinpoint unhealthy eating habits and identify the potential need for behavioral interventions to delay the onset of pre-diabetes and diabetes in at-risk patients (Rodríguez et al., 2023). Sensor-enabled insight generation on glucose, hunger, and possibly even sleep, mood, appetite, stress, and other aspects of eating behavior enables collecting real-world data on dietary choices and daily diet patterns through app and device data integration and combinations with image recognition and machine learning of daily food recall diaries. Data from questionnaires or app-based coding for meal events can further contextualize incoming combined data streams for full 24/7 activity data (Panza et al., 2018). In this way, it can help calculate discriminator onset hollows of individual eating events, identify incorrect insulin dosing associated with appetizing behavior, and flag hypoglycemia episodes and possible late-night eating behavior breaches. Based on these insight generation capabilities, we propose a smart age-, lifestyle-, and culture-sensitive intelligent tutor and user interface with nuanced tailored reminders sent as timely cues to action, in combination with contextual nudge reminders sent from user-selected friends, competent clinicians, and socially defined closed groups, that are flexible but structured during the user-specified preferred times throughout the day (Bak-Sosnowska, 2018).

5.2. Dietary Recommendations and Planning

Food planning and preparation are essential parts of a person's daily life. As user-generated diet data become ubiquitous, artificial intelligence (AI)-based dietary planning and analysis, which provide customized diet assistance, have garnered much attention. These systems are not simply food diary systems that users can easily use instead of conventional food diaries; they are complete dietary and nutritional assistance systems that use the latest computer vision and AI technologies to establish capabilities that were long thought impossible (Henderson & Alexander, 2012). They offer instructions for healthy diets that are customized for the individual by predicting the calorie or nutrition intake for everyday meal plans or detected meals in food diaries, and also create practical meal plans to follow. Traditional face-space-based diet analysis methods are based on the notion that there exists a global model that accurately represents the complicated mappings between food and its features. Such global representations are limited in flexibility; they are rare in diverse diet applications. Therefore, recent face-space-based methods have adopted a transfer-learning approach in which deep learning models are first trained on generic images and are fine-tuned to the target dataset. There are also sketch-based food image retrieval algorithms that search for food images similar to the user-uploaded sketch (Hwalla & Jaafar, 2021). These advanced technologies have been combined with other sensing technologies and data sources, such as smartphone camera sensors and location sensors, to build mobile food diary systems, semantic meal segmentation algorithms, and other user-diet-analyzing systems from crowdsourced food image datasets. However, from the previous discussion, we can see that food image retrieval capabilities have not reached the level of generic image retrieval methods, which are practical in diverse real-world applications (Porri et al., 2024). The current meal detection methods operate on the assumption that users record their foods using predefined food image categories, and there are limited daily-life applications of the suggested meal detection or meal analysis systems. Therefore, there are still gaps to be filled in AI-based dietary analysis methods, both regarding algorithm performance and the available application instances. However, considering that it has not been long since AI was first applied to the dietary analysis field, more sophisticated and diverse dietary analysis methods will be realized in the near future (Brończyk-Puzoń et al., 2015).

5.3. Exercise and Activity Monitoring

Artificial intelligence (AI) is modernizing nearly every area of our daily lives, including health, fitness, and nutrition. Every other day, we see news about innovative solutions and novel ideas using AI for a plethora of applications for better lifestyle management and surveillance. We are now talking about future homes, where AI and smart sensors will watch your every move, help you stay healthy, and nudge you in the right direction. Or intelligent wardrobe and clothing solutions that understand the type of activities you are doing and are aligned accordingly to maximize your progress and achieve your daily, weekly, and long-term activity goals (Hernández-Mijares et al., 2013). Or even healthcare wearables that monitor your vitals for day-to-day irregularities during various activities and through the course of different periods of time. A number of today's civilian and military wearable solutions deploy computer vision, AI, and smart image processing solutions, seamlessly recognizing various activities and returning meaningful real-time and long-term telemetry that aids users and professionals alike in their rehabilitation, recovery, and weights management. For example, the recently proposed constellation of smart clothing sensors that monitor the biomechanical characteristics of your body while exercising or carrying out other activities, such as walking, running, sit-to-stand and stand-to-sit, jogging, climbing stairs, and jumping. With the use of AI, these solutions can be positioned as the next-gen of effective wearable health monitoring and prevention therapy systems (Konishi et al., 2024). All this data can then be processed locally at the wearable device or uploaded to centralized servers, depending on the intended application and infrastructure.

6. AI AND PREDICTIVE MODELING IN OBESITY

Artificial intelligence (AI), particularly its sub-field machine learning (ML), has been used in various aspects of obesity research. Similar to its applications in diabetes research, a prominent domain in obesity research has been risk assessment models with either predicting risk for obesity occurrence, progression, or adverse effects, or a subtype of risk prediction with stratification or classification-related transformation of prediction values. Notably, hierarchical Bayesian methods have been used to model latent obesity classes among children, and achieved good prediction for changes in obesity category in subsequent years (Henderson & Alexander, 2012). However, ML-based risk assessment models usually focus on predicting weighting values or their classifications. For instance, neural networks and boosted or bagged decision trees have been used to build various prediction models to identify cases of obesity or overweight in adult populations. More recently, deep learning models, particularly deep convolutional neural networks (CNNs), have been proposed for predicting obesity in non-adult populations or non-obese adult cohorts. The primary focus has been either on using individual imaging data for model building or using the respective data for testing the trained models from external cohorts. Of note, the use of CNNs for structure analyses of imaging data allows for additional meta data extraction compared to DL/ML techniques based on the input data as a whole (Hwalla & Jaafar, 2021). Therefore, the applicability of systemically generated imaging meta data based on deep learning approaches needs to be further investigated in obesity data, even more in combination with clinical metadata than just unimodal evaluation of imaging data. On the other hand, DL/ML-based outcome prediction or classification has only recently been introduced in obesity research. Various outcomes related to weight and obesity have been predicted using ML for selected cohorts or populations, focusing on within- or multi-step long-term periods. Most of these studies have been conducted in pediatric cohorts, and use a mixture of non-invasively obtained datasets, but also address genotype data for prediction purposes (BALFOUR, 2021). While the applicability of ML for outcome prediction in obesity research seems promising, most of the available studies refer only to proof-of-concept work describing selected models based on exploratory data approaches.

6.1. Risk Assessment Models

The allure of machine learning in generating prognostic algorithms for diabetes and obesity management is partly because of the advancing predictive power of algorithms operating on big multidimensional data. However, risk assessment algorithms for T2DM and obesity are numerous, have been shown to identify at-risk individuals, and may serve as adjuncts to healthcare provider evaluations, as some algorithms rely on sparse and routinely collected data. The real value of machine learning is arguably the facilitation of refined risk assessment approaches to better define high-risk populations, through data mining of existing data, likely acting on a smaller number of patients (Porri et al., 2024). What separates what we know from what we can do, however, is the ability to generalize these algorithms or models across wider and diverse populations. There is a clear emerging need for machine learning models to develop enhanced, broad-based predictive capabilities, borrowing from the principles of data mining combined with transfer learning approaches and federated learning to overcome issues of statistical failures elsewhere (Brończyk-Puzoń et al., 2015). Machine learning approaches should also be able to converge on simplified or refined models able to deliver interpretable outputs or insights. Risk assessment should also evolve into forms that can address diverse population needs, including those with protection against T2DM risk but also those that allow selection of patients for early intervention and those that require more intensive follow-up, e.g., those that exhibit early trajectories of T2DM risk enhancement (Kaur et al., 2022). There is a distinct but related need for GDP-based modeling that could facilitate more direct application of risk assessment across health systems globally.

6.2. Long-term Outcome Predictions

Various anthropometric measures can be used to predict the development of long-term obesity-related complications, something that is currently practiced in clinical care. Longitudinal studies have demonstrated that adults with a high BMI (25–29.9 kg/m2) or a R-I at the time of obesity diagnosis have long-term dissatisfaction with the outcome. Utilizing more accurate tools that assess abdominal fat accumulation, such as R-ACT (or R-FOC), would enable surgeons to lower the threshold for surgical intervention in patients with a BMI of 25–29.9 kg/m2 or R-I that undergo concomitant reconstruction of a defect (Sefa-Yeboah et al., 2021). The risk of an unsatisfactory surgical weight loss outcome in patients with a compensatory defect is so high that it justifies all the concerns and criticism regarding the application of a low BMI threshold. We also demonstrated that the R-I score had higher predictive value than BMI alone. Consequently, we propose that adolescents with a BMI > 75th % percentile and an R-I value of 5 or more at the diagnosis of their obesity should be carefully followed up and considered for surgical treatment. Overtreatment with surgery always has implications for the patients and society on a larger scale. Accepting that the threshold for surgical obesity treatment is lower, most certainly implicates that a larger number of patients would undergo surgical therapy. It is reasonable to accept that the outcome for many selected patients is poor (Crompvoets et al., 2024). However, denying treatment to those patients healthy enough to undergo surgery may cause long-term detriment to them and society with respect to excess body weight, as presented in Table 2.

Table 2. AI in Obesity and Weight Management

AI Feature	Function	Impact on Obesity Management	Platform Example	Considerations	Reference
Smart Calorie Counters	Image recognition to log meals	Reduces manual food entry	Bite AI, Calorific	Accuracy of food detection	(Bak-Sosnowska, 2018)
AI Behavior Modeling	Analyzes habits and triggers	Tailor interventions for better results	Lark Health, Noom AI	May oversimplify psychological factors	(Panza et al., 2018)
Personalized AI Coaching	Recommends actions based on data	Improves adherence and outcomes	WW (Weight Watchers) AI Coach	Need for continued user engagement	(Henderson & Alexander, 2012)
Obesity Risk Classifiers	Classifies individuals by risk level	Enables preventive care	ML risk scoring at the Mayo Clinic	Ethical issues in labeling people	(Hwalla & Jaafar, 2021)
Virtual Nutritionists	Give AI-powered diet plans	Increases access to dietary advice	Nutrino, DietSensor	Generalization may not work for all groups	(Porri et al., 2024)
Emotion-Aware AI	Detects emotional eating patterns	Provides psychological insights	Wysa, Woebot + eating behavior tracking	Still experimental in clinical contexts	(Hernández-Mijares et al., 2013)
AI-Powered Sleep Trackers	Monitor sleep and suggest changes	Supports metabolic health and weight loss	SleepCycle + ML analytics	Sleep data may be affected by lifestyle variance	(Trouwborst et al., 2018)
Adaptive Exercise Plans	Create routines based on fitness level	Supports personalized physical activity	Freeletics AI Coach	Limited real-world condition modeling	(Konishi et al., 2024)
Genetics + AI Integration	Tailor's plans based on DNA	Precision nutrition for weight loss	Habit, Nutrigenomix	Privacy and cost of genetic testing	(Sefa-Yeboah et al., 2021)
Gut Microbiome + AI	Analyzes gut bacteria for diet matching	Promotes weight loss through gut balance	Viome AI	Scientific validity is still emerging	(Crompvoets et al., 2024)
Food Image AI	Tracks the type/ quantity of food via photo	Enhances the accuracy of food logs	SnapCalorie	Difficulty with mixed or ethnic dishes	(Zarkogianni et al., 2021)

continued on following page

Table 2. Continued

AI Feature	Function	Impact on Obesity Management	Platform Example	Considerations	Reference
AI Chat Support	Conversational tracking and feedback	Encourages daily progress tracking	Replika, Youper	May miss contextual emotional cues	(Power et al., 2024)
Long-Term Progress Prediction	Models weight loss trajectories	Helps set realistic goals	Fitbit Premium AI	Overreliance may reduce motivation	(Rodríguez et al., 2023)
Social AI Recommendation	Connects users with similar profiles	Fosters community and motivation	AI social matching in Noom	Privacy concerns in matching algorithms	(Bak-Sosnowska, 2018)

7. ETHICAL CONSIDERATIONS IN AI USE

The convergence of artificial intelligence with healthcare has brought to the forefront many non-technical considerations associated with the application of such systems into real-world scenarios. In the realm of diabetes management, AI has the potential to become a tool that revolutionizes preventive as well as corrective treatment of the condition. This potential can only be harnessed if patients or caretakers trust in AI systems is gained. Providers must utilize these systems in a way that is aligned with patient interests in advocating for safety and corrective care. If an AI-based diagnosis or treatment plan recommends a strategy contrary to prevailing standards, the question of liability will be paramount (Henderson & Alexander, 2012). Lawmakers must clearly define these liability statutes before society can fully embrace AI, which will likely exceed human capabilities. While these potential liability scenarios may seem insurmountable, they are no different than legal challenges posed by an autonomous vehicle or a new surgical robot. Diabetes management, be it through regulation of insulin levels in blood or maintenance of body mass index through a well-structured diet and physical regimen, relies heavily on the modes of data intake and interpretation. With this patient data, including blood glucose readings and probe results, being used during the algorithm development cycle, patient confidentiality and privacy must be ensured (Hwalla & Jaafar, 2021). Even if the collected data is stored anonymously on a server, a motivated entity can reverse-engineer actual patient identification based on contextual information or service used, prompting an ethical obligation on the part of system developers to safeguard patient integrity.

7.1. Data Privacy and Security

The rise of AI-enhanced technology in our everyday lives has intensified debates regarding data privacy and security. Many examples are given of purported invasions of privacy as people find AI-enhanced technology at the center of their lives. These discussions become even more deeply layered when looking at medical uses for AI-enhanced technology. The reader is invited to consider the privacy and data security concerns noted in the following paragraph, alongside the ethical discussions presented in the text. Technology for obtaining and using wearable physiological data is now ubiquitous, from basic smart watches to advanced wearable technology (Sefa-Yeboah et al., 2021). During data collection, sensitive physiological metrics are given in real-time, but what happens long-term to this data? Even in a hospital setting, such as data collection and analysis of abnormal heart variability given by vitals for diabetes patients undergoing surgery or the use of technology employing AI-enhanced technology for heart failure prediction, has vulnerabilities. The explicit use of technology to prevent cyber attacks on such hospital activity has also been invoked. As another potential example of a hospital implementation, that of AI-assisted CT scan COVID-19 assistance has been presented as providing acceptable downtime during paper dossier preparation, but what is the consequence of sensitive patient data going down without a secure path (Zarkogianni et al., 2021)? With the development of substantially novel technology and new approaches associated with AI-enhanced examination and monitoring of the human body, the real and potential issues surrounding data use, privacy, and sharing access are profound. Solutions for some of these issues are also considered, for example, technology for wearable devices. However, there is recognition that endeavoring to match various Privacy By Design goals, such as the centralization of data, may lead to compromise or conflict with others, such as use and disclosure. In addition, as collaborations between AI focus groups and healthcare academics, such as that of improving prediction of adverse outcomes, are noted for the ability to contribute substantial benefits, how this partnership evolves in terms of data sharing and access will reflect the advancement of AI with sufficient ethical governance (Panza et al., 2018).

7.2. Bias in AI Algorithms

Determining the causes of disease is essential for guiding proper treatment decisions and predicting clinical outcomes. However, despite growing interest in using AI and machine learning to identify the causes of chronic disease, such systems rarely provide insight into how decisions are made. Furthermore, many algorithms exist purely as "black boxes," creating unreliable detection modeling systems for symptoms. These valid and reliable assumptions have existed all along for detecting diabetes and obesity. These guidelines will allow AI systems to advance and achieve previously unattainable prediction and detection accuracy in diabetes and within other health topics (Henderson & Alexander, 2012). Bias is a concern in every area of AI research and development. This essay focuses on bias issues for health developers, researchers, and gives healthcare decision-makers considerations to reduce and remove algorithmic bias used by developers and researchers to further bias within AI systems. Some level of bias is unavoidable within algorithm-defined populations, including risk estimation, detection, or treatment decision populations. AI developers and researchers have biases or subjective assumptions when designing any AI algorithm (Porri et al., 2024). While it is commonly known that bias has a significant influence on how health-related 'crowds' make choices, it may or may not be used to change or remove algorithms for AI development. Algorithm bias originates from the data used in training. An AI algorithm only works as well as the data it receives for its input because datasets are not always fully representative of populations. Bias is introduced based on the proportions of subpopulations that were trained within a model (Hernández-Mijares et al., 2013). Model-reported clinical results only show the mean values from the entire population.

7.3. Patient Consent and Autonomy

With an increasing rollout of AI tools, it has become pertinent to consider how effectively AI tools may be incorporated into diabetes management and obesity care without a detriment to the patient-clinician relationship and mutual autonomy. Firstly, a major barrier to the effectiveness of these tools is patient consent. For predictive models to be effective, patients must consent to the model being invoked for high-risk stratification and must also consent to care pathways dictated by predicted diabetes or obesity risk scores (Bak-Sosnowska, 2018). Patients need to understand clearly how their data is being utilized and how scoring is ultimately beneficial to the management of diabetes or obesity risk. Additionally, cooperative goals between the patient and clinician should be developed that allow for shared decisions concerning health goals. Likewise, constant reinforcement of these AI use cases in the patient-provider interaction should be made to ensure continued patient buy-in, as an initial willingness to allow AI models into routine healthcare does not preclude a lapse in adherence to screening and monitoring protocols. Secondly, autonomy must be respected by AI tools in diabetes management and obesity care (Hwalla & Jaafar, 2021). We must contemplate how AI may factor into discussions regarding treatment selection. Tools must be developed that uphold the autonomy of diabetic patients in relation to their number of yearly A1c test monitoring. These tools should stimulate discussion between patient and clinician and allow for patient values to be heard in the context of these choices that dictate care. Additionally, we must strive for the equitable distribution of resources to control diabetes and obesity. Decision making regarding treatment initiation must be transparent, and current models should not disproportionately limit certain demographics of society from diabetes and obesity care or exacerbate already existent health disparities (Porri et al., 2024). Simultaneously, AI tools should seek to motivate participation in order to achieve diabetes and obesity goals with the least amount of participation on the part of the patient possible, as some demographics may not have the same access to technology and resources as the broader population.

8. CHALLENGES AND LIMITATIONS OF AI IN DIABETES AND OBESITY

AI is not without its challenges. These challenges cluster into three management categories: technical challenges, challenges of integrating AI into existing systems, and training challenges for healthcare providers. These challenges are described in three separate sections below. Technical challenges with AI in diabetes and obesity management arise in two primary areas: data-related challenges and AI engineering challenges. Data-related challenges arise from the management of large volumes of patient data generated by multiple devices, which will need to be securely stored long enough to test the validity of AI models and serve as ground truth for model training, and analyzed in real-time to provide decision support (Henderson & Alexander, 2012). These challenges are worsened by the fact that many of these devices use proprietary algorithms, meaning that not only are the physiological signals generated by different devices not transferable across devices, but also that the thresholds for abnormality (and by extension, action) likely differ by individual and are not clear. Furthermore, reliable, manageable explanations for the results that AI models provide are especially crucial in healthcare. Users will need to know that model predictions actually relate to and support clinically-meaningful hypotheses and are themselves generalizable, e.g., not based on a small, unrepresentative dataset of similar patients. Since model predictions need to be timely in order to be useful, challenges in AI engineering also require addressing (Porri et al., 2024). These challenges typically reside in the customized model inference pipelines that AI model developers create for each unique patient application context, each optimized multiple times. They involve training models on large datasets to perform well under changing application conditions and optimizing inference pipelines to meet demanding inference timing requirements on the small, ubiquitous devices that patients will carry to monitor their health. Even if AI solutions clear these technical hurdles, there are still barriers to adoption that will need to be overcome. For instance, AI solutions used in patient management need to be integrated with personalized management applications that deliver the model predictions to patients. These applications need to present predictions in an understandable and actionable manner so that patients trust and are motivated to use the predictions to inform their behavior (Brończyk-Puzoń et al., 2015). The applications also need to support the data communications protocols mandated by device management and monitoring regulations.

8.1. Technical Challenges

Although the area of AI in diabetic management and obesity has seen considerable growth in recent years, technical challenges remain. Data from disparate sources, such as medical health records, wearable sensors, and other heterogeneous digital environments, needs to be integrated. Many differences in existing data standards have resulted in significant challenges in the integration and interoperability of such data. In addition, the quality of the data can be poor, including incomplete or having numerous artifacts. There are issues of data privacy and selection bias, especially with data acquired from online communities (Hernández-Mijares et al., 2013). The area is still developing tools to conduct rigorous, generalizable research on unstructured datasets. The prediction of individual risk can present difficulties. For example, the majority of AI has been applied to prediction models detecting general associations, and may not be applicable to the individual. The prediction of cardiovascular disease, acute coronary syndrome, stroke, venous thromboembolism, and general COVID-related severity using AI offers great potential but considerable challenges, given the diversity of cause and effect underlying human illness. Outcomes of human disease are frequently found to be non-linear and affected by many factors at multiple levels; hence, the probability estimates for such predictions are often poor and not directly applicable at an individual level (Kaur et al., 2022; Konishi et al., 2024). In addition, serious legal and ethical issues can be associated with the application of AI algorithms in the personalization of risks.

8.2. Integration with Existing Systems

The integration of artificial intelligence (AI) and machine learning (ML) into existing healthcare systems is challenging but vital. AI-based tools will not be successful unless integrated with existing data flows. Healthcare providers deal with large amounts of health data every day. They track numerous clinical outcomes and population-level metrics. The success of AI/ML in clinical practice demands the integration of new predictive tools with dashboards that leverage ongoing data entry and monitoring. The commercial success of these new tools and models also depends upon their ability to interface with the existing and evolving electronic health record (EHR) and healthcare information technology (HIT) systems. Healthcare organizations have been slow in adopting novel AI technologies, primarily due to a lack of transparency, a lack of adequate validation, and an absence of proper implementation plans (Crompvoets et al., 2024). On one hand is the risk of 'AI effect,' where predictions of outcomes by AI tools are considered trivial once algorithms recognize AI tasks that require skills, perception, and cognition, mastered by healthcare professionals. Such premature success may lead to complacency instead of caution, discouraging continued investment and development in the field of health AI. On the other hand, there is a distrust of AI tools, especially deep learning algorithms, which do not provide explanations about how specific clinical decisions were derived. Given the high rate of litigation in some areas of healthcare practice, using a 'black box' AI tool to guide clinical decisions may be prone to medico-legal repercussions. At the same time, the increasing complexity of the AI pipeline and the difference in expertise between the AI engineers and engineers involved in installing, integrating, and interfacing AI technologies may lead to sub-optimal delivery, performance, and deployment of health AI tools (Zarkogianni et al., 2021).

8.3. Healthcare Provider Training

The role of healthcare providers is to reinforce key messages about diabetes management, motivate patients' behavior change, and provide support and advice through the process, guiding them toward resolution. The support of healthcare providers is paramount in the success of implementing digital technologies. So far, providers are not trained to make patients trust the technology. Lack of popularization generates fear towards how and what a patient can do with the tool and how it can be helpful. Nowadays, new technology can create distrust among some patients (Bak-Sosnowska, 2018). In order to have a good patient-provider relationship, both must trust each other. We believe that before training patients, providers should also receive some training about how it can help with diabetes management and obesity, training them to explain to patients the advantages that it brings to the synergy, that is that the patient is in constant monitoring with the healthcare provider where both make decisions in favor of the obesity problem or diabetes management. It can be an extra help, supporting both parts, helping them understand and anticipate micropatterns that otherwise would not be discovered without intelligence. Healthcare providers need to feel embraced by the tool and use its suggestions as an extra help during their decision process, and have full control of the decision process. There are already healthcare administration and management guidelines for controlling the amount of interference that technology should have during a medical consultation (Henderson & Alexander, 2012). Some guidelines explain that the decision should be the last resort during the consultation, but also that it has to suggest the right treatment in order for healthcare providers to accept its suggestions.

9. FUTURE DIRECTIONS IN AI FOR DIABETES AND OBESITY MANAGEMENT

The anticipated development of disruptive technologies, including wearables, microneedles, exosomes, and other nanotechnologies, augmented with AI, may help bridge many hurdles to treat diabetes and obesity. Large amounts of data coming from tamper-proof intelligent, non-invasive wearables/implants may lead to real-time symptom/crisis prediction and prevention, timely personalized therapeutics such as meal delivery/platforms paired with delivery devices, or even closed-loop personalized meal/drug delivery platforms combined with hypoglycemia prediction (BALFOUR, 2021). Technological and scientific advances in diabetes and obesity can be solved only by incorporating collective intelligence from scientists, regulators, industry, and patients, schools, universities, public health systems, and even corporations. A collaborative effort is essential to optimize people's health while keeping a balance with cultural, behavioral, and economic sustainability. All technological solutions should target the patients, minimizing the time, effort, and cost required for disease management. Patient-centred care must not include only patients, but relatives, caregivers, and clinicians, including all levels of health-complex care. Honest reward systems for health compliance must be embedded. By partially redistributing the benefits gained from the uptake of these technologies, the state could engage patients and families, who would also be rewarded for the improvements (Hernández-Mijares et al., 2013). Thus, companies should develop products not only to maximize their profit, but also to have a great impact on patients and the health system.

9.1. Emerging Technologies

Recent years have seen rapid advancements in technology innovations in medicine using Artificial Intelligence (AI). While AI has been used in the past to create algorithms for improved patient stratification using clinical data or to aid with prediction risk or prognosis, the future of AI in Medicine may focus on translational technology innovations such as Robotics integration into society or the use of ubiquitous sensors. The COVID-19 pandemic accelerated a host of these technologies, and some of these are now entering much of the fabric of society (Konishi et al., 2024). Continuous monitoring of patients using wearables is now possible through cost-effective sensors that patients can frequently reuse. While continuous glucose monitoring was already used for diabetes care, this technology is now being expanded to other analytes such as lactate, uric acid, and ketones. Similar systems have been developed for body composition analysis and blood pressure monitoring. Moreover, newer devices can now monitor sleep apnea through wearables, which is an important risk for MSD (Sefa-Yeboah et al., 2021). In tandem with wearables, improved AI-driven models for control systems are now being developed to better assess glycemia based on physiologic cues such as CGM, heart rate, breaths, body temperature, and circadian cycles. Parallelly, there have been improvements in the field of robotics, aided by AI. Robotics-assisted surgery, medical robots, and exoskeletons are becoming commonplace and show great promise in Supervise and Manage Diabetes (SMD) and other chronic diseases. While robotics-assisted surgery is used to lower morbidity and mortality for surgeries in diabetic patients, robotics-assisted physical rehabilitation is being explored not only to enhance rehabilitation for patients but also to augment glucose disposal through voluntary physical activities (Zarkogianni et al., 2021).

9.2. Collaborative Approaches

To optimize diabetes care in the technologically evolving healthcare landscape, we need to proactively foster collaborative practices for healthcare delivery that embrace novel technologies. With the rise of the participatory medicine movement, medical practice is moving from a paternalistic model of care towards a distributed and participatory model where the role of the patient is of equal importance with the healthcare team, assuming greater responsibility for their care – a model that may be suited both to controlling the chronicity of diabetes and to ultimately achieving a cure (Bak-Sosnowska, 2018). However, with growing concerns about burnout and moral injury of HCPs, it should not be a high expectation to consider patients as equal partners in the relationship throughout the whole course of diabetes. We should consider embedding people first, with thoughtful moments of shared decision-making built into a matrix of collaborative efforts, supported and nudged by AI-driven user-meaningful technologies to improve the already favorable collaborative participant-organization relationship further. Patient-clinician partnerships may be enabled, improved and supported by digitally designed interactive technologies predicting the patient's motivation, attitude, intent and factors associated, to synchronously trigger a virtuous cycle of engaging patients with tailored nudges and starting collaborative discussions about decisions for treatment selection, adherence and lifestyle modification aimed at harmonizing values, improving metabolic state and physical/mental outcomes (Rodríguez et al., 2023).

9.3. Patient-Centric Innovations

Emerging digital health technologies have the potential to increase patient engagement and self-management, and also to comply with healthcare pathways turned on patients. This last aspect is critical, as getting the trust of an engaged patient is very important for achieving successful digital transformations in healthcare and, therefore, linked to successful digital health solutions. Consumer acceptance, their level of trust, prior experiences, and their awareness towards health technology support systems are all factors that affect the change. Self-management of chronic diseases is the main focus of the new reshaping future of healthcare (Hwalla & Jaafar, 2021). Patients will be committed to managing their diseases in order to allow healthcare systems to manage scarce resources. To help patients share their outcomes with clinicians, sensing solutions have been proposed to provide continuous information over everyday activities, especially related to glycemic levels. Such experiences would create a collaborative care process, allowing clinicians to provide personalized care by continuously honing treatment choices and also by predicting diabetes risk. A patient-centered approach for designing digital solutions is key to favoring the adoption and later the adherence to the new technology. The unique needs, concerns, and abilities must be addressed. It is essential to partner with the end-users as they interact with the systems for the creation and optimization of the human-computer interaction design (Porri et al., 2024). By including patient feedback throughout the development cycle, the potential impact of biases that increase user frustration can be discovered early. Moreover, a patient-centered philosophy is essential to ensure potential user acceptance, improve usability, and assist self-management during the later-utilization phase. To further implement these principles during the system's design, the healthcare community must also be actively involved. This enables the establishment of respective conditions at the organizational level, which allow for a more seamless integration of the applications into a chronic care model. In addition, it helps to promote awareness about the opportunities offered by self-management solutions among the healthcare community and patients, which is important for their long-term use among patients suffering from diabetes and obesity (Bak-Sosnowska, 2018).

10. CASE STUDIES AND REAL-WORLD APPLICATIONS

This chapter features various implementations of AI in diabetes and obesity. The key development stages for AI to engage in medical use and therefore health system adoption are the scientific validation through clinical trials, regulatory approval, reimbursement, and integration into doctors' workflows. The approval or endorsement from health authorities increases the reliability of the technology and consequently the acceptance by the health system. Healthcare apps integrated into a healthcare system with proper data transfer protocols are likely to be used for a longer period. For doctors working with the personal health information of patients, the security and approval are important aspects as well (Panza et al., 2018). The chapter concludes with an outlook on future research-driven tools that utilize AI to increase the understanding of diseases substantially. Many private enterprises have already developed successful products by implementing them in daily clinical routines. One company won endorsement for predictive analytics about type 1 diabetes in children. Another helps adults and children alike to master their everyday life with type 2 diabetes along the lines of motivational interviews with feedback reminders and decision-making support. A promising watch has been developed to detect seizures in children who are affected by the health-threatening comorbidity, epilepsy (Rodríguez et al., 2023). Such predictive watches are not AI-driven per se, but rather rely on classical methods of machine learning. An explanation of machine learning has been given elsewhere in this essay. Another company targets adults for sensors attached to inhalers for asthma or COPD to gauge the health condition with sound clinical features, while not weighing the users down. Detecting respiratory health threats without active engagement of the users might be a game-changer. As for obesity, some companies try to capitalize on social features to further healthy nutrition in people who suffer from obesity (Power et al., 2024).

10.1. Successful AI Implementations

70% of adults in the US are overweight, and 40% are classified as obesity. With the rising costs of health care spending, where costs related directly to overweight and obesity are around 240 billion USD annually, there is a nationwide need for intervention. Major issues to consider when working with diabetes and obesity are self-care, motivation, support, and education. These can be improved with the use of artificial intelligence, virtual communities, and social networks. In the following sections, we present some successful interventions and applications using AI either as the major driving force behind the application or in conjunction with other forces. Weight loss apps provide real-time input to users regarding their activity, motivation, and education, feed them with healthy meal choices, and connect them with a support network (Henderson & Alexander, 2012). The apps may or may not be backed by expert counselors or psychologists. With such a plethora of apps, it isn't easy to decide which app to use and whether there are any benefits from one app over another. What is certain is that AI is already being increasingly used to improve older solutions and build new solutions to help manage diabetes and obesity. In 2015 alone, there were more than 313 million downloads of mobile apps to help manage obesity, diabetes, and other chronic diseases. To help steer diabetes technologies, it is necessary to share best and worst practices from a technology design, implementation, and business perspective. It is necessary to share how real-world data and conversations may help facilitate solution development (Hwalla & Jaafar, 2021). We show some successful examples from various options above, and hope that more examples will come in the future. Many AI-based solutions will never leave the pages of a research paper.

10.2. Lessons Learned from Failures

We present some common lessons learned from struggling systems. Early AI research struggled in curing diabetes, creating completely synthetic swine pancreas, building soft robots for diabetes tasks, and discovering molecular DNAs and elements invisible to lower microscopes. In many cases, no real-world systems or techniques were scalable and performed for every diabetes user. With hindsight, we found that such systems failed for reasons such as: problems were hard, real-world data was not available, prediction was too hard, using knowledge bases such as disease ontologies help, not all biological diabetic patients are the same, and the philosophies and human bottlenecks were not solved (Porri et al., 2024). With hindsight, we realize that some diabetes research problems were so hard that the correct representations of some problems, or the right solutions, mappings, transformations on the data, were so hard, or the algorithms, functions, or mappings were so hard that the task may be intrinsically very hard. For example, it would take a miracle in the correct understanding of what the correct representation is for discovering molecules and elements invisible to lower microscopes (Konishi et al., 2024). For any solution to scale in the real world, the solutions had to be good enough solutions, not only approximate, but also user-centered solutions. Also, any system had to work closely with humans while executing the problem tasks in actual human settings. Thus, a diabetes task-identifying system, solution, or AI agent had to be assistive or augmentative to humans and work seamlessly with humans in human-centered real-world tasks. Any prediction task would tend to be very hard to automate, as humans have their unique peculiarities and are unpredictable in many tasks (Crompvoets et al., 2024; Henderson & Alexander, 2012).

11. CONCLUSION

Among NCDs, diabetes is recognized as one of the major risk factors for obesity, and obesity is also a risk factor for other conditions, including type 2 diabetes. Obesity can be identified when there is excess fat accumulation. The most common measure of obesity is BMI, a ratio between weight and height, but fat distribution is also important. The wide availability of AI-based devices and apps suggests a promising convergence that has attracted international attention. Effective use of continuous glucose level data in diabetes management can help promote the dissemination of usage of AI usage. Furthermore, these devices often have other functions or are integrated with devices that measure steps, heart rate, sleep, etc. Obesity and diabetes management a multi-dimensional issues. Daily lifestyle factors, especially energy intake and exercise, play a critical role in the growing epidemic, while environmental factors limit interventions on both. Health institutions, the food industry, local governments, and society in general need to work together to find new solutions. AI technology is expected to facilitate the collection and sharing of vast amounts of data and to connect users to communities for mutual support. Innovative applications that quantify risks through intelligent environment-aided technologies in smart cities, embedded sensor networks, social participation networks, and smart wearable devices can help individuals and industries to break through the stagnation of available effective methods. Artificial intelligence has fueled hopes worldwide that novel AI-based strategies can, and will, lead us to solving tough-to-crack long-standing local-or-global-scale unattractive-and-serious problems and challenges in the evolving modern society, including massively-blacklisted impacts of overweight and obesity on poor-quality health and its long-term global implications. Society as a whole must deal with and combat the problem of the epidemic of overweight and obesity, using every possible approach.

REFERENCES

Aas, A. M., Axelsen, M., Churuangsuk, C., Hermansen, K., Kendall, C. W. C., Kahleova, H., Khan, T., Lean, M. E. J., Mann, J. I., Pedersen, E., Pfeiffer, A., Rahelić, D., Reynolds, A. N., Risérus, U., Rivellese, A. A., Salas-Salvadó, J., Schwab, U., Sievenpiper, J. L., Thanopoulou, A., & Uusitupa, E. M. (2023). Evidence-based European recommendations for the dietary management of diabetes. *Diabetologia*, *66*(6). Advance online publication. DOI: 10.1007/s00125-023-05894-8

Adesina, N., Dogan, H., Green, S., & Tsofliou, F. (2022). Effectiveness and usability of digital tools to support dietary self-management of gestational diabetes mellitus: A systematic review. In *Nutrients* (Vol. 14, Issue 1). https://doi.org/DOI: 10.3390/nu14010010

Ahmad, A., & Mehfuz, S. (2022). *Explainable AI-based early detection of diabetes for smart healthcare*. https://doi.org/DOI: 10.1049/icp.2022.0608

Alkhatib, A. (2020). Personalising Exercise and Nutrition Behaviours in Diabetes Lifestyle Prevention. *European Medical Journal*. Advance online publication. DOI: 10.33590/emj/19-00139

Andrès, E., Meyer, L., Zulfiqar, A. A., Hajjam, M., Talha, S., Bahougne, T., Ervé, S., Hajjam, J., Doucet, J., Jeandidier, N., & El Hassani, A. H. (2019). Telemonitoring in diabetes: evolution of concepts and technologies, with a focus on results of the more recent studies. *Journal of Medicine and Life, 2019*(3). https://doi.org/DOI: 10.25122/jml-2019-0006

Bak-Sosnowska, M. (2018). The level of anxiety in women seeking professional support in reduction of excessive weight. *Obesity Facts*, ●●●, 11.

BALFOUR, C. (2021). OBESITY IN AVIATION MEDICINE. *The Journal of the Australasian Society of Aerospace Medicine*, *12*(1). Advance online publication. DOI: 10.21307/asam-2020-001

Brończyk-Puzoń, A., Piecha, D., Nowak, J., Koszowska, A., Kulik-Kupka, K., Dittfeld, A., & Zubelewicz-Szkodzińska, B. (2015). Guidelines for dietary management of menopausal women with simple obesity. In *Przeglad Menopauzalny* (Vol. 14, Issue 1). https://doi.org/DOI: 10.5114/pm.2015.48678

Bul, K., Holliday, N., Bhuiyan, M. R. A., Clark, C. C. T., Allen, J., & Wark, P. A. (2023). Usability and Preliminary Efficacy of an Artificial Intelligence-Driven Platform Supporting Dietary Management in Diabetes: Mixed Methods Study. *JMIR Human Factors*, *10*. Advance online publication. DOI: 10.2196/43959

Crompvoets, P. I., Nieboer, A. P., van Rossum, E. F. C., & Cramm, J. M. (2024). Perceived weight stigma in healthcare settings among adults living with obesity: A cross-sectional investigation of the relationship with patient characteristics and person-centred care. *Health Expectations*, *27*(1). Advance online publication. DOI: 10.1111/hex.13954

Cushley, L. N., Krezel, A., Curran, K., Parker, K., Millar, S., & Peto, T. (2023). Influences on technology use and interpretation among young people living with type 1 diabetes. *Lifestyle Medicine*, *4*(1). Advance online publication. DOI: 10.1002/lim2.73

Dankwa-Mullan, I., Rivo, M., Sepulveda, M., Park, Y., Snowdon, J., & Rhee, K. (2019). Transforming Diabetes Care Through Artificial Intelligence: The Future Is Here. *Population Health Management*, *22*(3). Advance online publication. DOI: 10.1089/pop.2018.0129

Dewi Yudhani, R., Nurwening Sholikhah, E., Aris Agung Nugrahaningsih, D., & Primaningtyas, W. (2022). The bidirectional interaction between climate change and type 2 diabetes burden. *IOP Conference Series. Earth and Environmental Science*, *1016*(1). Advance online publication. DOI: 10.1088/1755-1315/1016/1/012054

Dimitriades, M. E., & Pillay, K. (2021). Dietary management practices for type 1 diabetes mellitus by dietitians in Kwazulu-Natal. *Health SA Gesondheid*, *26*. Advance online publication. DOI: 10.4102/hsag.v26i0.1506

Henderson, J., & Alexander, S. (2012). e-Learning – The future of child and adolescent obesity! *Obesity Research & Clinical Practice*, *6*. Advance online publication. DOI: 10.1016/j.orcp.2012.08.153

Hernández-Mijares, A., Bañuls, C., Gómez-Balaguer, M., Bergoglio, M., Víctor, V. M., & Rocha, M. (2013). Influence of obesity on atherogenic dyslipidemia in women with polycystic ovary syndrome. *European Journal of Clinical Investigation*, *43*(6). Advance online publication. DOI: 10.1111/eci.12080

Hwalla, N., & Jaafar, Z. (2021). Dietary management of obesity: A review of the evidence. In *Diagnostics* (Vol. 11, Issue 1). https://doi.org/DOI: 10.3390/diagnostics11010024

Hwalla, N., Jaafar, Z., & Sawaya, S. (2021). Dietary management of type 2 diabetes in the mena region: A review of the evidence. In *Nutrients* (Vol. 13, Issue 4). https://doi.org/DOI: 10.3390/nu13041060

Kaur, R., Kumar, R., & Gupta, M. (2022). Predicting risk of obesity and meal planning to reduce the obese in adulthood using artificial intelligence. *Endocrine*, *78*(3). Advance online publication. DOI: 10.1007/s12020-022-03215-4

Khattak, M., & Rehman, A. ur, Muqaddas, T., Hussain, R., Rasool, M. F., Saleem, Z., Almalki, M. S., Alturkistani, S. A., Firash, S. Z., Alzahrani, O. M., Bahauddin, A. A., Abuhussain, S. A., Najjar, M. F., Elsabaa, H. M. A., & Haseeb, A. (2024). Tuberculosis (TB) treatment challenges in TB-diabetes comorbid patients: A systematic review and meta-analysis. *Annals of Medicine*, *56*(1). Advance online publication. DOI: 10.1080/07853890.2024.2313683

Konishi, K., Nakagawa, H., Asaoka, T., Kasamatsu, Y., Goto, T., & Shirano, M. (2024). Brief communication: Body composition and hidden obesity in people living with HIV on antiretroviral therapy. *AIDS Research and Therapy*, *21*(1). Advance online publication. DOI: 10.1186/s12981-024-00599-3

Lakey, J. R., Casazza, K., Lernhardt, W., Mathur, E. J., & Jenkins, I. (2024). Machine Learning and Augmented Intelligence Enables Prognosis of Type 2 Diabetes Prior to Clinical Manifestation. *Current Diabetes Reviews*, *20*. Advance online publication. DOI: 10.2174/0115733998276990240117113408

Liu, Y., Yu, D., Luo, J., Cai, S., Ye, P., Yao, Z., Luo, M., & Zhao, L. (2022). Self-Reported Dietary Management Behaviors and Dietary Intake among Chinese Adults with Diabetes: A Population-Based Study. *Nutrients*, *14*(23). Advance online publication. DOI: 10.3390/nu14235178

Neblett, D. A., & Kennedy-Malone, L. (2024). Establishing and Affirming Social Connections: Recruiting Non-Hispanic Black Adults with Type 2 Diabetes. *Clinical Nursing Research*, *33*(5). Advance online publication. DOI: 10.1177/10547738231216530

Panza, G. A., Armstrong, L. E., Taylor, B. A., Puhl, R. M., Livingston, J., & Pescatello, L. S. (2018). Weight bias among exercise and nutrition professionals: a systematic review. In *Obesity Reviews* (Vol. 19, Issue 11). https://doi.org/DOI: 10.1111/obr.12743

Pongrac Barlovic, D., Harjutsalo, V., & Groop, P. H. (2022). Exercise and nutrition in type 1 diabetes: Insights from the FinnDiane cohort. In *Frontiers in Endocrinology* (Vol. 13). https://doi.org/DOI: 10.3389/fendo.2022.1064185

Porri, D., Morabito, L. A., Cavallaro, P., La Rosa, E., & Li, P. A., Pepe, G., & Wasniewska, M. (2024). Time to act on childhood obesity: the use of technology. In *Frontiers in Pediatrics* (Vol. 12). https://doi.org/DOI: 10.3389/fped.2024.1359484

Power, T. G., Baker, S. S., Barale, K. V., Aragón, M. C., Lanigan, J. D., Parker, L., Garcia, K. S., Auld, G., Micheli, N., & Hughes, S. O. (2024). Using Mobile Technology for Family-Based Prevention in Families with Low Incomes: Lessons from a Randomized Controlled Trial of a Childhood Obesity Prevention Program. *Prevention Science*, *25*(2). Advance online publication. DOI: 10.1007/s11121-023-01637-8

Rodríguez, N. R., Cote, L., Fuentes, C., Jaramillo, E., Arana, S., Castro, A., Behrens, E., Ramos, A., & Zerrweck, C. (2023). First National Consensus on the Safe Practice of Medical Tourism for Bariatric Surgery in Mexico. *Obesity Surgery*, *33*(4). Advance online publication. DOI: 10.1007/s11695-023-06468-8

Salinas Martínez, A. M., Juárez Montes, A. G., Ramírez Morado, Y., Cordero Franco, H. F., Guzmán de la Garza, F. J., Hernández Oyervides, L. C., & Núñez Rocha, G. M. (2023). Idealistic, realistic, and unrealistic expectations of pharmacological treatment in persons with type 2 diabetes in primary care. *Frontiers in Public Health*, *11*. Advance online publication. DOI: 10.3389/fpubh.2023.1058828

Sefa-Yeboah, S. M., Osei Annor, K., Koomson, V. J., Saalia, F. K., Steiner-Asiedu, M., & Mills, G. A. (2021). Development of a Mobile Application Platform for Self-Management of Obesity Using Artificial Intelligence Techniques. *International Journal of Telemedicine and Applications*, *2021*. Advance online publication. DOI: 10.1155/2021/6624057

Shamanna, P., Saboo, B., Damodharan, S., Mohammed, J., Mohamed, M., Poon, T., Kleinman, N., & Thajudeen, M. (2020). Reducing HbA1c in Type 2 Diabetes Using Digital Twin Technology-Enabled Precision Nutrition: A Retrospective Analysis. *Diabetes Therapy : Research, Treatment and Education of Diabetes and Related Disorders*, *11*(11). Advance online publication. DOI: 10.1007/s13300-020-00931-w

Steiner, G., Geissler, B., & Schernhammer, E. S. (2019). Hunger and obesity as symptoms of non-sustainable food systems and malnutrition. In *Applied Sciences (Switzerland)* (Vol. 9, Issue 6). https://doi.org/DOI: 10.3390/app9061062

Tang, T., Seddigh, S., Halbe, E., & Vesco, A. (2023). IDF2022-0929 TRIFECTA: Examining three digital health strategies to improve mental health outcomes in adults with type 1 diabetes. *Diabetes Research and Clinical Practice*, *197*. Advance online publication. DOI: 10.1016/j.diabres.2023.110357

Trouwborst, I., Verreijen, A., Memelink, R., Massanet, P., Boirie, Y., Weijs, P., & Tieland, M. (2018). Exercise and nutrition strategies to counteract sarcopenic obesity. In *Nutrients* (Vol. 10, Issue 5). https://doi.org/DOI: 10.3390/nu10050605

Udogadi, N. S., Onyenibe, N. S., & Abdullahi, M. K. (2019). Dietary Management of Diabetes Mellitus with Focus on Nigeria. *International Journal of Diabetes Research*, 2(1).

Vasiloglou, M. (2021). Comparison of novel and traditional dietary assessment methods in diabetes patients. *Diabetes Technology and Therapeutics, 23*(SUPPL 2).

Wilson, C. A., Newham, J., Rankin, J., Ismail, K., Simonoff, E., Reynolds, R. M., Stoll, N., & Howard, L. M. (2022). Systematic review and meta-analysis of risk of gestational diabetes in women with preconception mental disorders. In *Journal of Psychiatric Research* (Vol. 149). https://doi.org/DOI: 10.1016/j.jpsychires.2022.03.013

Yao, M., Lin, K., Fan, J., Ji, X., Wang, Y., Dong, A., Han, X., Qi, J., Chi, C., Haroon, S., Jackson, D., Cheng, K. K., & Lehman, R. (2024). Design and Development of Communication Skills Training in Diabetes Care for General Practitioners in China. *Chinese General Practice*, 27(7). Advance online publication. DOI: 10.12114/j.issn.1007-9572.2022.0900

Zarkogianni, K., Athanasiou, M., Mitsis, K., Chatzidaki, E., Polychronaki, N., Perakis, K., Vergeti, D., Antonopoulou, D., Papachristou, E., Chioti, V., Voutetakis, A., Kalafatis, E., Pervanidou, P., Kanaka-Gantenbein, C., & Nikita, K. (2021). A comprehensive approach to empower self-management of health in childhood obesity based on gamification mechanisms and biofeedback. *Diabetes Technology and Therapeutics, 23*(SUPPL 2).

Zheng, Y., Campbell Rice, B., Melkus, G. D., Sun, M., Zweig, S., Jia, W., Parekh, N., He, H., Zhang, Y. L., & Wylie-Rosett, J. (2023). Dietary Self-Management Using Mobile Health Technology for Adults With Type 2 Diabetes: A Scoping Review. In *Journal of Diabetes Science and Technology* (Vol. 17, Issue 5). https://doi.org/DOI: 10.1177/19322968231174038

KEY TERMS AND DEFINITIONS

AI in Nutritional Tracking: Tools using image recognition and machine learning to log and evaluate food intake.

AI-Powered Wearables: Smart devices that collect physiological data and use AI to interpret it for health insights.

Automated Insulin Delivery: AI-based closed-loop systems that calculate and deliver insulin doses in real time.

Behavioral Pattern Analysis: AI analysis of user behavior to optimize interventions for better weight and diabetes outcomes.

Clinical Decision Support Systems (CDSS): AI tools aiding healthcare professionals in making informed treatment decisions.

Digital Twin in Healthcare: Virtual replicas of patients created using AI to simulate metabolic behavior and disease progression.

Glucose Monitoring AI: AI systems are used to analyze glucose levels in real-time for personalized diabetes management.

Lifestyle Recommendations: AI-generated personalized advice on diet, sleep, and physical activity for weight and diabetes control.

Obesity Risk Prediction: AI algorithms trained to identify individuals at risk of obesity using biometric and lifestyle data.

Personalized Weight Loss Algorithms: AI models tailored to an individual's genetics, lifestyle, and metabolic profile for sustainable weight loss.

Predictive Analytics: AI-powered forecasting of blood sugar fluctuations and obesity risks based on historical and real-time data.

Telehealth Integration: The use of AI to support virtual diabetes and weight management consultations and monitoring.

Chapter 7
Role of Artificial Intelligence in Medical Imaging

Harmanpreet Kaur
https://orcid.org/0009-0002-3166-550X
Chitkara University, India

Gurwinder Singh
Panjab University, India

ABSTRACT

Artificial Intelligence (AI) is revolutionizing the world of computer science with its power and disruptive potential of completely changing the ways medical profession serves the humanity and healthcare sector. The use of AI in medicine has already begun changing the way the prevention, diagnosis, treatment, amelioration, and other physical and mental impairments are done. We may anticipate much more revolutionary developments as technology develops, which will significantly change the field of medical imaging and artificial intelligence in the years to come. The main goal addressed in this chapter is to acquaint researchers with the capacities of AI and its medical applications, as well as with the dangers that may lie ahead. This chapter presents recent advancements in the use of AI in healthcare, outlines challenges, legal/ethical considerations and future implications of AI in healthcare for creating safe and successful AI systems. In general, researchers might utilize the study as a reference manual for continuing advancements in research in pertinent realms of applications.

DOI: 10.4018/979-8-3373-3196-6.ch007

1. INTRODUCTION

Artificial Intelligence (AI) is the scientific and technological method of creating autonomous devices primarily by means of algorithms or rules that the machine obeys in order to simulate cognitive processes like acquiring knowledge and tackling issues that are common to humans. AI systems are capable of anticipating problems or addressing them as they arise, allowing them to function in a deliberate, intelligent, and adaptable way. The prowess of artificial intelligence lies in its capacity to acquire knowledge and identify correlations and configurations from extensive multidimensional and multimodal data sets. For instance, AI technology has the potential to transform a patient's comprehensive medical history into a singular value that encapsulates a probable diagnosis. Furthermore, AI systems are perpetually evolving and self-governing; they learn and adjust in response to new data and the study of AI, focuses on creating intelligent entities—machines that can decide how to comport themselves prudently and intelligently in a wide range of unanticipated surroundings(Hamet, 2017; Gupta, 2021).

With regard to prospective uses in illness identification, therapy suggestions, and feedback from patients, this chapter offers a thorough and current summary of the state of AI in healthcare. It also addresses the difficulties that come with it, including the necessity for human competence as well as ethical and legal issues. Thereby, it helps healthcare organizations use AI technology more successfully and raises awareness of the importance of AI in healthcare (Wubineh, 2023). As a result, the following primary research questions are established for this work:

1. What are the various ways in which AI technology is utilized in the healthcare sector?
2. How does the extensive integration of AI in the healthcare sector give rise to social, ethical, legal, and trust issues?
3. How much do the advantages and disadvantages of these methods rely on the particular situation in which they are used?
4. What are the main areas of research in healthcare that are currently under exploration or should be explored further?

The purpose of this chapter is to disseminate knowledge and increase public awareness of AI in the healthcare industry, with the goal of assisting decision systems in operating prospectively and giving patients an early prognosis. Thus, the following is a list of this chapter's primary contributions:

1. To help with the comprehension of the frontier concepts, an outline and historical context of AI technology are provided.

2. To help researchers expand their perspectives on AI techniques by highlighting the practicability of applications based on AI across multiple real-world application domains.
3. To offer a comprehensive evaluation of the efficacy and suitability of AI technology for healthcare applications in addition to a comparative review of all the latest works that apply the AI paradigm to a wide range of tasks in healthcare.
4. To discuss thoroughly the ethical, legal, and trust challenges in the context of AI in medical systems to enhance consumer comprehension and potentially boost confidence among citizens in the technology.
5. To identify and enumerate the possible research challenges that fall inside the purview of our investigation in order to guide future research, development, and optimization efforts.

Renowned archival sites like arXiv and reputable publishers like IEEE, Elsevier, PubMed, SpringerLink, Taylor & Francis, Nature are the sources of the references evaluated and discussed in this work. Additionally, the terms "artificial intelligence," "machine learning," "deep learning," "AI applications in healthcare," "AI ethics in healthcare," "computer vision," "AI for healthcare and medicine," "DL for healthcare and medicine," serve a purpose to identify the relevant references. Furthermore, only search results pertaining to the use of AI in healthcare were taken into account. The articles covering the previous couple of years of pertinent literature were chosen based on publications since 2017. This specific amount time frame was selected to encompass the absolute most current, thorough, and pertinent developments in artificial intelligence applications.

The rest of the chapter is structured in different sections. Section 2 provides the overview of artificial intelligence's history, understands the relation between Artificial Intelligence (AI), Machine learning (ML) and Deep learning (DL), and explores potential applications in the current study domain. Further, Section 3 explores several AI-powered applications to be promisingly deployed in the world of healthcare. Then an overview of AI's current research in the last 7 years' time frame is provided followed by a discussion on legal and ethical challenges of AI in healthcare. Then, the chapter discusses some possible future research directions for the development of AI in healthcare in Section 4. Finally, the last section concludes the chapter.

2. RELATION BETWEEN AI, ML AND DL

AI or machine intelligence (Sarker, 2022) encompasses the discipline of computer science focused on empowering machines to execute tasks requiring intelligence, typically performed by humans. AI technologies, such as specialized algorithms, enable computers and machines to comprehend, analyze, and derive insights from data. AI comprises various specialized areas like machine learning and deep learning, which enhance application intelligence either independently or synergistically. Machine learning (ML) (Sarker, 2021a), a subfield of computational intelligence involves algorithms that enable computer systems to enhance their performance autonomously based on experience. ML can be segmented into categories like supervised, unsupervised, and reinforcement learning (RL), with extensive ongoing research in sub-fields like semi-supervised, self-supervised, and multi-instance learning. Deep learning (DL) (Sarker, 2021b), a subset of machine learning, employs complex multilayer artificial neural networks to tackle intricate problems. "Deep" in deep learning signifies the utilization of multiple hierarchical stages to refine and enhance data, resulting in the creation of data-informed models. Deep learning algorithms find application in various domains such as autonomous vehicles, fraud prevention, healthcare, entertainment, language translation, and virtual personal assistants. Both Machine learning and deep learning are fundamental components of artificial intelligence that pave the way for creating intelligent systems and streamlining automated processes. Figure 1 shows the roles that machine learning and deep learning play in the field of artificial intelligence.

2.1 Historical perspective

AI in healthcare has changed considerably during the last five decades.

Advancements in ML and DL have led to the expansion of healthcare applications, enabling personalized medicine on top of algorithm-based approaches. Such models have prospective uses for diagnosing illnesses, treatment outcome prediction, and wellness prevention in the future thereby enhancing diagnostic accuracy, efficiency, disease monitoring, procedure accuracy, and patient outcomes (Kaul, 2020; Zhang 2021). The AI platform in medicine has evolved over time and is organized by key phases of transition as shown in Figure 2. During the 1930s, Alan Turing

Figure 1. Relation between Artificial Intelligence, Machine Learning and Deep Learning

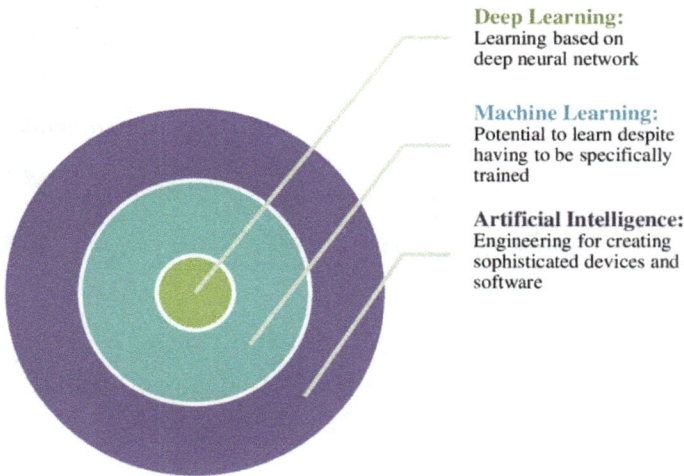

Deep Learning:
Learning based on deep neural network

Machine Learning:
Potential to learn despite having to be specifically trained

Artificial Intelligence:
Engineering for creating sophisticated devices and software

created the first Turing machines designed for automated intelligent mathematical computations, marking the initial steps towards the development of AI technology. The field of AI emerged as an academic discipline in the 1950s, sparking significant research in various areas such as natural language processing, learning, reasoning, and knowledge representation. In 1964, Joseph Weizenbaum introduced Eliza, the world's pioneering chatterbot, at the MIT AI Laboratory. Eliza operated by identifying keywords in the input text and formulating responses based on predefined reassembly rules, presenting text-based interactions that could simulate conversations with a human therapist.

The rise of AI with proven medical uses gained momentum in the 1970s. Saul Amarel at Rutgers University laid the groundwork for research resources on computers in medicine in 1971. The inception of INTERNIST-1 in the same year marked a significant milestone as the first artificial medical advisor globally. The tool used a search algorithm to determine therapeutic diagnoses by investigating the symptoms reported by patients. In 1986, the University of Massachusetts launched DXplain, a decision assistance system. This application generates a plurality of diagnoses based on the symptoms provided and functions as an electronic medical textbook, with thorough descriptions of ailments and extra references. The commencement of the contemporary era in the 2000s marked significant advancements in AI, particularly in its utilization in healthcare and everyday human activities. IBM's creation of the question-answering system, Watson, in 2007 showcased remarkable capabilities by outperforming leading contestants on the TV show Jeopardy. DeepQA, a component of Watson, employed language processing to analyze data across various contexts and extract information from diverse sources to formulate responses. This breakthrough expanded the scope of applications in healthcare, enabling inputs beyond mere symptoms and facilitating more intricate diagnostic outcomes.

Figure 2. Timeframe of the development and use of artificial intelligence in healthcare

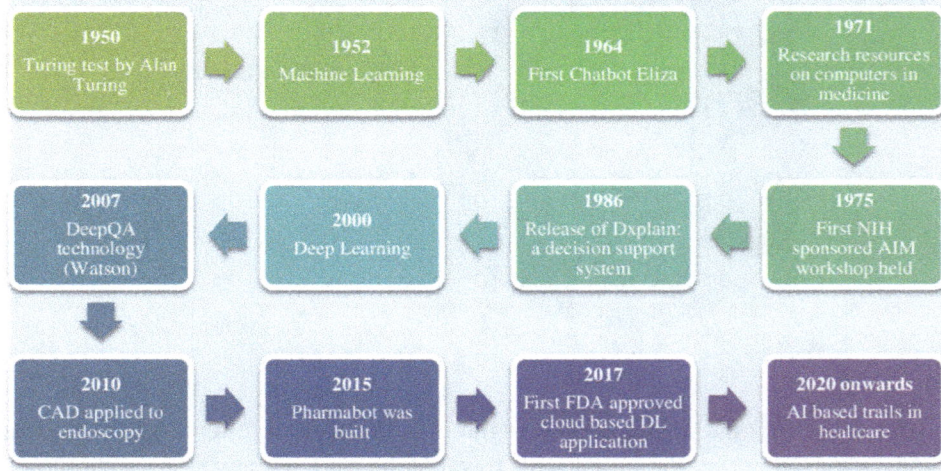

1950 Turing test by Alan Turing	1952 Machine Learning	1964 First Chatbot Eliza	1971 Research resources on computers in medicine
2007 DeepQA technology (Watson)	2000 Deep Learning	1986 Release of Dxplain: a decision support system	1975 First NIH sponsored AIM workshop held
2010 CAD applied to endoscopy	2015 Pharmabot was built	2017 First FDA approved cloud based DL application	2020 onwards AI based trails in healtcare

AI research further progressed, emphasizing Natural Language Processing (NLP) and computer vision, culminating in the development of virtual assistants like Apple's Siri (2011) and Amazon's Alexa (2014), capable of interpreting natural language and fulfilling user requests proficiently. Pharmabot was a chatbot built in 2015 to aid in understanding medications for paediatric patients as well as their guardians. In the year 2017, the Watson methodology succeeded in detecting RNA binding proteins which were connected alongside amyotrophic lateral sclerosis.A convolutional neural network (CNN) is a deep learning system that mimics the behaviour of linked neurones in the human brain. CNN algorithms now accessible include Le-NET, AlexNet, VGG, GoogLeNet, and ResNet. Hence, DL represented a significant leap in AI in healthcare as unlike ML, DL can automatically classify data without human intervention (Gupta, 2021; Kaul, 2020).

2.2 Types of AI

Artificial intelligence (AI) is predominantly concerned with understanding and executing intelligent tasks like cognition, learning new skills, and adjusting to novel circumstances and obstacles. AI is recognized as a field within science and engineering that concentrates on replicating a broad spectrum of aspects and operations found in human intelligence. Constructing a successful AI model poses a significant challenge due to the fluidity and heterogeneity of real-world scenarios and data. Nevertheless, an effective approach to comprehending the various types of AI is by analyzing three comprehensive classifications: AI based on capabilities, AI based on functionalities and AI based on usabilities (Sarker, 2022), with each type offering potential resolutions to diverse practical issues. Various types of AI explored in terms of computing and real-world services are shown in Figure 3.

Figure 3. Various categories of artificial intelligence

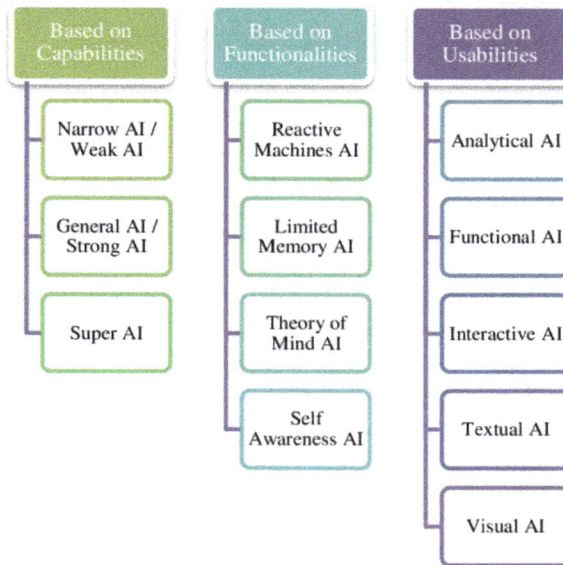

2.2.1 AI based on capabilities

- Narrow AI: Narrow AI, commonly referred to as artificial narrow intelligence (ANI) or weak AI and pertains to AI systems that are specifically programmed to execute precise tasks or instructions. These technologies are focused on excelling in a single cognitive function and are unable to autonomously acquire proficiencies beyond their predefined scope. Typically, they employ machine learning and neural network algorithms to accomplish these designated assignments.For example, natural language processing is a form of narrow AI since it can understand and react to spoken commands yet fails to execute additional tasks. AI virtual assistants, self-driving cars, and visual recognition application software are a few instances of narrow AI.

- General AI: General AI, known as artificial general intelligence (AGI) or strong AI refers to AI systems that possess the capacity to learn, reason, and execute a diverse set of tasks akin to human beings. The primary objective behind developing AGI is to produce machines that can competently handle a variety of functions and function as human-like, highly intelligent aids in day-to-day activities.

- Super AI: Super intelligent artificial intelligence or Super AI surpasses human intellect in problem-solving, creativity, and various skills, and has the capacity to cultivate its own emotions, desires, needs, and beliefs, enabling it to autonomously make decisions and address challenges.

2.2.2 AI based on functionalities

- Reactive Machine AI: Reactive machines, considered as AI systems with lacking memory, are programmed for precise tasks, relying solely on current input due to their inability to store past interactions. These systems, rooted in statistical mathematics, excel in processing extensive datasets to generate outputs that mimic intelligent responses. IBM Deep Blue (Chess-playing supercomputer AI) and Netflix Recommendation Engine are examples of Reactive Machine AI.

- Limited Memory AI: Unlike Reactive Machine AI, this type of AI has the capability to remember previous occurrences and results while observing particular items or circumstances continuously. With the help of past and present data, LM AI can make decisions on the best course of action that is expected to lead to a favorable result. Generative AI tools (such as ChatGPT, Bard and DeepAI), Virtual assistants and chatbots (such as Siri, Alexa, Google Assistant, Cortana and IBM Watson) and Self-driving cars are examples of Limited Memory AI.

- Theory of mind AI: The idea of AI that can sense and discern other people's emotions is known as theory of mind. The phrase, which comes from psychology, refers to people's capacity to discern the emotions of others and make predictions about their future behavior based on that perception. With the ability to deduce human intentions and objectives, Theory of Mind AI could tailor its interactions with people to reflect their psychological requirements and goals. Additionally, it would be capable of contextualizing and understanding writings and artwork, something that current generative AI tools are not. Senior AI researcher Rafael Tena of the insurance provider Acrisure gave the following scenario to show how a successful theory of mind application will transform the field: Due to the lack of human error, a self-driving automobile might outperform a human driver in most situations. However, as a driver, you will naturally slow down when crossing your neighbor's house as you know that their child likes to play near to the roadside after school. This is something that an AI car with rudimentary memory is unlikely to be able to achieve.

- Self-awareness AI: Self-Aware AI, like theory of mind AI, is purely hypothetical. Self-aware AI, sometimes known as the AI point of singularity, is the level beyond theory of mind and constitutes one of the long-term goals in the advancement of artificial intelligence. When artificial intelligence (AI) reaches self-awareness, it is believed that robots will become uncontrollable due to their capacity to comprehend not only human emotions and thoughts, but also their own internal conditions and characteristics. Sophia, a robot created by Hanson Robotics, is arguably the most well-known example of self-aware AI. Although Sophia isn't self-aware in the strict sense, her sophisticated use of existing AI technologies offers a preview of what AI can become in the future.

2.2.3 AI based on usabilities

- Analytical AI: Analytics commonly pertains to the identification, interpretation, and communication of significant data patterns. Analytical AI is geared towards uncovering novel insights, patterns, and connections within data, facilitating data-informed decision-making. Analytical AI applications include forecasting consumer needs, inventory optimization, sentiment modeling, and manufacturer risk assessment and mitigation.
- Functional AI: Functional artificial intelligence operates in a manner comparable to analytical artificial intelligence by examining extensive datasets to identify patterns and relationships. In contrast, functional AI is characterized by its ability to perform tasks instead of merely offering suggestions. Robotics and Internet of Things applications might benefit from a functioning AI model to make quick decisions.
- Interactive AI: Interactive artificial intelligence commonly facilitates effective and interactive automation of communication, a technology widely integrated into various facets of our everyday routines, notably within the business realm. Intelligent personal assistants, or chatbots, can serve as excellent illustrations of interactive AI. Another typical application of interactive AI is dialogue and workflow authentication.
- Textual AI: Textual AI commonly encompasses textual analysis or natural language processing, enabling businesses to utilize functions such as text

identification, speech-to-text conversion, machine translation, and content creation. Examples of text AI include text identification, autonomous translation, speech-to-text alteration, and multimedia creation platforms.

- Visual AI: Visual AI can often identify, categorize, and arrange objects in addition to creating insights from photos and videos. As a result, visual AI is a field of artificial intelligence that teaches robots to comprehend and interpret visual information similarly to how humans might. This kind of AI is frequently applied in domains like augmented reality (AR) and visual computing.

3. CATEGORIZATION OF ML AND DL MODELS

Machine Learning (ML) has become increasingly significant in scientific studies, ranging from interpreting enormous amounts of data to making precise predictions and supporting researchers in their work to enable them to make discoveries more efficiently. Nowadays, the main purpose of ML applications in the healthcare industry is to analyze vast volumes of data in order to help physicians alongside other healthcare providers make better decisions. Physicians can use this technology to help detect patterns, tendencies, and abnormalities while minimizing error rates. As explained beneath, numerous approaches to machine learning can be applied for modeling in a given field based on their learning methods and characteristics (Javaid, 2022; Aggarwal, 2023). The machine learning techniques are described in Figure 4, with a focus on model building tasks and procedures.

Figure 4. Different kinds of machine learning methods alongside examples

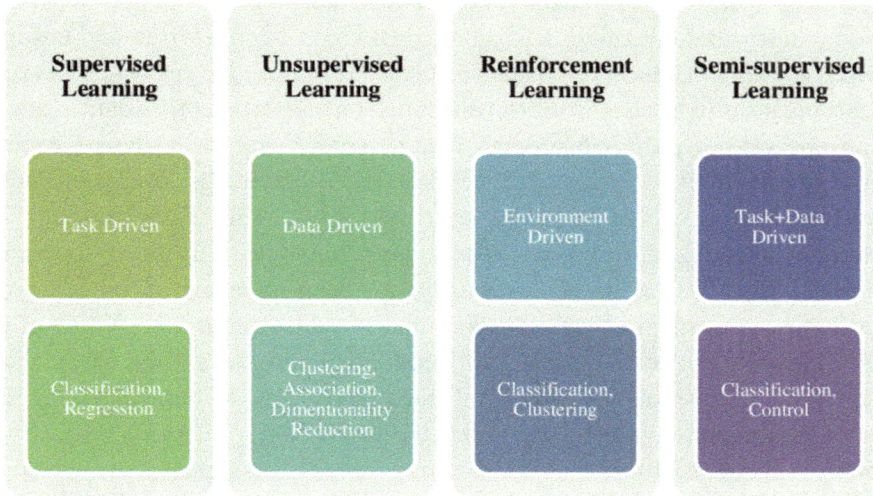

1. Supervised Learning: This process occurs when certain objectives have been optimized to be efficiently attained via an ensemble of inputs; for instance, a task-oriented methodology that employs labeled data to learn algorithms to categorize data or predict results, like identifying spam-like emails. Classification and regression analysis constitute the two most frequently encountered supervised learning tasks. K-nearest neighbors, Support Vector Machines, Ensemble learning, Linear regression are recognized as popular methods that ought to be applied to a multitude of supervised learning tasks, depending on the type of data provided in a specific application area.
2. Un-Supervised Learning: It is a data driven methodology with a main objective to extract sequences and hierarchies from unlabeled data. Among the most popular unsupervised tasks include clustering, lowering dimensionality, identifying relationships, and recognizing anomalies. Clustering algorithms like K-means, K-Mediods, CLARA, hierarchical clustering, single or complete linkage, association learning algorithms like AIS, Apriori-TID and Apriori-Hybrid, FP-Tree, and RARM, as well as feature selection and extraction techniques like Pearson Correlation, principal component analysis, etc., are popular methods for completing unsupervised learning tasks.
3. Reinforcement Learning: It is an environment-driven approach. Reinforcement learning (RL) main features are (i) handling sequential decision-making; (ii) no supervisor—just a scalar reward—and (iii) significantly delayed feedback. Some

typical instances of reinforcement learning models include temporal-difference learning, Q-learning, and deep reinforcement learning.

4. Semi-supervised Learning: It is an amalgamation of supervised and unsupervised learning methods. For instance, it can be employed to perform supervised learning tasks like classification even though only a portion of the data is labeled (unsupervised learning). In order to obtain a larger dataset with labels, the model is trained on an inadequately, labeled dataset. Post-training, the created dataset and the original dataset of images are combined to train the final model.

5. Self-supervised Learning: One kind of unsupervised learning is self-supervised learning, in which a machine learns feature representations through a proxy task that uses supervisory signals and data. Once learn-representation has concluded, the annotated data is utilized to further refine it. One advantage of self-supervised learning is that it eradicates the requisite for human data tagging, which eliminates instances in which the technology effectively extracts the embodied context from the data, resulting in metadata signals that correspond to the representations. Since both systems learn representations without labels, this system is comparable to unsupervised learning. The main distinction is that self-supervised learning in this context does not entail learning the data's inherent structure and is not centered on clustering, discovering anomalies, reduction of dimensionality, and determination of density.

6. Weakly-supervised Learning: Weak supervision, which is a subfield of machine learning, can be defined as the process of classifying unlabeled data through the use of sparse, noisy sources that produce a supervision signal, which actually results in the labeling of a lot of training data in a supervised manner. While the imprecise supervised data in "weakly-supervised learning" refers to the newly labeled data, a very strong prediction model, however, can be built with it. Image-level annotations and weak annotations, such as by using dots and scribbles, help to identify the objects in the weakly supervised approach.

Figure 5. Basic categories of deep learning models

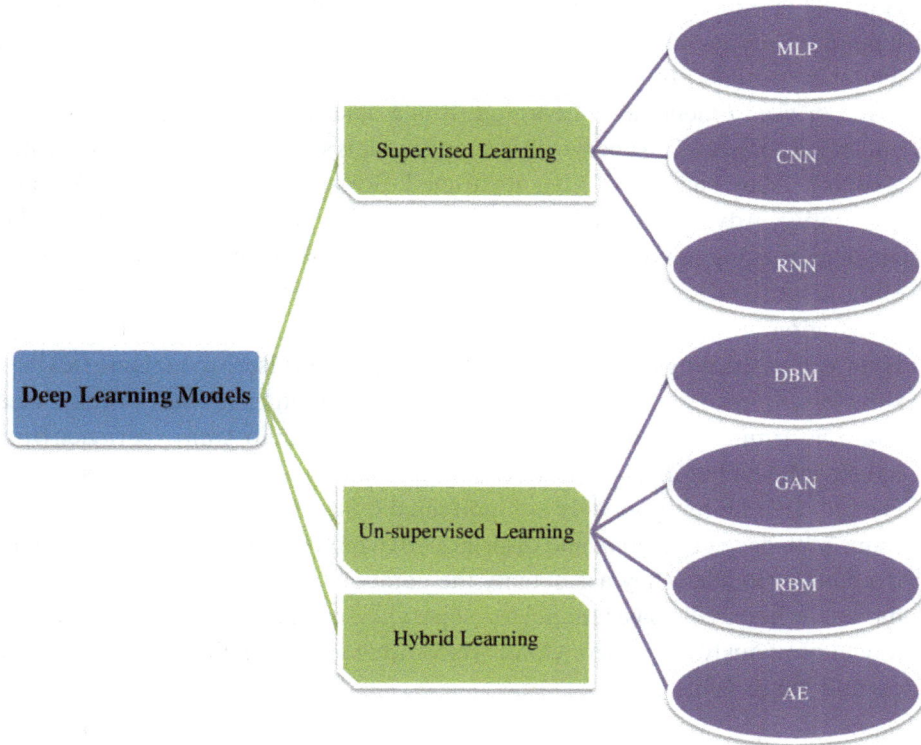

In healthcare, DL methodologies can be deployed for a multitude of tasks, including obtaining medical images and identifying abnormalities in them. In particular, these methods are used to effectively and efficiently identify problematic signals within these images, in addition to improving the quality of images acquired using different modalities. Deep learning models are extremely complicated and employ multiple algorithms. Even while no network is impeccable, quite a few algorithms function better for particular applications than others. Convolutional neural networks (CNNs), recurrent neural networks (RNNs), attention models, and transformer structures are the leading categories of DL methods utilized in medical imaging that are covered in this section (Miotto, 2017; Piccialli, 2020; Aggarwal, 2023). Prior to delving into the specifics of these DL models, it is helpful to go over the different kinds of learning tasks (shown in Figure 5) that exist, particularly:

1. Supervised / Discriminative Learning: It is a task-driven method which employs labeled training data. Multi-Layer Perceptrons (MLP), Convolutional Neural Networks (CNN or ConvNet), Recurrent Neural Networks (RNN), and their

variations are the most prominent representations of discriminative models. A model is trained via supervised learning through the utilization of both the input data and its target label. Typically, supervised learning is used to train a neural network to produce the corresponding label for a specific sample.

2. Unsupervised / Generative Learning: It is a data-driven method that inspects unlabeled datasets. Unsupervised learning models such as Deep Belief Networks (DBNs), Auto encoders (AE), Restricted Boltzmann Machine (RBM) and Generative Adversarial Networks (GANs) have been applied to numerous medical imaging applications, including surveillance of motion, general modeling, classification enhancement, artifact reduction, alongside medical imaging registration.

3. Hybrid deep learning models: The generative (unsupervised) models are flexible; showing the potential to acquire knowledge from either labeled or unlabeled data. Discriminative (supervised) models, however, cannot gain experience from unlabeled data but instead, they are superior to their generative in these tasks. Hybrid deep learning models are motivated by the fact that a framework that trains both deep generative and discriminative models concurrently can benefit from both models. They are notably the combination of several deep learning models, wherein the basic model is a supervised or unsupervised deep learning model previously discussed. Comparison among various DL-based models is carried out in Table 1.

Table 1. Comparison among various DL-Based models

DL Model	Description	Advantages	Disadvantages	Application
MLP	A supervised feed forward NN with leastwise three layers (a input image, an undetected layer, and an output layer).	Can resolve problems that are not linearly separable and that are organized to approximate all continuous functions	Insufficient training data or an overly complex model could make them susceptible to over-fitting and hyper-parameter optimization.	Visual and auditory recognition, natural language processing, and time-series prediction.
CNN	Utilize a sequence of convolutional layers for obtaining information from the input image, and then one or more fully connected layers to determine the outcome.	Automatically learn relevant features from raw input data, are very prevalent in practical applications since they are resistant to noise and distortion in the input data.	High computational requirement, claim large amounts of labeled training data, susceptible to over-fitting whilst the training data is controlled or noisy.	Image and video recognition tasks, image classification and segmentation, object detection.
RNN	It is a neural network whereupon each subsequent step receives its input from the previous step's output and can be used to model sequence data.	Handle sequential data effectively, Process inputs of any length, distribute weights among time stages to improve training effectiveness	Prone to vanishing and exploding gradient problems, Computationally slower, can be difficult to train, particularly for lengthy sequences.	Speech recognition, machine translation, natural language processing and text generation
DBM	It is a sort of generative model that is made to find complex structures inside big datasets by learning to replicate the input data that is provided.	Competency to learn intricate patterns and correlation in data, capacity to produce latest information that is comparable to the training set.	Training is slow and computationally expensive, Utilizing the model in practical applications may be challenging due to the complexity of interpreting the correlations and patterns that have been discovered.	Image recognition, bioinformatics, language modeling and text generation.
GAN	By training two neural networks to compete using an already-existing training dataset, to yield more authentic information.	Can be trained using unlabeled data, generate data similar to real data	Complexity of the training process can lead to over fitting, utilized to produce counterfeits, hard to maintain quality control over the produced data	Generating realistic images, human-like text generation, data augmentation, anomaly detection, simulate complex systems and predict future behavior
RBM	Is a kind of generative model that can be trained over an ensemble of input variables to learn a probabilistic distribution.	To improve performance, additional models can benefit from including the activations of the hidden layer accurately determined and sufficiently precise to represent distribution.	Training is more difficult, Weight Adjustment, RBM's CD-k algorithm is less popular than the back propagation method.	Image and video processing, financial modeling, Anomaly detection, Collaborative
AE	Are NN that use back propagation algorithm for feature learning and learn data without supervision	Do not require labelled data during training, dimensionality reduction in complex high-dimensional data, trained to eliminate noise from input data, automatically extract pertinent features from the data	Sensitive to the choice of hyper-parameters, lack of robustness, exposed to over-fitting when trained on limited data	Feature detection, image coloring, dimensionality reduction, anomaly detection and watermark removal.

4. POTENTIAL APPLICATIONS OF AI

More recently, AI has undergone a transformation in its research scope encompassing not just computer science but also fields like psychology, linguistics, and philosophy. Its applications span diverse sectors including education, e-commerce, healthcare, robotics, navigation, agriculture, military, marketing, and gaming. Examples of widely utilized AI applications include search engines like Google, recommender systems such as Netflix, self-driving vehicles like Tesla, and human speech recognition systems including Siri and Alexa. AI, along with its related fields like robotics, the internet of things, and machine learning, can profoundly impact our societies. Technology has the potential to enhance human life by simplifying tasks, boosting safety, and increasing productivity. Various AI applications, such as facial recognition for security, industrial automation, natural language processing for translation, household robotics, machine learning, and visual processing for healthcare, are making our lives more convenient (Lu, 2019; Zhang, 2021). Figure 6 shows multiple prospective real-world AI application areas. However, technological skeptics debate whether AI is truly necessary in our daily lives. AI can have a detrimental impact on society, including unfavorable societal change, layoffs, income disparity, and online criminal activity. As a result, the application of artificial intelligence in various sectors of our community continues to be a topic of active research. On that topic, this paper provides insight into the application of AI in the healthcare sector.

Figure 6. Possible applications of artificial intelligence

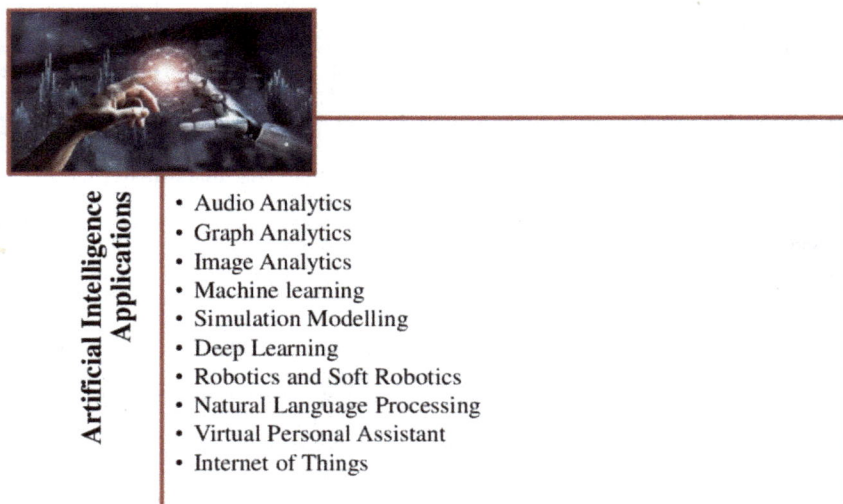

Artificial Intelligence Applications

- Audio Analytics
- Graph Analytics
- Image Analytics
- Machine learning
- Simulation Modelling
- Deep Learning
- Robotics and Soft Robotics
- Natural Language Processing
- Virtual Personal Assistant
- Internet of Things

4.1 AI in Healthcare

Artificial Intelligence (AI), an emerging discipline that is rapidly advancing and gaining additional roles in healthcare, replicates human intelligence to precisely automate assignments. To autonomously complete an endeavor, it employs distinct algorithms, guidelines, and directives. AI tools have been applied in medicine to diagnose infections, provide treatments tailored to each patient, anticipate implant sizes, and assess the clinical results of various pre- and post-operative procedures. Figure 7 shows multiple prospective application areas of AI in healthcare that could revolutionize the medical industry. Like the magnifier, phonendoscope, and an electrocardiogram, AI systems must be viewed as a tool that has been created throughout time to make up for the limits in doctors' perceptual abilities (Piccialli, 2020; Alowais, 2023).

Figure 7. Applications of AI in Healthcare That Could Change the Industry

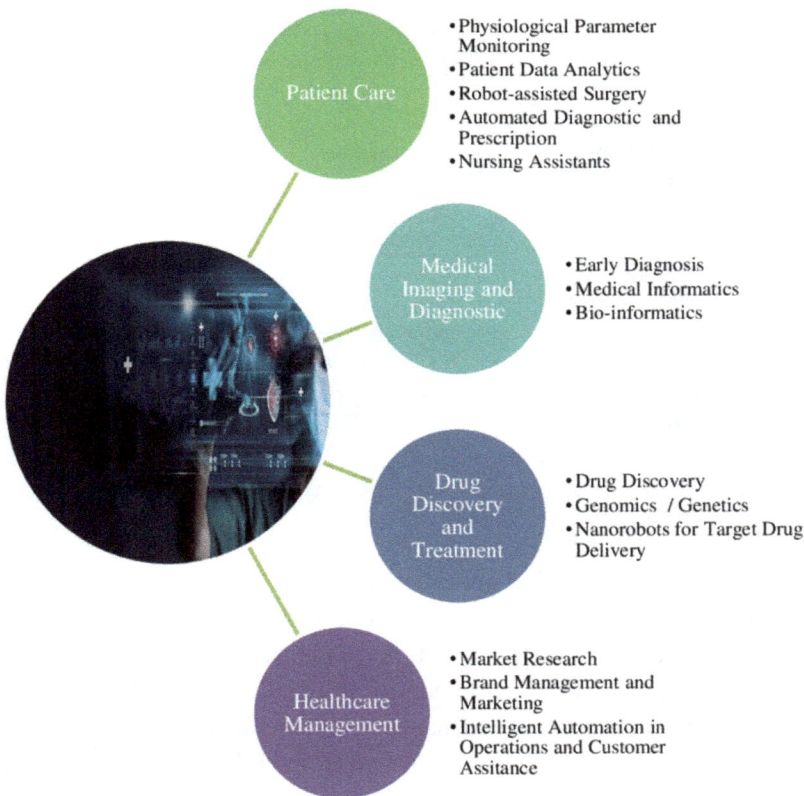

Figure 7. Applications of AI in Healthcare That Could Change the Industry

Patient Care
- Physiological Parameter Monitoring
- Patient Data Analytics
- Robot-assisted Surgery
- Automated Diagnostic and Prescription
- Nursing Assistants

Medical Imaging and Diagnostic
- Early Diagnosis
- Medical Informatics
- Bio-informatics

Drug Discovery and Treatment
- Drug Discovery
- Genomics / Genetics
- Nanorobots for Target Drug Delivery

Healthcare Management
- Market Research
- Brand Management and Marketing
- Intelligent Automation in Operations and Customer Assitance

4.2 Processing steps for AI in healthcare

There are various processes involved in using AI in healthcare, and these may change based on the particular application and conditions. A conceptual schematic that depicts the relationships amongst the various steps in the application of AI in healthcare is shown in Figure 8. Interactions occur between various elements during this process, including the information being processed, the AI model, and the individuals engaged in developing it. An AI model, for instance, may be trained using the data that humans have gathered and pre-processed. This model could then be used to produce inferences or predictions that physicians could employ when determining their therapeutic solutions. Various stages in the process of AI in healthcare are as follows:

Figure 8. Process of AI in healthcare

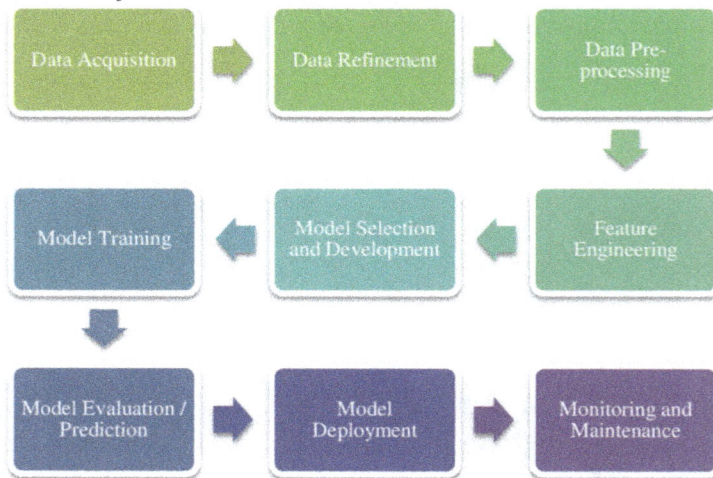

1. Data Acquisition: Acquiring pertinent data is the initial stage in the process of AI. Real-time data streams, unorganized information involving text or images, and organized information from relational databases might all qualify under this category. Since the quality and quantity of data accessible have a significant impact on the AI system's performance, exquisite data is the cornerstone of an AI model's effectiveness. Data is collected from various sources like electronic health records, clinical trials and wearable devices.
2. Data Refinement and Pre-processing: Following collection, the data must be cleaned and pre-processed, including missing value handling, duplicate removal,

anonymization of AI data, standardization of the data format, and any necessary data normalization or transformation to make it accessible to artificial intelligence algorithms. This constitutes a significant stage in the AI process that ensures the training set is void of biases and noise, which can have a detrimental influence on the model's accuracy.

3. Feature Engineering: In this step, the most pertinent factors (or attributes) in the dataset that may affect the AI model's predictions are identified. Feature engineering might entail either developing novel attributes or identifying the most instructive ones among the available data. AI models' precision as well as productivity can be greatly increased by meticulously selecting their attributes.

4. Model Selection and Development: In this stage, data analysts choose the most effective artificial intelligence algorithm (e.g., neural networks, support vector machines, decision trees etc) for the assigned task. Because distinct tasks involve various methodologies to attain optimal outcomes, model selection is an essential aspect of the AI process. The process may be streamlined, expenses can be decreased, and errors can be eliminated by choosing the appropriate AI process automation solution.

5. Model Training: The selected model will be trained on the prepared dataset. In this step, the model goes through the data and looks for patterns and relations to learn. Training is defined as modifying the model's parameters to get the lowest prediction errors. If the model is complex, as it would be in case of deep learning networks, this step may require a lot of computational resources and time. Hyperparameter optimization is usually performed after the training to improve the model's performance. The usage of diverse AI tools can boost the training process and raise the model's accuracy level.

6. Model Evaluation / Prediction: Post-training, the model should be critically evaluated to see how accurate it is when dealing with new and unobserved data. First, the data should be split into training and testing sections. Metrics like accuracy, precision, recall, and F1 score are then applied to measure its performance. The assessment part at the end of the AI workflow step confirms that the model does not exhibit the AI over-fitting and AI under-fitting problems and has good generalization ability.

7. Model Deployment: Following training and validation, the model is deployed to the real-world setting and prepared for its application in making decisions or making predictions in real time. Making sure the model is compliant with the production environment involves connecting it to application platforms before deploying it. The transition of the model from the training to the testing phase is an illustration of a significant stage in AI processes encountered in sectors like healthcare where decisions must be made in real time.

8. Monitoring and Maintenance: Once the AI model has been deployed, the model requires constant monitoring to ensure that the model continues to produce good results over time. Moreover, the model's performance can be downgraded due to the changes in data patterns, in this case running updates and retraining the model are necessary. In this stage of the AI workflow, the model's predictions are monitored, hyper parameters are retuned, and the model is retrained with new data to ensure its accuracy and trustworthiness, which is done by the data scientists in most cases.

4.3 Benefits of AI in Healthcare

Despite the ethical concerns raised by the implementation of artificial intelligence in healthcare, it is essential to acknowledge the remarkable opportunities that AI brings in this area. These advantages could improve patient outcomes, streamline the delivery of healthcare, and solve current issues in the healthcare system. Comprehending and valuing these benefits can aid in placing the ethical ramifications in perspective and direct the prudent and advantageous application of AI in healthcare (Piccialli, 2020; Ali, 2023).

1. More Precise Diagnoses: AI systems have proven to be remarkably adept in identifying illnesses and ailments. Large volumes of patient data, involving genetic histories, hospital documentation, and clinical images, can be analyzed using machine learning algorithms to find trends and possible diagnoses. Using AI diagnostic tools, healthcare professionals can get not only correct but quick insights to make their diagnoses, as a result, the frequency of diagnosis that are wrong is likely to be reduced, and treatment strategies would be better.
2. Personalized Therapy: AI systems allow personalized and precision medicine to be adopted. AI systems possess the ability of creating individualized treatment regimens by analyzing patient data, including genetic information and medical history. The made-to-measure methodology will not only boost the effectiveness of therapy but also minimize the possibility of unwanted reactions. Furthermore, with AI, the healthcare team is able to give the patients the therapy that is the most appropriate for their individual needs.
3. Prognostics: AI is capable of interpreting massive amounts of data In order to locate commonalities and anticipate clinical results. AI models can predict the course of an illness, mortality rates, and possible complications by scrutinizing previous statistics. This predictive nature of AI encourages the doctors to take preventive measures that will include treatment, disease status can be detected, and the patient can be managed effectively even in the long-term. Healthcare

workers can use these forecasts to act and conduct individual patient care, which will make the service more effective and cheaper.

4. Advanced Clinical Judgment: By offering scientific recommendations and proven suggestions, machines with AI can help medical practitioners make well-informed decisions. Large amounts of clinical information, therapeutic manuals, and the scientific literature can all be analyzed by AI algorithms to provide perceptions and aid in the clinical judgment performed by healthcare practitioners. This increase in clinical judgment has the potential to improve the efficiency of care, decrease practitioner variability, and support scientifically supported medicine.

5. Research and pharmacological Exploration: AI is essential for speeding up pharmacological and health care research. Large volumes of scientific literature, clinical trials, and genomic data can be analyzed by machine learning algorithms to uncover novel pharmaceutical methods, locate possible therapeutic targets, and expedite the creation of medications. AI-powered analyzers can reveal relationships and insights that skilled investigators might not perceive, which could result in more rapid clinical application of study findings as well as improved treatments.

6. Telemedicine and Remote Monitoring: AI technologies also make it easier to conduct distant monitoring of patients and e-health, especially in marginalized or inaccessible regions. Wearable technology and monitoring devices can gather clinical information in real time that AI algorithms can interpret to identify mutations while offering early warnings. The AI-equipped telemedicine platforms have the capability to facilitate remote consultations where people can access healthcare services much more easily, save themselves the traveling pain, and enjoy the utmost comfort of being treated.

7. Workflow Efficiency and Easement: The AI area has the ability to boost managerial effectiveness within healthcare applications, promote the disposition of resources, and boost managerial effectiveness within healthcare applications. AI-driven chatbots and virtual assistants can take care of mundane questions and appointment booking, freeing up medical staff members to work on more difficult assignments. AI-powered solutions may additionally computerize testimony procedures, which frees up extra hours for assisting patients and lessens the workload associated with paperwork.

These advantages could revolutionize healthcare delivery, enhance patient outcomes, and solve systemic issues if AI's potential is fully realized. To guarantee that these advantages are accomplished prudently, ethically, and in a way that preserves the dignity of patients, anonymity, and fair access to treatment, it is imperative to manage the ethical ramifications of AI implementation. Some of the most intriguing and recent studies on the application of AI in the medical industry are summarized in Table 2.

Table 2. A review of a few recently published papers on the application of AI in healthcare

Author	Application	Application area	AI approach	Conclusion
Al-Waisyetal. (2021)	For identifying COVID-19 virus in chest X-ray images	Chest radiography imaging	DBN + *CDBN	Is capable of being applied in a genuine clinical setting for COVID-19 early diagnosis and therapy monitoring in less than three seconds per image.
Sundar et al. (2021)	To discover the gene signature that serves as a preliminary prognostic biomarker for the benefits of the chemotherapy drug.	Oncology	Random Forest Machine Learning Model	Capable of anticipating which patient subgroup would benefit from the chemotherapy drug for gastric tumors
Liu et al. (2022)	To use EHRs to depict a medical event that is closely related to the prediction task	Medical event prediction (MEP)	Multi-channel *LSTM	Is an efficient task-wise approach for modeling the unpredictable temporal and diverse features of medical time series data.
Jianget al. (2022)	To investigate the effect of low-dose *CTE in the diagnosis of ulcerative colitis and Crohn's disease	Gastrointestinal diseases	Guided Image Filtering	Enhanced diagnostic precision in cases of inflammatory bowel disease with complicated appearances
Dipro et al. (2022)	To detect Parkinson's disease through Federated Learning	Brain	CNN	Utilizes little processing power and is quite accurate at eliminating privacy concerns, making the framework quicker and effective.
Yin et al. (2022)	To differentiate *TNBC from fibroadenoma	Breast Cancer	Deep learning models	The integrated assessment of MRI-based models demonstrated outstanding accuracy in distinguishing between fibroadenoma and TNBC.
Piette et al. (2022)	AI-Powered Patient-oriented Pain Management with Mobile Health Devices	Chronic pain	Reinforcement Learning	Cognitive behavior therapy (CBT) powered by AI is more successful than conventional CBT.

continued on following page

Table 2. Continued

Author	Application	Application area	AI approach	Conclusion
Menzies et al. (2023)	To identify and treat pigmented skin lesions.	Skin Cancer	Mobile phone-powered AI instruments	AI powered by mobile phones is precise in prognosis but needs to be used carefully when making managerial choices.
Nam et el. (2023)	To examine how AI-based CAD software might increase the frequency of actionable lung nodule diagnosis on chest radiographs	Actionable lung nodules	Commercial AI-CAD system	AI enhanced the identification of both malignant and actionable lung nodules; false-referral rates were similar to those of manual evaluation.
Sun L et al. (2023)	To investigate lightweight AI systems for processing AIS patients' magnetic resonance imaging (MRI) images	Acute ischemic stroke (AIS)	CNN	AIS lesions were precisely detected and segregated by an AI model; initial therapy changed the amounts of inflammatory factors and *EPC mobilization.

*CDBN=Convolutional DBN, LSTM=Long Short-Term Memory, CTE = CT Enterography, TNBC = Triple-negative breast cancer, EPC = endothelial progenitor cell

5. ETHICAL AND LEGAL CONSIDERATIONS

When it comes to technology, legal and ethical issues are particularly prominent in aspects like privacy, surveillance, bias, and discrimination, and also in the realm of philosophical questions around the role of human judgment. It is in case of the spreading use of the latest digital technologies as a source of error and unsafe data channels that the problem of inaccuracy appeared. Inaccuracies in a specific health-care field's fundamental procedure are among the most fatal to happen because they may harm the victims the most. This is important to keep in mind in a setting like the hospital, when the individuals interact with physicians at a moment when they are most susceptible. At present, no clearly defined regulations are addressing the legal and ethical aspects of the use of AI in health care settings. However, this review attempts to highlight issues such as the need for more transparent algorithms, privacy, and protection of all the beneficiaries on one hand and the cyber security of associated vulnerabilities on the other (Rodrigues, 2020). Figure 9 highlights some ethical and legal issues related to the application of AI in healthcare environments.

5.1 Ethical Concerns in AI Healthcare Applications

The introduction of artificial intelligencein healthcare is of enormous advantages, besides being accompanied by a wide array of ethical concerns among them. The issues need to be handled respectfully by considering patients' well-being as well as upholding moral values (Rodrigues, 2020; Kumar, 2023). Below are the primary ethical issues related to AI healthcare applications:

Figure 9. Ethical and Legal considerations associated with the application of AI to healthcare.

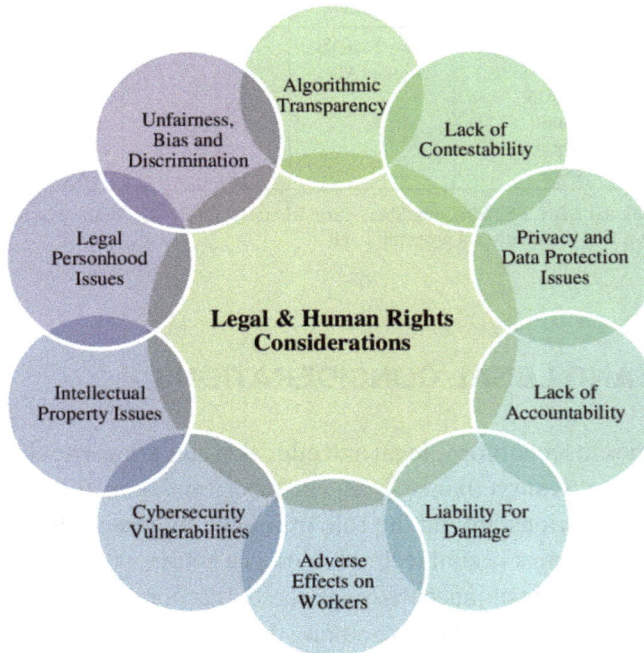

1. Privacy and Data Security: The implementation of AI in healthcare demands the patient's data as a source, but these data are highly sensitive including personally identifiable data, prescriptions, and even the entire human genome. Safeguarding the confidentiality of information and guaranteeing confidentiality of patient information are of utmost significance.It is necessary to have effective data governance models, strong access regulations, encrypted storage spaces, and data impersonalizing protocols for eliminating or at least minimizing the

potential of records violations, illicit utilization, and manipulation of personally identifiable health data.

2. Transparency and Explicability: Accountability, transparency, and the capacity to elucidate the logic underpinning AI-generated suggestions are all impacted by the opaqueness of AI algorithms, which is sometimes referred to as the black box dilemma. To promote trust and allow for critical review, both patients and healthcare providers should be competent to understand the process by which AI makes its decisions. Therefore, ensuring AI algorithms is transparent and explicable implies both the general acceptance and the promotion of well-informed decision-making.

3. Informed authorization and patient independence: Medical decisions could be influenced by AI technologies, which would raise ethical questions about informed authorization and individual freedom. The patients are entitled to know how AI will be used in their treatment, the constraints of suggestions made by AI, and whether they can give informed authorization or choose to opt out. To preserve the dignity of patients, open dialogue and patient participation in decision-making are extremely important.

4. Effects on physicians: The workforce of physicians and medical experts may be impacted by the use of AI in healthcare. There are issues with deficient skills, job relocation, and the possible loss of interpersonal skills. Human-AI conjunction should be given top priority in ethical utilization of AI, providing physicians with the knowledge, assistance, and educational resources they need to successfully incorporate AI into their professional lives. It's critical to make sure AI enhances healthcare workers rather than completely replaces them.

5. Integrity and Prejudice: AI systems that have been trained on partial or biased datasets run the risk of exacerbating or maintaining current healthcare inequities. Bias can take many different forms, such as socioeconomic, racial, gender, or regional bias. Addressing and reducing prejudice in AI algorithms is essential to ensuring that everyone receives equal and impartial healthcare. This calls for thorough algorithm testing, varied and comprehensive testing information, and constant bias scrutiny.

6. Accountability and Responsibility: The application of AI in healthcare raises issues regarding responsibility and obligation as a consequence of inaccuracies unfavourable outcomes, or harm prompted by automated systems. Identifying accountability and conferring responsibility can be difficult because AI algorithms and methodologies for making decisions are multifaceted. To address these issues and guarantee that trustworthy individuals can be held accountable, it is essential to establish specific regulations and policies for accountability.

7. Regulatory and Ethical Guidelines: The swift growth of artificial intelligence in healthcare calls for the creation of strong regulatory and ethical guidelines.

These frameworks ought to cover aspects involving transparency, prejudice remediation, openness, and confidentiality, along with informed consent. In order to create ethical norms and guidelines that match AI technologies with moral values and patient-centered services, cooperation between physicians, legislators, ethical philosophers, and technological professionals is essential.

Medical professionals can successfully navigate the legally appropriate and accountable application of AI in healthcare by recognizing and resolving these ethical issues. To guarantee that the potential advantages of AI are achieved while preserving patient rights, confidentiality, and fair execution of treatment, ethical considerations ought to be incorporated into the planning, development, and execution of AI systems.

5.2 Medical Imaging Datasets

Numerous advancements have arisen through machine learning public challenges. These initiatives provided supporting materials in the form of datasets (which are often expensive and time consuming to collect) and, at times, baseline algorithms, contributing to the facilitation of various research studies aimed at the development and evaluation of novel algorithms (Pinto-Coelho, 2023; Khalifa 2024). The promotion of a competitive objective was pivotal for promoting the development of a scientific community around a given topic. In Table 3, some popular datasets are presented.

Table 3. Medical Image Datasets

Dataset	Organ	Description	Publisher
BRATS	Brain	Multimodal Brain Tumor Segmentation Benchmark (BRATS) is a yearly challenge for comparing several brain tumor segmentation methods. It includes preliminary multimodal MRI scans of lower-grade glioma and glioblastoma along with mortality information and ground- truth labels which assist participants in segmenting and predicting the malignant cells.	University of Pennsylvania
MedPix	Multiple	It provides free access to healthcare data including clinical subjects, instructional scenarios, and medical images with over 59,000 indexed and curated images from over 12,000 patients	National Library of Medicine
KiTS	Kidney	Kidney Tumor Segmentation Benchmark (KiTS) is an evaluation and comparison dataset for kidney tumor segmentation algorithms. A total of 300 CT scans of the kidneys and kidney cancers make up the dataset. Worldwide, a number of healthcare centers supply the data and segmentations.	ZENODO

continued on following page

Table 3. Continued

Dataset	Organ	Description	Publisher
LiTS	Liver	An evaluation and comparison dataset for liver tumor segmentation algorithms is the Liver Tumor Segmentation Benchmark (LiTS). With 130 scans in the training set and 70 scans in the test set, the dataset includes CT scans of the liver and liver tumors. Worldwide, plenty of healthcare institutions distribute the data and segmentations.	TUM Graduate School
ADNI	Brain	Brain scans and associated information from patients with Alzheimer's disease are gathered into the Alzheimer's Disease Neuro Imaging Initiative (ADNI) image collections. Accommodates CSV file formats and includes both MRI and PET modalities.	Private-Public partnership
MURA	Bone X-rays	The Musculoskeletal Radiographs (MURA is a large dataset of musculoskeletal radiographs comprising 40,561 images from 14,863 investigations. Radiologists manually classify each investigation as normal or abnormal.	Stanford ML Group
NIH Chest X-rays	Chest X-ray	A large dataset of chest X-ray images containing over 112,000 images from more than 30,000 unique patients. The images are labeled with 14 common disease labels.	NIH Clinical Center
TCAI	Multiple	comprises medical images from clinical investigations and 22 modalities spanning 54 different organs, displaying both healthy and significantly damaged conditions of body organs (from cancer), kept in DICOM files.	National Cancer Institute
OASIS	Brain	OASIS (Open Access Series of Imaging Studies) aims to make neuroimaging publicly accessible to the scientific community with four variations: OASIS-1, OASIS-2, OASIS-3, and OASIS-4.	Howard Hughes Medical Institute
Kaggle	Multiple	For use in AI applications, Kaggle medical image datasets are compilations of medical images which are arranged and labelled. The databases are usually classified into classes or categories containing a huge number of images such as CT, MRI, and X-ray scans.	Google LLC
COVID-19 X-ray	Chest X-ray	This dataset includes cleaned images from patients with COVID-19, as well as images of different viral pneumonia along with certain normal chest X-ray images no pneumonia / COVID-positive symptoms.	Darwin Labs

6. CHALLENGES AND CONSIDERATIONS

Numerous facets of healthcare could be revolutionized by AI developments, opening the door to a more individualized, accurate, predictive, and portable future. The broader integration and application of AI in healthcare systems, nonetheless, is plagued with difficulties. In addition to safety and regulatory issues, these obstacles encompass, but aren't exclusive to, technological capabilities, organizational resources, moral and ethical behaviours, along with information quality and availability. Over the past decade, the implementation of digitization in health records has been an epitome of efficiency, especially in healthcare systems that involve billing and reimbursement. Nevertheless, the next 10 years will be about society seeing the benefits of these digital assets which cannot be observed right now and how this can be done toward better clinical outcomes with the help of artificial intelligence and the subsequently created novel data assets and tools. One thing here is that medical practice and technology are getting to a convergence point. While there are many opportunities, there are also significant obstacles that must be addressed in the real world and the scope of implementing such innovation. Moreover, we must bring in advanced skills and feature in technology-enabled training of healthcare workers and the future leaders ensuring these individuals are conversant with technology instead of apprehensive from the possibility of an AI-augmented healthcare system (Rajpurkar, 2022; Saw, 2022).The following constitute a handful of the major challenges (Figure 10) that need to be resolved whilst AI is fully included into the healthcare sector:

Figure 10. Challenges to be addressed before practical use of AI systems in medical imaging

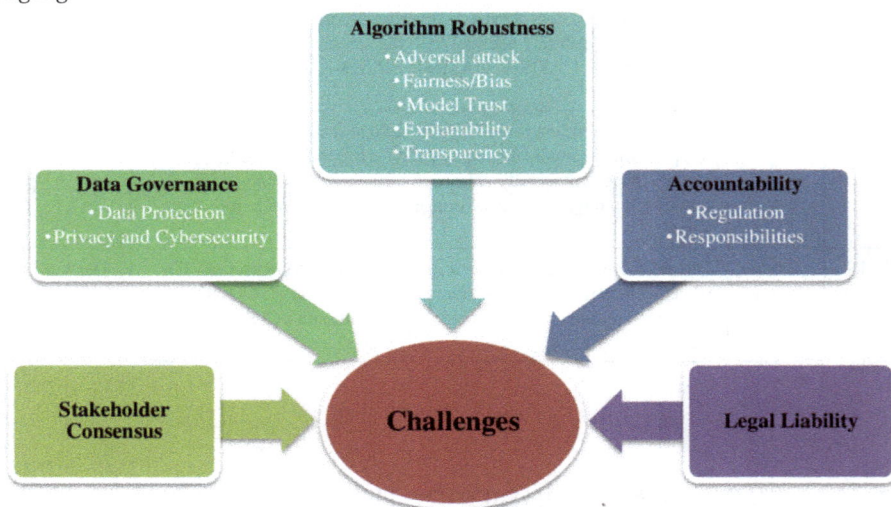

1. To promote enhancement in the healthcare system and societal advantages, it is crucial to comprehend the requirements and concerns of various stakeholders, including radiologists, clinicians, and healthcare workers. Findings show that

different stakeholders had varying perspectives on the difficulties posed by AI; nevertheless, in order to advance AI technology into clinical settings, all stakeholders must work together to create a comprehensive strategy for creating appropriate legal AI regulations and policies that protect equity and people's autonomy.

2. Numerous AI techniques necessitate a lot of data to interpret. A variety of formats and sources, including images, three-dimensional video patterns, medical imaging, and numerical data, can be used to gather medical data. However, due to ethical concerns, gathering patient data can occasionally be challenging. Additionally, algorithms may produce exceptional accuracy when applied to minimal amounts of data, but this may not be useful or practicable. Consequently, one of the challenges in healthcare data analysis is gathering reliable, clean, and effective data.

3. Privacy concerns constitute a significant barrier to data collecting and sharing because AI technologies depend on enormous databases. Data pertaining to medical conditions is exceedingly challenging to distribute and manage across several databases since patient records comprise sensitive data. This implies that software developers have to abide by confidentiality laws that could impede the advancement of AI. Thus, it is necessary to converse about the policies and standards that AI technology must adhere to, including those pertaining to ethics, the law, and personal values that influence how individuals in society respond.

4. Artificial intelligence algorithms are susceptible to misconceptions and could generate inaccurate forecasts. An adversarial attack occurs when images are subjected to inconsistencies, resulting in the AI model's prediction to produce contradictory classifications. This adversarial attack in the field of healthcare could have disastrous results, endanger patient lives, and enable the creation of fake treatment claims/payments, or other misleading situations.

5. It is beneficial for AI systems to be dependable, practical, and simple to incorporate into healthcare process as long as they come with concise, understandable instructions outlining their proper usage and timing. The improved explainability would not only increase user trust but also enable engineers to more completely inspect models for faults and confirm the extent to which AI decision-making resembles skilled human approaches.

6. Prior to training the AI model, data frequently has to be pre-processed in the AI development stage. Data is often divided into training and testing datasets, with the testing dataset being used to assess the model's efficacy. To guarantee adequate transparency, precise explanations of the data source, data attributes, and data governance procedure are essential as physicians will also be able to evaluate the dependability of the algorithms' output with unambiguous model transparency,

7. Safety and accountability procedures that are functioning globally aren't yet amended taking into consideration possible consequences patient may suffer from judgments made by an AI-based clinical tool. As part of any advanced healthcare system, medical professionals and organizations unintentionally promise patients that they will use good judgment, perform their jobs competently, and aid with the patient's recuperation. By holding people to a higher standard of moral accountability, expert complacency may be prevented. But it's important to differentiate between legal liability and moral accountability.

8. The practice of assigning and recognizing tasks is a must for creating the optimal possible liability structure. To create the best possible liability structure, work assignment and recognition are essential practices. Since patients who suffer losses by the negligence of medical professionals may sue for financial damages, doctors must adhere to a set of ethical guidelines and administer their patients with the utmost care. Clinicians must therefore accept AI as a helpful tool to assist their current decision-making procedures and avoid medical malpractice claims, in order to support their present decision-making processes and prevent medical malpractice claims, clinicians must embrace AI as a supportive tool.

When preparing to use AI for health, healthcare executives should take the following concerns into account (Miotto, 2017; Khalifa, 2024):

1. Procedures for moral and responsible data access: medical records are extremely private, erratic, compartmentalized, and not ideally suited for the creation, assessment, application, and implementation of machine learning

2. Having access to enough processing power for rendering recommendations in real time, which is being revolutionized by cloud computing

3. Having domain-specific knowledge or previously acquired knowledge to comprehend and develop a portion of the standards that must be executed to the datasets

4. Developing trustworthy AI algorithms that are integrated into suitable workflows requires careful consideration, investigation, and study of the problems that occur when algorithms are applied in the real world.

7. CONCLUSION

Rapid advancements in artificial intelligence have the potential to revolutionize health care imaging and prognosis in previously unheard-of ways. An unprecedented amount of activity has been sparked by the enormous potential that AI holds for precision medicine. The combination of AI with medical imaging has significantly improved healthcare. From early detection to accurate assessment, artificial intelligence has significant promise for enhancing medical imaging diagnosis. Medical practitioners can use AI to provide precise diagnoses, customize treatment regimens, and enhance patient outcomes by utilizing the abundance of information found in medical imaging. To further improve AI's potential in medical imaging, researchers are always investigating new algorithms, structures, and techniques. In addition to updating practitioners and lowering professional expenses, it can help physicians obtain impartial consensus imaging and enhance quality assurance in experimental research and patient care. Additionally, in order to translate research discoveries into useful applications that can help patients all across the world, partnerships between physicians, mathematicians, alongside business professionals are essential.

There are several obstacles that must be overcome in order to successfully integrate AI into healthcare. One of the most important of these is that all stakeholders must provide consistent support, which is made more difficult by their interdependencies. A change that seems good to one stakeholder could really make another less supportive. Numerous obstacles to the adoption and application of AI have been found which includes computational aversion, accessibility, guidelines for research and approval, perceived risks to self-reliance, liabilities, data privacy and effectiveness, and unbalanced financial aid. However, theoretical, empirical, laboratory, and field research are required to fully analyse these obstacles.In conclusion, as AI becomes an integral part of the healthcare, the integration of AI into healthcare will soon significantly alter the field of medical diagnosis both academically and professionally due to the enormous computational resources and intriguing learning techniques that are becoming widely accessible.

DECLARATION OF COMPETING INTEREST

The authors of the manuscript declare no conflict of interest.

FUNDING

This research did not receive any specific grant from funding agencies in the public, commercial, or not-for-profit sectors.

AUTHOR'S CONTRIBUTION

All authors contributed equally in the preparation of the chapter.

ACKNOWLEDGEMENT

The authors extend their appreciation to anonymous referees for their constructive recommendations and useful suggestions

REFERENCES

Aggarwal, N., Saini, B. S., & Gupta, S. (2023). Role of artificial intelligence techniques and neuroimaging modalities in detection of Parkinson's Disease: A Systematic review. *Cognitive Computation*, *16*(4), 2078–2115. DOI: 10.1007/s12559-023-10175-y

Al-Waisy, A. S., Mohammed, M. A., Al-Fahdawi, S., Maashi, M. S., Garcia-Zapirain, B., Abdulkareem, K. H., Mostafa, S. A., Kumar, N. M., & Le, D. (2021). COVID-DeepNet: Hybrid multimodal deep learning system for improving COVID-19 pneumonia detection in chest x-ray images. *Computers, Materials & Continua/Computers. Materials & Continua (Print)*, *67*(2), 2409–2429. DOI: 10.32604/cmc.2021.012955

Ali, O., Abdelbaki, W., Shrestha, A., Elbasi, E., Alryalat, M. A., & Dwivedi, Y. K. (2023). A systematic literature review of artificial intelligence in the healthcare sector: Benefits, challenges, methodologies, and functionalities. *Journal of Innovation & Knowledge*, *8*(1), 100333. DOI: 10.1016/j.jik.2023.100333

Alowais, S. A., Alghamdi, S. S., Alsuhebany, N., Alqahtani, T., Alshaya, A. I., Almohareb, S. N., Aldairem, A., Alrashed, M., Saleh, K. B., Badreldin, H. A., Yami, M. S. A., Harbi, S. A., & Albekairy, A. M. (2023). Revolutionizing healthcare: The role of artificial intelligence in clinical practice. *BMC Medical Education*, *23*(1). Advance online publication. DOI: 10.1186/s12909-023-04698-z PMID: 37740191

Dipro, S. H., Islam, M., Al, N. A., Sharmita, A. M., Chakrabarty, A., & Reza, T. (2022). A federated learning based privacy preserving approach for detecting Parkinson's disease using deep learning. International Conference on Computer and Information Technology (ICCIT), 139 144.https://doi.org/DOI: 10.1109/ICCIT57492.2022.10055787

Gupta, R., Srivastava, D., Sahu, M., Tiwari, S., Ambasta, R. K., & Kumar, P. (2021). Artificial intelligence to deep learning: Machine intelligence approach for drug discovery. *Molecular Diversity*, *25*(3), 1315–1360. DOI: 10.1007/s11030-021-10217-3 PMID: 33844136

Hamet, P., & Tremblay, J. (2017). Artificial intelligence in medicine. *Metabolism: Clinical and Experimental*, *69*, S36–S40. DOI: 10.1016/j.metabol.2017.01.011 PMID: 28126242

Javaid, M., Haleem, A., Singh, R. P., Suman, R., & Rab, S. (2022). Significance of machine learning in healthcare: Features, pillars and applications. *International Journal of Intelligent Networks*, *3*, 58–73. DOI: 10.1016/j.ijin.2022.05.002

Jiang, F., Fu, X., Kuang, K., & Fan, D. (2022). Artificial Intelligence Algorithm-Based Differential Diagnosis of Crohn's disease and Ulcerative colitis by CT Image. *Computational and Mathematical Methods in Medicine*, 1–12. DOI: 10.1155/2022/3871994 PMID: 35419083

Kaul, V., Enslin, S., & Gross, S. A. (2020). History of artificial intelligence in medicine. *Gastrointestinal Endoscopy*, *92*(4), 807–812. DOI: 10.1016/j.gie.2020.06.040 PMID: 32565184

Khalifa, M., & Albadawy, M. (2024). AI in diagnostic imaging: Revolutionising accuracy and efficiency. *Computer Methods and Programs in Biomedicine Update*, *5*, 100146. DOI: 10.1016/j.cmpbup.2024.100146

Kumar, P., Chauhan, S., & Awasthi, L. K. (2023). Artificial Intelligence in Healthcare: Review, Ethics, Trust Challenges & Future Research Directions. *Engineering Applications of Artificial Intelligence*, *120*, 105894. DOI: 10.1016/j.engappai.2023.105894

Liu, S., Wang, X., Xiang, Y., Xu, H., Wang, H., & Tang, B. (2022). Multi-channel fusion LSTM for medical event prediction using EHRs. *Journal of Biomedical Informatics*, *127*, 104011. DOI: 10.1016/j.jbi.2022.104011 PMID: 35176451

Lu, Y. (2019). Artificial intelligence: A survey on evolution, models, applications and future trends. *Journal of Management Analytics*, *6*(1), 1–29. DOI: 10.1080/23270012.2019.1570365

Menzies, S. W., Sinz, C., Menzies, M., Lo, S. N., Yolland, W., Lingohr, J., Razmara, M., Tschandl, P., Guitera, P., Scolyer, R. A., Boltz, F., Borik-Heil, L., Chan, H. H., Chromy, D., Coker, D. J., Collgros, H., Eghtedari, M., Forteza, M. C., Forward, E., & Kittler, H. (2023). Comparison of humans versus mobile phone-powered artificial intelligence for the diagnosis and management of pigmented skin cancer in secondary care: A multicentre, prospective, diagnostic, clinical trial. *The Lancet. Digital Health*, *5*(10), e679–e691. DOI: 10.1016/s2589-7500(23)00130-9 PMID: 37775188

Miotto, R., Wang, F., Wang, S., Jiang, X., & Dudley, J. T. (2017). Deep learning for healthcare: Review, opportunities and challenges. *Briefings in Bioinformatics*, *19*(6), 1236–1246. DOI: 10.1093/bib/bbx044 PMID: 28481991

Nam, J. G., Hwang, E. J., Kim, J., Park, N., Lee, E. H., Kim, H. J., Nam, M., Lee, J. H., Park, C. M., & Goo, J. M. (2023). AI improves nodule detection on chest radiographs in a health screening population: A randomized controlled trial. *Radiology*, *307*(2). Advance online publication. DOI: 10.1148/radiol.221894 PMID: 36749213

Piccialli, F., Di Somma, V., Giampaolo, F., Cuomo, S., & Fortino, G. (2020). A survey on deep learning in medicine: Why, how and when? *Information Fusion*, *66*, 111–137. DOI: 10.1016/j.inffus.2020.09.006

Piette, J. D., Newman, S., Krein, S. L., Marinec, N., Chen, J., Williams, D. A., Edmond, S. N., Driscoll, M., LaChappelle, K. M., Kerns, R. D., Maly, M., Kim, H. M., Farris, K. B., Higgins, D. M., Buta, E., & Heapy, A. A. (2022). Patient-Centered pain care using artificial intelligence and mobile health tools. *JAMA Internal Medicine*, *182*(9), 975. DOI: 10.1001/jamainternmed.2022.3178 PMID: 35939288

Pinto-Coelho, L. (2023). How Artificial intelligence is shaping medical Imaging Technology: A survey of Innovations and applications. *Bioengineering (Basel, Switzerland)*, *10*(12), 1435. DOI: 10.3390/bioengineering10121435 PMID: 38136026

Rajpurkar, P., Chen, E., Banerjee, O., & Topol, E. J. (2022). AI in health and medicine. *Nature Medicine*, *28*(1), 31–38. DOI: 10.1038/s41591-021-01614-0 PMID: 35058619

Rodrigues, R. (2020). Legal and human rights issues of AI: Gaps, challenges and vulnerabilities. *Journal of Responsible Technology*, *4*, 100005. DOI: 10.1016/j.jrt.2020.100005

Sarker, I. H. (2021a). Machine learning: Algorithms, Real-World applications and research directions. *SN Computer Science*, *2*(3). Advance online publication. DOI: 10.1007/s42979-021-00592-x PMID: 33778771

Sarker, I. H. (2021b). Deep Learning: A comprehensive overview on techniques, taxonomy, applications and research directions. *SN Computer Science*, *2*(6). Advance online publication. DOI: 10.1007/s42979-021-00815-1 PMID: 34426802

Sarker, I. H. (2022). AI-Based modeling: Techniques, applications and research issues towards automation, intelligent and smart systems. *SN Computer Science*, *3*(2). Advance online publication. DOI: 10.1007/s42979-022-01043-x PMID: 35194580

Saw, S. N., & Ng, K. H. (2022). Current challenges of implementing artificial intelligence in medical imaging. *Physica Medica*, *100*, 12–17. DOI: 10.1016/j.ejmp.2022.06.003 PMID: 35714523

Sun, L., Zhang, H., Yang, Y., & Wang, X. (2023). Exploration of the influence of early rehabilitation training on circulating endothelial progenitor cell mobilization in patients with acute ischemic stroke and its related mechanism under a lightweight artificial intelligence algorithm. *PubMed*, *27*(12), 5338–5355. DOI: 10.26355/eurrev_202306_32768 PMID: 37401269

Sundar, R., Kumarakulasinghe, N. B., Chan, Y. H., Yoshida, K., Yoshikawa, T., Miyagi, Y., Rino, Y., Masuda, M., Guan, J., Sakamoto, J., Tanaka, S., Tan, A. L., Hoppe, M. M., Jeyasekharan, A. D., Ng, C. C. Y., De Simone, M., Grabsch, H. I., Lee, J., Oshima, T., & Tan, P. (2021). Machine-learning model derived gene signature predictive of paclitaxel survival benefit in gastric cancer: Results from the randomised phase III SAMIT trial. *Gut*, *71*(4), 676–685. DOI: 10.1136/gutjnl-2021-324060 PMID: 33980610

Wubineh, B. Z., Deriba, F. G., & Woldeyohannis, M. M. (2023). Exploring the opportunities and challenges of implementing artificial intelligence in healthcare: A systematic literature review. *Urologic Oncology Seminars and Original Investigations*, *42*(3), 48–56. DOI: 10.1016/j.urolonc.2023.11.019 PMID: 38101991

Yin, H., Jiang, Y., Xu, Z., Jia, H., & Lin, G. (2022). Combined diagnosis of multiparametric MRI-based deep learning models facilitates differentiating triple-negative breast cancer from fibroadenoma magnetic resonance BI-RADS 4 lesions. *Journal of Cancer Research and Clinical Oncology*, *149*(6), 2575–2584. DOI: 10.1007/s00432-022-04142-7 PMID: 35771263

Zhang, C., & Lu, Y. (2021). Study on artificial intelligence: The state of the art and future prospects. *Journal of Industrial Information Integration*, *23*, 100224. DOI: 10.1016/j.jii.2021.100224

Chapter 8
Advanced Image Encryption Framework for Securing Gray and Color Medical Images

Santhosh Kumar Veeramalla
https://orcid.org/0000-0002-0560-7130
BVRIT HYDERABAD College of Engineering for Women, India

Roshan Bodile
National Institute of Technology, Jalandhar, India

B. Jailsingh
https://orcid.org/0000-0002-6268-2188
National Institute of Technology, Calicut, India

ABSTRACT

This study presents a secure image encryption method designed specifically for grayscale and color medical images, aimed at maintaining security and integrity during transmission and storage. The system utilizes a hybrid encryption method that integrates symmetric and asymmetric cryptography alongside image processing techniques. A specialized preprocessing step, optimized for medical image characteristics, improves both speed and encryption quality. The method facilitates the processing of color images via color space transformation, maintaining diagnostic integrity after decryption. A secure key management protocol effectively addresses the challenges associated with key generation and distribution. The system will undergo testing across various medical image datasets, assessing encryption and

DOI: 10.4018/979-8-3373-3196-6.ch008

decryption speed, key sensitivity, attack resistance, and computational efficiency. This study enhances secure medical image processing applicable to telemedicine, cloud diagnostics, and electronic health record systems.

I. INTRODUCTION

Medical imaging stands at the forefront of modern healthcare, driving advancements in diagnosis, treatment planning, and patient management. The integration of digital technologies into medical imaging has transformed the way healthcare providers capture, store, and transmit medical data. This digital transition has not only improved the efficiency and precision of diagnostic practices but also facilitated the widespread sharing of critical medical information across different healthcare systems. However, with these advancements comes an increased responsibility to protect sensitive patient data from potential breaches and cyber threats (Li & Zheng, 2002).

The digital nature of modern medical images—encompassing modalities such as X-rays, CT scans, and MRIs—makes them particularly vulnerable to unauthorized access and exploitation. Ensuring the confidentiality, integrity, and availability of medical images is essential, not only to comply with stringent regulatory standards but also to preserve the trust and privacy of patients (Kamal et al., 2021). The potential consequences of compromised medical data underscore the critical need for advanced security measures.

In this context, encryption emerges as a vital strategy for safeguarding medical images. However, traditional encryption techniques often fall short when applied to medical images, which are characterized by unique attributes such as high pixel correlation and the need for accurate diagnostic information preservation. The complexities introduced by color medical imaging further complicate the encryption process, requiring algorithms that can adapt to the specific requirements of both grey and color images (Liu & Xiao, 2020).

Driven by the imperative to enhance the security of medical imaging, this research introduces a novel encryption algorithm specifically designed for grey and color medical images. The algorithm is built on a foundation of robust cryptographic principles, tailored to address the distinctive challenges posed by medical images. Grey images, such as X-rays, are crucial for accurate diagnostics, while color images, increasingly used in advanced medical imaging techniques, add layers of complexity due to their multi-channel data structure (Chen et al., 2008; Wang et al., 2015; Baptista, 1998; Fridrich, 1998).

Traditional encryption methods often struggle with the high correlation between adjacent pixels in medical images, which can lead to vulnerabilities. This research proposes a cutting-edge solution that integrates multiple stages, including image splitting, pixel scrambling, chaotic key generation, and diffusion. By employing these techniques, the proposed algorithm effectively disrupts the pixel correlation, ensuring that the encrypted images are highly secure and resistant to cryptographic attacks. Furthermore, the algorithm is designed to maintain the integrity of diagnostic information, ensuring that the security measures do not compromise the utility of the medical images (Zhang et al., 2016; Veeramalla et al., 2023; Bharat Babu et al., 2023; Gali et al., 2023; Khan & Shah, 2014; Behnia et al., 2008; Pareek et al., 2006; Kanso & Smaoui, 2009).

This study not only advances the field of medical image encryption but also sets a new standard for how sensitive medical data should be protected in an increasingly digital healthcare landscape. We provide a cutting-edge method for dividing images that serves as the foundation of our encryption algorithm. This novel technique starts by partitioning the picture into separate blocks, and then applying a random permutation on these pieces. This permutation process reorganizes the blocks in an apparently disorderly fashion, further intensified by pixel replacement inside each block. These procedures are carefully crafted to disturb the high association that usually occurs between adjacent pixels in medical pictures, which are often vulnerable to possible assaults.

In order to enhance the encryption process, a logistic map is used to disperse the distorted picture. The beginning condition for this chaotic map is exclusively determined by the plain picture, guaranteeing that the encryption process is tightly linked to the precise content of the image. By adding this requirement, an extra level of protection is implemented, greatly increasing the difficulty for attackers to decipher the encryption without having the original picture (Kanso & Smaoui, 2009; Ye & Huang, 2017; Kaur & Kaur, 2011; Fu et al., 2013; Liu & Wang, 2011; Belazi et al., 2016).

The combination of these strategies produces an algorithm that is very resistant to differential attacks, which aim to exploit small variations in the input to get knowledge about the encryption key. Our technique has undergone a thorough investigation, which shows that it outperforms current encryption methods in terms of both speed and security. This is especially apparent in its capacity to preserve the integrity of the encrypted picture while efficiently thwarting illegal access.

The results of our work demonstrate that the method we have developed is very efficient in encrypting medical pictures, effectively maintaining the secrecy of the images without sacrificing their diagnostic usefulness. Our technique establishes a new standard for medical picture encryption by providing exceptional security and performance. This makes it an essential tool for safeguarding sensitive medical data.

II. LITERATURE REVIEW

With the increasing need to secure sensitive medical data, various approaches to image encryption and steganography have emerged. Liao et al. proposed a novel method (Liao et al., 2018) in their study that aimed at preserving the privacy of medical JPEG images by concealing sensitive information. Unlike traditional steganographic techniques that modify discrete cosine transform (DCT) coefficients and potentially disrupt inter-block relationships, this method emphasizes maintaining the dependencies between DCT coefficients across adjacent blocks. By dynamically allocating cost values during the embedding process, the method clusters changes, ensuring minimal disruption and improved performance over previous techniques. The experimental results confirm that this method enhances privacy without significantly altering the image structure.

In another effort to secure medical data, Usman et al. introduced a steganographic approach (Usman & Usman, 2018) that utilizes image steganography to safeguard patient information. Their paper presents a method where swapped Huffman tree coding is applied to compress and encrypt data before embedding it into cover images. By focusing on the edge regions of the image for data embedding, this technique offers high imperceptibility, ensuring that the hidden data is not easily noticeable. The method combines lossless compression and manifold encryption to maintain the confidentiality of sensitive medical data while ensuring that the embedded information blends seamlessly with the cover image.

Further addressing the security needs of medical data, Vengadapurvaja et al. in their paper (Vengadapurvaja et al., 2017) explored the use of homomorphic encryption in the healthcare sector. With the growing adoption of Electronic Health Records (EHR) and the integration of cloud services, there is a pressing need to secure data during transmission and storage. Homomorphic encryption enables the performance of operations on encrypted data without compromising its confidentiality. The authors proposed an efficient homomorphic encryption scheme that allows medical images to be securely stored and manipulated in cloud environments while maintaining high levels of security and performance.

Ke et al. (2019), in their paper, tackled the problem of reversible data hiding in medical images. The paper proposes an algorithm that utilizes Most Significant Bit (MSB) prediction to identify and correct prediction errors before encrypting the image. This method leverages the local correlation between adjacent pixel values to predict errors, storing them in a binary map to ensure accurate reconstruction. The proposed high-capacity reversible data hiding method enables secure encryption and retrieval of medical images, with simulation results showing superior performance over existing algorithms in maintaining image quality while offering robust security.

Hua et al. (2018) presented a new medical image encryption scheme in their paper which aims to enhance security while maintaining efficiency. The algorithm introduces random data into the image and then performs two rounds of high-speed pixel scrambling and adaptive diffusion, dispersing the data across the entire image. The encryption scheme supports bitwise XOR and modulo arithmetic, offering adaptability to both hardware and software platforms. Experimental results demonstrate that this method provides high security, fast processing, and resilience to impulse noise and data loss, outperforming several state-of-the-art encryption techniques.

Chen et al. (2020) introduced a technique designed to safeguard medical images during transmission and storage. The framework utilizes Shearlet transform, known for its ability to effectively characterize texture information in images, which is critical for medical diagnostics. The image is decomposed into sub-images, shuffled, and synthesized before being encrypted with double random phase encoding (DRPE). The proposed framework allows flexibility in adjusting parameters and offers improved security through simulation results, proving to be an effective solution for securing medical data while preserving critical image details.

Lastly, Cao et al. (2017) proposed an encryption algorithm that derives edge maps from the source image to enhance security. The method involves bit-plane decomposition, random sequence generation, and pixel permutation, offering flexibility in terms of image type, edge detection, and permutation techniques. The algorithm's large key space and strong key sensitivity make it highly resistant to various attacks. Experimental evaluations reveal that the method provides superior security and performance, especially for images with fuzzy edge maps, outperforming other contemporary encryption algorithms.

III. THE PROPOSED METHOD

The proposed encryption algorithm is a comprehensive and robust solution tailored to address the unique challenges associated with securing grey and color medical images. This method is structured into several key stages, each meticulously designed to ensure the confidentiality, integrity, and resilience of medical images against various cryptographic attacks. Below is an in-depth exploration of the entire encryption and decryption process.

1. Encryption Process

The encryption process is the core of the proposed method, consisting of four critical stages: Image Splitting, Confusion (Scrambling), Key Generation, and Diffusion. Each stage contributes uniquely to transforming a plain image into a highly secure encrypted image.

Image Splitting

The first step in the encryption process involves dividing the plain image into smaller, non-overlapping blocks. This step is essential as it disrupts the spatial correlation typically found in medical images, which is a known vulnerability. The algorithm offers flexibility in the size of these blocks (e.g., 16x16, 32x32, 64x64), allowing the user to adjust the level of security and computational load according to specific needs.

Once the image is divided into blocks, each block is subject to a further subdivision into smaller sub-blocks, depending on a random number generated for each block. This additional subdivision is crucial for introducing randomness into the encryption process, ensuring that even if two blocks contain identical or similar content, their encryption will differ significantly due to the random sub-block configuration. This randomness is a key feature of the algorithm, enhancing its ability to resist statistical and pattern-based attacks.

Confusion (Scrambling)

After splitting the image, the algorithm enters the confusion stage, where the pixel arrangement within each block and sub-block is altered to create a scrambled version of the image. This stage is designed to obscure the original structure of the image, making it unintelligible to unauthorized viewers. The confusion process is carried out through several distinct operations:

Zigzag Pattern Application: A zigzag scanning pattern is applied to both the undivided blocks and the sub-blocks. This pattern rearranges the pixels in a non-linear fashion, breaking the original order and introducing a level of unpredictability.

Block Rotation: Following the zigzag pattern, each block and sub-block undergoes a 90-degree rotation. This rotation further scrambles the pixel arrangement, ensuring that even neighboring pixels within the same block are no longer in their original positions relative to each other.

Random Permutation: To add an additional layer of complexity, a random vector rrr is generated, dictating a permutation sequence for the blocks. This random permutation is applied across all blocks, effectively disrupting any remaining spatial correlation between blocks. The combination of these scrambling techniques makes it extremely difficult for an attacker to deduce the original image without the correct decryption key.

Key Generation

One of the most important parts of the suggested method is key generation as it ensures the encryption procedure is secure. Deriving the key from the logistic map, a chaotic system famous for its sensitivity to beginning conditions—a trait often desired in cryptography applications—is the process.

Initial Condition Calculation: The initial condition Y_0 for the logistic map is computed based on the pixel values of the plain image. This ensures that the key is uniquely tied to the specific image being encrypted, further enhancing security.

Iterative Sequence Generation: The logistic map is iterated multiple times to produce a sequence. The initial sequence is discarded (often referred to as the transient period) to remove any predictability that might be present at the start.

Key Formation: In the diffusion step, the last key sequence is generated from the processed remaining sequence. Ensuring that even a little alteration to the plain image will produce an entirely new key is included into the key generation process. This provides strong defense against known plaintext and differential attacks. Figure 3 displays the logistic map's bifurcation diagram.

Diffusion

In the last step of encryption, known as diffusion, the created key is used to change the pixel values of the encrypted picture. This is an essential stage because it ensures that the encrypted picture is very sensitive to changes in either the key or the plain image, and that each bit of the key has a considerable impact on the whole image.

Diffusion Process: The picture vector that has been jumbled up and the key sequence K(i) are subjected to a bitwise exclusive OR (XOR) operation in order to facilitate the diffusion process. Achieving strong security requires this procedure to inject a layer of non-linearity. By radically differing from the plain and scrambled images, the encrypted picture becomes almost unintelligible without the right key, thanks to the XOR process.

To make matters more complicated, the diffusion step adds a regulated amount of noise to the picture, making it much more difficult to reverse-engineer the encryption process. Along with key-driven diffusion, this noise makes sure the encrypted picture is safe and won't be broken by cryptography

2. Decryption Process

The decryption process is the reverse of the encryption process and requires the correct key to successfully retrieve the original image. Each stage of decryption is carefully designed to undo the transformations applied during encryption, restoring the image to its original state.

Inverse Diffusion

The first step in decryption involves reversing the diffusion process. This is achieved by applying a bitwise XOR operation between the encrypted image vector and the same key sequence K(i) used during encryption. This step effectively removes the noise and other alterations introduced during the diffusion process, yielding the scrambled image.

Reverse Permutation

The next step is to reverse the random permutation applied to the blocks during the confusion stage. Using the same random vector r that was generated during encryption, the blocks are permuted back to their original positions. This step is crucial for restoring the spatial arrangement of the image blocks.

Inverse Rotation and Zigzag Pattern

Following the reverse permutation, the blocks and sub-blocks are rotated back by 90 degrees to undo the rotation applied during encryption. After this, the inverse of the zigzag pattern is applied to return the pixels within each block and sub-block to their original order. These operations are essential for accurately reconstructing the original image.

Block Merging

The last step in restoring the original picture is to combine all of the blocks and sub-blocks. At this point, you'll put the pieces together in the right order to create the final picture. The decoded picture will be an identical match for the original plain picture if everything is done well and the right key is utilized.

It is our intention that the decryption procedure will be just as safe as the encryption process. Data security is maintained throughout its lifespan since it is difficult to get the raw picture by reversing the modifications without the right key.

Figure 1 depicts the whole procedure. The suggested encryption algorithm's flowchart graphically depicts the sequential steps of encrypting and decrypting a medical picture, starting with a plain image and ending with its original form. The two primary components of the flow diagram are the encryption and decryption processes.

Flowchart Description

Start: The process begins with loading the plain medical image, which can be either a grey or a color image.

Plain Image Splitting

The loaded image is divided into non-overlapping blocks. Each block may be further subdivided into smaller sub-blocks based on a randomly generated value. This step prepares the image for subsequent scrambling and diffusion operations.

Confusion (Scrambling)

Zigzag Pattern Application: The pixels within each block and sub-block are rearranged using a zigzag scanning pattern.

Rotation: Each block and sub-block is rotated by 90 degrees to further obscure the pixel arrangement.

Random Permutation: A random permutation is applied to the blocks using a randomly generated vector r, resulting in a scrambled image.

Key Generation

Initial Condition Calculation: The initial condition Y_0 for the logistic map is calculated based on the pixel values of the plain image.

Logistic Map Iteration: The logistic map is iterated to generate a chaotic sequence, which is then processed to form the key sequence $K(i)$.

Diffusion: Bitwise XOR Operation: The scrambled image vector undergoes a bitwise XOR operation with the key sequence $K(i)$, resulting in the final encrypted image. This operation ensures that the encrypted image is significantly different from the original and scrambled images.

Output Encrypted Image: The encrypted image, which is now highly secure and resistant to attacks, is stored or transmitted.

Decryption Process (Reverse of Encryption): The decryption process begins with loading the encrypted image.

Inverse Diffusion: The encrypted image is processed by performing a bitwise XOR operation with the same key sequence $K(i)$, yielding the scrambled image.

Reverse Permutation: The blocks of the scrambled image are permuted back to their original positions using the vector r from the encryption process.

Inverse Rotation and Zigzag: The blocks and sub-blocks are rotated back, and the zigzag pattern is undone, restoring the original pixel arrangement within each block.

Block Merging: The blocks and sub-blocks are merged to reconstruct the original plain image.

Output Decrypted Image: The final output is the decrypted image, which should be an exact replica of the original plain image if the correct key was used throughout the decryption process.

End: The process concludes, ensuring that both the encryption and decryption were performed successfully.

Figure 1. Flowchart

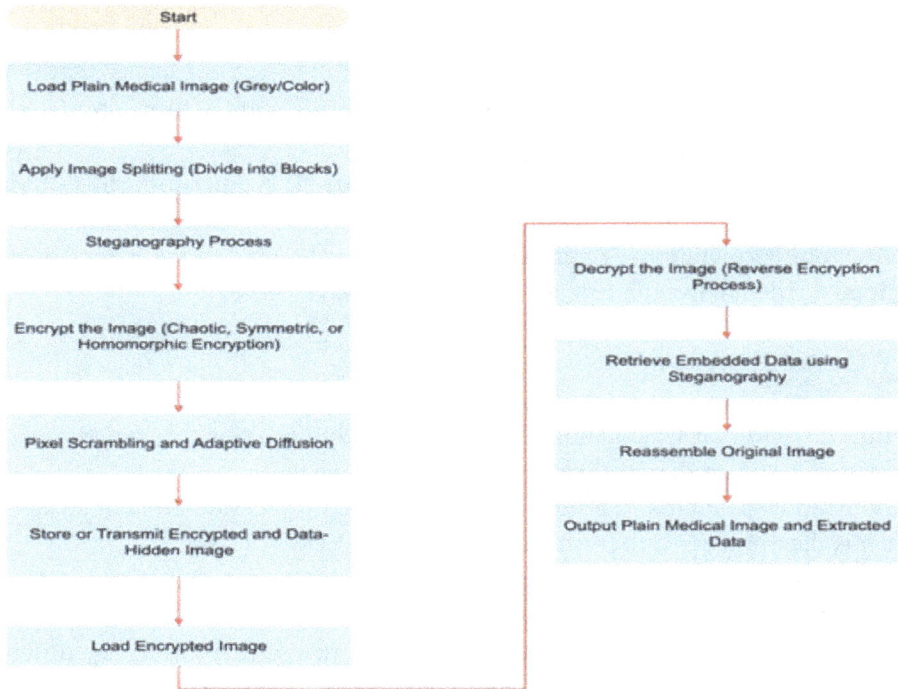

IV. SIMULATION RESULTS

Figure 2 shows the user interface for selecting and uploading a basic picture. The picture upload and histogram may be seen in figure 2.a. The histogram will then appear underneath the uploaded picture. The distribution of picture pixels is shown by the histogram. Image 1 in greyscale is this.Here we can see the histogram that was generated after the picture upload. Figure 2.b shows the key generation together with its related histogram. Figure 2.c shows the encrypted picture with its accompanying histogram. Figures 2.a and 2.c indicate that the encrypted and plain images' histograms should be different. The decrypted picture and histogram are shown in figure 2.d.The histograms of the plain picture and the encrypted image are identical, as seen in the figure below. Table 1 displays the image-related characteristics and their associated determined values.

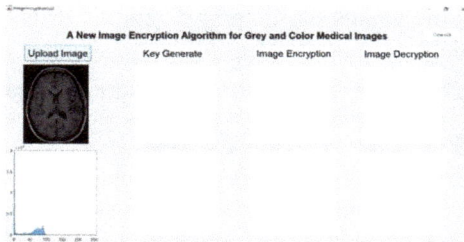

Fig 2.a : Uploading image

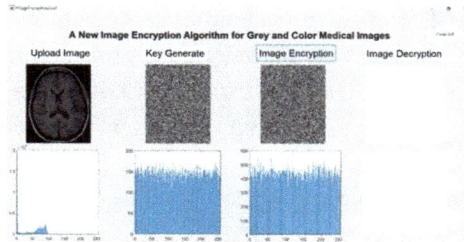

Fig 2.c : Encrypted Image

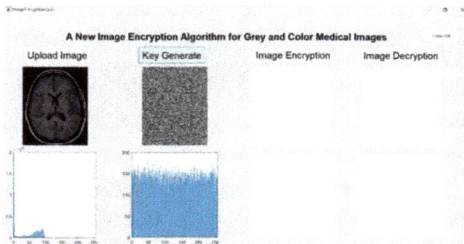

Fig 2.b : Key Generation

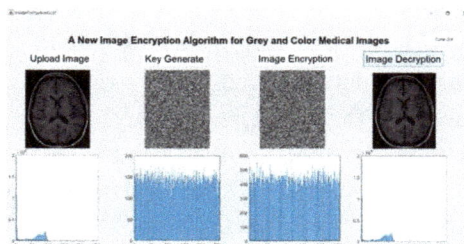

Fig 2.d : Decrypted Image

Table 1. Calculated parameters of the Image

PARAMETERS	VALUES
Mean-squared error	31.50
Peak-SNR	-41.17
SNR(signal-to-noise ratio)	2.1819
SSIM Score(structural similarity index measure)	-0.0011
MSSIM Score(mean structural similarity index measure)	0.0000
Entropy for Encrypted image	0.4018

continued on following page

Table 1. Continued

PARAMETERS	VALUES
Entropy for Decrypted image	0.6562
NPCR Score(number of pixel change rate)	99.58
UACI Score(unified average changing intensity)	36.76

MSE:

The average squared difference between the values predicted by a model or estimator and the actual values observed may be measured using the Mean Squared Error (MSE). The formula for it is the sum of the squares of the discrepancies between the expected and observed values.

Peak-SNR:

An image or video's reconstructed signal may be evaluated for quality using the Peak Signal-to-Noise Ratio (PSNR), which compares the reconstructed signal to the original signal. It measures how much corrupting noise may degrade a signal's fidelity relative to the signal's maximum potential power. dB is the unit of measurement for PSNR.

The structural similarity index metric known as the SSIM score is:

By comparing the structural information in the original and distorted pictures, the Structural Similarity Index Measure (SSIM) may be used to evaluate the perceived quality of digital photos or movies. Images' structural information, brightness, and contrast are considered by SSIM, in contrast to more conventional measures such as Mean Squared Error (MSE).

Three factors—structure, contrast, and brightness—are combined to form the SSIM index. A number between -1 and 1 represents this, with 1 indicating that the photos are quite similar to one other.

Score for the MSSIM (mean structural similarity index):

A composite metric for evaluating picture quality, the Mean Structural Similarity metric Measure (MSSIM) is an expansion of the Structural Similarity Index Measure (SSIM). In contrast to MSSIM, which computes the average SSIM value over the whole picture, SSIM determines how similar two separate image patches are.

A popular measure in image processing and computer vision applications, MSSIM offers a comprehensive evaluation of picture quality by taking the average similarity across several patches into account. The greater the MSSIM value, the more similar the photos are to one another.

NPCR(number of pixel change rate):

To measure how well cryptographic methods work, especially when encrypting images, one might look at the Number of Pixel Change Rate (NPCR). It quantifies the fraction of an image's pixels that undergo a cryptographic operation (like encryption) and hence change.

As a percentage, NPCR shows how much of a difference there is between the original and encrypted pictures. A larger number indicates a more significant difference. This statistic is crucial

to evaluate the diffusion property of cryptographic algorithms, whereby the security is guaranteed by making sure that even a tiny modification to the input changes the output significantly.

Unified Average Changing Intensity (UACI):

One measure used to assess the efficacy of cryptographic methods, especially those dealing with picture encryption, is the Unified Average Changing Intensity (UACI). Comparing the original and encrypted (or decrypted) photos, it finds the average intensity change between matching pixels in both sets of images.

A higher UACI value indicates a more significant shift in intensity between the two pixels in question. It's a crucial measure for evaluating the confusion and diffusion qualities of cryptographic algorithms, which are designed to guarantee security by making sure that changes to the input cause unexpected and substantial changes to the output.

Analysis of Information Entropy:

Information entropy quantifies the degree to which the picture is chaotic. Entropy is defined mathematically as:

$$H\left(m\right) = \sum_{i=1}^{w} p\left(m_i\right) \log_2 \frac{1}{p\left(m_i\right)}$$

Analysis of Image Histogram:

The histogram shows how the image's pixels are distributed. To make it impossible for attackers to decipher encrypted images, the histogram should be flat. Additionally, there should be no similarity in the histogram of the encrypted and plain images.

Figure 3. Encryption and Decryption of another medical image

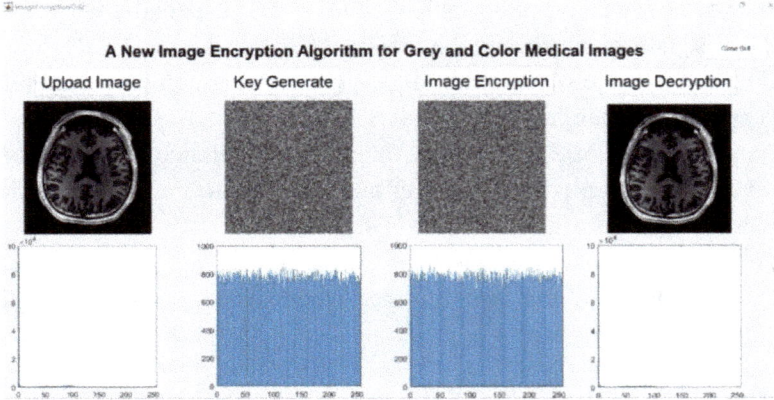

Histograms of both unencrypted and encrypted medical photos are shown in Figure 3. Our approach produces uniformly distributed histograms for encrypted photos, which differ significantly from the histograms of the equivalent plain images.

Analysis of Correlation Coefficient

Since the values of neighboring pixels are almost equal, there is a strong connection between them, especially in the simple picture. An encrypted picture with little connection between neighboring pixels is the foundation of an efficient encryption technique. Coefficients of horizontal (H), vertical (V), and diagonal (D) correlation for encrypted test pictures and their gray counterparts. The correlation coefficient values for the encrypted photos are close to zero, in contrast to the near-one values for all the test images. The approaches that are based on Img1 are compared and detailed. Experiment results show that suggested approach successfully lowers encrypted image's neighboring pixels' correlation.

The correlation coefficient of grey image 1 is
1.0000 0.0008
0.0008 1.0000
The correlation coefficient of grey image 2 is
1.0000 0.0004
0.0004 1.0000
The correlation coefficient of color image 1 is
1.0000 0.0023
0.0023 1.0000
The correlation coefficient of color image 2 is

1.0000 0.0044
0.0044 1.0000

Results of Color Medical Image Testing

Color medical pictures have become more common in illness diagnosis as a result of the technological advancements in medical instruments. Color medical photos may also be encrypted using our suggested approach. Because there are three possible values for each pixel in a color image—red, green, and blue—these pictures often have more detail than their grey counterparts. Figure 4 shows one possible method for encrypting color images: first, divide the picture into its RGB channels. Then, use the algorithm to encrypt each channel separately.

Figure 4. Color image encryption and decryption

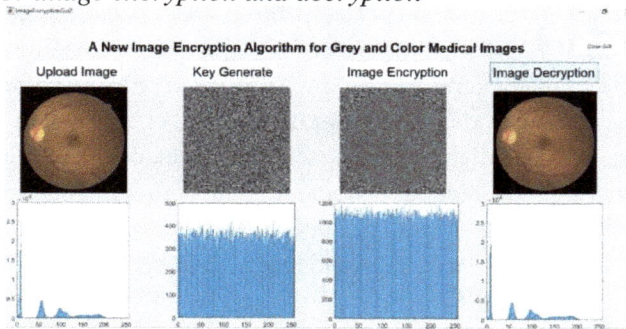

Table 2. Performance metrics for color images

PARAMETERS	VALUES
Mean-squared error	40.11
peak-SNR	-40.75
SNR(signal-to-noise ratio)	2.61
SSIM score(structural similarity index measure)	0.0002
MSSIM Score(mean structural similarity index measure)	0.000
Entropy for Encrypted image	0.036
Entropy for Decrypted image	0.3178
NPCR(number of pixel change rate)	99.60
UACI(unified average changing intensity)	34.96

The efficiency with which the suggested picture encryption method protects both black-and-white and color medical images is shown by the findings. Reliable indications of strong encryption quality and durability include performance measurements such as Mean-Squared Error (MSE), Peak Signal-to-Noise Ratio (PSNR), Structural Similarity Index Measure (SSIM), entropy, Number of Pixel Change Rate (NPCR), and Unified Average Changing Intensity (UACI). There is a lot of distortion between the original and encrypted photographs because there is a high Mean Squared Error (MSE) and a negative Peak Signal-to-Noise Ratio (PSNR). The encrypted pictures also show little structural similarity to the originals, as shown by the low values of the Structural Similarity Index (SSIM) and Multi-Scale Structural Similarity (MSSIM). With UACI and NPCR scores that are so precise, the system can better resist differential attacks since even little changes to the original image will result in encrypted pictures that are drastically different from one another. In addition, histogram analysis reveals that the encrypted photographs have an equal distribution of pixels, which destroys statistical attacks.

As a consequence of the method's effectiveness, the correlation between adjacent pixels dropped sharply, and their values are now very close to zero. Disrupting the inherent structure of medical images requires this. Even after encryption, there was still no correlation between the three color channels in either the grayscale or color medical images. Additionally, this method ensures the confidentiality of sensitive medical data, making it an excellent choice for encrypting medical photos without compromising diagnostic information. In conclusion, the results show that the proposed method is very effective and dependable in protecting medical images inside electronic healthcare systems.

V. CONCLUSION

The proposed image encryption algorithm successfully addresses the challenges of securing both grey and color medical images, offering robust protection without compromising the integrity of diagnostic data. Through the use of sophisticated methods including diffusion, chaotic key generation, pixel scrambling, and picture splitting, the algorithm guarantees that encrypted images are very resilient to cryptographic assaults. Evaluations of the algorithm's performance using a variety of metrics, including as MSE, PSNR, SSIM, entropy, NPCR, and UACI, show that it significantly increases encryption quality and randomness while removing the structural correlations present in medical pictures.

Additionally, uniform histograms and nearly-zero pixel correlation coefficients demonstrate how well the system protects sensitive medical data against statistical and differential assaults. The encryption technique is flexible and consistently works well for medical photos in both grayscale and color. All things considered, this study offers a very effective and safe way to safeguard medical pictures in healthcare systems, which makes it a vital instrument for maintaining patient privacy and guaranteeing adherence to data security guidelines.

REFERENCES

Belazi, A., El-Latif, A. A. A., & Belghith, S. (2016). A novel image encryption scheme based on substitution-permutation network and chaos. *Signal Processing Image Communication*, *28*(3), 292–300. DOI: 10.1016/j.sigpro.2016.03.021

Cao, W., Zhou, Y., Chen, C. L. P., & Xia, L. (2017). Medical image encryption using edge maps. *Signal Processing*, *132*, 96–109. DOI: 10.1016/j.sigpro.2016.10.003

Chen, C. K., Lai, J. L., & Chang, C. C. (2008). Efficient watermarking method based on significant difference of wavelet coefficient quantization. *IEEE Transactions on Multimedia*, *10*(5), 746–757. DOI: 10.1109/TMM.2008.922839

Chen, G., Ma, M., Tang, C., & Lei, Z. (2020). Generalized optical encryption framework based on shearlets for medical image. *Optics and Lasers in Engineering*, *128*, 106026. Advance online publication. DOI: 10.1016/j.optlaseng.2020.106026

Fridrich, J. (1998). Symmetric ciphers based on two-dimensional chaotic maps. *International Journal of Bifurcation and Chaos in Applied Sciences and Engineering*, *8*(6), 1259–1284. DOI: 10.1142/S021812749800098X

Fu, C., Meng, W., Zhan, Y., & Qi, C. (2013). An efficient and secure medical image protection scheme based on chaotic maps. *Computers & Electrical Engineering*, *39*(5), 1606–1622. DOI: 10.1016/j.compeleceng.2013.05.005

Gali, R. L., Manne, P., & Veeramalla, S. K. (2023). Structuring hybrid model using bilateral and guided filters for image denoising. In *2023 International Conference on Next Generation Electronics (NEleX)*. IEEE. https://doi.org/DOI: 10.1109/NEleX59773.2023.10421518

Hua, Z., Yi, S., & Zhou, Y. (2018). Medical image encryption using high-speed scrambling and pixel adaptive diffusion. *Signal Processing*, *144*, 134–144. DOI: 10.1016/j.sigpro.2017.10.004

Kamal, S. T., Hosny, K. M., Elgindy, T. M., Darwish, M. M., & Fouda, M. M. (2021). A new image encryption algorithm for grey and color medical images. *IEEE Access : Practical Innovations, Open Solutions*, *9*, 37855–37865. DOI: 10.1109/ACCESS.2021.3063237

Kanso, A., & Smaoui, N. (2009). Logistic chaotic maps for binary numbers generations. *Chaos, Solitons, and Fractals*, *40*(5), 2557–2568. DOI: 10.1016/j.chaos.2007.10.049

Kaur, M., & Kaur, R. (2011). Image encryption techniques: A selected review. *Journal of Theoretical and Applied Information Technology*, *30*(1), 1–12.

Ke, G., Wang, H., Zhou, S., & Zhang, H. (2019). Encryption of medical image with most significant bit and high capacity in piecewise linear chaos graphics. *Measurement*, *135*, 385–391. DOI: 10.1016/j.measurement.2018.11.074

Khan, M., & Shah, T. (2014). A literature review on image encryption techniques. *3D Research*, *5*(4), Article 29. https://doi.org/DOI: 10.1007/s13319-014-0029-0

Liao, X., Yin, J., Guo, S., Li, X., & Sangaiah, A. K. (2018). Medical JPEG image steganography based on preserving inter-block dependencies. *Computers & Electrical Engineering*, *67*, 320–329. DOI: 10.1016/j.compeleceng.2017.08.020

Liu, H., & Wang, X. (2011). Color image encryption using spatial bit-level permutation and high-dimension chaotic system. *Optics Communications*, *284*(16–17), 3895–3903. DOI: 10.1016/j.optcom.2011.04.001

Liu, Z., & Xiao, D. (2020). Medical image encryption using a novel chaos-based encryption algorithm. *IEEE Access : Practical Innovations, Open Solutions*, *8*, 172894–172905. DOI: 10.1109/ACCESS.2020.2991420

Pareek, N. K., Patidar, V., & Sud, K. K. (2006). Image encryption using chaotic logistic map. *Image and Vision Computing*, *24*(9), 926–934. DOI: 10.1016/j.imavis.2006.02.021

Usman, M. A., & Usman, M. R. (2018). Using image steganography for providing enhanced medical data security. In *Proceedings of the 2018 15th IEEE Annual Consumer Communications & Networking Conference (CCNC)* (pp. 1–4). IEEE. https://doi.org/DOI: 10.1109/CCNC.2018.8319263

Veeramalla, S. K., & Kumar, S. (2023). Segmentation of MRI images using a combination of active contour modeling and morphological processing. *Journal of Mechanics in Medicine and Biology*, *23*(4), 2340002. Advance online publication. DOI: 10.1142/S021951942340002X

Vengadapurvaja, A. M., Nisha, G., Aarthy, R., & Sasikaladevi, N. (2017). An efficient homomorphic medical image encryption algorithm for cloud storage security. *Procedia Computer Science*, *115*, 643–650. DOI: 10.1016/j.procs.2017.09.150

Wang, X., Zhang, Y., & Bao, X. (2015). A novel chaotic block image encryption algorithm based on dynamic random growth technique. *Optics and Lasers in Engineering*, *66*, 10–18. DOI: 10.1016/j.optlaseng.2014.08.005

Ye, G., & Huang, K. (2017). An efficient symmetric image encryption algorithm based on an intertwining logistic map. *Neurocomputing*, *251*, 45–53. DOI: 10.1016/j.neucom.2017.04.016

Zhang, X., Wang, Y., & Gu, Z. (2016). A novel image encryption scheme based on a linear hyperbolic chaotic system of partial differential equations. *Journal of Electronic Imaging*, *25*(2), 023014. Advance online publication. DOI: 10.1117/1. JEI.25.2.023014

Chapter 9
Decoding the Invisible:
AI and Radiomics for Predictive and Personalized Imaging

Shubham Gupta
https://orcid.org/0000-0003-1202-2779
Parul University, India

Vishnu Vinod
https://orcid.org/0009-0001-8866-181X
NAMO College of Allied Health Sciences, India

ABSTRACT

Artificial intelligence (AI) and radiomics are fundamentally transforming the future of medical imaging by uncovering therapeutically significant information that traditional interpretation methods often overlook. This chapter delves into their expanding roles in healthcare, radiology, and metabolic medicine, highlighting how AI-driven radiomic analysis can be seamlessly integrated into clinical workflows to enhance diagnostic precision. Radiomics enables predictive modeling and personalized diagnostics by extracting and analyzing subtle imaging features and complex patterns from common modalities such as CT, MRI, and PET. Utilizing advanced AI techniques to decode microscopic textural variations, metabolic activity trends, and early indicators of disease progression, radiologists are evolving into sophisticated data interpreters. The chapter explores the revolutionary impact of AI in improving diagnostic accuracy, stratifying patient risk, and tailoring treatment strategies—especially critical in metabolic diseases where early detection is vital for effective intervention.

DOI: 10.4018/979-8-3373-3196-6.ch009

1 INTRODUCTION

1.1 Overview of Radiomics and its Emergence in the Medical Field

Radiomics represents a rapidly advancing field within medical imaging, characterized by the extraction and computational analysis of a vast array of quantitative features from conventional radiological images. The fundamental principle underpinning radiomics is that medical imaging harbours information that extends beyond visual interpretation, and that such data can be systematically quantified to identify imaging biomarkers indicative of the underlying pathophysiological processes of disease.

With the advancement and widespread adoption of radiological imaging modalities such as computed tomography (CT), magnetic resonance imaging (MRI), and positron emission tomography (PET), high-resolution and standardized images began to be routinely generated across diverse patient populations. This resulted in the accumulation of large, uniform datasets amenable to in-depth analysis. The growing demand for objective and reproducible metrics catalysed the emergence of quantitative imaging, wherein characteristics such as tumour size, shape, and texture are measured (Gillies et al., 2016).

Advancements in high-performance computing and machine learning have enabled the extraction of numerous quantitative features from medical images, supporting the shift toward personalized medicine. Radiomics has emerged as a key method for developing non-invasive imaging biomarkers to predict disease phenotypes and treatment outcomes. Its integration with genomic and clinical data has given rise to radio genomics, highlighting radiomics' role in multi-omics research and translational medicine.(Parmar et al., 2015).

1.2 Role of Artificial Intelligence (AI) in Transforming Diagnostic Radiology

Artificial Intelligence (AI), especially through machine learning (ML) and deep learning (DL), has revolutionized diagnostic radiology by enhancing radiologists' interpretation capabilities and optimizing imaging workflows. Deep learning models, particularly convolutional neural networks (CNNs), are central to this progress, enabling accurate image classification, segmentation, and anomaly detection. Trained on large annotated datasets, these models support identifying pathologies like tumors, fractures, haemorrhages, and pulmonary nodules with high sensitivity and specificity, ultimately improving diagnostic accuracy, efficiency, and clinical decision-making.(Anwar et al., 2018).

AI has also enabled the development of computer-aided detection (CADe) and computer-aided diagnosis (CADx) tools. These systems provide secondary reads or diagnostic suggestions, reducing oversight errors and inter-reader variability. Both computer-aided diagnosis (CAD) systems and radiomics leverage computational tools to enhance medical imaging analysis, but they differ in purpose and methodology. CAD systems are designed as standalone applications to support clinicians in detecting or diagnosing specific pathologies, with early success in screening for breast carcinoma (Dromain et al., 2013). These systems generally aim to deliver a binary output, such as the presence or absence of disease. In contrast, radiomics represents a workflow focused on the extraction of quantitative imaging features and their subsequent storage. These can then be analysed to uncover patterns and build predictive models. Radiomics also integrates imaging biomarkers with other patient-specific data, thereby enhancing the accuracy and personalization of diagnostic and therapeutic strategies (Arimura et al., 2018).

AI has also been instrumental in image acquisition and reconstruction. Algorithms can optimize scan parameters, reduce noise, and reconstruct high-quality images from low-dose data, which is particularly beneficial in modalities such as CT and MRI. This not only reduces radiation exposure but also enhances patient comfort and throughput (Jo et al., 2023; Tian et al., 2022).

1.3 Importance of Personalized Medicine in Modern Healthcare

Personalized medicine goes beyond the conventional one-size-fits-all approach by customizing treatment based on unique genetic, environmental, and lifestyle factors. It enhances diagnosis, treatment effectiveness, and minimizes adverse effects by discovering patient-specific biomarkers; this is particularly noticeable in cancer with targeted medicines like EGFR and HER2 inhibitors (Chen et al., 2022; Rossi et al., 2021).

Identification of high-risk individuals for diseases like cancer and cardiovascular disease is aided by developments in risk models and genetic screening. Healthcare efficiency and illness knowledge are improved by the integration of machine learning, electronic health records, and high-throughput technology (Ji et al., 2025). The importance of AI and radiomics in cancer treatment and tailored diagnostics is highlighted in this chapter, along with new developments like federated learning and multi-omics integration.

2 FUNDAMENTALS OF RADIOMICS

2.1 Definition and Principles of Radiomics

Radiomics is an interdisciplinary and data-intensive field involving medical imaging, computational science, and precision medicine. The workflow includes extraction and analysis of a large number of quantitative features from standard-of-care medical images—most commonly computed tomography (CT), magnetic resonance imaging (MRI), and positron emission tomography (PET)—using algorithmic and statistical techniques (Kumar et al., 2012).

Pathologies such as cancer, inflammation, or fibrosis induce measurable changes in tissue architecture and physiology, which in turn alter the intensity, texture, and spatial distribution of signals captured in radiological images. These alterations are often subtle but can be systematically quantified through mathematical descriptors such as variations in intratumoural texture which may correspond to differences in cell density, necrosis, vascularization, or stromal content—all of which are linked to tumour aggressiveness and therapeutic response (Zhou et al., 2024).

Radiomics translates these imaging patterns into high-dimensional quantitative data, producing what are known as *radiomic features*. These features enable medical images to act as repositories of spatial, functional, and textural information. These features can be used to construct imaging biomarkers that support a wide range of clinical tasks, such as disease detection and classification, tumour grading or staging, prediction of molecular or histopathologic subtypes, prognostic modelling (e.g., survival analysis) and response assessment to systemic therapies or radiotherapy (Lee et al., 2022).

By transforming images into structured data, radiomics enables data mining and pattern recognition within medical imaging, aligning it with the broader objectives of artificial intelligence in healthcare. Moreover, as it is non-invasive, repeatable, and based on existing clinical imaging workflows, radiomics holds significant promise for longitudinal monitoring and personalized treatment planning.

Radiomics is also increasingly being integrated into the field of precision oncology, where its ability to capture spatial and temporal heterogeneity at the whole-tumour level complements traditional tissue biopsies, which may suffer from sampling bias. In addition, radiomics supports radiogenomic research, where imaging phenotypes are linked to genetic and transcriptomic profiles, providing a bridge between genotype and phenotype in a clinical context. Figure 1 illustrates a generalized radiomics workflow.

Figure 1. Sequence of Processes in Radiomics

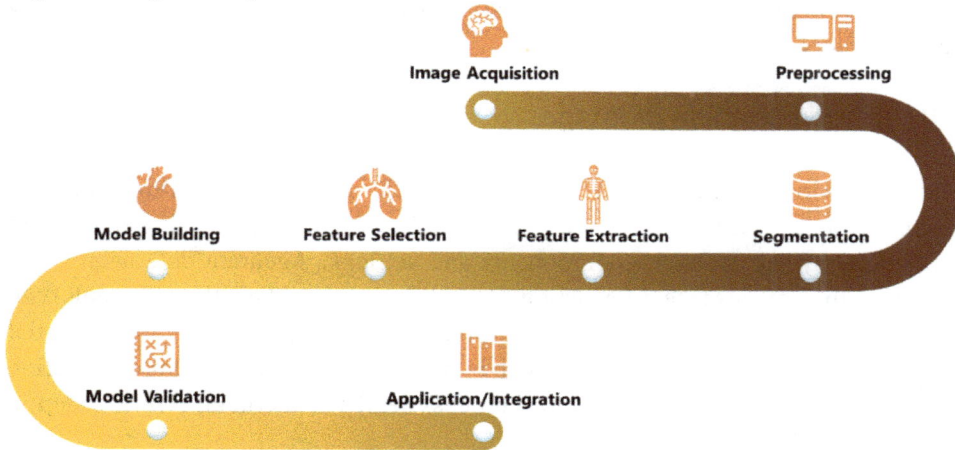

2.2 Image Acquisition

Radiomics involves extracting quantitative features from high-quality medical images obtained through modalities like CT, MRI, and PET. CT is commonly used in thoracic and cancer imaging due to its high spatial resolution, enabling analysis of texture, shape, and intensity. MRI allows multi-parametric analysis through various sequences, while PET captures metabolic activity, enabling SUV-based feature extraction. However, radiomic features are highly sensitive to variations in scanner hardware, acquisition settings (e.g., slice thickness, FOV, pixel spacing), and reconstruction algorithms. These inconsistencies can lead to significant variability, affecting the reliability and reproducibility of radiomic models (Zhao, 2021).

To enhance consistency and reproducibility in medical imaging, various strategies have been implemented across modalities. In CT, phantoms are used to evaluate reconstruction protocol consistency, with noise reduction as an initial step. In MRI, Diffusion-Weighted Imaging (DWI) and Dynamic Contrast-Enhanced (DCE) protocols are valuable for assessing tissue cellularity and vascular flow, respectively. PET acquisition variability can be minimized by following guidelines from the Society of Nuclear Medicine and the European Association of Nuclear Medicine. Standardization efforts by QIBA and the Image Biomarker Standardisation Initiative (IBSI) promote consistent acquisition and preprocessing techniques. Multi-center studies benefit from adopting uniform protocols recommended by The Cancer Imaging Archive (TCIA) and the American College of Radiology Imaging Network (ACRIN) to reduce inter-site variability. Additionally, harmonization algorithms like ComBat—originally developed for genomics—are used to correct scanner or site-related batch effects in radiomic data, further improving data comparability across centers.

2.2.1 Reconstruction of Image

Medical images are created by mathematically reconstructing raw data from scanners into grayscale visuals. The quality and characteristics of these images are influenced by the scanner's components and settings. Accurate data acquisition preserves the object's true information, but reconstruction algorithms (kernels) can introduce variability. These algorithms affect key image attributes—like spatial resolution and anatomical detail—which in turn impact radiomic feature extraction and analysis. Thus, the reconstruction process serves as a crucial filtering step in medical imaging.

2.3 Preprocessing

Radiomics exhibits a high sensitivity to various parameters that can influence the extracted features and, consequently, the reproducibility and comparability of radiomic analyses across different imaging protocols. Hence, pre-processing techniques aim to reduce the variability introduced by those parameters, thereby making the images more consistent for radiomic evaluation (Scapicchio et al., 2021).

Some major techniques in preprocessing are described as follows:

- Resampling
- Intensity Normalization
- Discretization
- Filtering of Images
- Image Co-registration
- Bias Field Correction

2.3.1 Resampling

Resampling standardizes the voxel size of images by interpolating the original image data onto a new, standard grid, such as 1 mm^3. There are multiple methods of interpolation such as linear, spline, and nearest Neighbor. Different imaging devices and protocols produce images with varying voxel dimensions (e.g., 0.5×0.5×1 mm vs. 1×1×5 mm). Many radiomics features, especially texture-based ones (e.g., GLCM, GLRLM), are sensitive to spatial resolution. Without resampling, radiomics features may capture differences due to acquisition settings, instead of true biological heterogeneity. Upsampling increases resolution but may introduce artifacts, whereas downsampling reduces resolution to limit computational complexity.

2.3.2 Intensity Normalization

It is also known as min-max normalization and is useful in CT imaging, where pixel values represent Hounsfield Units (HU). For instance, in a 12-bit CT image, pixel values range from 0 to 4095, so normalization involves dividing each pixel intensity by 4095. In contrast, MRI images benefit more from standardization, also known as Z-score normalization, since their intensity values do not have a fixed scale.

2.3.3 Discretization

Discretization also known as gray-level discretization, quantization, or binning—is the process of converting continuous voxel intensity or density values into a limited number of discrete levels or bins. This simplifies the image structure and facilitates feature extraction. It is essential for calculating statistical second-order texture features from matrices like the Gray-Level Co-occurrence Matrix (GLCM) and Gray-Level Run Length Matrix (GLRLM), which require images with discrete gray levels. Discretization is defined by three parameters: the data range, the number of bins, and the bin width, as shown in fig 2. The product of bin number and bin width will give the range of data; hence, it is possible to control only two of the parameters (van Timmeren et al., 2020). There are two main types of discretization methods:

1. **Range**: The original data range is generally retained during processing.
2. **Fixed Bin Size (FBS)**: A predefined bin width is used. If bin size is 25 HU, then intensities 0 - 24 are integrated in bin 1, 25–49 in bin 2 and so on. This method is appropriate for reproducibility by normalizing the intensities of various images across different scanners.
3. **Fixed Bin Number (FBN)**: A set number of bins divides the image intensity range into equal-width intervals (e.g., range 0–1000 with 50 bins means each bin is width 20). Choosing between a fixed number of bins or fixed bin width affects texture feature extraction: fewer bins can obscure details, while too many bins may amplify noise. Different discretization methods impact the reproducibility and robustness of radiomic features by helping to reduce noise and variability between scanners (Cè et al., 2024).

Figure 2. Discretized Values of a Normal Histogram

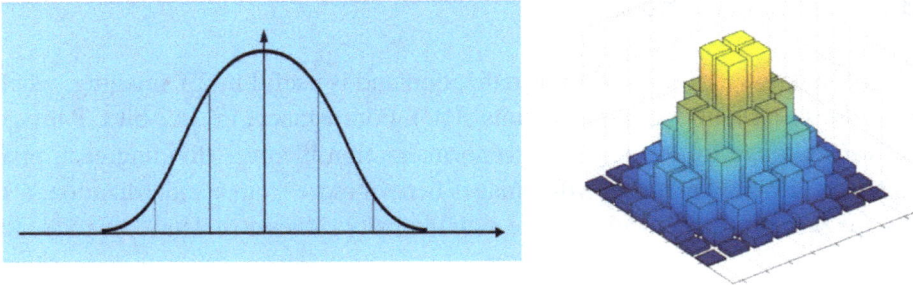

2.3.4 Filtering of Images

Image filtering is a key preprocessing step in radiomics that reduces noise and enhances important image features like edges, textures, and structural patterns. By using specific filters, different frequency components can be targeted—low-frequency filters highlight broad structures, while high-frequency filters emphasize fine details. This process improves the accuracy of feature extraction and significantly enhances the reliability and predictive performance of radiomic models (Demircioğlu, 2022). A summary of different types of filters in radiomics and their characteristics is provided in the Table 1.

Table 1. Different filters and their descriptions

Filter Type	Purpose	Emphasis	Characteristics
Wavelet Decomposition	Multiscale frequency analysis	Both low- and high-frequency components	Produces multiple sub-bands capturing structure and texture at different scales
High-pass Filter	Enhance fine detail by removing low-frequency content	Fine textures, small structures	May increase noise if not applied cautiously
Low-pass Filter	Emphasize smooth, large-scale structures	Homogeneous regions and broad shapes	Used to suppress fine noise and retain overall structure
Laplacian of Gaussian (LoG)	Edge enhancement with scale control	Edges, blobs, fine spatial features	Controlled by σ (sigma); larger σ highlights broader edges

continued on following page

Table 1. Continued

Filter Type	Purpose	Emphasis	Characteristics
Gaussian Filter	Noise reduction through smoothing	General image structure; reduces high-frequency noise	May cause slight blurring; suitable for denoising prior to analysis
Gabor Kernel	Texture and orientation analysis	Directional textures and fine patterns	Tuned to specific frequencies and orientations
Sobel or Prewitt Filter	Edge detection via intensity gradient analysis	Directional edges and contours	Sensitive to changes in intensity; good for shape-based features

2.3.5 Image Co-Registration

Variations in patient positioning, imaging protocols, or equipment can cause spatial misalignment between medical images. Co-registration corrects this by aligning all images to a common coordinate system, ensuring anatomical consistency and accurate region-of-interest (ROI) mapping across datasets. This process is especially crucial in longitudinal studies, multi-scanner data, or multi-modal imaging. In neuroimaging, co-registration often involves aligning images to a standard reference like the MNI template to account for individual brain differences. However, while this enhances anatomical consistency, it may compromise the quality of radiomic features (Stefano et al., 2021).

There are several approaches, depending on the type of images:

- **Rigid Registration**: aligns images by rotation and translation (no shape change)
- **Deformable registration**: allows local warping to match anatomical differences (e.g., breathing motion)
- **Affine Registration**: adds scaling and shearing to the rigid transformation

2.3.6 Bias Field Correction

This method is used specifically in Magnetic Resonance Imaging (MRI) to correct bias fields—low-frequency intensity variations across the image caused by magnetic field inhomogeneities, coil non-uniformities, patient positioning, or hardware issues. These variations affect radiomic features (e.g., first-order statistics, texture, and shape features) by introducing false intensity differences. Bias field correction algorithms estimate and remove these variations by modeling the bias as a smooth field and subtracting it (in the log domain) from the image, resulting in uniform tissue intensities. Newer techniques have further improved homogeneity and reduced noise (Mishro et al., 2020). Some common algorithms used for the purpose are outlined in Table 2

Table 2. Common algorithms used for bias field correction

Algorithm	Characteristics	Correction Method	Use Cases
N3 - Nonparametric Nonuniform Intensity Normalization	Classic method-Nonparametric	Iterative histogram sharpening via entropy minimization	Brain MRI, neuroimaging pipelines
N4ITK - from Insight Toolkit	Extension of N3- Uses B-spline fitting	Iterative B-spline-based bias field estimation	Brain, prostate, and breast MRI (widely used in radiomics
SPM Unified Segmentation	Bayesian framework-Tissue probability maps	Simultaneous bias correction and tissue segmentation	Brain MRI (especially T1-weighted)
ANTS N4 - N4 in Advanced Normalization Tools	Same algorithm as N4ITK-Better integration with ANTs workflows	B-spline approximation	Neuroimaging, multi-modal MRI studies
BCUNet (Deep Learning-based)	Deep learning approach-Data-driven	Trained CNN predicts and removes bias field	Research: emerging for general MRI correction

Pre-processing in radiomics involves image transformations and adjustments before extracting quantitative features from medical images, ensuring robust, reproducible, and comparable radiomic features across different protocols and modalities. Techniques and methods are discussed in a table 3.

Table 3. Various filtering methods and their descriptions

Task	Description
Resampling	Adjust the pixel/voxel size to a uniform spacing across all images
	Ensures features are not biased due to differing image resolutions
	Common methods: linear, spline, nearest-neighbor interpolation
Intensity Normalization	Standardizes the pixel/voxel intensity range
	Facilitates comparison across methods and parameters
	Methods: Z-score, Min-max normalization, Histogram matching
Discretization	Converts continuous values into finite categories or bins
	Three parameters: data range, number of bins, and bin width
	Reduces the impact of inter-scanner variability

continued on following page

Table 3. Continued

Task	Description
Filtering / Noise Reduction	Removes artifacts and reduces high-frequency noise
	Improves the quality of texture features
	Common filters: wavelet, Laplacian of Gaussian
Image Co-registration	Aligns images from different time points, modalities, or patients
	Useful for multi-modality radiomics (e.g., PET/CT fusion)
	Involves rigid or deformable transformations
Bias Field Correction	Specifically for MRI neuroimaging applications
	Corrects for intensity non-uniformity
	Algorithms: N3, N4ITK, BCUNet

2.4 Segmentation

Segmentation is the process of separating a region of interest (ROI) in a medical image, such as tumours, lesions, organs, or anatomical structures, from which radiomic features are extracted. This process is technically challenging due to the often-indistinct boundaries of many tumors and anatomical regions. It also raises a point of disagreement regarding the balance between achieving objective truth and ensuring consistency (Kumar et al., 2012).

There are multiple approaches to segmentation, such as manual, semi-automated, and automated methods, which are also described in METRICS (Kocak et al., 2024). Manual segmentation, a time-consuming process involving expert outlining of ROI/VOI, is susceptible to observer bias and inter-operator variability, potentially impacting feature reproducibility.

Semi-automated segmentation uses user input for seed points or contours, expanding to ROI segmentation but requiring manual correction. Techniques include region growing, thresholding, graph-cut, and level set using tools like ITK-SNAP, 3D Slicer, or MITK.

In automated segmentation, deep learning algorithms such as CNNs, especially U-Net architectures, are trained on annotated datasets and perform segmentation without human intervention. These algorithms are still being developed, as they have varied instances of accuracy and generalizability (Cè et al., 2024; van Timmeren et al., 2020). A list of widely used software and tools for segmentation is listed in the following table 4:

Table 4. Common software used for segmentation

Software	Type	Key Features	Use Case Scenario
3D Slicer	GUI-based	Multi-modality, manual/semi-auto segmentation, script support (Python)	Research, prototyping
ITK-SNAP	GUI-based	manual + semi-auto segmentation; good for volumetric labelling	Manual contouring
nnU-Net	Deep learning	DL model with automatic configuration	Auto segmentation (academic + clinical)
MONAI	Deep learning	PyTorch-based	Customizable AI pipelines
MITK	GUI-based	Integrated with ITK/VTK; real-time interaction	Clinical tool development
Fiji (ImageJ)	Classical	Simple image analysis + plugins (segmentation macros)	2D segmentation tasks
SimpleITK	Library	Supports classic algorithms; C++ and Python bindings	Programmatic segmentation

2.5 Feature Extraction

Feature extraction is a method of quantitatively analyzing medical images to extract measurable features that describe tumor characteristics. It converts images into mineable data by extracting predefined features from specific regions of interest (ROIs) or volumes of interest (VOIs). Radiomic features can be classified into histogram-based, texture-based, model-based, transform-based, and shape-based categories.

2.5.1 Histogram-Based Features

First-order features, or first-order statistics, describe the distribution of voxel intensities within a region of interest (ROI) without considering spatial relationships. They include mean, median, variance, entropy, kurtosis, and skewness. These statistics can be biologically or clinically relevant, such as homogeneous tissues having narrow histograms and heterogeneous or abnormal tissues having broad, skewed, or multimodal distributions (Rizzo et al., 2018).

2.5.2 Texture-Based Features

Radiomics uses texture features to quantify patterns, variations, and heterogeneity in gray-level intensities across a region of interest. These features assess spatial distribution and relation to each other, helping identify tissue heterogeneity, disease aggressiveness, tumor grade, fibrosis, necrosis, or treatment response. Several statistical matrices describe texture.(Mayerhoefer et al., 2020). Most commonly used matrices and the features included in them are described as follows:

Gray Level Co-occurrence Matrix (GLCM)

It is a matrix where each element (i, j) represents the number of times that a voxel with intensity level 'i' is found adjacent to a voxel with intensity 'j', at a defined distance and direction. Common directions include $0°, 45°, 90°, 135°$ and a common distance being 1 voxel. Features included in this matrix are contrast, entropy, energy, among others. For instance, if the contrast difference between Neighboring values is high, it shows more texture variation, indicating heterogeneous tumors. Similarly, high energy shows uniformity, indicating homogenous tissues like fibrosis.

Gray Level Run Length Matrix (GLRLM)

GLRLM counts the number of runs (i.e., consecutive voxels with the same gray level) in a specified direction. Each element (i, j) of the matrix is the number of runs with gray level 'i' and run length 'j'. Different types of features in this matrix include Short Run Emphasis (SRE) which emphasizes fine textures; Long Run Emphasis (LRE) which emphasizes coarse textures; Gray Level Non-Uniformity (GLNU) which denotes variation in gray levels; Run Percentage (RP) that shows texture compactness among others. These features can be clinically correlated as high SRE: indicating fine-grained texture (e.g., healthy tissue) or high LRE indicating coarse, possibly necrotic or fibrotic texture.

Gray Level Size Zone Matrix (GLSZM)

GLSZM measures the size of homogeneous zones, connected regions of neighboring pixels/voxels with the same gray level in any direction. It counts these zones, and larger, uniform areas with the same gray level result in larger zones. GLSZM considers all directions by default, allowing 2D pixels to have 8 neighbors and 3D voxels up to 26 neighbors. Common features include Small Area High Gray Level, Small Area Low Gray Level, and Large Area High Gray Level.

Neighborhood Gray Tone Difference Matrix (NGTDM)

NGTDM describes how much each pixel or voxel differs from its neighbors in intensity. For each pixel or voxel, NGTDM takes the intensity (gray level), calculates the average intensity of its neighbors (within a certain distance, like 1 or 2 pixels) and measures the difference between the pixel and this average. It repeats this across the whole image or ROI and sums the results that indicates how much each pixel "stands out" compared to its surroundings. Commonly used features include coarseness, busyness, complexity and strength among others.

Gray Level Dependence Matrix (GLDM)

GLDM is a texture matrix that compares a central pixel to surrounding pixels based on their gray levels. It counts neighboring pixels if their gray level is close enough to the central pixel's, determined by a dependence criterion. Central pixels are grouped by intensity and their dependent neighbors, storing the number of times a central pixel with intensity i has j dependent neighbors. Features extracted include Large Dependence Emphasis, Small Dependence Emphasis, and Dependence Entropy.

Higher-order Features

Higher-order features are a sophisticated class of radiomic features that capture complex patterns, textures, and frequency-based information. These features are extracted after applying mathematical or frequency-based transformations to the original medical image. They capture multi-scale texture patterns, directional or frequency-specific signals and subtle variations not evident in original images. Common Filters and transforms used include wavelet transform, Laplacian of Gaussian (LoG) Filtering, Fractal Analysis, Minkowski Functionals among others.

2.5.3 Model-Based Features

Model-based analyses analyze the geographical distribution and correlations of pixel intensities using mathematical or statistical models to describe the textures of images. By fitting parameterized equations to picture data, these models, which include autoregressive, fractal, and Markov random fields, produce radiomic characteristics. Conversely, transform-based features use mathematical transformations, such as wavelet, Fourier, and Gabor filters, to draw attention to particular patterns, textures, and frequencies in pictures. These transformations are useful for sophisticated texture analysis because they make it possible to identify subtle, directional, and multi-scale differences. Both feature classes are essential for creating predictive imaging models and are frequently provided by radiomics libraries. (Mayerhoefer et al., 2020).

2.5.4 Shape-Based Features

Shape-based features describe the geometric properties of a region of interest (ROI), typically a tumor, lesion, or organ. These features are derived independently of image intensity values and quantify the size, outline, and dimensional characteristics of an object, providing important information about tumor heterogeneity, growth patterns, and invasiveness. They can be broadly divided into 2D, which is extracted from a single slice, and 3D extracted from volumetric data.

Features such as volume and area measure the overall extent of the tumor or structure and are clinically useful for tracking tumor growth or shrinkage during treatment. Features like sphericity, compactness, elongation or flatness describe the geometric complexity and regularity of the ROI (Zwanenburg et al., 2020).

2.6 Feature Selection and Dimensionality Reduction

Each region of interest in radiomics datasets frequently has a significant number of quantitative features, many of which may be unnecessary or duplicated, which could impair model performance. Feature selection and dimensionality reduction are two crucial preprocessing stages used to create efficient and broadly applicable models. By removing redundancy and noise, the feature selection techniques of Filter, Wrapper, and Embedded aid in preserving the most informative features(Cè et al., 2024). On the other hand, dimensionality reduction uses methods such as PCA, LDA, t-SNE, and UMAP to convert data into new, lower-dimensional representations. t-SNE and UMAP are mostly utilized for visualization rather than predictive modeling, whereas PCA and LDA are used for compression and classification (Scapicchio et al., 2021).

Figure 3. Various Methods of Feature Extraction

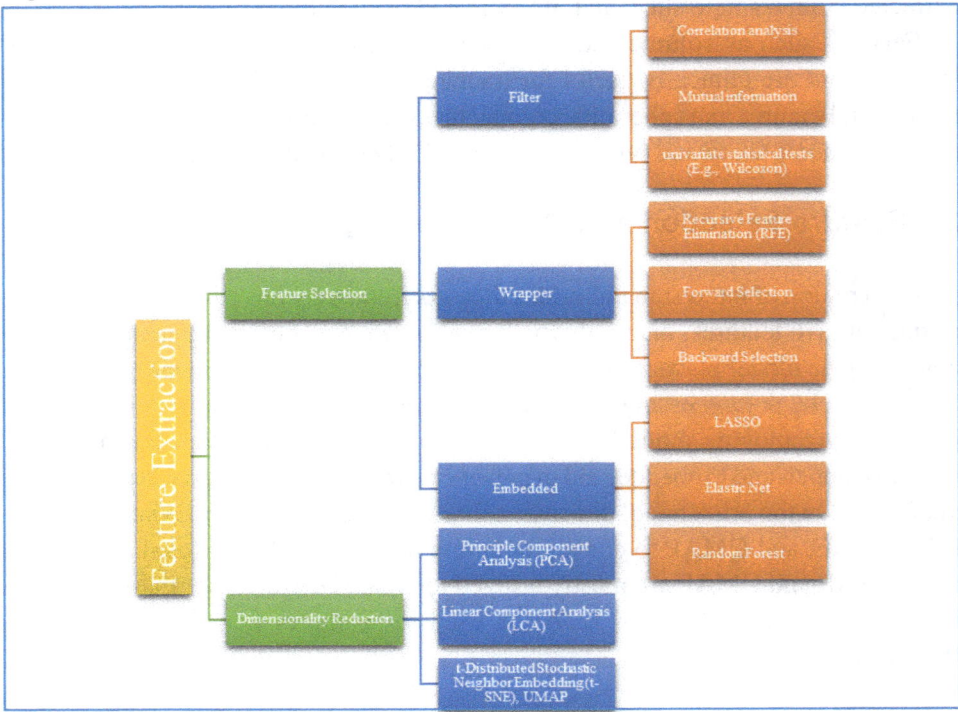

2.7 Model Building

The radiomics workflow involves building a model using machine learning or statistical methods to classify disease types, predict treatment response, and stratify patient risk. Machine learning is increasingly preferred for model building, as it feeds labelled or unlabelled data to algorithms that identify patterns and recognize radiomic features, shown in Figure 4. Supervised learning trains the model on labelled data, resulting in known labels like malignant/benign or survival time.

Supervised learning is categorized by the type of target variable: regression predicts continuous values (e.g., survival time), while classification predicts categories (e.g., benign vs. malignant tumors). Classification can be binary or multiclass. In contrast, unsupervised learning analyzes unlabelled data to find patterns or groupings, aiding in tasks like patient phenotyping and subgroup discovery when predefined labels are not available (Cè et al., 2024). The main tasks in radiomics model building include:

- **Classification** uses algorithms like SVM, Random Forest, Logistic Regression, XGBoost, and k-nearest neighbour to predict discrete categories, such as brain tumors.
- **Regression** uses algorithms like Linear Regression, LASSO, Ridge, and SVR to predict continuous outcomes, such as patient survival or tumor growth rate.
- **Clustering** uses K-Means, Hierarchical Clustering, or DBSCAN to group similar data points based on features without labels.

Figure 4. Common methods of building a Radiomics Model

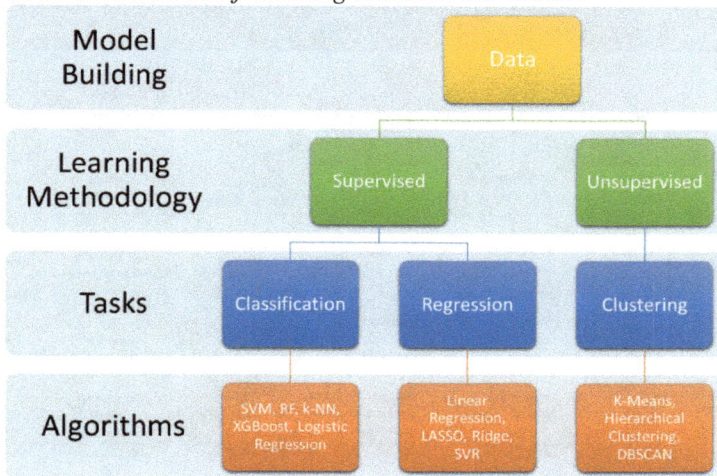

2.7.1 Model Validation

Validation is a crucial process that assesses a model's performance and generalizability by evaluating its predictive accuracy using a trained or independent dataset, ensuring its ability to generalize to new patient data, assess clinical reliability, enable reproducibility, prevent overfitting, and meet regulatory standards.(Moons et al., 2015).

They may be classified into Internal and external validation methods are used to assess performance within a training dataset, while external validation tests a model on an independent dataset, but requires access to external data, which can be challenging due to privacy and standardization issues (Nicoletti et al., 2024).

2.8 Radiomics Workflow and Pipeline Overview

The radiomics workflow is a structured process that converts standard medical images into high-dimensional quantitative data for clinical and research applications. It starts with image acquisition, pre-processing to standardize features, segmentation to isolate the region of interest, feature extraction to compute quantitative descriptors, feature selection and dimensionality reduction to eliminate redundancy, and model development and validation using machine learning or statistical techniques to correlate radiomic features with clinical endpoints shown in Figure 5.

Figure 5. Summary of a Radiomics Workflow

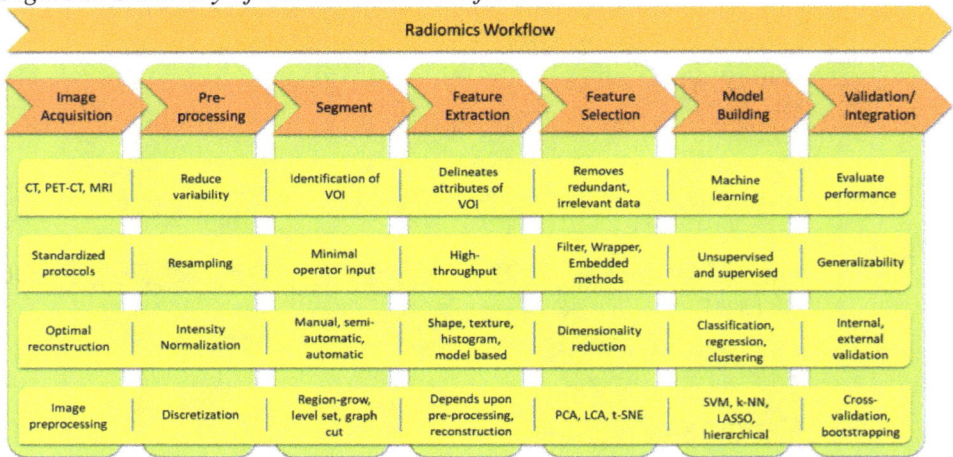

Image Acquisition	Pre-processing	Segment	Feature Extraction	Feature Selection	Model Building	Validation/ Integration
CT, PET-CT, MRI	Reduce variability	Identification of VOI	Delineates attributes of VOI	Removes redundant, irrelevant data	Machine learning	Evaluate performance
Standardized protocols	Resampling	Minimal operator input	High-throughput	Filter, Wrapper, Embedded methods	Unsupervised and supervised	Generalizability
Optimal reconstruction	Intensity Normalization	Manual, semi-automatic, automatic	Shape, texture, histogram, model based	Dimensionality reduction	Classification, regression, clustering	Internal, external validation
Image preprocessing	Discretization	Region-grow, level set, graph cut	Depends upon pre-processing, reconstruction	PCA, LCA, t-SNE	SVM, k-NN, LASSO, hierarchical	Cross-validation, bootstrapping

The radiomics workflow is illustrated in the schematic diagram below, which outlines the major sequential steps involved in the process, highlighting how raw imaging data is transformed into clinically actionable insights shown in Figure 6

Figure 6. Schematic Diagram of Radiomics Workflow

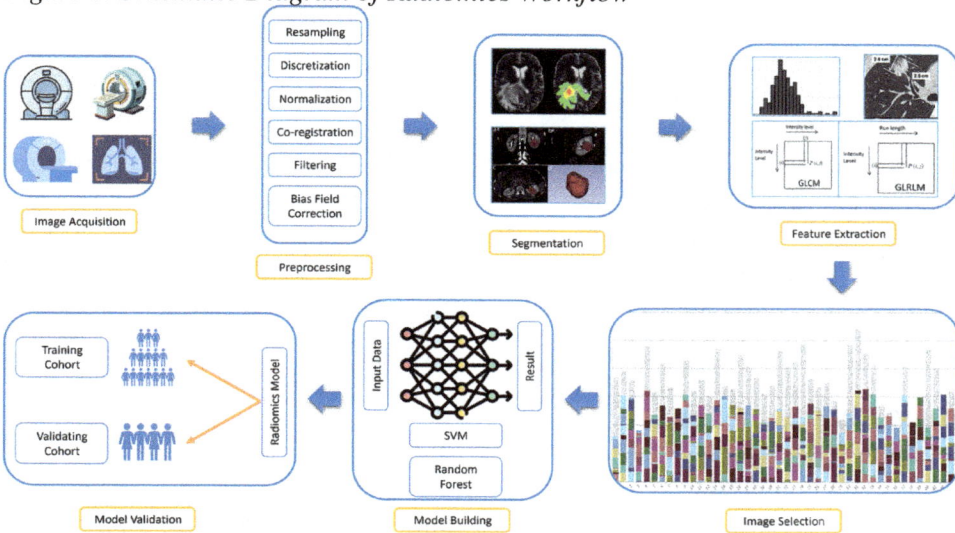

3 ROLE OF ARTIFICIAL INTELLIGENCE IN IMAGING

Artificial intelligence (AI) has emerged as a game changer in the field of medical imaging, providing powerful computational tools for automating, improving, and accelerating clinical operations. From image acquisition and preprocessing to interpretation and decision assistance, AI is changing the way radiologists and imaging professionals work with medical data. As the volume and complexity of imaging data grow, AI facilitates a shift toward precision medicine by enhancing diagnostic accuracy, lowering inter-observer variability, and predicting disease outcomes more accurately than ever before. The fundamental differences between Artificial Intelligence delves into the most influential AI architectures used in medical imaging; discusses the growing importance of explainability and interpretability in clinical adoption; and investigates the integration of AI within the radiomics framework for improved pattern recognition and predictive analytics (Pinto-Coelho, 2023).

3.1 AI vs ML vs DL in Medical Imaging

AI is a vast subject of computer science that seeks to develop systems capable of doing activities that would ordinarily need human intelligence. In medical imaging, AI refers to algorithms that interpret images, assist with diagnosis, optimize imaging methods, and even anticipate treatment response. AI simulates cognitive capabilities like reasoning, perception, learning, and problem solving.

Machine Learning (ML)

Machine learning (ML) is an area of AI that allows machines to learn from data. Rather of being explicitly written, ML algorithms recognize patterns in data and improve their performance over time. In imaging, machine learning is utilized for tasks such as tissue classification, organ localization, and disease detection. There are three major paradigms in machine learning: supervised, unsupervised, and reinforcement (Pinto-Coelho, 2023).

Deep Learning (DL)

DL is a subset of ML that uses multi-layered neural networks, particularly deep neural networks (DNNs), to automatically learn features from raw data. DL reduces the need for human feature engineering and is particularly good at spotting complicated patterns in huge datasets, making it perfect for imaging applications. Deep learning promotes breakthroughs in image categorization, segmentation, synthesis, and registration. In summary, although AI is the overarching concept, ML is the methodology by which AI learns, and deep learning is the most powerful and scalable approach within ML, particularly when dealing with unstructured visual data (Taye, 2023).

3.2 Key AI Models Used in Medical Imaging

Several deep learning architectures have demonstrated remarkable performance across several modalities and clinical use cases, driving the utility of AI in imaging.

1. **CNNs:** Convolutional Neural Networks are the most commonly used DL models in medical imaging. They excel at learning spatial hierarchies in images using layers of convolutions, pooling, and non-linear activations.
2. **RNNs:** Recurrent Neural Networks are intended to process sequential data while retaining memory of earlier inputs. Though less common in static imaging, RNNs are useful in dynamic imaging (for example, functional MRI) and time-series tasks.
3. **GANs:** Generative Adversarial Networks are made up of two neural networks: the generator and the discriminator, which are trained adversarially. The generator creates realistic visuals, and the discriminator determines their veracity.

4. **Transformers**: Attention-based Deep Networks, which were originally developed for natural language processing, have lately been repurposed for imaging using architectures such as Vision Transformers (ViTs) (Kshatri & Singh, 2023).

Table 5. AI models: Core functionalities and use cases in medical imaging

AI Model	Core Function	Applications in Medical Imaging
CNN	Spatial pattern recognition	Lesion detection, organ segmentation, abnormality classification (CT, MRI, X-ray)
RNN	Sequential data processing	Functional MRI, cardiac imaging, and Tumor progression tracking
GAN	Image generation/ enhancement	Image synthesis, denoising, modality conversion (CT - MRI)
Transformer	Long-range dependency modeling	Image classification, multi-modal fusion, and report generation

3.3 Explainability and Interpretability of AI in Clinical Settings

The so-called "black-box" aspect of deep learning models poses a significant barrier to mainstream clinical adoption of AI in imaging. While these models frequently exceed traditional methods in terms of accuracy, they typically do not provide explicit reasons for their judgments, which raises serious problems in high-risk contexts such as healthcare (Nittas et al., 2023).

Explainability is the ability of an AI model to convey how it arrived at a specific outcome.

Interpretability relates to a human user's ability to understand and trust the model's output, such as that of a radiologist or clinician.

Clinical Requirements for Explainable AI (XAI):

1. Accountability: Clinicians must justify AI-assisted diagnosis.
2. Regulatory compliance: Explainable models make it easier to get permission from regulatory authorities like the FDA and EMA.
3. Ethical transparency: Patients and providers must grasp the ethical implications of AI decision-making.

There are some Enhancing Technique with application in medical imaging shown in table 6.

Table 6. Common Techniques for Enhancing Explainability

Technique	Description	Application in Medical Imaging
Saliency Maps & Grad-CAM	Visual overlays that highlight key regions in the input image that influenced the AI's decision.	Identifying tumors, lesions, or areas of abnormality detected by AI.
Layer-wise Relevance Propagation (LRP)	Traces the relevance of input features through the network layers to explain decisions.	Dissecting how deep models reach diagnostic conclusions.
SHAP & LIME	Model-agnostic tools that assign importance scores to features contributing to predictions.	Explaining predictions of complex models, especially in radiomics analysis.
Case-Based Reasoning (CBR)	Displays similar past cases to support the AI's current decision.	Supporting radiologists with examples from historical imaging databases.

3.4 Integration of AI in Radiomics for Pattern Recognition and Prediction

Radiomics is the high-throughput extraction of quantitative features from medical pictures, converting visual data into mineable, organized information. It works on the assumption that medical photographs include a plethora of information that is not visible to the human eye shown in Table 7 (Tian, J; 2018).

Table 7. Radiomics Models Demonstrating Pattern Recognition and Predictive Capabilities

Component	Description	Applications in Clinical Practice
Enhanced Feature Extraction	Traditional radiomics uses handcrafted features (shape, texture, intensity). Deep learning (DL)-based radiomics uses CNNs/autoencoders to extract abstract, high-dimensional features.	Improves correlation with tumour biology and enables more robust image representation.
Pattern Recognition and Disease Characterization	Enables precise tissue characterization (e.g., benign vs malignant). Predictive models analyze tumour heterogeneity, vascularity, and perfusion.	Aids in early diagnosis, risk stratification, and prognosis estimation.
Radio genomics	Correlates imaging features with genetic or molecular profiles (e.g., EGFR mutations). Enables non-invasive tumour phenotyping.	Reduces need for repeated biopsies; supports targeted therapy decisions.

continued on following page

Table 7. Continued

Component	Description	Applications in Clinical Practice
Predictive Modeling	Models predict treatment response (e.g., to immunotherapy), recurrence, and survival. Supports individualized prognosis estimation.	Enhances personalized medicine by tailoring treatment to patient-specific phenotypes.
Workflow Integration	Radiomics platforms now integrate with PACS, EHR, and clinical decision support systems. Real-time dashboards deliver actionable insights.	Enables seamless integration of radiomics into routine clinical workflows.

4 PREDICTIVE RADIOMICS: APPLICATIONS AND CASE STUDIES

4.1 Early Disease Detection and Progression Modelling

Radiomics facilitates the preclinical detection of disease by quantifying imaging biomarkers that may precede radiological or clinical manifestations. Through high-dimensional feature extraction from conventional imaging modalities such as CT, MRI, and PET, radiomics captures variations in texture, shape, and intensity that are indicative of early pathological processes. These quantitative features can be leveraged to train machine learning algorithms capable of identifying subtle abnormalities with improved temporal sensitivity. This methodology enables non-invasive, data-driven screening workflows, enhances diagnostic precision in indeterminate or borderline cases, and supports high-throughput implementation in population-level screening initiatives.

These models have been mainly used in the early detection of carcinoma and other benign tumors. Their applications are elaborated in the following Table 8:

Table 8. Studies encompassing the prediction of various diseases or conditions

Study	Disease/ Condition	Modality	Cohort / Sample Size	Radiomic Features	Feature Selection	Software / Tools	Performance Metrics
(Cao et al., 2024)	Nasopharyngeal Carcinoma	MRI	train: n=154 validate: n=65	Shape, first-order, GLDM, GLCM, GLRLM, GLSZM, NGTDM	LASSO	Slicer 5.0.3, PyRadiomics	AUC - 0.936
(Lu et al., 2023)	Non-small cell lung cancer	CT	train: n=190 validate: n=80	histogram, geometry and texture features (GLCM, GLRLM)	univariate Cox proportional regression	MATLABR2022a	AUC - 0.75
(Bao et al., 2022)	Nasopharyngeal Carcinoma	MRI	train: n=119 validate: n=52	intensity, shape, textural features, wavelet features	LASSO	PyRadiomics V2.1.2	AUC - 0.808 C-index - 0.651
(Yang et al., 2022)	Non-Small Cell Lung Cancer	CT	train: n=68 validate: n=28	first-order, texture, and transformation-based features	mRMR (minimum Redundancy Maximum Relevance), LASSO	ITK-SNAP, PyRadiomics	AUC - 0.88
(Xie et al., 2022)	Rectal carcinoma	MRI	train: n=110 validate: n=56	GLSZM	LASSO Cox regression	PyRadiomics	C-index 0.627
(B. Zhang et al., 2020)	Radiation-induced brain injury in nasopharyngeal carcinoma	MRI	train: n=194 validate: n=48	Volume, size, solidity, eccentricity, GLCM, GLRLM, GLSZM, NGTDM	imbalance-adjusted bootstrap resampling	ITK-SNAP, MATLAB 2014a	AUC - 0.830
(Shen et al., 2020)	Nonmetastatic Nasopharyngeal Carcinoma	MRI	train: n=230 validate: n=97	Shape, first-order, GLDM, GLCM, GLRLM, GLSZM, NGTDM	LASSO, Recursive feature elimination (RFE)	Slicer 5.0.3 PyRadiomics	AUC - 0.936
(Du et al., 2019)	Nonmetastatic Nasopharyngeal Carcinoma	MRI	train: n=217 validate: n=60	First-order texture-based shape-based	Hierarchal clustering analysis	ITK-SNAP, PyRadiomics SciPy, scikit-learn, SHAP	AUC - 0.80

Through these studies radiomics has shown promise in early disease detection and disease progression modeling across a range of conditions, particularly in oncology. Radiomic models have successfully distinguished between benign and malignant lesions or predicted early treatment-related damage before clinical symptoms arise. Radiomics can forecast outcomes such as progression-free survival, recurrence, and disease evolution over time. Methods used across studies include classical machine learning algorithms (e.g., random forest, Cox regression), deep learning approaches, and sometimes integration with clinical features to enhance performance.

4.2 Predicting Treatment Response (e.g., Chemoradiotherapy, Immunotherapy)

Using pre-treatment and in some instances intra- or post-treatment imaging, it is possible to build models that can forecast whether a tumor will respond well, poorly, or not at all to a planned treatment such as chemotherapy, radiotherapy, immunotherapy, or targeted therapy. Radiomics quantifies tumor phenotype and microenvironmental features from imaging, which often correlate with molecular characteristics and treatment sensitivity. These features may capture heterogeneity, shape or margins, density and intensity patterns. Tumors with high textural irregularity are often less responsive to uniform therapies and irregular or spiculated tumors may behave more aggressively or resist treatment. Changes in grayscale histograms can reflect necrosis, fibrosis, or active tumor regions which can be captured using radiomic workflows.

Some prominent studies that have employed radiomics for treatment prediction have been elaborated in the following table 9:

Table 9. Representative studies employing radiomics for treatment response prediction

Study	Disease / Condition	Modality	Cohort / Sample Size	Radiomic Features	Feature Selection	Software / Tools	Performance Metrics
(Xu et al., 2025)	Hepatocellular carcinoma	CT	train: n=315 validate: n=80	Shape, first-order, texture	ICC, LASSO, RFECV	ITK-SNAP	AUC - 0.883
(Louis et al., 2024)	Non-small cell lung carcinoma	CT	train: n=401 validate: n=33	Shape, first-order, texture (GLCM, GLDM, GLRLM, GLSZM)	mRMR	PyRadiomics	AUC - 0.65
(Sozutok et al., 2024)	Hepatocellular carcinoma	MRI	train: n=65 validate: n=20	first-order, second-order	LASSO	Rstudio	AUC - 0.850

continued on following page

Table 9. Continued

Study	Disease / Condition	Modality	Cohort / Sample Size	Radiomic Features	Feature Selection	Software / Tools	Performance Metrics
(Kang et al., 2024)	Pancreatic ductal adeno-carcinoma	FDG-PET/CT	train: n=194 validate: n=48	intensity features, intensity histogram, GLCM, GLRLM, GLSZM, NGTDM	LASSO	LIFEx 7.4.0	C-index - 0.681
(Sherminie et al., 2023)	Glioma	MRI	train: n=77 validate: n=33	minor and major axis length, area and volume density, least axis length, volume voxel and mesh	LASSO	MATLAB 2014a	AUC - 0.91
(B. Y. Chen et al., 2022)	Rectal Carcinoma	MRI	train: n=91 validate: n=46	first-order, GLCM, GLRLM, GLSZM, GLDM, NGTDM	LASSO	ITK-SNAP, PyRadiomics v3.0	AUC - 0.838
(Zhuang et al., 2021)	Rectal Carcinoma	MRI	train: n=113 validate: n=64	first-order, GLCM, GLRLM, GLSZM, GLDM	mRMR, LASSO	ITK-SNAP, PyRadiomics	AUC - 0.88

4.3 Prognostic Models in Oncology (Lung, Breast, Brain, Prostate, etc.)

Prognostic models in radiomics refer to predictive frameworks that utilize quantitative imaging features extracted from standard-of-care medical images (like CT, MRI, PET) to forecast the future clinical outcome of a patient, such as overall survival, progression-free survival, disease-free survival, time to recurrence and likelihood of metastasis. These models help stratify patients by risk, optimize clinical decision-making, and personalize treatment plans. Some key studies that have developed prognostic models have been listed as Table 10 below.

298

Table 10. Representative studies employing radiomics models for prognosis

Study	Disease/ Condition	Modality	Cohort / Sample Size	Radiomic Features	Feature Selection	Software/Tools	Performance Metrics
(Cepeda et al., 2025)	Glioblastoma	USG	train: n=114	Shape, first-order, texture (GLCM, GLDM, GLRLM, GLSZM, NGTDM)	mRMR	ITK-SNAP	C-index - 0.87
(Mansouri et al., 2024)	Head and Neck cancer	CT	train: n=240	50 first-order, 136 texture based (GLCM, GLRLM, GLSZM, GLDZM, NGTDM)	mRMR	MatLab IBM	C-index - 0.73
(Philip et al., 2024)	Head and Neck Squamous Cell Carcinoma	PET	train: n=232 validate: n=102	Shape, first-order, texture (GLCM, GLDM, GLRLM, GLSZM, NGTDM)	LIFEx	LIFEx	C-index - 0.70
(Tang et al., 2023)	Non-Small Cell Lung Cancer	CT	train: n=352 validate: n=102	Shape, first-order, texture (GLCM, GLDM, GLRLM, GLSZM, NGTDM)	Eclipse	3D slicer, Pyradiomics	AUC - 0.949
(Yolchuyeva et al., 2023)	Non-Small Cell Lung Cancer	CT	train: n=223 validate: n=162	Intensity, shape, texture, filter-based	ReliefF-based	Pyradiomics	C-index - 0.57
(Lee et al., 2022)	Breast Cancer	MRI	train: n=111 validate: n=44	Shape, first-order, texture (GLCM, GLDM, GLRLM, GLSZM, NGTDM)	LASSO	3D slicer, Pyradiomics	C-index - 0.63

Radiomics-based prognostic models have emerged as powerful tools in oncology. in non-small cell lung cancer (NSCLC), radiomics features derived from radiotherapy planning CT images, when integrated with clinical variables, improved 1-year survival prediction with an AUC as high as 0.949. Similar integrative models in NSCLC patients treated with immunotherapy yielded consistent predictive performance (C-index ~0.63), highlighting their generalizability across treatment types. Thus, these prognostic tools are well-positioned for seamless clinical integration, offering scalable and cost-effective solutions for precision oncology.

4.4 Risk Stratification and outcome Prediction Using AI-Driven Radiomics

Risk stratification and outcome prediction using radiomics refers to the process of categorizing patients into different risk groups like low, intermediate or high and forecasting specific clinical outcomes like recurrence, metastasis, complications or treatment failure based on quantitative features extracted from medical images. This application is seen as parallel to prognosis, but it focuses more on individualizing clinical pathways by identifying which patients are at higher risk of poor outcomes and require more aggressive or tailored interventions. Some models that have been developed for the purpose are listed in the following table 11.

Table 11. Representative studies employing radiomics for risk stratification and prediction

Study	Disease/ Condition	Modality	Cohort / Sample Size	Radiomic Features	Feature Select	Software / Tools	Performance Metrics
(Z.-Y. Wei et al., 2024)	Endometrial cancer	MRI	train: n=79 validate: n=33	first-order, texture (GLCM, GLDM, GLRLM, GLSZM, NGTDM)	LASSO	3D Slicer 5.2.1, PyRadiomics	AUC - 0.82
(Y. Lin et al., 2024)	Endometrial cancer	MRI	train: n=287 validate: n=69	First-order, 3D shape-based	LASSO	Matlab	Rad-Score Train: 71.1% Validate: 71.0%
(P. Wang et al., 2024)	Non-small Cell Lung Cancer	CT	train: n=122 validate: n=30	intensity, shape, textural features, wavelet features	LASSO	PyRadiomics V2.1.2	AUC Train: 0.972 Validate: 0.937

continued on following page

Table 11. Continued

Study	Disease/ Condition	Modality	Cohort / Sample Size	Radiomic Features	Feature Select	Software / Tools	Performance Metrics
(L. Wang et al., 2023)	Gastric Cancer	CT	train: n=166 validate: internal, n=83, external, n=34	first-order, texture, shape-based	Boruta	ITK-SNAP, Syngo.via Frontier	C-index Train: 0.83 Validate: internal - 0.75, external - 0.76
(X. Zhang et al., 2022)	Lung adeno-carcinoma	CT	train: n=131 validate: n=41	first-order, shape, texture-based	Boruta	Syngo.via Frontier	C-index Train: 0.78 Validate: 0.72
(T. Wang et al., 2022)	Non–Small Cell Lung Cancer		train: n=381 validate: internal n=163, external n=48	first-order, shape, texture (GLCM, GLDM, GLSZM, GLRLM, NGTDM)	Spearman correlation analysis, Univariable Cox regression	3D-Slicer, PyRadiomics 3.7	C-index Train: 0.83 Validate: internal - 0.78, external - 0.75
(J. Chen et al., 2020)	Endometrial Cancer	MRI	train: n=70 validate: n=32	first-order, histogram, GLCM, GLRLM, GLSZM	LASSO	ITK-SNAP, Artificial Intelligent Kit-A.K	AUC Train: 0.756 Validate: 0.704

5 PERSONALIZED IMAGING AND PRECISION MEDICINE

The future of medical imaging lies in its integration with precision medicine, which tailors illness prevention, diagnosis, and therapy to each patient's unique traits. Radiology is transitioning from solely anatomical visualization to a data-rich science capable of providing patient-specific insights using modern computational approaches. AI-powered imaging, particularly when combined with radiomics, genomes, and clinical biomarkers, is critical to this change.

5.1 Linking Radiomics with Genomics and Clinical Biomarkers (Radiogenomics)

Radio genomics is a fast-evolving discipline that combines imaging data (radiomics) with genetic, proteomic, and clinical indicators. It offers non-invasive profiling of tumors and other diseases, allowing for a more in-depth understanding of disease at the molecular level. Radio genomics provides a gateway to individualized, non-invasive diagnoses and allows for the selection of targeted therapies based on a tumour's expected genetic subtype (Nandakumar, S et al, 2022). Some of the clinical application listed in table 12.

Table 12. Overview of Radio genomics – Components and Clinical Applications

Aspect	Description	Applications
Radiomics	Extraction of phenotypic features from medical images, such as shape, texture, and intensity.	CT-derived features are used to assess tumour heterogeneity or margins.
Genomics	Includes genetic mutations (e.g., EGFR, KRAS), gene expression levels, and copy number variations.	EGFR and ALK mutations predicted from lung CT radiomics.
Clinical Biomarkers	Includes blood tests, histopathology, immunohistochemistry, and clinical lab findings.	MGMT methylation and IDH mutation are linked with MRI features in glioblastoma.
Integration	Combines radiomics with biopsy and laboratory data to enhance predictive accuracy and biological insight.	Cross-validation of imaging features with molecular and clinical markers.
Clinical Value	Enables non-invasive tumour phenotyping and stratification, guiding personalized therapy decisions.	Reduces the need for repeat biopsies and supports targeted treatment planning.

5.2 Patient-Specific Imaging Biomarkers for Treatment Planning

AI-driven imaging has given clinicians the possibility to extract quantitative, patient-specific biomarkers that guide treatment regimens. Once approved, these biomarkers serve as surrogate indicators for medication response, prognosis, and disease aggressiveness (Jyothi, N. M. ;2023) as listed in Table 13 below.

Table 13. AI models trained on these imaging biomarkers can forecast patient-specific outcomes such as progression-free survival (PFS) and overall survival (OS).

Biomarker Category	Description	Clinical Applications
Morphological	Features like size, shape, and boundary irregularities. Example: Irregular tumor margins indicate invasiveness.	Assess tumour resectability Guide surgical planning
Textural	Measures of intratumoral heterogeneity, such as entropy and kurtosis. Correlates with microenvironment features like hypoxia and necrosis.	Predict aggressiveness and prognosis. Identify high-risk tumour regions
Functional	Dynamic features such as perfusion, diffusion, and metabolic activity derived from imaging modalities like DCE-MRI, PET.	Evaluate suitability for radiotherapy/chemotherapy. Monitor treatment response

5.3 Dynamic Radiomics and Longitudinal Imaging Analysis

Traditional radiomics has been largely concerned with extracting features from static medical pictures captured at a single point in time. While this approach is useful in capturing tumour shape, heterogeneity, and intensity characteristics, it ignores a fundamental aspect of disease progression: time. Diseases like cancer are essentially dynamic, with changing biological and phenotypic characteristics (Jyothi, N. M.;2023). This issue is addressed by dynamic radiomics, which, when paired with longitudinal imaging analysis, assesses temporal changes in radiomic characteristics over serial imaging sessions, some of the traditional radiomics listed in Table 14.

Table 14. Illustration of Traditional Radiomics and Image Analysis Methods

Aspect	Description	Clinical Significance / Applications
Traditional Radiomics	Captures static imaging features at a single time point, providing a snapshot of tumor characteristics.	Limited in detecting subtle changes or disease evolution; may miss early progression or treatment response.
Dynamic Radiomics	Involves sequential extraction of radiomic features over time from follow-up imaging studies.	Enables continuous monitoring of disease trajectory and tumor response to therapy.
Longitudinal Imaging Analysis	Evaluates trends, patterns, and temporal changes in tumor morphology and function across multiple scans.	Detects early signs of recurrence, metastasis, or therapeutic resistance.
Time-Series Modeling	Utilizes AI algorithms such as RNNs and LSTM networks to model temporal feature progression.	Forecasts future tumor behavior based on historical imaging data, supporting predictive and adaptive care.

continued on following page

Table 14. Continued

Aspect	Description	Clinical Significance / Applications
Biomarker Evolution Tracking	Measures variation in size, texture, shape, and perfusion across time points.	Identifies early imaging biomarkers of progression before morphological changes become evident.
Immunotherapy Use Case	Dynamic CT radiomics helps differentiate between true progression and pseudo-progression due to immune cell infiltration in the early response phase.	Prevents premature discontinuation of effective immunotherapy, improving outcome assessment accuracy.
Support for Adaptive Therapy	Feedback-driven modification of treatment plans based on real-time imaging feature changes.	Optimizes therapy intensity and duration; reduces unnecessary toxicity.

5.3.1 Clinical Application Example: Immunotherapy Monitoring

Standard radiographic criteria in immunotherapy patients may misread early tumor expansion as disease progression, a condition known as pseudo-progression. This is caused by immune cell infiltration, not Tumor growth. The working of Dynamic radiomics is shown in Figure 7 and Step can be:

- Evaluating textural changes and functional imaging markers might help you distinguish between actual progression and pseudo progression.
- Reduce false positives and wasteful cessation of useful treatments.
- Provide a more comprehensive, biology-informed response evaluation than size-based criteria alone. Example of clinical application: monitoring response to immunotherapy shown in table 15

Table 15. Benefits of Longitudinal Imaging Analysis in Clinical Workflow

Advantage	Clinical Value
Adaptive Therapy Planning	Allows dynamic modification of treatment based on updated imaging feedback.
Non-Invasive Disease Surveillance	Reduces dependence on invasive procedures such as serial biopsies.
Personalized Prognostic Assessment	Models disease trajectory unique to the individual, improving prognostic accuracy.
Treatment Response Evaluation	Captures real-time changes in tumor biology, supporting more timely interventions.

Figure 7. Dynamics Radiomics

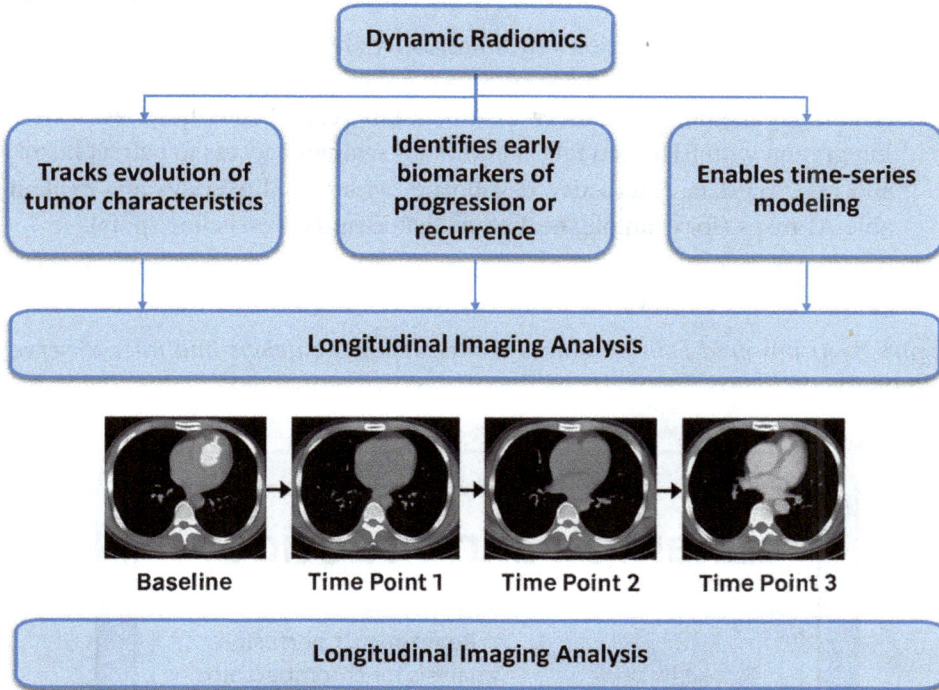

5.3.2 Future Directions

1. Integrating wearable biosensors and liquid biopsies to deliver multi-modal temporal health data.
2. Development of automated platforms for real-time longitudinal feature extraction and decision support in PACS and EHR systems.
3. Expansion into dynamic radio genomics, which links temporal imaging aspects to developing molecular profiles.

5.4 Real-time AI-assisted decision support systems in imaging

AI-integrated imaging technologies have made it possible to make real-time decisions at the point of care. These technologies process & interpret images in real time, providing therapeutically useful information while increasing the speed & accuracy of radiologic assessments shown in figure 8

Real-Time Decision Support Systems (DSS) provide

- Instant image interpretation and abnormality alarms, such as for acute stroke detection.
- Risk rating methods for cancer, treatment failure, and consequences.
- Integration with EHR and PACS allows for seamless access to patient history and imaging data. Interactive dashboards with visual overlays and explainable AI maps (for example, heat maps that identify worrisome spots).

Figure 8. AI-powered DSS platforms reduce reporting delays and inter-observer variability.

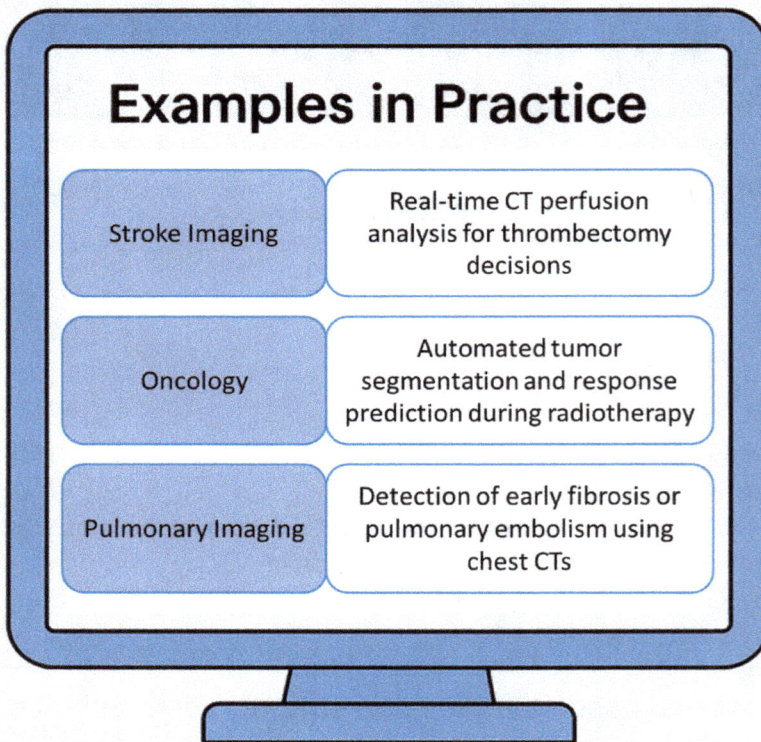

Examples in Practice

Stroke Imaging	Real-time CT perfusion analysis for thrombectomy decisions
Oncology	Automated tumor segmentation and response prediction during radiotherapy
Pulmonary Imaging	Detection of early fibrosis or pulmonary embolism using chest CTs

6 CHALLENGES AND LIMITATIONS

Despite promising advances in Artificial Intelligence (AI) in imaging and radiomics, a number of difficulties and limits prevent seamless clinical translation. These difficulties cover technical, regulatory, and ethical dimensions.

6.1 Data Quality and Heterogeneity

Issue: Medical imaging data is frequently gathered from several institutions utilizing various scanners, protocols, and reconstruction techniques. This variability may bring noise and bias into AI algorithms.

Impact: AI systems trained on a single dataset may underperform when applied to photos from different institutions, reducing generalizability.

Solution Strategies

- Using multi-center datasets with heterogeneous populations.
- Preprocessing techniques (such as image normalization and harmonization algorithms).
- Domain adaptation and transfer learning techniques.

6.2 Standardization and Reproducibility.

Issue: There are no globally acknowledged techniques for image acquisition, segmentation, or feature computation in radiomic feature extraction.

Impact: Inconsistent results across studies and platforms undermine clinical trust and impede validation efforts.

Solution Strategies

- The creation of standard operating procedures (SOPs).
- Adoption of open-source toolkits that comply with the Image Biomarker Standardization Initiative (IBSI).
- Automated segmentation technologies help to reduce inter-observer variability.

6.3 Overfitting and Validation Concerns

Issue: Deep learning algorithms are prone to overfitting when trained on tiny or unrepresentative datasets. Performance may appear to be outstanding during internal testing but fail in real-world deployment.

Impact: This leads to incorrect conclusions and dangerous clinical decision support.

Solution Strategies

- Use cross-validation and external validation cohorts.
- Apply regularization techniques and data augmentation.
- Prefer explainable AI (XAI) frameworks for improved interpretability and transparency.

6.4 Regulatory and Ethical Considerations

Issue: Clinical use of AI tools necessitates demanding regulatory permissions (e.g., FDA, EMA). Furthermore, AI judgments must be understandable, accountable, and equitable.

Impacts include rollout delays, liability concerns, and clinician opposition.

Solution Strategies

- Design prospective clinical studies to assess AI-assisted workflows.
- Ensure that AI systems follow data privacy rules (e.g., GDPR, HIPAA).
- Encourage multidisciplinary collaboration among radiologists, data scientists, and ethicists.

7 EMERGING TRENDS AND FUTURE DIRECTIONS

7.1 Federated Learning and Privacy-Preserving AI

Federated learning is a machine learning technique where multiple devices or servers collaboratively train a shared model without sharing their raw data. Instead of centralizing all the data in one, each participant trains the model locally using their own data and then shares only model updates (like gradients or weights) with a central server. It has particularly strong potential in radiomics, where privacy, data volume, and variability across institutions are critical concerns as illustrated in Figure 9.

The sequence of steps involves a central coordinator defining a model architecture (e.g., CNN for image classification or segmentation) in the initial phase. Participating institutions use their own radiomics data to train the model locally. These locally trained models send encrypted or anonymized updates to a central server, which combines updates using methods like Federated Averaging (FedAvg) to create a new global model. The improved model is sent back to participants for the next training round and the cycle is repeated (Raza et al., 2025).

Figure 9.

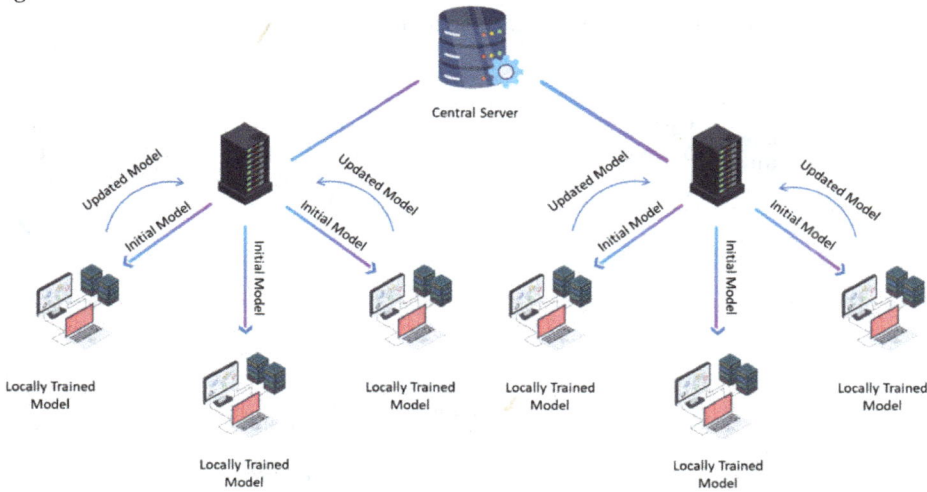

Based on the types of architecture described in the literature, they can be divided into three major types:

- Horizontal Federated Learning
- Vertical Federated Learning
- Federated Transfer Learning

Horizontal Federated Learning (sample-based) – Clients have datasets with the same feature space, which could be the same type of variables like age, tumor size or CT radiomic features, but different data samples. It is applicable in situations when multiple centres each have scan data of different patients, but all use the same imaging modality and annotation protocols as shown in Figure 10.

Vertical Federated Learning (feature-based) – Participants have datasets with the same patient samples or overlapping IDs, but different features. When multiple organizations or clients have differing data, a radiology department has imaging data and a genetics lab has gene expression data for the same patients, they may be combined to form a comprehensive feature set for the patients.

Federated Transfer Learning (cross-domain) – It is applicable when the clients have different feature spaces and data samples. A small clinic having limited patient imaging data may combine the data or benefit from a larger hospital that has a vast labeled dataset. The shared model can be fine-tuned or adapted using transfer learning but can have challenges like aligning model structures and semantics across domains.

Figure 10. Overlap and differences in federated learning architectures

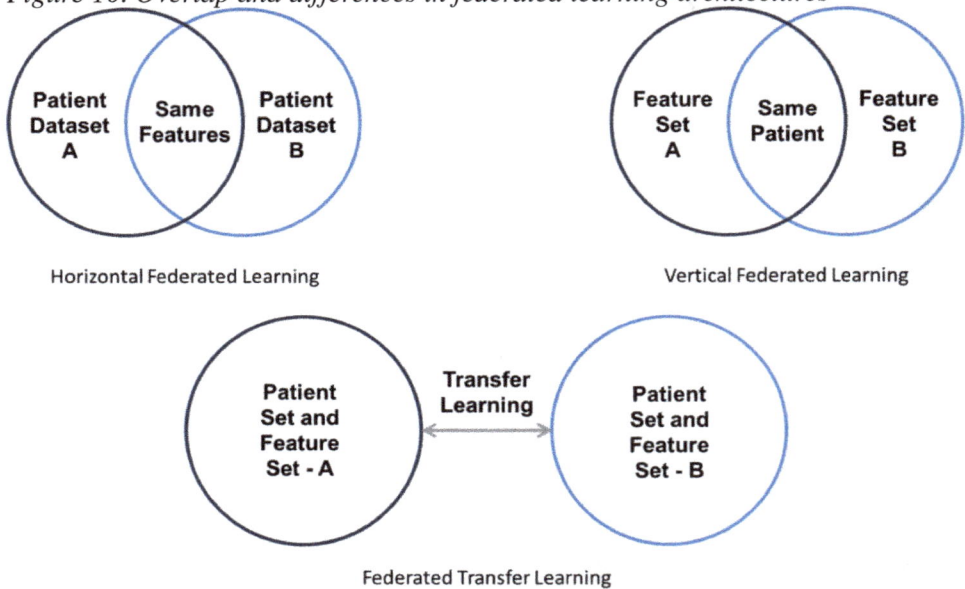

Horizontal Federated Learning

Vertical Federated Learning

Federated Transfer Learning

7.1.1 Federated Aggregation

Federated aggregation is a technique that greatly affects model performance, convergence, resilience, and privacy by integrating locally trained model updates from several clients into a single global model. FedProx, which adapts FedAvg by adding a proximal term to handle non-IID data and reduce model divergence; Fed-Nova, which normalizes updates by learning rate and training steps to address client drift and enhance stability; and Federated Averaging (FedAvg), which averages local model weights and works well with IID data, are important aggregation techniques. Encrypting client updates so that the server can only see the aggregated output is how Secure Aggregation (SecAgg) protects data privacy. (Ntantiso et al., 2023).

7.2 Multi-Omics Integration With Radiomics

Multomics refers to the integrated analysis of multiple "omics" datasets that capture different layers of biological information. It's a systems biology approach that aims to provide a more comprehensive view of how molecular processes interact and affect human health, disease, and treatment responses. Each "omics" layer captures a specific aspect of biological data such as genomics, transcriptomics, proteomics, microbiomics among others. It enables comprehension of complex disease mechanisms, diagnostics, prognosis, and treatment strategies by combining two or more omics datasets from the same individual or cohort. The most commonly integrated omics datasets with radiomics are those that provide complementary biological insights to imaging phenotypes such as genomics, transcriptomics and proteomics.

7.2.1 Radio Genomics

The interdisciplinary field of radio genomics blends genomics, which examines genetic mutations and variations like EGFR, KRAS, or VHL, with radiomics, which extracts quantitative features from medical imaging. This integration improves cancer diagnosis, prognosis, and treatment tailoring by enabling non-invasive molecular feature prediction. Gene mutation prediction, tumor categorization, prognosis, and radiation planning are all supported by radio genomics, which correlates imaging characteristics (such as tumour margins) with genomic profiles and uses machine learning to find predictive radiomic signals (Liu et al., 2023). Applications include classifying patients with brain and lung cancer according to risk and survival by combining MRI radiomics with genomic data, and using CT to predict VHL mutations or venous invasion in hepatocellular carcinoma (Shui et al., 2021).

7.2.2 Radiomics with Transcriptomics

The integration of radiomics and transcriptomics bridges macroscopic imaging features with molecular gene expression profiles, enabling non-invasive insights into tumour biology. This enhances cancer diagnosis, prognosis, and therapeutic strategies by correlating quantitative imaging patterns with transcriptomic pathways. Transcriptomic profiling involves gene expression and signature derivation among others. Gene expression involves analysis in which microarrays or RNA sequencing quantify mRNA levels, identifying pathways like cell cycle or immune response and molecular subtypes. Stable transcriptomic signatures differentiate malignant vs. non-malignant tissue and predict outcomes.

The approach has been used for predicting immunotherapy response. In HOT/COLD tumor classification, CT radiomics has been shown to predict PD-L1 expression, T-cell infiltration, and IFN-γ pathway activity, stratifying tumors into immunologically "hot" (responsive) or "cold" (resistant) categories. Combining radiomics with transcriptomic HOT scores can also improve prediction of 3-month progression-free survival in NSCLC patients on anti-PD-1 therapy. In Tumor Microenvironment (TME) Decoding, radiomic signatures correlate with CD8+ T-cell density and extracellular matrix organization, offering non-invasive TME assessment. PET radiomics in head-neck cancer reflects DNA repair, metabolism, and signal transduction pathways, validated via Reactome analysis (Tixier et al., 2020).

7.2.3 Radiomics with Proteomics

The integration of radiomics and proteomics is a significant advancement in precision oncology. It combines quantitative imaging features with protein expression profiles to identify pathways linked to tumor aggressiveness. This approach has been used in ovarian cancer to characterize tumors, with high stromal NNMT in CT scans predicting platinum resistance and poor survival by altering histone methylation in cancer-associated fibroblasts. Protein imaging correlations can be made, with MAGEA4a linked to supradiaphragmatic lymphadenopathy and reduced levels of CRIP2 linked to mesenteric disease. Radiomic prognostic vectors in epithelial ovarian cancer correlate with fibronectin abundance, a driver of tumor invasion. The integration of multiomics with radiomics offers a microscopic view of tumor biology, including genetic mutations, gene expression, protein regulation, and metabolic pathways. This enables fused models to outperform unimodal approaches in predicting tumor subtypes, genetic mutations, survival outcomes, and treatment responses. Machine learning and deep learning algorithms have also enabled complex data fusion and pattern recognition for integrative modelling.(Beer et al., 2020).

7.3 Quantum Computing and Next-Gen AI Models in Imaging

Quantum computing is a new paradigm of computing based on the principles of quantum mechanics and shows promise of having an impact on molecular simulations, precision medicine, DNA sequencing, medical imaging, and optimization problems in treatment planning, healthcare operations and supply chain optimization. Quantum algorithms can significantly accelerate MRI and CT image reconstruction, reducing scan times while improving resolution. Conventional imaging techniques struggle with massive datasets, but quantum computing enables parallel processing, refining images faster and more efficiently. It can also enhance segmentation accuracy by leveraging quantum-inspired clustering techniques, improving diagnostic precision. Optimization of storage and retrieval through quantum data encoding, makes it easier to manage and analyze large-scale medical imaging datasets.

7.3.1 Image Reconstruction and Quality

Quantum algorithms like the Quantum Fourier Transform (QFT) enable faster processing of raw imaging data, particularly in MRI and CT scans. By analysing entire datasets simultaneously, QFT reduces reconstruction times from hours to minutes, enabling real-time imaging for urgent clinical decisions. For complex linear systems in iterative reconstruction, the Harrow-Hassidim-Lloyd (HHL) algorithm offers exponential speedups over classical methods.

Quantum computing improves diagnostic accuracy through noise reduction, improving resolution, and adapting the imaging parameters. Quantum algorithms filter artefacts in MRI and CT scans, which improves signal-to-noise ratios and reduces noise. Quantum sensors detect minute magnetic fields, capturing finer soft-tissue details while optimizing MRI parameters in real-time based on patient anatomy, shortening scan times by 30-50% while maintaining clarity.

Although current quantum hardware remains experimental, hybrid quantum-classical systems show promise in clinical trials. As error-correction and qubit stability improve, quantum-enhanced medical imaging is poised to become standard practice (L. Wei et al., 2023).

7.4 Fully Autonomous Diagnostic Imaging Systems

Fully autonomous diagnostic imaging systems use artificial intelligence (AI) and deep learning to automate image acquisition, analysis, and reporting, enhancing diagnostic accuracy and workflow efficiency. These systems address challenges like human error, interpretation variability, and resource limitations in healthcare settings. Core technologies include AI-driven image analysis, robotic automation, simulation, and validation. AI algorithms have shown superior sensitivity in detecting malignancies, while deep learning models can reduce false negatives by 27% compared to radiologists. AI can also detect subtle anomalies, such as tumors or fractures, with higher accuracy than traditional methods. These systems can also forecast disease progression or health risks, enabling proactive interventions. Fully automatic systems can capture and reconstruct 3D images with <1% volume measurement error, reducing operator dependency. Robotic automation systems, like the auto-RUSS system, can demonstrate reproducibility and minimize operator-dependent variability. Virtual testing platforms like NVIDIA Isaac for Healthcare ensure safety and efficacy before real-world deployment (X.-X. Lin et al., 2025).

These systems offer multiple advantages and operation benefits like improved diagnostic accuracy, gains in efficiency and overall reduction in the costs. Automated systems can reduce misinterpretation rates in emergency departments, critical for time-sensitive conditions like stroke with automated triaging systems reducing report turnaround times significantly.

These advances also have their own challenges like data heterogeneity, ethical concerns and regulatory hurdles. Very few AI models are validated on multi-ethnic cohorts, risking algorithmic bias and multiple institutions lack protocols for AI transparency. Due to this FDA-cleared AI tools are much less in number and even those show degraded performance in real-world settings due to dataset shift (Khalifa & Albadawy, 2024).

8 CONCLUSION

To summarize, the integration of artificial intelligence (AI) and radiomics constitutes a paradigm shift in medical imaging, providing unparalleled prospects for predictive, personalized, and precision medicine. Significant findings include AI's capacity to automate image processing, identify complicated patterns, and give therapeutically relevant insights that are frequently beyond human vision. Radiomics adds to this by quantifying imaging features in high-dimensional data, which improves diagnostic, prognostic, and therapeutic predictions. Together, they have the potential to revolutionize accuracy, efficiency, and patient outcomes in a variety of clinical contexts. To realize this promise, interdisciplinary collaboration between radiologists, computer scientists, doctors, and biomedical engineers is required. Furthermore, strong translational research frameworks must be developed to test AI-powered technologies in clinical settings, ensuring their safety, reliability, and ethical use.

REFERENCES

Anwar, S. M., Majid, M., Qayyum, A., Awais, M., Alnowami, M., & Khan, M. K. (2018). Medical Image Analysis using Convolutional Neural Networks: A Review. In *Journal of Medical Systems* (Vol. 42, Issue 11). Springer New York LLC. https://doi.org/DOI: 10.1007/s10916-018-1088-1

Arimura, H., Soufi, M., Ninomiya, K., Kamezawa, H., & Yamada, M. (2018). Potentials of radiomics for cancer diagnosis and treatment in comparison with computer-aided diagnosis. In *Radiological Physics and Technology* (Vol. 11, Issue 4, pp. 365–374). Springer Tokyo. https://doi.org/DOI: 10.1007/s12194-018-0486-x

Bao, D., Liu, Z., Geng, Y., Li, L., Xu, H., Zhang, Y., Hu, L., Zhao, X., Zhao, Y., & Luo, D. (2022). Baseline MRI-based radiomics model assisted predicting disease progression in nasopharyngeal carcinoma patients with complete response after treatment. *Cancer Imaging; the Official Publication of the International Cancer Imaging Society*, 22(1). Advance online publication. DOI: 10.1186/s40644-022-00448-4 PMID: 35090572

Beer, L., Sahin, H., Bateman, N. W., Blazic, I., Vargas, H. A., Veeraraghavan, H., Kirby, J., Fevrier-Sullivan, B., Freymann, J. B., Jaffe, C. C., Brenton, J., Miccó, M., Nougaret, S., Darcy, K. M., Maxwell, G. L., Conrads, T. P., Huang, E., & Sala, E. (2020). Integration of proteomics with CT-based qualitative and radiomic features in high-grade serous ovarian cancer patients: An exploratory analysis. *European Radiology*, 30(8), 4306–4316. DOI: 10.1007/s00330-020-06755-3 PMID: 32253542

Cao, X., Wang, X., Song, J., Su, Y., Wang, L., & Yin, Y. (2024). Pretreatment multiparametric MRI radiomics-integrated clinical hematological biomarkers can predict early rapid metastasis in patients with nasopharyngeal carcinoma. *BMC Cancer*, 24(1). Advance online publication. DOI: 10.1186/s12885-024-12209-6 PMID: 38589858

Cè, M., Chiriac, M. D., Cozzi, A., Macrì, L., Rabaiotti, F. L., Irmici, G., Fazzini, D., Carrafiello, G., & Cellina, M. (2024). Decoding Radiomics: A Step-by-Step Guide to Machine Learning Workflow in Hand-Crafted and Deep Learning Radiomics Studies. *Diagnostics (Basel)*, 14(22), 2473. DOI: 10.3390/diagnostics14222473 PMID: 39594139

Cepeda, S., Esteban-Sinovas, O., Singh, V., Moiyadi, A., Zemmoura, I., Del Bene, M., Barbotti, A., DiMeco, F., West, T. R., Nahed, B. V., Giammalva, G. R., Arrese, I., & Sarabia, R. (2025). Prognostic Modeling of Overall Survival in Glioblastoma Using Radiomic Features Derived from Intraoperative Ultrasound: A Multi-Institutional Study. *Cancers (Basel)*, *17*(2). Advance online publication. DOI: 10.3390/cancers17020280 PMID: 39858063

Chen, B. Y., Xie, H., Li, Y., Jiang, X. H., Xiong, L., Tang, X. F., Lin, X. F., Li, L., & Cai, P. Q. (2022). MRI-Based Radiomics Features to Predict Treatment Response to Neoadjuvant Chemotherapy in Locally Advanced Rectal Cancer: A Single Center, Prospective Study. *Frontiers in Oncology*, *12*. Advance online publication. DOI: 10.3389/fonc.2022.801743 PMID: 35646677

Chen, J., Gu, H., Fan, W., Wang, Y., Chen, S., Chen, X., & Wang, Z. (2020). MRI-based radiomic model for preoperative risk stratification in stage I endometrial cancer. *Journal of Cancer*, *12*(3), 726–734. DOI: 10.7150/jca.50872 PMID: 33403030

Chen, Y., Wang, Z., Yin, G., Sui, C., Liu, Z., Li, X., & Chen, W. (2022). Prediction of HER2 expression in breast cancer by combining PET/CT radiomic analysis and machine learning. *Annals of Nuclear Medicine*, *36*(2), 172–182. DOI: 10.1007/s12149-021-01688-3 PMID: 34716873

Demircioğlu, A. (2022). The effect of preprocessing filters on predictive performance in radiomics. *European Radiology Experimental*, *6*(1). Advance online publication. DOI: 10.1186/s41747-022-00294-w PMID: 36045274

Dromain, C., Boyer, B., Ferré, R., Canale, S., Delaloge, S., & Balleyguier, C. (2013). Computed-aided diagnosis (CAD) in the detection of breast cancer. *European Journal of Radiology*, *82*(3), 417–423. DOI: 10.1016/j.ejrad.2012.03.005 PMID: 22939365

Du, R., Lee, V. H., Yuan, H., Lam, K. O., Pang, H. H., Chen, Y., Lam, E. Y., Khong, P. L., Lee, A. W., Kwong, D. L., & Vardhanabhuti, V. (2019). Radiomics model to predict early progression of nonmetastatic nasopharyngeal carcinoma after intensity modulation radiation therapy: A multicenter study. *Radiology. Artificial Intelligence*, *1*(4). Advance online publication. DOI: 10.1148/ryai.2019180075 PMID: 33937796

Gillies, R. J., Kinahan, P. E., & Hricak, H. (2016). Radiomics: Images are more than pictures, they are data. *Radiology*, *278*(2), 563–577. DOI: 10.1148/radiol.2015151169 PMID: 26579733

Ji, C., Ge, W., Zhu, C., Shen, F., Yu, Y., Pang, G., Li, Q., Zhu, M., Ma, Z., Zhu, X., Fu, Y., Gong, L., Wang, T., Du, L., Jin, G., & Zhu, M. (2025). Family history and genetic risk score combined to guide cancer risk stratification: A prospective cohort study. *International Journal of Cancer*, *156*(3), 505–517. DOI: 10.1002/ijc.35187 PMID: 39291673

Jo, G. D., Ahn, C., Hong, J. H., Kim, D. S., Park, J., Kim, H., Kim, J. H., Goo, J. M., & Nam, J. G. (2023). 75% radiation dose reduction using deep learning reconstruction on low-dose chest CT. *BMC Medical Imaging*, *23*(1). Advance online publication. DOI: 10.1186/s12880-023-01081-8 PMID: 37697262

Jyothi, N. M. (2023). AI-Enabled Genomic Biomarkers: The Future of Pharmaceutical Industry and Personalized Medicine. *Seybold Report Journal*, *18*(08), 54–72.

Kang, Y. K., Ha, S., Jeong, J. B., & Oh, S. W. (2024). The value of PET/CT radiomics for predicting survival outcomes in patients with pancreatic ductal adenocarcinoma. *Scientific Reports*, *14*(1). Advance online publication. DOI: 10.1038/s41598-024-77022-4 PMID: 39578496

Khalifa, M., & Albadawy, M. (2024). AI in diagnostic imaging: Revolutionising accuracy and efficiency. In *Computer Methods and Programs in Biomedicine Update* (Vol. 5). Elsevier B.V., DOI: 10.1016/j.cmpbup.2024.100146

Kocak, B., Akinci D'Antonoli, T., Mercaldo, N., Alberich-Bayarri, A., Baessler, B., Ambrosini, I., Andreychenko, A. E., Bakas, S., Beets-Tan, R. G. H., Bressem, K., Buvat, I., Cannella, R., Cappellini, L. A., Cavallo, A. U., Chepelev, L. L., Chu, L. C. H., Demircioglu, A., deSouza, N. M., Dietzel, M., & Cuocolo, R. (2024). METhodological RadiomICs Score (METRICS): A quality scoring tool for radiomics research endorsed by EuSoMII. *Insights Into Imaging*, *15*(1). Advance online publication. DOI: 10.1186/s13244-023-01572-w PMID: 38228979

Kshatri, S. S., & Singh, D. (2023). Convolutional neural network in medical image analysis: A review. *Archives of Computational Methods in Engineering*, *30*(4), 2793–2810.

Kumar, V., Gu, Y., Basu, S., Berglund, A., Eschrich, S. A., Schabath, M. B., Forster, K., Aerts, H. J. W. L., Dekker, A., Fenstermacher, D., Goldgof, D. B., Hall, L. O., Lambin, P., Balagurunathan, Y., Gatenby, R. A., & Gillies, R. J. (2012). Radiomics: The process and the challenges. *Magnetic Resonance Imaging*, *30*(9), 1234–1248. DOI: 10.1016/j.mri.2012.06.010 PMID: 22898692

Lee, J., Kim, S. H., Kim, Y., Park, J., Park, G. E., & Kang, B. J. (2022). Radiomics Nomogram: Prediction of 2-Year Disease-Free Survival in Young Age Breast Cancer. *Cancers (Basel)*, *14*(18). Advance online publication. DOI: 10.3390/cancers14184461 PMID: 36139620

Lee, J. Y., & Lee, K. sig, Seo, B. K., Cho, K. R., Woo, O. H., Song, S. E., Kim, E. K., Lee, H. Y., Kim, J. S., & Cha, J. (2022). Radiomic machine learning for predicting prognostic biomarkers and molecular subtypes of breast cancer using tumor heterogeneity and angiogenesis properties on MRI. *European Radiology*, *32*(1), 650–660. DOI: 10.1007/s00330-021-08146-8 PMID: 34226990

Lin, X.-X., Li, M.-D., Ruan, S.-M., Ke, W.-P., Zhang, H.-R., Huang, H., Wu, S.-H., Cheng, M.-Q., Tong, W.-J., Hu, H.-T., He, D.-N., Lu, R.-F., Lin, Y.-D., Kuang, M., Lu, M.-D., Chen, L.-D., Huang, Q.-H., & Wang, W. (2025). Autonomous robotic ultrasound scanning system: A key to enhancing image analysis reproducibility and observer consistency in ultrasound imaging. *Frontiers in Robotics and AI, 12*. Advance online publication. DOI: 10.3389/frobt.2025.1527686 PMID: 39975565

Lin, Y., Wu, R. C., Lin, Y. C., Huang, Y. L., Lin, C. Y., Lo, C. J., Lu, H. Y., Lu, K. Y., Tsai, S. Y., Hsieh, C. Y., Yang, L. Y., Cheng, M. L., Chao, A., Lai, C. H., & Lin, G. (2024). Endometrial cancer risk stratification using MRI radiomics: Corroborating with choline metabolism. *Cancer Imaging; the Official Publication of the International Cancer Imaging Society*, *24*(1). Advance online publication. DOI: 10.1186/s40644-024-00756-x PMID: 39182135

Liu, Z., Duan, T., Zhang, Y., Weng, S., Xu, H., Ren, Y., Zhang, Z., & Han, X. (2023). Radiogenomics: a key component of precision cancer medicine. In *British Journal of Cancer* (Vol. 129, Issue 5, pp. 741–753). Springer Nature. https://doi.org/DOI: 10.1038/s41416-023-02317-8

Louis, T., Lucia, F., Cousin, F., Mievis, C., Jansen, N., Duysinx, B., Le Pennec, R., Visvikis, D., Nebbache, M., Rehn, M., Hamya, M., Geier, M., Salaun, P. Y., Schick, U., Hatt, M., Coucke, P., Lovinfosse, P., & Hustinx, R. (2024). Identification of CT radiomic features robust to acquisition and segmentation variations for improved prediction of radiotherapy-treated lung cancer patient recurrence. *Scientific Reports*, *14*(1). Advance online publication. DOI: 10.1038/s41598-024-58551-4 PMID: 38641673

Lu, C. F., Liao, C. Y., Chao, H. S., Chiu, H. Y., Wang, T. W., Lee, Y., Chen, J. R., Shiao, T. H., Chen, Y. M., & Te Wu, Y. (2023). A radiomics-based deep learning approach to predict progression free-survival after tyrosine kinase inhibitor therapy in non-small cell lung cancer. *Cancer Imaging; the Official Publication of the International Cancer Imaging Society*, *23*(1). Advance online publication. DOI: 10.1186/s40644-023-00522-5 PMID: 36670497

Mansouri, Z., Salimi, Y., Amini, M., Hajianfar, G., Oveisi, M., Shiri, I., & Zaidi, H. (2024). Development and validation of survival prognostic models for head and neck cancer patients using machine learning and dosiomics and CT radiomics features: A multicentric study. *Radiation Oncology (London, England)*, *19*(1). Advance online publication. DOI: 10.1186/s13014-024-02409-6 PMID: 38254203

Mayerhoefer, M. E., Materka, A., Langs, G., Häggström, I., Szczypiński, P., Gibbs, P., & Cook, G. (2020). Introduction to radiomics. *Journal of Nuclear Medicine*, *61*(4), 488–495. DOI: 10.2967/JNUMED.118.222893 PMID: 32060219

Mishro, P. K., Agrawal, S., Panda, R., & Abraham, A. (2020). Novel fuzzy clustering-based bias field correction technique for brain magnetic resonance images. *IET Image Processing*, *14*(9), 1701–1709. DOI: 10.1049/iet-ipr.2019.0942

Moons, K. G. M., Altman, D. G., Reitsma, J. B., Ioannidis, J. P. A., Macaskill, P., Steyerberg, E. W., Vickers, A. J., Ransohoff, D. F., & Collins, G. S. (2015). Transparent reporting of a multivariable prediction model for individual prognosis or diagnosis (TRIPOD): Explanation and elaboration. *Annals of Internal Medicine*, *162*(1), W1–W73. DOI: 10.7326/M14-0698 PMID: 25560730

Nandakumar, S., Khan, S. A., Ganesan, P., Sweety, P., Francis, A. P., Sekar, M., ... & Meenakshi, D. U. (2022). Deep Learning and Precision Medicine: Lessons to Learn for the Preeminent Treatment for Malignant Tumors. *Deep Learning for Targeted Treatments: Transformation in Healthcare*, 127-169.

Nicoletti, G., Mazzetti, S., Maimone, G., Cignini, V., Cuocolo, R., Faletti, R., Gatti, M., Imbriaco, M., Longo, N., Ponsiglione, A., Russo, F., Serafini, A., Stanzione, A., Regge, D., & Giannini, V. (2024). Development and Validation of an Explainable Radiomics Model to Predict High-Aggressive Prostate Cancer: A Multicenter Radiomics Study Based on Biparametric MRI. *Cancers (Basel)*, *16*(1). Advance online publication. DOI: 10.3390/cancers16010203 PMID: 38201630

Nittas, V., Daniore, P., Landers, C., Gille, F., Amann, J., Hubbs, S., & Blasimme, A. (2023). Beyond high hopes: A scoping review of the 2019–2021 scientific discourse on machine learning in medical imaging. *PLOS Digital Health*, *2*(1), e0000189. PMID: 36812620

Ntantiso, L., Bagula, A., Ajayi, O., & Kahenga-Ngongo, F. (2023). A Review of Federated Learning: Algorithms, Frameworks and Applications. In *Lecture Notes of the Institute for Computer Sciences* (pp. 341–357). Social Informatics and Telecommunications Engineering., DOI: 10.1007/978-3-031-34896-9_20

Parmar, C., Grossmann, P., Bussink, J., Lambin, P., & Aerts, H. J. W. L. (2015). Machine Learning methods for Quantitative Radiomic Biomarkers. *Scientific Reports, 5*. Advance online publication. DOI: 10.1038/srep13087 PMID: 26278466

Philip, M. M., Watts, J., McKiddie, F., Welch, A., & Nath, M. (2024). Development and Validation of Prognostic Models Using Radiomic Features from Pre-Treatment Positron Emission Tomography (PET) Images in Head and Neck Squamous Cell Carcinoma (HNSCC) Patients. *Cancers (Basel), 16*(12). Advance online publication. DOI: 10.3390/cancers16122195 PMID: 38927901

Pinto-Coelho, L. (2023). How Artificial Intelligence Is Shaping Medical Imaging Technology: A Survey of Innovations and Applications. *Bioengineering (Basel, Switzerland), 10*(12), 1435. DOI: 10.3390/bioengineering10121435 PMID: 38136026

Raza, A., Guzzo, A., Ianni, M., Lappano, R., Zanolini, A., Maggiolini, M., & Fortino, G. (2025). Federated Learning in radiomics: A comprehensive meta-survey on medical image analysis. In *Computer Methods and Programs in Biomedicine* (Vol. 267). Elsevier Ireland Ltd., DOI: 10.1016/j.cmpb.2025.108768

Rizzo, S., Botta, F., Raimondi, S., Origgi, D., Fanciullo, C., Morganti, A. G., & Bellomi, M. (2018). Radiomics: the facts and the challenges of image analysis. In *European Radiology Experimental* (Vol. 2, Issue 1). Springer. https://doi.org/DOI: 10.1186/s41747-018-0068-z

Rossi, G., Barabino, E., Fedeli, A., Ficarra, G., Coco, S., Russo, A., Adamo, V., Buemi, F., Zullo, L., Dono, M., de Luca, G., Longo, L., Dal Bello, M. G., Tagliamento, M., Alama, A., Cittadini, G., Pronzato, P., & Genova, C. (2021). Radiomic Detection of EGFR Mutations in NSCLC. *Cancer Research, 81*(3), 724–731. DOI: 10.1158/0008-5472.CAN-20-0999 PMID: 33148663

Scapicchio, C., Gabelloni, M., Barucci, A., Cioni, D., Saba, L., & Neri, E. (2021). A deep look into radiomics. In *Radiologia Medica* (Vol. 126, Issue 10, pp. 1296–1311). Springer-Verlag Italia s.r.l. https://doi.org/DOI: 10.1007/s11547-021-01389-x

Shen, H., Wang, Y., Liu, D., Lv, R., Huang, Y., Peng, C., Jiang, S., Wang, Y., He, Y., Lan, X., Huang, H., Sun, J., & Zhang, J. (2020). Predicting Progression-Free Survival Using MRI-Based Radiomics for Patients With Nonmetastatic Nasopharyngeal Carcinoma. *Frontiers in Oncology, 10*. Advance online publication. DOI: 10.3389/fonc.2020.00618 PMID: 32477932

Sherminie, L. P. G., Jayatilake, M. L., Hewavithana, B., Weerakoon, B. S., & Vijithananda, S. M. (2023). Morphometry-based radiomics for predicting therapeutic response in patients with gliomas following radiotherapy. *Frontiers in Oncology*, *13*. Advance online publication. DOI: 10.3389/fonc.2023.1139902 PMID: 37664038

Shui, L., Ren, H., Yang, X., Li, J., Chen, Z., Yi, C., Zhu, H., & Shui, P. (2021). The Era of Radiogenomics in Precision Medicine: An Emerging Approach to Support Diagnosis, Treatment Decisions, and Prognostication in Oncology. In *Frontiers in Oncology* (Vol. 10). Frontiers Media S.A., DOI: 10.3389/fonc.2020.570465

Sozutok, S., Piskin, F. C., Balli, H. T., Yucel, S. P., & Aikimbaev, K. (2024). Predicting treatment responses using magnetic resonance imaging-based radiomics in hepatocellular carcinoma patients undergoing transarterial radioembolization. *Revista da Associação Médica Brasileira*, *70*(11). Advance online publication. DOI: 10.1590/1806-9282.20240721 PMID: 39630762

Stefano, A., Leal, A., Richiusa, S., Trang, P., Comelli, A., Benfante, V., Cosentino, S., Sabini, M. G., Tuttolomondo, A., Altieri, R., Certo, F., Barbagallo, G. M. V., Ippolito, M., & Russo, G. (2021). Robustness of pet radiomics features: Impact of co-registration with mri. *Applied Sciences (Switzerland)*, *11*(21). Advance online publication. DOI: 10.3390/app112110170

Tang, F. H., Fong, Y. W., Yung, S. H., Wong, C. K., Tu, C. L., & Chan, M. T. (2023). Radiomics-Clinical AI Model with Probability Weighted Strategy for Prognosis Prediction in Non-Small Cell Lung Cancer. *Biomedicines*, *11*(8). Advance online publication. DOI: 10.3390/biomedicines11082093 PMID: 37626590

Taye, M. M. (2023). Understanding of Machine Learning with Deep Learning: Architectures, Workflow, Applications and Future Directions. *Computers*, *12*(5), 91. DOI: 10.3390/computers12050091

Tian, Q., Li, X., Li, J., Cheng, Y., Niu, X., Zhu, S., Xu, W., & Guo, J. (2022). Image quality improvement in low-dose chest CT with deep learning image reconstruction. *Journal of Applied Clinical Medical Physics*, *23*(12). Advance online publication. DOI: 10.1002/acm2.13796 PMID: 36210060

Tian, J., Dong, D., Liu, Z., Zang, Y., Wei, J., Song, J., ... & Zhou, M. (2018). Radiomics in medical imaging—detection, extraction and segmentation. Artificial intelligence in decision support systems for diagnosis in medical imaging, 267-333.

Tixier, F., Cheze-le-Rest, C., Schick, U., Simon, B., Dufour, X., Key, S., Pradier, O., Aubry, M., Hatt, M., Corcos, L., & Visvikis, D. (2020). Transcriptomics in cancer revealed by Positron Emission Tomography radiomics. *Scientific Reports*, *10*(1). Advance online publication. DOI: 10.1038/s41598-020-62414-z PMID: 32221360 van Timmeren, J. E., Cester, D., Tanadini-Lang, S., Alkadhi, H., & Baessler, B. (2020). Radiomics in medical imaging—"how-to" guide and critical reflection. In *Insights into Imaging* (Vol. 11, Issue 1). Springer. https://doi.org/DOI: 10.1186/s13244-020-00887-2

Wang, L., Zhu, L., Yan, J., Qin, W., Wang, C., Xi, W., Xu, Z., Chen, Y., Jiang, J., Huang, S., Yan, C., Zhang, H., Pan, Z., & Zhang, J. (2023). CT-Based Radiomic Score: A Risk Stratifier in Far-Advanced Gastric Cancer Patients. *Academic Radiology*, *30*, S220–S229. DOI: 10.1016/j.acra.2022.12.034 PMID: 36610930

Wang, P., Luo, Z., Luo, C., & Wang, T. (2024). Application of a Comprehensive Model Based on CT Radiomics and Clinical Features for Postoperative Recurrence Risk Prediction in Non-small Cell Lung Cancer. *Academic Radiology*, *31*(6), 2579–2590. DOI: 10.1016/j.acra.2023.11.028 PMID: 38172022

Wang, T., She, Y., Yang, Y., Liu, X., Chen, S., Zhong, Y., Deng, J., Zhao, M., Sun, X., Xie, D., & Chen, C. (2022). Radiomics for Survival Risk Stratification of Clinical and Pathologic Stage IA Pure-Solid Non-Small Cell Lung Cancer. *Radiology*, *302*(2), 425–434. DOI: 10.1148/radiol.2021210109 PMID: 34726531

Wei, L., Liu, H., Xu, J., Shi, L., Shan, Z., Zhao, B., & Gao, Y. (2023). Quantum machine learning in medical image analysis: A survey. *Neurocomputing*, *525*, 42–53. DOI: 10.1016/j.neucom.2023.01.049

Wei, Z.-Y., Zhang, Z., Zhao, D.-L., Zhao, W.-M., & Meng, Y.-G. (2024). Magnetic resonance imaging-based radiomics model for preoperative assessment of risk stratification in endometrial cancer. *World Journal of Clinical Cases*, *12*(26), 5908–5921. DOI: 10.12998/wjcc.v12.i26.5908 PMID: 39286374

Xie, F., Zhao, Q., Li, S., Wu, S., Li, J., Li, H., Chen, S., Jiang, W., Dong, A., Wu, L., Liu, L., Huang, H., Xu, S., Shao, Y., Liu, L., Li, L., & Cai, P. (2022). Establishment and validation of novel MRI radiomic feature-based prognostic models to predict progression-free survival in locally advanced rectal cancer. *Frontiers in Oncology*, *12*. Advance online publication. DOI: 10.3389/fonc.2022.901287 PMID: 36408187

Xu, J., Li, J., Wang, T., Luo, X., Zhu, Z., Wang, Y., Wang, Y., Zhang, Z., Song, R., Yang, L. Z., Wang, H., Wong, S. T. C., & Li, H. (2025). Predicting treatment response and prognosis of immune checkpoint inhibitors-based combination therapy in advanced hepatocellular carcinoma using a longitudinal CT-based radiomics model: A multicenter study. *BMC Cancer*, *25*(1). Advance online publication. DOI: 10.1186/s12885-025-13978-4 PMID: 40181337

Yang, H., Wang, L., Shao, G., Dong, B., Wang, F., Wei, Y., Li, P., Chen, H., Chen, W., Zheng, Y., He, Y., Zhao, Y., Du, X., Sun, X., Wang, Z., Wang, Y., Zhou, X., Lai, X., Feng, W., & Xu, Y. (2022). A combined predictive model based on radiomics features and clinical factors for disease progression in early-stage non-small cell lung cancer treated with stereotactic ablative radiotherapy. *Frontiers in Oncology*, *12*. Advance online publication. DOI: 10.3389/fonc.2022.967360 PMID: 35982975

Yolchuyeva, S., Giacomazzi, E., Tonneau, M., Ebrahimpour, L., Lamaze, F. C., Orain, M., Coulombe, F., Malo, J., Belkaid, W., Routy, B., Joubert, P., & Manem, V. S. K. (2023). A Radiomics-Clinical Model Predicts Overall Survival of Non-Small Cell Lung Cancer Patients Treated with Immunotherapy: A Multicenter Study. *Cancers (Basel)*, *15*(15). Advance online publication. DOI: 10.3390/cancers15153829 PMID: 37568646

Zhang, B., Lian, Z., Zhong, L., Zhang, X., Dong, Y., Chen, Q., Zhang, L., Mo, X., Huang, W., Yang, W., & Zhang, S. (2020). Machine-learning based MRI radiomics models for early detection of radiation-induced brain injury in nasopharyngeal carcinoma. *BMC Cancer*, *20*(1). Advance online publication. DOI: 10.1186/s12885-020-06957-4 PMID: 32487085

Zhang, X., Lu, B., Yang, X., Lan, D., Lin, S., Zhou, Z., Li, K., Deng, D., Peng, P., Zeng, Z., & Long, L. (2022). Prognostic analysis and risk stratification of lung adenocarcinoma undergoing EGFR-TKI therapy with time-serial CT-based radiomics signature. *European Radiology*, *33*, 825–835. DOI: 10.1007/s00330-022-09123-5/ Published PMID: 36166088

Zhao, B. (2021). Understanding Sources of Variation to Improve the Reproducibility of Radiomics. In *Frontiers in Oncology* (Vol. 11). Frontiers Media S.A., DOI: 10.3389/fonc.2021.633176

Zhou, T., Yang, M., Xiong, W., Zhu, F., Li, Q., Zhao, L., & Zhao, Z. (2024). The value of intratumoral and peritumoral radiomics features in differentiating early-stage lung invasive adenocarcinoma (≤3 cm) subtypes. *Translational Cancer Research*, *13*(1), 202–216. DOI: 10.21037/tcr-23-1324 PMID: 38410219

Zhuang, Z., Liu, Z., Li, J., Wang, X., Xie, P., Xiong, F., Hu, J., Meng, X., Huang, M., Deng, Y., Lan, P., Yu, H., & Luo, Y. (2021). Radiomic signature of the FOWARC trial predicts pathological response to neoadjuvant treatment in rectal cancer. *Journal of Translational Medicine*, *19*(1). Advance online publication. DOI: 10.1186/s12967-021-02919-x PMID: 34112180

Zwanenburg, A., Vallières, M., Abdalah, M. A., Aerts, H. J. W. L., Andrearczyk, V., Apte, A., Ashrafinia, S., Bakas, S., Beukinga, R. J., Boellaard, R., Bogowicz, M., Boldrini, L., Buvat, I., Cook, G. J. R., Davatzikos, C., Depeursinge, A., Desseroit, M.-C., Dinapoli, N., Dinh, C. V., & Löck, S. (2020). The Image Biomarker Standardization Initiative: Standardized Quantitative Radiomics for High-Throughput Image-based Phenotyping. *Radiology*, *295*(2), 328–338. DOI: 10.1148/radiol.2020191145 PMID: 32154773

Chapter 10
Healthcare Text–Mining Approach to Detect Metabolic Syndrome by Analyzing User-entered Symptoms in Natural Language

Kunj Bihari Meena

(iD) https://orcid.org/0000-0001-8159-9024

Jaypee University of Engineering and Technology, Guna, India

Kunal Kumar Singh

Jaypee University of Engineering and Technology, Guna, India

Manan Jain

(iD) https://orcid.org/0009-0002-6868-0498

Jaypee University of Engineering and Technology, Guna, India

Shreyash Sundarrao Dhande

Jaypee University of Engineering and Technology, Guna, India

Vipin Tyagi

(iD) https://orcid.org/0000-0003-4994-3686

Jaypee University of Engineering and Technology, Guna, India

DOI: 10.4018/979-8-3373-3196-6.ch010

ABSTRACT

Metabolic syndrome involves abdominal adiposity, raised blood pressure, and lipid abnormalities. Early detection is essential, as timely intervention reduces future cardiometabolic risk. However, conventional diagnosis depends on structured clinical data, which is slow to collect and often incomplete. This chapter presents an AI-based prediction system that identifies metabolic syndrome from free-text patient descriptions. The approach uses NLP to convert symptom narratives into structured medical features. The pipeline includes preprocessing, feature engineering, named entity recognition, clinical term mapping, and classification using logistic regression, random forest, and XGBoost. Model performance was evaluated using accuracy and AUC-ROC. XGBoost achieved the best results, with 0.8732 accuracy and 0.9608 AUC.

1. INTRODUCTION

Metabolic syndrome is a serious health concern affecting many people today. It increases the chances of cardiovascular disease. The primary contributing factors include excess waist circumference, increased fasting plasma glucose, high blood pressure, hypertriglyceridemia and low value of HDL cholesterol. As per (World Health Organization, 1999), if a person has any two symptoms out of blood pressure, high triglycerides, low HDL, obesity, and microalbuminuria along with Insulin resistance, then it is considered as metabolic syndrome. Similarly, another definition states that if a person has three or more of these risk factors simultaneously then it is considered as metabolic syndrome (National Cholesterol Education Program, 2001). Around the globe this is an important public health problem these days.

The WHO estimates that about 20-25 percent of adults in the world are having some form of metabolic syndrome, especially in the urbanized and industrialised parts of the globe (Aggoun, 2007). Globalization has led to increased obesity, physical inactivity, and unhealthy eating patterns, these results in an increase of metabolic syndrome across the globe. Also, this is more common among older people but due to modern socio-culture, it also affecting younger population (Alberti et al., 2009). Metabolic syndrome is generally overlooked especially in developing countries with limited resources. The syndrome can be prevented and managed by detecting it and taking some timely actions and lifestyle modifications.

International Diabetes Federation (IDF) and the National Cholesterol Education Program (NCEP) have laid down the clinical and biochemical criteria for detecting metabolic syndrome. These include blood pressure, various anthropometric measurements, fasting blood glucose, lipid profile, and other relevant laboratory and clinical examinations. Mostly, clinical and biochemical criteria for diagnosing metabolic syndrome are too complex, expensive, slow, and prone to inaccurate results. Moreover, rural and underdeveloped areas usually lack the infrastructure and resources to conduct such elaborate evaluations. Many people remain undiagnosed until serious life-threatening health complications start to occur. There is a need of low-cost, rapid, and easy solution that can identify individuals with metabolic syndrome at the initial stages.

Artificial Intelligence (AI) can analyze large volumes of complex data, uncover hidden patterns and can also provide predictive insights with accuracy and efficiency surpassing traditional statistical methods. There are several applications of AI and ML (Machine Learning) in every step of life. For example in digital image forensics ML is used for detecting tampered or fake images (Meena & Tyagi, 2021). ML is widely used in financial fraud detection, in autonomous vehicles for real-time decision-making and navigation, and in smart agriculture for optimizing crop yield through predictive analytics (Tomar et al., 2022).

In clinical settings, ML has been successfully used for a variety of tasks including image analysis, disease classification, patient risk assessment, and treatment recommendation systems. By integrating AI into healthcare, it becomes possible to streamline time-consuming processes, ease the burden on medical professionals and improve diagnostic accuracy which is ultimately leading to better outcomes. AI-powered tools can benefit users greatly that enable disease detection and risk prediction process more accessible, smooth and cost efficient also.

However, one major challenge in using AI for detecting conditions like metabolic syndrome is the nature of healthcare data itself. As the healthcare data is often highly unstructured therefore it becomes very difficult to work with such unstructured data. The Unstructuredness of healthcare data also creates same challenge while applying AI for metabolic syndrome detection. Often clinical notes, patient complaints and other symptom descriptions exist as free text in the medical record, making it difficult for standard ML models that don't work with unstructured text but rather with structured numerical data. Natural Language Processing (NLP), a subfield of AI, aims to overcome this difficulty by allowing computers to process human language input in order to extract useful information (Kreimeyer et al., 2017). NLP methods can help us to convert text to structured, quantifiable features, which can be fed into ML models for prediction. This development decreases the requirements of manual data input process and allows for great diversity of patient information to be introduced in diagnosis system.

AI and ML models are shown to be useful in prediction of metabolic syndrome and its complications by various studies in last few years. In the field of medical research, supervised machine learning algorithms such as Logistic Regression, Random Forests, Decision Trees, Support Vector Machine (SVM), and Extreme

Gradient Boosting (XGBoost) have been widely explored (Shehab et al., 2022). Among these, the XGBoost algorithm has gained particular attention. Researchers appreciate it for its strong ability to handle high-dimensional complex data, manage missing values effectively and its built-in regularization features that help to reduce the risk of overfitting (Nielsen, 2016). Due to its efficiency and accuracy, XGBoost has become a popular choice for clinical applications.

This chapter presents an AI-powered metabolic syndrome prediction system designed to assess the likelihood of metabolic syndrome using NLP and ML based algorithms. The system accepts text input containing symptoms from the user. Then, it processes through NLP pipeline to clean and tokenize it. After that, it recognizes the entity and transforms the entities into proper value of clinical indicators. Finally, the prediction is made using the trained ML model. Publicly available clinical data are utilized to train and validate the proposed models.

The main aim of the work in this chapter is to show capabilities of NLP and ML techniques for metabolic syndrome prediction. Furthermore, the study aims to show how such AI-based diagnostic systems can perform better-than conventional ones. Finally, the chapter highlights how AI-based systems can facilitate disease prevention. The system minimizes delays in diagnosis, reduces healthcare provider workload, and makes risk prediction tools accessible to clinicians as well as non-clinicians by automating extraction of clinical indicators from unstructured text inputs and analyzing them.

2. LITERATURE REVIEW

In last few years, the rising use of AI and ML techniques in healthcare services has been observed. These technologies are showing great promise in improving the diagnosis of diseases, predicting risks and managing patients. ML algorithms can discover deep-rooted patterns in clinical datasets that humans would not likely ever be able to find. Multiple studies demonstrate the effectiveness of AI models in automating diagnostics and clinical decision-making. Since, metabolic syndrome is becoming a pressing global public health issue; investigators are very much interested in obtaining advanced, reliable prediction techniques. This literature review primarily highlights three aspects: (1) survey of existing ML based diagnostic systems; (2) past research on prediction of metabolic syndrome using ML, and (3) the applications of NLP in healthcare diagnostics. The objective of this section is to provide an overview of the current research trends, identify existing limitations, and position the proposed system within the present research scenario.

2.1 Existing ML-Based Medical Diagnostic Systems

Numerous diagnostic frameworks have been developed focusing on specific disease identification powered by ML techniques. Recently, many studies have employed ML algorithms to predict diseases such as cardiovascular diseases, diabetes, breast cancer, liver disease and even COVID-19. Rajkomar et al. (2018) used the deep learning algorithms on Electronic Health Records (EHR) for predicting in-hospital mortality, readmissions and diagnosis of the patients. Esteva et al. (2017) also introduced a technique to classify images of skin cancer. The study suggests that their proposed method can detect skin cancer with almost same accuracy as a dermatologist.

Supervised machine learning techniques like Logistic Regression, Decision Trees, Random Forest, SVM can be used to classify medical data. Chicco & Jurman (2020) utilized a Random Forest model to predict heart failure in patients by relying on structural clinical data. The authors conclude that their proposed method demonstrates higher accuracy than conventional statistical methods. Chen & Guestrin (2016) proposed the XGBoost algorithm, which has become very popular because it provides promising results for various classification problems in general. The XGBoost method can handle missing data and also has built-in regularization. The XGBoost can be effectively used in the situation where dataset is having small sample sizes and high dimensionality.

2.2 Studies on Metabolic Syndrome Prediction

Machine Learning has been studied quite extensively for many diseases however; very few studies have focused on the prediction of metabolic syndrome. To the best of our knowledge, (Aggoun et al., 2007) was one of the first large-scale studies with significant analysis of risk factors for metabolic syndrome and why they should be detected early as it causes cardiovascular and metabolic diseases.

Worachartcheewan et al. (2015) used ensemble techniques of Random Forest to predict metabolic syndrome. They reported better accuracy and sensitivity of these ensemble methods over baseline classifier. Shin et al. (2023) proposed a noninvasive predictive model for early detection of metabolic syndrome using decision tree classifiers. The authors used a Korean health dataset of 70,370 samples for model evaluation. This model achieved 0.889 AUC, 0.855 recall, and 0.773 specificity. However this work does not include blood biomarkers, which might affect detection accuracy in borderline cases. Yang et al. (2022) developed metabolic syndrome risk prediction model. This work introduced Differential State Features (DSFs) and Differential Numerical Features (DNFs) to capture changes over time in clinical variables like Body Mass Index (BMI), Triglycerides (TG), and Waist Circumference

(WC). This model achieved an AUC of 0.930 and accuracy of 0.849. However, this model shows lower performance in terms of the precision and F1 score.

Choe et al. (2018) proposed a metabolic syndrome prediction model that employed Naïve Bayes ML model. This method achieved AUC of 0.69. The study highlights that adding genetic markers improves performance slightly over clinical data alone. The drawback of this method is that this model performs poorly under sensitivity and recall. Gutiérrez-Esparza et al. (2020) discussed an approach to identify optimal prognostic variables for metabolic syndrome using random forest classifier. Further, chi-squared and Correlation-based Feature Selection (CFS) was also used. The results suggest that best performance was achieved using waist-to-height ratio as a key feature. Perveen et al. (2019) designed a method based on J48 decision tree to detect metabolic syndrome. The combination of Naïve Bayes and K-medoids under-sampling achieved the best AUC of 0.79.

Yu et al. (2020) applied decision tree algorithms to predict metabolic syndrome. The authors explored several tree-based ML models such as CART and Random Forest. The Random Forest obtained the highest AUC of 0.904. Hosseini-Esfahani et al. (2021) proposed a data mining-based approach using the Random Forest algorithm to identify metabolic syndrome. Kim et al. (2022) used nine machine learning algorithms, including XGBoost and Random Forest, to predict metabolic syndromes. The XGBoost classifier achieved AUC = 0.851 and F1 score = 0.851. This study concluded that waist-to-hip ratio and BMI were the most important features.

Trigka & Dritsas (2023) explored various supervised ML techniques to predict the metabolic syndrome. Their method achieved accuracy of 89.35% and F1 score values of 0.898 on the dataset from National Health and Nutrition Examination Survey (NHANES).

Although such systems are being built, a large gap remained for the building of systems employing unstructured descriptions of symptoms or patient narratives as input. Many of the existing studies are based solely on numerical inputs and do not incorporate information from clinical notes and patient symptoms. Currently, there are few prediction systems that can produce real-time and risk-based predictions using natural language inputs. The proposed system addresses these issues by using NLP techniques for numeric feature extraction from unstructured data and machine learning for classification for metabolic syndrome prediction.

2.3 Applications of Natural Language Processing (NLP) in Healthcare

NLP has become a significant healthcare analytics tool that can turn unstructured text into structured information that can be utilized for decision making. Clinical notes, patient Narratives, discharge summaries and consultation notes contain many key health indicators that are generally not processable by standard ML systems. NLP methods like Named Entity Recognition (NER), Parts of Speech (POS) tagging and text classification allow extracting the clinical features, symptoms and diagnosis from unstructured text.

Kreimeyer et al. (2017) provided an overview of NLP systems in clinical research and argued that these NLP-based systems can be used for disease surveillance, adverse event detection and phenotyping. Zhou et al. (2024) provided an extensive survey of NLP based techniques, mainly designed for smart healthcare. The authors introduced a pipeline of NLP approaches to solve healthcare problems. Then, they explained how NLP can play a vital role in COVID-19 pandemic and mental health.

Essentially NLP based systems have the major advantage of utilizing unstructured data source for enabling wide variety of input for clinical decision making. NLP improves predictive model performance and diagnostic accuracy by translating verbal symptom descriptions into numerical indicators. Despite its advantages, very little research has been done in predicting the metabolic syndrome through use of NLP-based ML methods. The proposed system in this chapter has novelty and significant impact because of this gap.

The reviewed literature discusses the use of ML and AI in healthcare, particularly for disease classification and risk prediction. While several studies have proved the effectiveness of ML techniques in diagnosing chronic diseases, limited research has focused specifically on metabolic syndrome prediction, especially using free-text symptom descriptions. Existing systems such as (Trigka & Dritsas, 2023), predominantly rely on structured clinical data and overlook valuable unstructured patient inputs. Although NLP has proven valuable in healthcare applications, its integration with metabolic syndrome prediction models remains underdeveloped. This chapter addresses these gaps by suggesting an AI-powered metabolic syndrome prediction system that combines NLP-based feature extraction with machine learning classifiers, offering a comprehensive, scalable solution for early risk detection.

3. PROPOSED METHOD

This chapter provides a system that can predict the likelihood of metabolic syndrome in individuals using both structured data (like lab results and health parameters) and unstructured, natural language input (like symptom descriptions by a patient). This dual approach not only makes the system flexible but also more user-friendly, especially for non-technical users where structured data is not always available. Figure 1 shows the steps of the proposed model.

Figure 1. Main steps of the proposed model

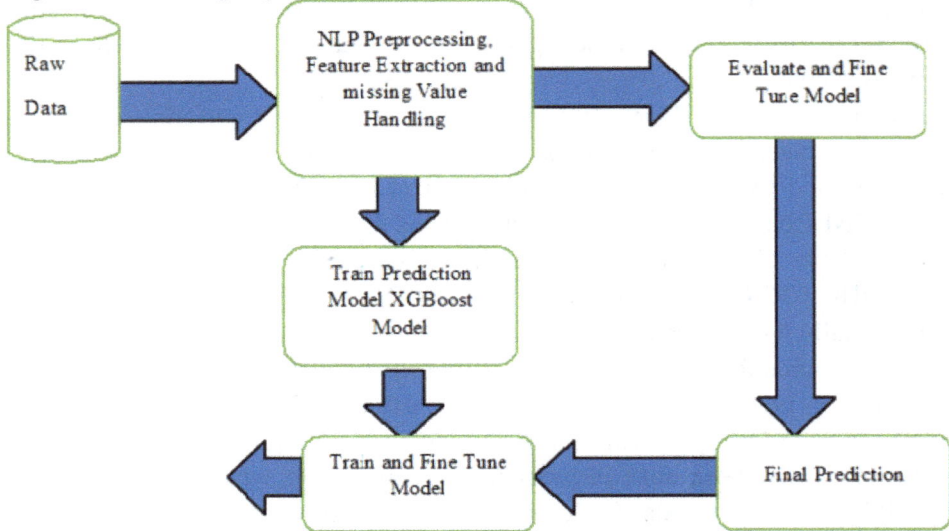

At a high level, the system works in several stages. First, it receives a symptom description written in plain English e.g., "a 45-year-old female with waist 95 cm, BMI 28.3 and blood sugar." This input is passed through a NLP pipeline that extracts meaningful clinical features like age, gender, BMI, blood glucose, HDL (High-Density Lipoprotein), triglycerides, etc. These features are then preprocessed and used to make predictions using a trained XGBoost machine learning model.

The proposed system is designed to be scalable, interpretable and easy to integrate with electronic health records or mobile applications in the future.

3.1 Preprocessing

Proper cleaning and preparation of data before feeding it to machine learning models is important. Healthcare data is mostly a raw clinical data, which contains missing values, mixed types and different scales having an impact on model accuracy. For delivering clean data, a preprocessing pipeline was built in this work so that models can work properly. The stages include: handling missing values, feature engineering, scaling numerical values and encoding categorical data. The same process was applied both during training and while predicting in real-time so as to maintain synchronization in the model's learning.

3.1.1. Handling Missing Values

Like many real-world datasets, the dataset used in this work also contains some missing values in some of the features; for example waist circumference, marital status, and BMI shows some missing values. One of the solutions may be to remove these rows but it leads to loss of valuable information. So, *SimpleImputer* from Scikit-learn was used which replaces missing values with the mean of each numerical column. This approach is not only straightforward but often effective also in healthcare datasets where missing values are random or minimal. During deployment, the imputer was saved as a .pkl file to ensure the same logic was applied during the prediction. It can be noted that some features such as marital status have non-numeric values. These features are first converted into numerical form using LabelEncoder (as discussed in Section 3.1.4), after which SimpleImputer is applied to handle missing values.

3.1.2 Feature Engineering

Five clinically significant derived features were engineered to enhance the discriminative power of the proposed model. The *Waist_BMI_Ratio* was computed using:

$$Waist\_BMI\_Ratio = \frac{WaistCirc(cm)}{BMI(kg/m^2)}$$

This ratio quantifies central adiposity, a key diagnostic criterion for metabolic syndrome. The *Glucose_Triglycerides* interaction term:

$$Glu\cos e\_Triglycerides = BloodGlu\cos e(mg/dL) \times Triglycerides(mg/dL)$$

captures synergistic effects between hyperglycemia and dyslipidemia. The lipid profile marker *HDL_Triglycerides_Ratio*:

$$HDL\_Triglycerides\_Ratio = \frac{HDL(mg/dL)}{Triglycerides(mg/dL)}$$

reflects atherogenic risk, with lower values indicating poorer lipid metabolism. *BMI_Category* was discretized per WHO standards:

$$BMI\_Category = \begin{cases} 0 & if\, BMI < 18.5 \\ 1 & if\, 18.5 \leq BMI < 25 \\ 2 & if\, 25 \leq BMI < 30 \\ 3 & if\, BMI \geq 30 \end{cases}$$

The binary feature *WaistCirc_High* implemented International Diabetes Federation (IDF) metabolic syndrome criteria:

$$WaistCir c_{High} = \begin{cases} WaistCirc > 102cm \\ 0 \ otherwise \end{cases}$$

These features provide additional insights into each patient's condition and improved model accuracy and were added as new columns in the dataset and the same was done during real-time prediction.

3.1.3 Scaling and Normalization

In medical datasets, the value for glucose can range in the hundreds while values of features like BMI or HDL are much smaller. Without normalization, these imbalances can skew model performance. Hence, numerical features were standardized to zero mean with unit variance via:

$$z = \frac{x - \mu}{\sigma}$$

where μ and σ represent the training set's feature-wise mean and standard deviation, respectively.

Standardization was performed using StandardScaler from Scikit-learn to ensure that all the numerical values have a mean of 0 and standard deviation of 1.

3.1.4. Encoding Categorical Variable

The dataset contains many categorical variables like Sex, Marital Status and Race. ML models can not interpret text values directly, so Label Encoding was applied to convert these strings into numeric codes. For example "Male" and "Female" are encoded as 0 and 1 respectively. During the prediction also, the system fills missing values in the new data using the same medians learned during training. This helped ensure smooth prediction even when partial data was entered.

3.2. User Input Processing using NLP

The system accepts input in plain English (natural language) form from the users making it more user-friendly, especially for non-technical users or situations where structured data is not available. The system allows users to type descriptions like: "A 45-year-old female with BMI 29.5, high blood sugar and waist 98cm".

In order to obtain suitable numeric values from the descriptive input, a custom NLP pipeline is developed using regular expressions and keyword mapping. This module analyses the user's input and extracts the relevant medical indicators like age, BMI, blood glucose, HDL and more. The extracted values are then mapped to features required by the machine learning model, completing the data preprocessing loop in real time.

The main motivation to enable system to take descriptive text as input is that in the real world, especially in primary care or rural clinics, numeric well-structured data is not always available easily. Patients usually express their symptoms in natural language. An NLP–based module is created that understands these descriptions to reduce the efforts of manual data entry by clinicians. Further, this also increases the usability of the proposed metabolic syndrome detection system. Moreover, from a machine learning standpoint, enabling text-to-feature conversion unlocks new opportunities for dynamic, on-the-fly predictions, which is particularly valuable for preventive care and early detection strategies.

3.2.1 Named Entity Recognition (NER)

The concept of named entity recognition lies at the core of the NLP pipeline. The process begins with basic preprocessing steps, including lowercasing text for case insensitivity and using regular expressions to detect meaningful clinical terms and values especially pattern and hidden insights such as numbers followed by units (e.g., "150 mg/dL").

Keywords like "BMI", "blood glucose", "waist" and "HDL" are captured along with their associated values. In this study, the NLP pipeline mainly depends on regular expression (regex)-based text extraction to identify key clinical terms and symptom descriptions from unstructured input. This rule-based approach was selected for its simplicity, interpretability, and efficiency in processing short, domain-specific clinical texts. It allows direct mapping of symptom expressions to structured clinical features required by the ML model.

Custom regular expressions are written to match clinical indicators. For example, if the input text has "blood glucose is 145 mg/dL" the parser would extract the value "145" and assign it to the feature named BloodGlucose. The system accounts for different wording so it will understand that blood sugar and blood glucose are the same. Like this, an interpretation of high BMI and low HDL is made against a clinical threshold. Due to this, the input does not need to be in a particular format for the NLP component to act.

3.2.2 Feature Mapping

Once the system has identified and extracted the entities that are input by the user, the next step involves feature mapping. Feature mapping is transforming those recognized values into a structured format so that it matches what the machine learning model expects.

For numeric inputs like "BMI 29.5" or "waist 98 cm", the values are directly mapped with the corresponding feature of model. But, when the quantitative data is not given and qualitative or descriptive phrases are given like "low HDL" or "high blood sugar", then the system applies predefined clinical thresholds. For example, if "low HDL" is detected then the value of HDL is automatically set to 40 mg/dL in context with metabolic syndrome diagnostic standards.

These mapping rules are defined with the help of a Python dictionary. And these are applied programmatically during preprocessing step. This ensures that the model takes consistent, structured input without depending on the fact whether user enters exact numerical values or descriptive clinical phrases. This feature mapping step is crucial in maintaining compatibility between free-text input and the trained machine learning model.

3.3 Model Selection

In the design of a prediction system, different machine learning models were used for the prediction of the result. Selection of best machine learning model is an important part of any prediction system. In this study, three different supervised machine learning algorithms: Random Forest, Logistic Regression and XGBoost are used. Different models have their own strengths and weaknesses. The objective is to compare the results of multiple models and check how well these models can predict whether a person is likely to have metabolic syndrome or not. Each model was trained using the same dataset and then evaluated and compared their performances. For performance comparison, standard metrics like accuracy, AUC-ROC curves and confusion matrix, precision, recall, and F1 score were used. This comparison helped to select the most reliable and accurate model for the deployment.

Logistic Regression performs well when the dataset is small to medium sized, its feature have linear relationships, when features are not highly correlated and dataset is cleaned, Random Forest works well with high-dimensional data, as it avoids overfitting due to bagging and random feature selection and it handles non-linear relationships, complex pattern in a better way. XGBoost is considered when high predictive accuracy is required. It works well with large datasets. It can handle mixed data types (numeric and categorical).

3.3.1 Logistic Regression

Logistic Regression (LaValley, 2008) estimates the probability of an event occurring. There are three categories of logistic regression models: Binary logistic, Multinomial logistic and Ordinal logistic regression. Logistic regression belongs to the family of supervised machine learning models. The evaluation began with Logistic Regression which is a classic algorithm for binary classification. It is a simple, interpretable machine learning model that works well when the relationship between features and the outcome is linear. Logistic Regression gave a solid baseline to compare more advanced models against. During testing, it achieved decent accuracy and was very fast to train. However, it struggled with complex, non-linear patterns that are common in healthcare data. For example, it could not effectively capture interactions between features like the Triglycerides/HDL ratio or BMI x WaistCircumference. While useful, it was clear that a more sophisticated model could offer better predictive power for this particular use case.

3.3.2 Random Forest

Random Forest (Schlenger, 2024) combines the output of multiple decision trees in order to give a single output result and is easy to use and flexible also and hence it's widely adopted by the developers. Random Forest algorithm is capable of handling both classification and regression problems. Unlike Logistic Regression, Random Forest can handle non-linear relationships and interactions between variables without requiring extensive feature engineering. It also offers built-in feature importance scores, which was helpful during analysis. The model performed better than Logistic Regression in terms of both accuracy and recall. However, Random Forest models tend to be larger and slightly slower during prediction, which was a concern for real-time web applications. While it was a strong contender and gave consistent results, it still fell a bit short as compared with the results of XGBoost.

3.3.3 XGBoost

XGBoost (Chen & Guestrin, 2016) is an algorithm which is a part of ensemble learning category. It uses decision tree as base learner and employs regularization techniques to enhance the generalization of the model. In boosting, the trees are built sequential so each subsequent tree targets to reduce the errors. In contrast to bagging approaches like Random Forest, boosting uses tree with lesser number of splits. If the number of trees is more, then it can lead to overfitting. So, it is always a tricky part to select the stopping criteria for boosting.

After comparing the previous two models, XGBoost model was evaluated which is an advanced boosting machine learning algorithm. XGBoost builds decision trees sequentially and focuses on correcting the errors of previous trees that make it more powerful than bagging methods like Random Forest. It also includes regularization, which reduces the risk of overfitting which is a common issue in small or noisy healthcare datasets. In testing, it was found that XGBoost consistently outperformed the other models across all metrics. It achieved the highest accuracy, best AUC-ROC score and lowest false negatives which is especially important in health diagnostics. Based on these results, XGBoost was selected as final model for deployment. A summary of all three models' comparison is shown in Table 1.

Table 1. Comparison of various ML models under different aspects

Feature/Aspect	Logistic Regression	Random Forest	XGBoost
Model Type	Linear model	Ensemble of Decision Trees	Gradient Boosted Decision Trees
Handling Non-linearity	Poor (only linear relationships)	Good (captures non-linear patterns)	Excellent (captures complex patterns)
Interpretability	Very high	Medium	Lower
Training speed	Very fast	Moderate	Slightly slower than Random Forest
Overfitting Risk	Low	Medium	Low
Hyperparameter Sensitivity	Low	Medium	High
Memory Usage	Very Low	High	Moderate
Performance on Small Data	Good	Good	Good
Performance on Complex Data	Poor	Good	Excellent
Suitability for Healthcare Data	Good for baseline models	Good for medium complex problems	Excellent for complex patterns and high-stakes prediction

XGBoost gives the best balance across all these metrics. It gives high AUC-ROC which indicates that it performs well at distinguishing between patients with and without metabolic syndrome, even when the decision boundary was unclear.

4. EXPERIMENTAL RESULTS

This section gives information about the dataset, performance metrics and comparison of performance of different algorithms that are used to train model.

4.1 Dataset Description

For experiments, a publicly available dataset "Metabolic Syndrome Prediction Dataset" is used. The dataset is publicly available at https://data.world/informatics -edu/metabolic-syndrome-prediction. This dataset is created by NHANES (National Health and Nutrition Examination Survey) which is a health-related program conducted by the National Center for Health Statistics (NCHS) to provide information on the health and nutritional status of the non-institutionalized civilian resident population of the United States. Note that this same dataset is also used by (Trigka & Dritsas, 2023). This dataset is chosen because of its comprehensive coverage of clinical and demographic variables relevant to metabolic syndrome prediction. It provides a solid foundation for training and evaluating the machine learning models. The dataset is in a CSV format due to which it becomes easy for integration into data processing pipeline. The dataset contains multiple records each representing an individual with various health-related attributes. There are 2402 rows and 15 columns in the CSV file that contains dataset. Where first row indicates the names of the features hence there are total 2401 samples for evaluating the model. Among 15 columns listed in Table 2 first column is used for sequence number hence 14 columns represent the feature. Last column indicates the target variable whereas 13 columns are used as input variables.

Table 2. Overview of dataset features and their corresponding descriptions for the metabolic syndrome prediction model.

Column Name	Description
Seqn	Sequential identification number
Age	Age of the individual
Sex	Gender (e.g., Male, Female)
Marital	Marital status of the individual
Income	Income level or income-related information
Race	Ethnic or racial background of the individuals
WaistCirc	Waist circumference measurement
BMI	Body Mass Index, a measure of body composition

continued on following page

Table 2. Continued

Column Name	Description
Albuminuria	Measurement related to albumin in urine
UrAlbCr	Urinary albumin-to-creatinine ratio
UricAcid	Uric acid levels in the blood
BloodGlucose	Blood glucose levels which is an indicator of diabetes risk
HDL	High density Lipoprotein cholesterol levels (the good cholesterol)
Triglycerides	It gives the information about the triglyceride level in someone's blood
Metabolic Syndrome	Binary variable indicating the presence (1) or absence (0) of metabolic syndrome

The features reported in Table 2 align with the criteria commonly used to diagnose the metabolic syndrome. It makes the dataset suitable for predictive modelling objectives. The dataset holds the details about the people who got affected by metabolic syndrome which is a challenging health condition linked to several risk factors that increase the likelihood of heart disease. Categorization of features by demographic, anthropometric, clinical, and lifestyle domains for metabolic syndrome prediction is shown in Table 3.

Table 3. Categorization of features by demographic, anthropometric, clinical, and lifestyle domains for metabolic syndrome prediction.

Category	Features
Demographics	Age, Sex, Marital, Income, Race
Anthropometric Measurements	Waist circumference and BMI
Clinical Measurements	Albuminuria, UrAlbCr, UricAcid, BloodGlucose, HDL, Triglycerides
Lifestyle factors	Income
Target variable	Metabolic Syndrome

Upon initial examination, the dataset appeared well structured; however, following challenges were also there:

Missing Data: Some entries were missing in critical fields like waist circumference, marital status, and BMI. During preprocessing, the issue was handled by applying imputation techniques and ensuring that missing or incomplete data was properly handled before further analysis.

Class Imbalance: The distribution of the target variables was slightly imbalanced with a higher proportion of individuals not diagnosed with metabolic syndrome. In particular, there exist a total of 1579 samples for non-metabolic syndrome class where as 822 for metabolic syndrome class. In order to mitigate this, stratified sampling and evaluation metrics were used that account for the resulting imbalance.

Feature Correlation: Some of the features exhibited multicollinearity which can affect the model performance. Therefore, by applying feature engineering additional five features were created as discussed in section 3.1.2. By acknowledging and addressing these challenges, it can be ensured that the dataset was adequately prepared for training robust and reliable machine learning models.

4.2 Performance Metrics

To find the effectiveness of the proposed machine learning models in predicting the metabolic syndrome whether a patient has the syndrome or not, the performance of models are evaluated using several widely accepted classification metrics (Meena & Tyagi, 2021), (Meena & Tyagi, 2020). These metrics helps in measuring how well a model distinguishes between individuals with and without the syndrome and how reliable the predictions of the models are in context of real-world medical.

- **Precision**: It is the proportion of positive predictions that were actually correct. In case, it tells how many patients predicted are having metabolic syndrome truly had it. Precision is calculated as:

$$Precision = \frac{TP}{TP + FP}$$

- **Recall (Sensitivity)**: It is the ability of the model to correctly identify all actual positive cases. High recall is critical in healthcare to ensure that no high-risk patients are missed. It is computed as:

$$Recall = \frac{TP}{TP + FN}$$

- **F1 score**: It gives a balanced measure of precision and recall. It becomes useful when the distribution of class is uneven. It can be determined as:

$$F1\ score = 2*\frac{Precision*Recall}{Precision + Recall}$$

- **Accuracy**: It is the proportion of total correct predictions made by the model. Accuracy is considered as a good starting point. But, if the classes are imbalanced then it is mislead. It is calculated as:

$$Accuracy = \frac{TP + TN}{TP + TN + FP + FN}$$

- **Area under the Curve:** The AUC represents ability of the model to distinguish between positive and negative classes. A higher AUC mean better separability. It can be calculated as:

$$AUC - ROC = \int_0^1 TPR\, dFPR$$

- **Log Loss (Logarithmic Loss):** Log Loss measures the uncertainty of the model's predictions. A lower log loss value reflects higher confidence in predicted probabilities. It can be computed as:

$$Log\ Loss = -\frac{1}{N} \sum_{i=1}^{N} [yi\ \log(pi) + (1 - yi)\log(1 - pi)]$$

- **Matthews Correlation Coefficient (MCC):** MCC is a balanced metric that considers true and false positives and negatives. It is especially informative when dealing with imbalanced datasets. MCC can be calculated as:

$$MCC = \frac{TP.TN - FP.FN}{\sqrt{(TP + FP)(TP + FN)(TN + FP)(TN + FN)}}$$

- **Balanced Accuracy:** The metric provides the average of sensitivity (recall) and specificity, which helps when classes are not evenly distributed.

$$Balanced\ Accuracy = \frac{1}{2} \left(\frac{TP}{TP + FN} + \frac{TN}{TN + FP} \right)$$

- **Specificity (True Negative Rate):** Specificity refers to how well a model identifies negative instances. It can be calculated as:

$$Specificity(True\ Negative\ Rate) = \frac{TN}{TN + FP}$$

- **Confusion Matrix**: In addition to standard performance metrics, models were also evaluated using the confusion matrices which provide a detailed breakdown of the prediction outcomes.

For classifying samples as metabolic (positive class) or non-metabolic (negative class) the terms can defined as:

- **TP** = (metabolic predicted as metabolic) True Positives
- **TN** = (non-metabolic predicted as non-metabolic) True Negatives
- **FP** = (non-metabolic predicted as metabolic) False Positives

- **FN** = (metabolic predicted as non-metabolic) False Negatives

4.3 Experimental Setup

The model training process was conducted using python programming on the Jupyter Notebook. This notebook is an open-source interactive computing environment where the dataset was loaded, preprocessing was performed, multiple machine learning models (Random Forest, Logistic Regression, and XGBoost) were trained and the final components were saved for deployment. Jupyter notebook made the process easier to visualize data at every single step, test the individual code blocks and iterate quickly based on the model performance.

Initially required Python libraries to complete the proposed system include pandas, numpy and Scikit-learn. The Scikit-learn library is used to import the machine learning models. Then loading of the dataset was done using pandas library.

Then, the missing values were handled using SimpleImputer and also applied LabelEncoder for categorical features and scaled numerical features with StandardScaler. These steps ensured that the dataset was clean, consistent and ready for training the machine learning models. Then, engineered features like Triglycerides / HDL and WaistCircumference X BMI were created which are known to improve predictive power in metabolic health contexts. Then, the process continued with splitting the dataset into training and testing sets. Scikit-learn library of python has a function named 'train-test-split()' function which helps in splitting the dataset into two parts training set and testing set. By using train_test_split() function, the dataset was split into 80:20 ratio. 80% split part of the dataset was used for training the model and 20% split part was used for testing the trained model. This ensured that dataset had unseen data to evaluate the models after training. As already discussed, there are three different models that have been used – Logistic Regression, Random Forest and XGBoost using the training data. All three models were evaluated using the test set and performance metrics such as accuracy, precision, recall and AUC-ROC curves, etc as discussed in section 4.2. The result comparison was done to compare all the performance metrics in order to check their effectiveness. The comparison of these metrics helped in selecting the best model not only based on accuracy but also on how well they identified true positives and avoided the false negatives.

After testing, it became clear that XGBoost consistently outperformed and other two models in all key metrics. It handled complex, non-linear relationships better and also allowed to tune various parameters like learning rate, depth and regularization terms. Once model was finalized, the XGBoost model was saved using Python's pickle model as model.pkl. The scaler, imputer and encoders used during preprocessing were saved to make sure that the same transformations could be applied to live user inputs during the prediction. In order to maintain the consistency among the deployment environments, .pkl files played an important role.

Machine learning models require careful adjustment of hyperparameters to perform well. These settings control how the model learns from data. Without proper tuning, models may overfit (memorize training data) or underfit (fail to learn patterns). For medical predictions like metabolic syndrome, accurate models are crucial. Hyper-parameter tuning helps find the best balance between complexity and performance.

Several methods exist for tuning hyperparameters: Grid Search: Tests all possible combinations in a given range. It's thorough but slow for large parameter spaces. Random Search: Tests random combinations within ranges. Bayesian Optimization: Uses past results to guide future searches. More advanced but complex to implement. Manual Tuning: Relies on expert knowledge, however, this is time-consuming and less systematic approach. We used Randomized Search for three key reasons: first, it is faster than grid search when testing many parameters; second, it works very well with medium-sized dataset like we used; third, it finds good enough solutions without exhaustive searching.

Table 4. Hyperparameter settings using randomized search for each of three ML models used for metabolic syndrome prediction.

Model	Hyperparameters Searched	Best Parameters
Logistic Regression	C: [0.01, 0.1, 1, 10, 100] solver: ['lbfgs', 'liblinear']	C: 0.1 solver: liblinear
RandomForest	n_estimators: [100, 200, 300, 500] max_depth: [5, 10, 15, None] min_samples_split: [2, 5, 10] min_samples_leaf: [1, 2, 4]	n_estimators: 200 max_depth: 15 min_samples_split: 2 min_samples_leaf: 1
XGBoost	n_estimators: [100, 200, 300, 500] max_depth: [3, 5, 7, 9] learning_rate: [0.01, 0.05, 0.1, 0.2] subsample: [0.6, 0.8, 0.9, 1.0]	n_estimators: 200 max_depth: 7 learning_rate: 0.2 subsample: 0.9

Table 4 presents various parameters setting along with best settings of hyper-parameters. The best parameters showed interesting patterns: Logistic Regression worked best with mild regularization (C=0.1). This prevents overfitting while keeping useful patterns. Random Forest performed well with moderately deep trees (max_depth=15). This captures complex relationships without being too specific. XGBoost benefited from a higher learning rate (0.2) and some randomness (sub-sample=0.9). This combination helped it learn quickly while avoiding overfitting. Both Random Forest and XGBoost models used relatively small ensemble sizes (200 trees/estimators). This suggests data patterns could be captured without extremely complex models. The tuning process took about 2 hours for all models, showing good efficiency. These results prove that careful hyperparameter tuning improves model performance. The chosen settings make the models both accurate and reliable for medical use.

5. EXPERIMENTAL RESULT COMPARISON

In this section, result obtained via all three models (Random Forest, Logistic Regression and XGBoost are compared. The comparison is done based on the performance metrics like AUC-ROC curves, Confusion Matrix and also the results are compared under quantitative metrics.

5.1 Experimental Results Under AUC-ROC Curves

The evaluation of machine learning models for metabolic syndrome prediction reveals critical differences in their diagnostic capabilities, as demonstrated by their AUC-ROC (Area under the Receiver Operating Characteristic Curve) scores. The AUC-ROC curve is a fundamental metric in medical diagnostics which measures the ability of a machine learning model to differentiate between a healthy individual and one who is suffering from metabolic syndrome. If the AUC value comes to be higher than 0.5 it indicates that model is learning the patters. If the AUC value ranges between 0.9-1.0 then it is considered as excellent, if it ranges between 0.8-0.9 then it is considered as good, if it lies below 0.8 then it is assumed to be suboptimal in medical use. If the AUC value comes as exact 1.0 then it means the perfect prediction and if it is exact 0.5 then it is considered as random guessing.

5.1.1 AUC-ROC Curve for Logistic Regression

Figure 2 shows the AUC-ROC curve of Logistic Regression. From the Figure 2 it can be noticed that the AUC value for Logistic Regression is 0.91. ROC curve also shows good separation ability between positive and negative classes. However, in comparison to XGBoost and Random Forest, the performance of Logistic Regression was slightly lower at lower threshold values. The phenomenon indicates a reduced tendency of Logistic Regression to capture true positives in the early prediction range.

Figure 2. ROC curve of the Logistic Regression model indicating an AUC value of 0.91.

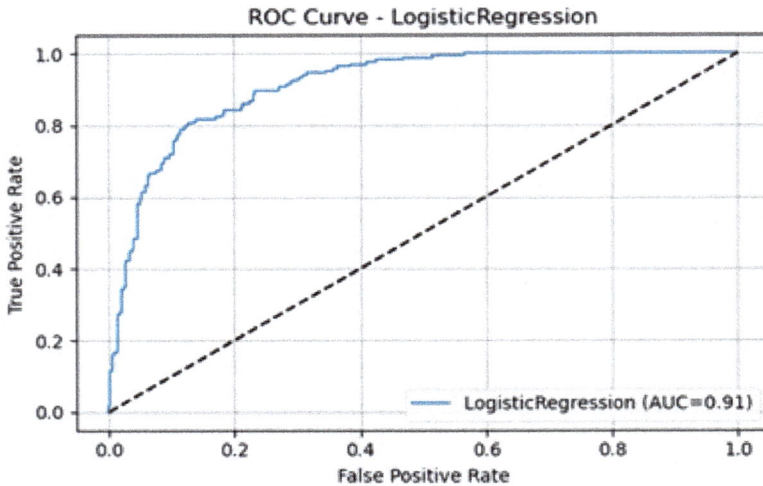

5.1.2 AUC- ROC Curve for Random Forest

Figure 3 shows the AUC-ROC curve of the Random Forest model. From this figure it can be observed that it gives good results and achieved an AUC of 0.95. The ROC curve shape is very similar to that of XGBoost which clearly indicates that Random Forest is highly effective at classification. However, its AUC value is not able to reach the AUC value of XGBoost model.

Figure 3. ROC curve of the Random Forest model indicating an AUC value of 0.95.

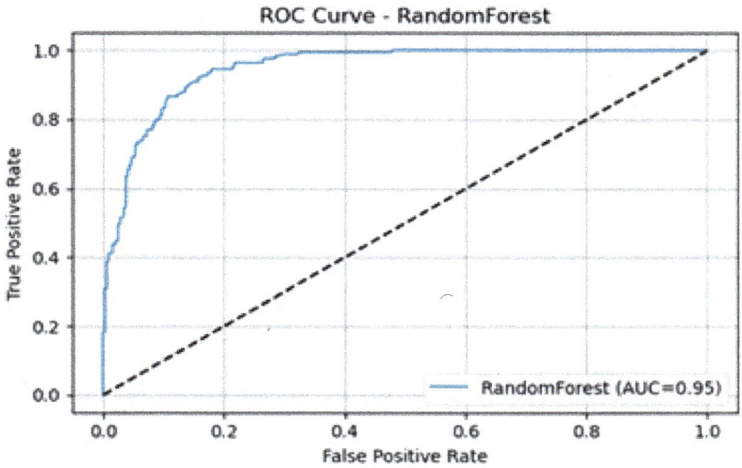

5.1.3 AUC- ROC Curve for XGBoost

The ROC curve for the XGBoost shows (Figure 4) a sharp rise towards the top-left corner of the plot which clearly show it's excellent performance. The AUC value of the XGBoost model is 0.96 which demonstrates that this model is highly capable of correctly distinguishing between individuals with or without metabolic syndrome. It has a strong balance between sensitivity and specificity, minimizing both false positives and false negatives.

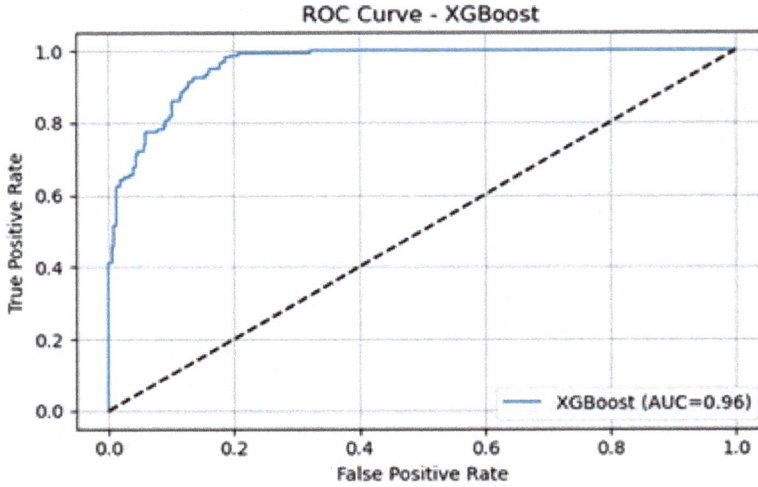

5.2 Experimental Results under Confusion Matrix

A Confusion Matrix is a performance evaluation metric that can test the accuracy of a classification model. The Confusion Matrix discusses about of number of correct or incorrect predictions by comparing the predicted labels against the actual (true) labels.

5.2.1 Confusion Matrix for Logistic Regression

Figure 5 shows confusion matrix of Logistic Regression. The model correctly identified 267 true negatives and 135 true positives. Whereas, the model is misclassifying 49 false positives and 30 false negatives. These results indicate strong overall predictive accuracy. It showed a decent performance but not satisfactory performance in correctly distinguishing between healthy individuals and those at risk.

Figure 5. Confusion matrix of the Logistic Regression model illustrating its classi-fication performance on the test dataset.

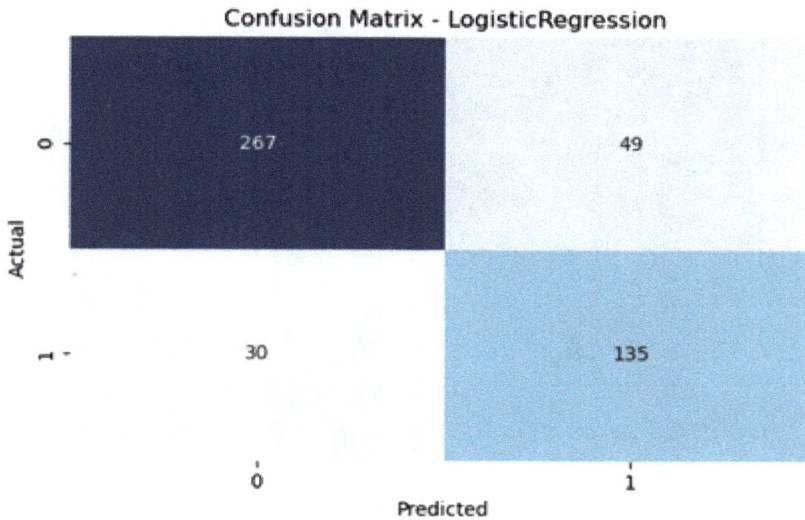

Confusion Matrix - LogisticRegression

5.2.2 Confusion Matrix for Random Forest

Confusion matrix for Random Forest is shown in Figure 6.

The model correctly predicted 276 true negatives and 144 true positives, while producing 40 false positives and 21 false negatives, demonstrating slightly improved accuracy and sensitivity compared to Logistic Regression. The Random Forest model achieved slightly higher number of true positives compared to XGBoost but it also produced more false positives. This clearly indicates that while Random Forest is slightly better in identifying at-risk individuals but at the same time it also increased the number of healthy people incorrectly flagged as positive cases.

Figure 6. Confusion matrix of the Random Forest model illustrating its classification performance on the test dataset.

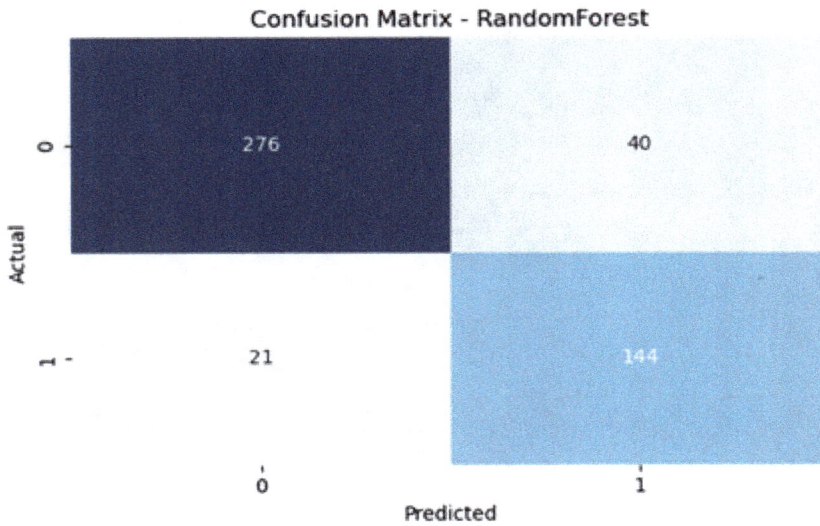

Confusion Matrix - RandomForest

5.2.3 Confusion Matrix for XGBoost

Confusion matrix of the XGBoost model is highlighted in Figure 7. It can be seen from the matrix that, the XGBoost model correctly identified 287 true negatives and 133 true positives. On the other hand, it is misclassifying 29 false positives and 32 false negatives. These results indicate that XGBoost achieved a balanced trade-off between sensitivity and specificity, with strong overall predictive performance.

Figure 7. Confusion matrix of the XGBoost model illustrating its classification performance on the test dataset.

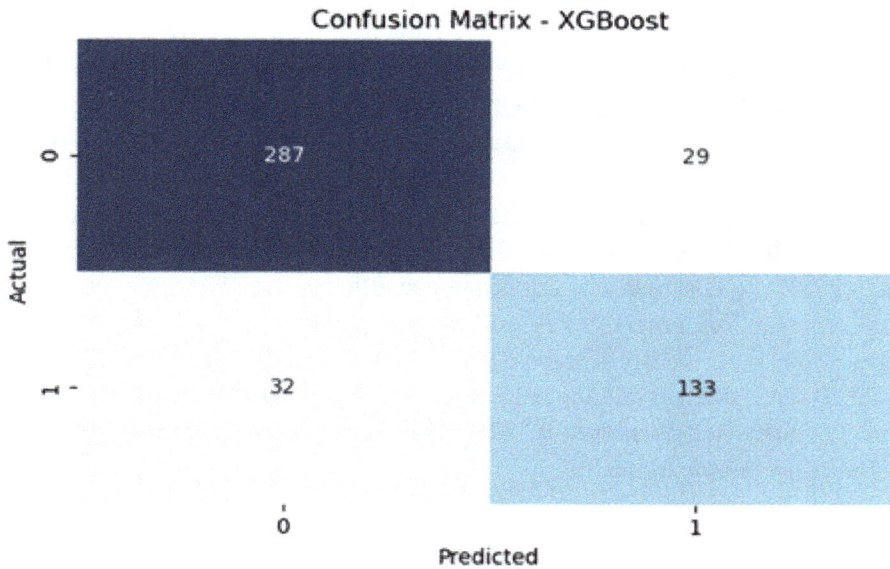

Confusion Matrix - XGBoost

5.3 Results Comparison Using Quantitative Metrics

Table 5 reports the experimental results that were obtained from the three models under a total of ten metrics. The results show that all three models performed well and Random Forest and XGBoost are equally good (87.32% accuracy). Logistic Regression is slightly behind at 83.58% accuracy. This means that if 100 patients are considered, the tree-based models will correctly classify around 87 patients while Logistic Regression will get around 84 correct results. It can be observe that, the XGBoost is the best in precision (82.10%). This means when XGBoost indicates that a patient has metabolic syndrome, it is correct 82 times out of 100. Random Forest was close behind at 78.26%, while Logistic Regression was lowest at 73.37%. So XGBoost gives fewer false alarms which are important. In terms of recall performance, Random Forest performed best with 87.27%. This means it correctly identifies 87 out of 100 actual metabolic syndrome cases. XGBoost identified only 80 out of 100 cases (80.61% recall). So for finding all sick patients, Random Forest is better. F1 score balances precision and recall. Random Forest scored highest in terms of precision and recall (82.52%), meaning it gives the best overall balance between finding real cases and avoiding false alarms.

XGBoost performs best in terms of AUC score (96.08%). This shows its best performance at separating healthy and sick patients. Performance of Random Forest is 94.80% in terms of AUC score. A value of AUC score above 90% is considered excellent in medical tests. Random Forest has the lowest log loss (0.2862), meaning its predictions are most confident and accurate. Lower log loss means more reliable probability scores. Matthews Correlation Coefficient (MCC) measures overall model quality. Random Forest scored highest MCC of 0.7288, showing it makes the most balanced predictions overall. Again, Random Forest led in terms of Balanced Accuracy (87.31%). This metric is important because data may have unequal classes. It confirms Random Forest works well for both healthy and sick patients. Under Average Precision, XGBoost is best and achieves Average Precision of 92.69%, meaning it is excellent at ranking patients correctly from high to low risk. XGBoost in terms of Specificity achieved 90.82%. This means it correctly identifies 91 out of 100 healthy people as healthy.

Table 5. Comparative analysis of classification performance metrics for Logistic Regression, Random Forest, and XGBoost models. The best-performing model for each metric is highlighted.

Metric	Logistic Regression	Random Forest	XGBoost	Best
Accuracy	0.8358	0.8732	**0.8732**	XGBoost, Random Forest
Precision	0.7337	0.7826	**0.8210**	XGBoost
Recall	0.8182	**0.8727**	0.8061	Random Forest
F1 score	0.7736	**0.8252**	0.8135	Random Forest
AUC	0.9119	0.9480	**0.9608**	XGBoost
Log Loss	0.4042	**0.2862**	0.2923	Random Forest
MCC	0.6477	**0.7288**	0.7175	Random Forest
Balanced Accuracy	0.8316	**0.8731**	0.8571	Random Forest
Average Precision	0.8199	0.8981	**0.9269**	XGBoost
Specificity	0.8449	0.8734	**0.9082**	XGBoost

From a practical implementation perspective, the results reported in sections 5.1, through 5.3 carry significant implications for healthcare deployment strategies. In hospital settings where diagnostic certainty is paramount and resources exist for follow-up testing, XGBoost's precision-focused performance would minimize unnecessary patient anxiety and optimize resource utilization. On the other hand, public health screening initiatives prioritizing comprehensive case identification would benefit more from Random Forest's recall-oriented capabilities, even if this requires accepting marginally more false positives for subsequent verification. The consistent performance gap between these ensemble methods and Logistic Regression across all metrics justifies their additional computational complexity. However, Logistic Regression retains value in resource-constrained environments or preliminary analyses due to its simplicity and interpretability.

5.4 Feature Importance Estimation using SHAP Method

SHAP (SHapley Additive exPlanations) (Lundberg & Lee, 2017) is a powerful method for interpreting machine learning models. SHAP provides interpretation by assigning each feature an importance value based on game theory principles. It calculates Shapley values that fairly distribute the contribution of each feature to the prediction of model by considering all possible feature combinations. Bar and beeswarm plots are the two popular ways of visualizing the feature importance. As results reported in the previous section indicates that XGBoost is best performer hence SHAP method is applied on this model. TreeExplainer is used for efficient SHAP value computation. The bar plot ranks features by their mean absolute impact, where as the beeswarm plot reveals how feature values influence predictions across the dataset.

Figure 8. SHAP-based feature importance plot for the XGBoost model, showing BloodGlucose as the most influential feature.

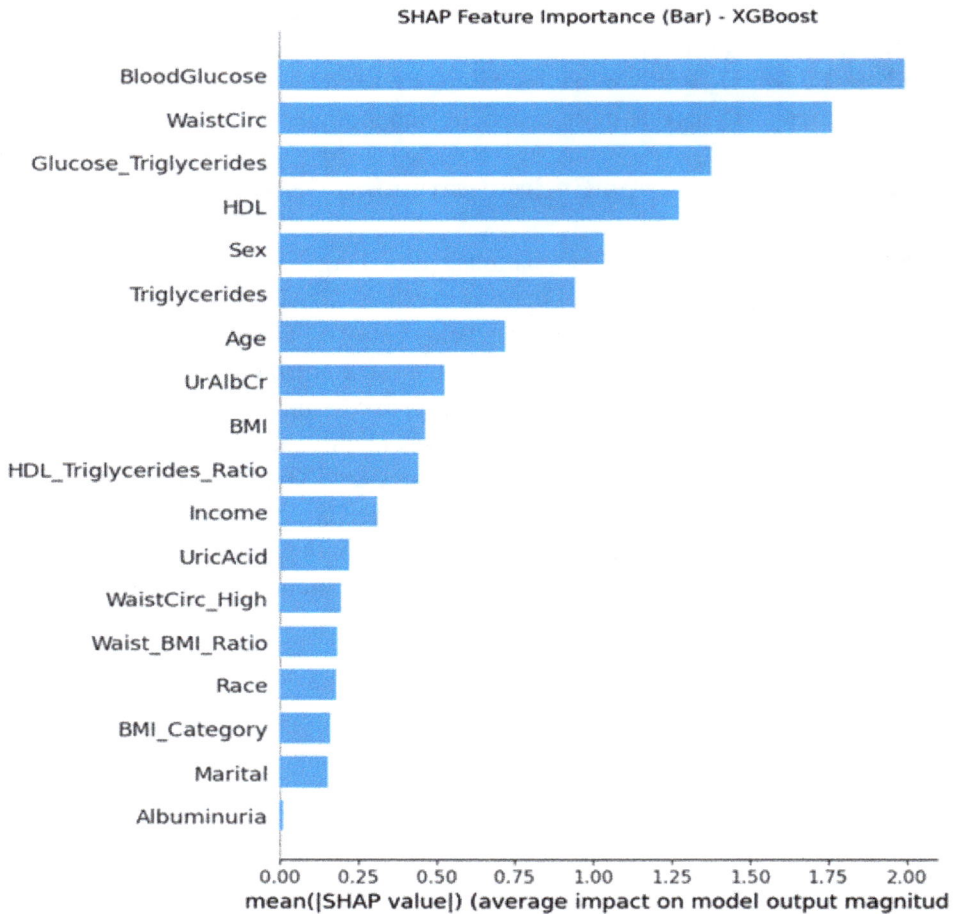

SHAP Feature Importance (Bar) - XGBoost

Figure 8 shows SHAP bar plot which highlights the feature importance of XG-Boost model. From the Figure it can be noticed that BloodGlucose emerges as the dominant predictor. Higher mean absolute SHAP value of BloodGlucose is indicating that variations in blood sugar levels have the strongest influence on the predictions. This fact is also validated from the research article that concludes that glucose metabolism is a prime factor in metabolic disorder diagnosis. Next, WaistCirc and Glucose_Triglycerides also show substantial impact. These two features indicate that XGBoost model focuses on central obesity and lipid-glucose interactions which are key factors in conditions like diabetes and cardiovascular disease.

It can also be noticed that features like HDL, Sex, Triglycerides, and Age are categorized as moderately important features. These are the well-established predictors in metabolic and cardiovascular health models. However, plot also suggests that UrAlbCr and BMI features contribute with relatively lower influence. On the other hand, demographic and biochemical factors such as Income, UricAcid, Race, BMI_Category, Marital Status, and Albuminuria show minimal impact. Note that Albuminuria is least important feature. Hence, removing this feature will not affect the performance of the model significantly. In short, this SHAP analysis provides transparent, model-agnostic insights into key drivers of predictions. These interpretations are valuable in healthcare applications where interpretability is crucial for clinical and stakeholder decision-making.

5.5 DISCUSSION

Building an intelligent system to predict metabolic syndrome was a challenge. Through this work, demonstration of how machine learning, especially advanced models like XGBoost can assist in early health risk detection using basic clinical and demographic features was done. The results showed strong performance in multiple evaluation metrics. One of the major strengths of the system was it was able to handle the user input in natural language format also. Unlike traditional systems that require highly structured data, the proposed model can process natural language descriptions entered by users. This was made possible through a lightweight text processing pipeline using regular expression and clinical mapping. It allows the system in becoming more user-friendly and accessible also to a wider range of users.

Another merit of the proposed system is its robust predictive power. XGBoost consistently outperformed both Logistic Regression and Random Forest in accuracy, precision, and AUC-ROC scores. The relatively low number of false negatives observed in the confusion matrix was particularly encouraging. In healthcare applications, missing a true case can have serious consequences and model's focus on minimizing such errors makes it highly valuable for real-world deployment.

There are some scopes of improvement, for example, the regex-based feature extraction has limited adaptability to variations in language, context, and phrasing. It may not work properly when model has to deal with semantically equivalent expressions that differ in wording or structure. Hence, advanced NLP methods such as spaCy-based named entity recognition, transformer architectures, or BERT-based clinical models could improve generalization and understanding of contextual nuances in free-text input.

Another limitation of the proposed work is that the single dataset is used for model evaluation. As discussed in section 4.1, the dataset used was derived from the National Health and Nutrition Examination Survey (NHANES), a U.S. population-based study. The dataset includes samples from various race and demographics. For example 40% of samples are from White race, 23% from Black, 14.7% from Asian, 9.9% Hispanic, 9.9% from Mexican-American, and remaining 2.5% belongs to other race. Still the dataset represents a single population source with specific regional, lifestyle, and healthcare characteristics. As a result, potential biases related to geography, socioeconomic conditions, and healthcare access may affect performance of models. This limits the generalizability of the proposed system to populations outside the U.S. or to data collected under different clinical requirements. In future, the proposed system can be validated using external datasets from different countries or healthcare systems to ensure broader applicability and robustness.

Additionally, symptom extraction pipeline relied heavily on specific keyword patterns. In reality, patients may describe their symptoms much differently than through the current language of the text processing logic.

Hyperparameter optimization can also be improved to further increase the robustness. Even though Randomized search based hyperparameter tuning was performed for XGBoost and the other models, techniques such as Grid search or Bayesian Optimization could be an even better method to find the best hyperparameters. In addition, widening the system to predict the risk of metabolic syndrome and risk levels for each component (hypertension, diabetes) will provide a more elaborate health profile for the users. In future, the incorporation of this system into mobile apps or hospital management systems would prove to be very effective. Providing custom health recommendations would become a decision support system for health care providers.

All things considered, the potential of machine learning and AI in preventive healthcare is massive as per this work. There is still plenty of room for improvement that can make the solutions powerful, scalable and effective in the practical medical environment, even though solution is a good first step.

Ethical considerations like data privacy and model explainability are critical for AI-based healthcare systems. The dataset NHANES is publicly available for research; however, it is required to follow proper data protection law during the deployment in the real-world scenarios. It can be noticed that, to enhance transparency, SHAP-based feature importance was used to explain model decisions. Ensuring privacy, interpretability, and accountability will be essential for building trust and promoting responsible use of AI in healthcare.

In real-world, clinical deployment of the proposed system presents several practical challenges. For instance, integrating the model with Electronic Health Record (EHR) systems requires interoperability with diverse data formats. It also may require a secure data exchange, and compliance with hospital IT policies. Further, physician adoption depends on the usability, transparency, and ability of the system to provide actionable insights without disrupting clinical workflows.

5.6 CONCLUSION

In this chapter, a natural language processing and machine learning based system is developed that can predict metabolic syndrome based on the symptoms available in text input. The aim is to make a tool that can help in early diagnosis and preventive healthcare in an easily accessible manner. A natural language processing driven framework is developed to transfer pre-existing free-text user symptoms into structured format that can handle anything from a one-word answer to a detailed clinical essay.

The current study explored various machine learning models such as Random Forest, Logistic Regression, and XGBoost. After careful performance analysis using evaluation metrics precision, recall, accuracy, F1 score and AUC-ROC, XGBoost turned out as the best. It achieved the highest accuracy (0.8732) and AUC score (0.9608) showing that it has excellent predictive power and striking a balance between sensitivity and specificity, which are both important in healthcare.

A key feature of this system is its ability to extract clinical features from the unstructured natural language that a normal user or patient will enter as an input. It can be used by providers and patients easily.

The results are quite encouraging, yet there is a lot of future work to be done. The performance and adaptability of the system can be further enhanced by augmenting the dataset with more representative patient profiles, integrating sophisticated NLP techniques for Name-Entity Recognition. The actual use of a system in the clinic can provide important insight to improve the system. Further, future improvements like the automatic inclusion of real-time data from wearable health devices such as continuous glucose monitors and smartwatches can be done. These integrations will improve diagnostic accuracies and also help to dynamically assess the risks on a continuous basis.

REFERENCES

Aggoun, Y. (2007). Obesity, metabolic syndrome, and cardiovascular disease. *Pediatric Research, 61*(6), 653–659. DOI: 10.1203/pdr.0b013e31805d8a8c PMID: 17426660

Alberti, K. G. M. M., Eckel, R. H., Grundy, S. M., Zimmet, P. Z., Cleeman, J. I., Donato, K. A., & Smith, S. C. (2009). Harmonizing the metabolic syndrome: A joint interim statement of the international diabetes federation task force on epidemiology and prevention; National heart, lung, and blood institute; American heart association; World heart federation; International. *Circulation, 120*(16), 1640–1645. DOI: 10.1161/CIRCULATIONAHA.109.192644 PMID: 19805654

Chen, T., & Guestrin, C. (2016). XGBoost: A scalable tree boosting system. *Proceedings of the ACM SIGKDD International Conference on Knowledge Discovery and Data Mining, 13-17-Augu*, 785–794. DOI: 10.1145/2939672.2939785

Chicco, D., & Jurman, G. (2020). Machine learning can predict survival of patients with heart failure from serum creatinine and ejection fraction alone. *BMC Medical Informatics and Decision Making, 20*(1), 1–16. DOI: 10.1186/s12911-020-1023-5 PMID: 32013925

Choe, E. K., Rhee, H., Lee, S., Shin, E., Oh, S.-W., Lee, J.-E., & Choi, S. H. (2018). Metabolic Syndrome Prediction Using Machine Learning Models with Genetic and Clinical Information from a Nonobese Healthy Population. *Genomics & Informatics, 16*(4), e31. DOI: 10.5808/gi.2018.16.4.e31 PMID: 30602092

Esteva, A., Kuprel, B., Novoa, R. A., Ko, J., Swetter, S. M., Blau, H. M., & Thrun, S. (2017). Dermatologist-level classification of skin cancer with deep neural networks. *Nature, 542*(7639), 115–118. DOI: 10.1038/nature21056 PMID: 28117445

Gutiérrez-Esparza, G. O., Vázquez, O. I., Vallejo, M., & Hernández-Torruco, J. (2020). Prediction of metabolic syndrome in a Mexican population applying machine learning algorithms. *Symmetry, 12*(4), 1–16. DOI: 10.3390/SYM12040581

Hosseini-Esfahani, F., Alafchi, B., Cheraghi, Z., Doosti-Irani, A., Mirmiran, P., Khalili, D., & Azizi, F. (2021). Using machine learning techniques to predict factors contributing to the incidence of metabolic syndrome in tehran: Cohort study. *JMIR Public Health and Surveillance, 7*(9), 1–12. DOI: 10.2196/27304 PMID: 34473070

Informatics Education. (2019). *Metabolic Syndrome Prediction* [Dataset]. data. world. Retrieved October 28, 2025, https://data.world/informatics-edu/metabolic-syndrome-prediction

Kim, J., Mun, S., Lee, S., Jeong, K., & Baek, Y. (2022). Prediction of metabolic and pre-metabolic syndromes using machine learning models with anthropometric, lifestyle, and biochemical factors from a middle-aged population in Korea. *BMC Public Health*, *22*(1), 1–11. DOI: 10.1186/s12889-022-13131-x PMID: 35387629

Kreimeyer, K., Foster, M., Pandey, A., Arya, N., Halford, G., Jones, S. F., & Botsis, T. (2017). Natural language processing systems for capturing and standardizing unstructured clinical information: A systematic review. *Journal of Biomedical Informatics*, *73*, 14–29. DOI: 10.1016/j.jbi.2017.07.012 PMID: 28729030

LaValley, M. P. (2008). Logistic regression. *Circulation*, *117*(18), 2395–2399. DOI: 10.1161/CIRCULATIONAHA.106.682658 PMID: 18458181

Lundberg, S. M., & Lee, S. I. (2017). A unified approach to interpreting model predictions. *Advances in Neural Information Processing Systems*, 4766–4775.

Meena, K. B., & Tyagi, V. (2020). A copy-move image forgery detection technique based on tetrolet transform. *Journal of Information Security and Applications*, *52*. Advance online publication. DOI: 10.1016/j.jisa.2020.102481

Meena, K. B., & Tyagi, V. (2021). A deep learning based method for image splicing detection. In *Journal of Physics: Conference Series* (Vol. 1714). IOP Publishing Ltd. DOI: 10.1088/1742-6596/1714/1/012038

National Cholesterol Education Program. (2001). Third Report of the NCEP Expert Panel on Detection, Evaluation, and Treatment of High Blood Cholesterol in Adults (Adult Treatment Panel III). *Circulation*, *106*(25), 3143–3421. PMID: 12485966

Nielsen, D. (2016). Tree Boosting With XGBoost Why Does XGBoost Win "Every" Machine Learning Competition? *Master of Science in Physics and Mathematics*, *3*(1), 24–34. DOI: 10.1111/j.1758-5899.2011.00096.x

Perveen, S., Shahbaz, M., Keshavjee, K., & Guergachi, A. (2019). Metabolic Syndrome and Development of Diabetes Mellitus: Predictive Modeling Based on Machine Learning Techniques. *IEEE Access : Practical Innovations, Open Solutions*, *7*, 1365–1375. DOI: 10.1109/ACCESS.2018.2884249

Rajkomar, A., Oren, E., Chen, K., Dai, A. M., Hajaj, N., Hardt, M., & Dean, J. (2018). Scalable and accurate deep learning with electronic health records. *Digital Medicine*, *1*(1), 1–10. DOI: 10.1038/s41746-018-0029-1 PMID: 31304302

Schlenger, J. (2024). Random Forest. *Computer Science in Sport*, 201–207. DOI: 10.1007/978-3-662-68313-2_24

Shehab, M., Abualigah, L., Shambour, Q., Abu-Hashem, M. A., Shambour, M. K. Y., Alsalibi, A. I., & Gandomi, A. H. (2022). Machine learning in medical applications: A review of state-of-the-art methods. *Computers in Biology and Medicine, 145*. Advance online publication. DOI: 10.1016/j.compbiomed.2022.105458 PMID: 35364311

Shin, H., Shim, S., & Oh, S. (2023). Machine learning-based predictive model for prevention of metabolic syndrome. *PLoS ONE, 18*(6 June), 1–28. DOI: 10.1371/journal.pone.0286635

Tomar, J. S., Mishra, P., Gupta, A., Meena, K. B., & Tyagi, V. (2022). A Proposed Model for Precision Agriculture. *Communications in Computer and Information Science, 1614 CCIS*, 430–441. DOI: 10.1007/978-3-031-12641-3_35

Trigka, M., & Dritsas, E. (2023). Predicting the occurrence of metabolic syndrome using machine learning models. *Computation (Basel, Switzerland), 11*(9), 170.

Worachartcheewan, A., Shoombuatong, W., Pidetcha, P., Nopnithipat, W., Prachayasittikul, V., & Nantasenamat, C. (2015). Predicting metabolic syndrome using the random forest method. *The Scientific World Journal, 2015*. Advance online publication. DOI: 10.1155/2015/581501 PMID: 26290899

World Health Organization. (1999). *Definition, Diagnosis and Classification of Diabetes Mellitus and its Complications*. WHO.

Yang, H., & Yu, B., OUYang, P., Li, X., Lai, X., Zhang, G., & Zhang, H. (2022). Machine learning-aided risk prediction for metabolic syndrome based on 3 years study. *Scientific Reports, 12*(1), 1–11. DOI: 10.1038/s41598-022-06235-2 PMID: 34992227

Yu, C. S., Lin, Y. J., Lin, C. H., Te Wang, S., Lin, S. Y., Lin, S. H., & Chang, S. S. (2020). Predicting metabolic syndrome with machine learning models using a decision tree algorithm: Retrospective cohort study. *JMIR Medical Informatics, 8*(3), 1–18. DOI: 10.2196/17110 PMID: 32202504

Zhou, B., Yang, G., Shi, Z., & Ma, S. (2024). Natural Language Processing for Smart Healthcare. *IEEE Reviews in Biomedical Engineering, 17*, 4–18. DOI: 10.1109/RBME.2022.3210270 PMID: 36170385

Chapter 11
Transforming Preventive Medicine Through Artificial Intelligence

Richa Singh

https://orcid.org/0009-0007-0196-4919

Lovely Professional University, India

Lovleen Marwaha

Lovely Professional University, India

ABSTRACT

However, AI has greatly changed the way that healthcare proceeds, making it possible to detect disease early and predict the risk of happening. Blood tests, MRI's, CT scans, X-rays and any other clinical, genetic and imaging data is used along with machine learning and deep learning models to detect diseases before the symptoms show up. For diseases such as cancer, cardiovascular and neurological etc., CNNs and NLP techniques help analyze scans, pathology slides, electronic health records. Risk models based on the patient's history, lifestyle or genetics are evaluated using AI technology. Despite this, they face ethical and validation issues, risks regarding data privacy, and validation needs. To bring guaranteed and proper AI solutions, effective collaboration between medical professionals, AI researchers and policymakers is pivotal. This chapter focuses on the discussion of AI's applications, advantages and restrictions, future potential, for the benefit of clinicians and researchers to optimize patient outcomes and advance precision medicine.

DOI: 10.4018/979-8-3373-3196-6.ch011

INTRODUCTION

AI is playing a great role in analyzing and diagnosing diseases in today's society by providing new ways of risk assessment (Aamir *et al.,*2024)). Thanks to technological developments and finding techniques such as machine learning, deep learning and data analytics, there are possibilities of identifying various diseases at its preliminary stages leading to good results for the patients and lessor burden to healthcare systems. AI deepens a diagnosis by processing large and diverse data sets, reducing the errors, and offering an individualized approach to a patient (Harry., 2023). The article also underscores the importance of the early detection of the disease for an early treatment to be administered. As mentioned earlier, the conventional diagnostic techniques and approaches are load bearing on the human knowledge and evaluation. Smart technologies like CNN in diagnosis through imaging and NLP in analysis of electronic health records have eliminated time barriers and precision of disease diagnoses. These technologies are notably useful in the screening of diseases such as cancer, cardiovascular diseases, and neurological diseases in which early identification of the diseases can go a long way in increasing the likelihood that the disease can be treated (Gupta & Pandey., 2024).

Likewise, preventive risk assessment models are AI based, of which the goal is to predict the probability of one getting a specific disease taking grounds like the medical history of the individual, genetics, and lifestyle, and the environment in which the individual resides (Rane, Choudhary, &Rane.,2023a). These models assist the healthcare wise professionals in the diagnosis of high risk patients in anticipation of developing the actual disease symptoms using massive datasets and predictive analytics. It helps to save money on health care and extend the quality of patients' life by changing the concept of a medical management paradigm from an episodic model to the one of prevention (Aminizadeh *et al.,* 2024). Nonetheless, this advancement comes with significant concerns when in use in clinical practice. Issues such as privacy of data, issue of fairness in the algorithms, and the need to regulate AI are still other challenges that make implementation difficult. Moreover, in many cases the AI models are still in development thus they must be validated and updated periodically for better reliability and relevance to the healthcare field. Meeting these challenges requires the input of AI scientists dealing with the issues, doctors, and the policy makers, with the core aim of developing AI solutions that are ethical, understandable and, responsive to the patient needs (Mennella *et al.,* 2024).

In this chapter, information about the concept of AI in early diagnosis and prediction of risks is presented, including the effectively of the idea, its strengths and weaknesses, as well as its possible further development. When the role of AI in healthcare is understood, researchers as well as clinicians will be in a position to determine the ways and means about how they can best develop healthcare in the areas of precision medicine diagnostics and preventative measures (Amann *et al.,* 2020).

2. BASIC IDEAS OF AI IN MEDICAL SCIENCE

Artificial intelligence is used in health care in a way that adopts machine learning, deep learning and predictive analysis of complicated data sets. The disease identification and patient surveillance can be done through working with different algorithms such as decision trees, support vector machines (SVM), and random forests. Modern deep learning models such as the CNN are thus proven to enhance the performance of medical imaging analysis in that they are able to diagnose anomalies proficiently (Tsuneki., 2022). Some of these algorithms include artificial neural networks (ANNs), recurrent neural networks (RNNs), and generative adversarial networks (GANs) to predict the state of a patient's health and determine an ideal treatment process for a patient. Through the use of big data and predictive analytics, it is capable of analyzing large amounts of medical data and making analysis on risks and providing the clinicians with real-time data with efficiency in healthcare (Alowais *et al.,* 2023).

2.1 Introduction to Learning models in Healthcare

ML, DL are a part of AI wherein the computer gets the ability to decide for itself from data patterns scraped out from raw data. 8 Real ML algorithms get better with exposure and employs the methods based on statistical measures like decision trees-SMVs, random forests, and k-NN (Arinez et al., 2020). These techniques assist in the medical diagnostics as they make possible ability of particular program to execute the pattern recognition in the clinical data. Deep learning, an even more sophisticated form of ML, employs the artificial neural models to analyze big data in the medical field. CNN has redeemed medical imaging by accurately detecting anomalies in radiological scans including X-ray, MRI and CT since the discoveries of the CNN. On the other hand, recurrent neural networks (RNNs) are very useful in the analysis of sequential medical data; this kind of data is particularly important in patient management concerning time-series information related to the advancement of diseases (Luo., 2017).

When implementing ML and DL in healthcare diagnostics, medical image analysis is automated, technologies of NLP are used to process the EHRs, and AI predicted models to forecast disease outcomes. Of the four discussed AI technologies discussed above, all of them increase the diagnostic speed, accuracy and efficiency thus improving the patient's outcome (Agrawal & Jain., 2020).

Table 1. Comparison of Machine Learning and Deep Learning

Feature	Machine Learning (ML)	Deep Learning (DL)
Definition	Performance improvement occurs through statistical processing of available data.	Optimizes the processing efficiency of big data in healthcare.
Data Requirement	Operates efficiently with reduced amounts of input data.	Uses vast amounts of structured and unstructured data for training.
Processing Type	Needs manual selection and transformation of data attributes for better learning.	Learns data features directly from unprocessed information.
Application in Healthcare	Patient history analysis to classify possible illness.	Improves cancer diagnosis by examining pathology slides.

2.2 Major AI Algorithms Applied in Medical Diagnosis

Using a number of algorithms, artificial intelligence systems that are used for diagnostics work more accurately and have better predictability. Some of the commonly applied AI models are as follows:

- **Artificial Neural Networks (ANNs):** Imitating the human brain, there is an ability of ANNs in the identification of patterns in vast medical data (Goel, Goel, & Kumar., 2023).
- **Recurrent Neural Networks (RNNs):** In the process of time series analysis disease dynamics are tracked and patient's health prognosis is predicted with RNNs (Morid, Sheng, & Dunbar., 2023).
- **Generative Adversarial Networks (GANs):** Such synthesized medical images assist in AI training in both the training phase as well as in arriving at accurate diagnosis (Nie *et al.,* 2018).
- **Convolutional Neural Networks (CNNs):** The purpose-built image-processing system CNN finds critical application in disease detection during early stages for radiology, pathology, and dermatology (Yu *et al.,* 2021).
- **Decision Trees and Random Forests:** Interpretability enables the clinical decision-making process since it means that the available patient data is formulated for constructing diagnostics routes (Rane, Choudhary, & Rane., 2023b).
- **Gradient Boosting Machines (GBMs):** XGBoost and LightGBM are algorithms that enhance the predictive modeling in aspects of risk evaluation and prognosis on the treatment outcome (Shehadeh *et al.,* 2021).

When these AI models are incorporated in practicing health care delivery, diagnostic precision is achieved as a result of minimising human predispositions and mistakes.

2.3 Making Medical Prediction Using Vast Patient Information

The technology depends heavily on extensive amounts of medical information known as big data that comes from different original sources (Dash *et al.,* 2019).

- **Electronic Health Records (EHRs):** AI extracts valuable insights from patient histories, clinical notes, and lab results (Adomson *et al.,* 2023).
- **Genomic Data:** It looks for disease indicators and inherited disease susceptible regions, etc.
    Medical Imaging Databases: X-ray, MRI, and CT scans are diagnosed through the help of artificial intelligence for the early identification of diseases (Ghaffar Nia, Kaplanoglu, & Nasab., 2023).
- **Wearable Health Devices:** Health monitoring through smartwatches and biosensors to check is another activity that can be mal-practiced because it allows the divergence detection of abnormal vital signs in the real time (Sharma *et al.,* 2021).
- **Clinical Trial Data:** AI helps in discovering drugs and weighs the needs and tendencies toward a treatment (Ashiwaju, Orikpete, & Uzougbo., 2023).

It converts these datasets into usable information, by assisting the healthcare professionals in:

- **Identify Disease Risk Factors:** This places AI into the context of assessing the probability of an individual being affected by a disease due to inherited genes, style of living and the physical surrounding (Singh *et al.,* 2024).
- **Enhance Early Disease Detection:** The patient data patterns reportable by machine learning algorithms allow healthcare professionals to intervene early to alter the course of the disease (Javaid *et al.,* 2022).
- **Optimize Treatment Plans:** AI makes a flexible treatment plan in accordance with the patient's characteristics, optimizes the outcome, and reduces the side effects (Yogeshappa., 2024).
- **Improve Healthcare Resource Management:** AI identifies patient admission patterns, schedules the proper use of resources in a hospital and manages supplies consistently (Munavalli *et al.,* 2021).

- **Support Epidemiological Surveillance:** Big data identities track diseases to help in planning and managing the outbreak to contain the spread within the population (Wu *et al.,* 2020).

The continued use of big data in health care makes the use of AI as a tool the beginning of more accurate and personalized medicine, where interventions are given depending on the data gathered to enable improvement of patient care and organization of health care service delivery.

3. AI'S ROLE IN PREVENTIVE DISEASE DIAGNOSIS

AI plays a substantial role in the early disease detection since it boosts performance of diagnostics and offers predictive analysis. This is been done using big data applied on medical records to discover that there are symptoms that are displayed before the onset of certain diseases. Machine learning is used in imaging technologies to diagnose and predict cancer, heart diseases, and neurological disorders through radiology images, histological slides, and bio-markers respectively (Amir *et al.,* 2022). Besides, AI-based timeless evaluate one's genetic profile, life style factors, and environment correlate to have anclinical indicators to take early actions. Integrating artificial intelligence into early disease diagnosis then goes a long way in improving the situation as far as improving the patient's management and health status is concerned, as well as in sparing the health care systems from unnecessary costs that comes with an avalanche of late presentations (Rane, Choudhary, & Rane., 2023a).

3.1 AI-Powered Radiological and Pathological Diagnosis

Advancements in artificial intelligence have brought about immense innovation in radiology and pathology since it has helped in improving on image interpretation and lowering the chances of human error and incrementing the overall accuracy. Deep learning, of which convolution neural networks (CNNs) are a part, has received high appreciation for its efficiency when it comes to cancerous lesion detection in Mammograms, CT scans, and MRI. These models work on pixel level, and examine the instances that might not be discernable even by a physician. Image recognition using artificial intelligence helps to point out such regions for the attention of radiologists, reduce false negatives and provide an option for early diagnosis, thus improving disease detection rates among patients (Bi *et al.,* 2019).

In pathology, AI has the significant function of histopathological slide analysis in automating them. This implies that by the usage of high-end image processing,

AI models determine the geometry of cells, diagnose ailments, and even differentiate a malignancy type and severity to match human pathologists. This leads to minimization of one examiner's subjectivity, thus making the diagnostics as consistent as possible and allowing other, more complex and truly important, cases be handled. It also helps in the tissue sample segmentation and gives details of the tumor grading and its progression, which is crucial for management. In addition, it has been established that the AI-pathology applications are compatible with both, LIS and non LIS systems, thus increasing the scalability and improving TAT (Cui and Zhang., 2021).

Figure 1.

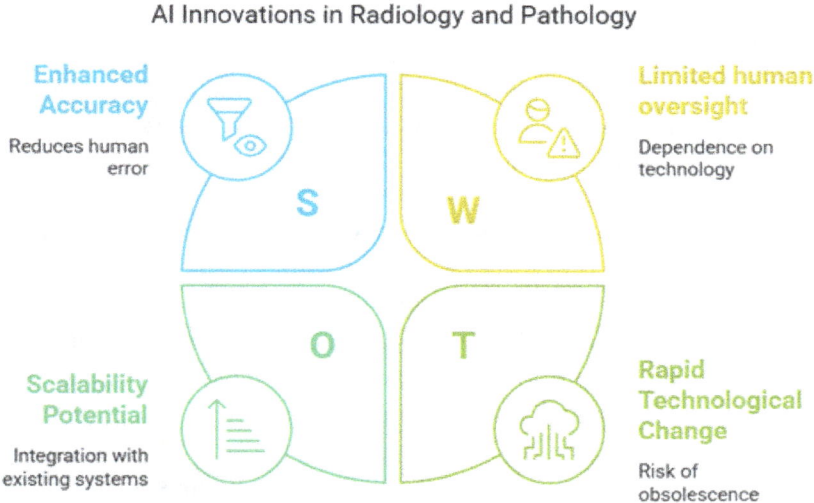

AI Innovations in Radiology and Pathology

Enhanced Accuracy
Reduces human error

Limited human oversight
Dependence on technology

Scalability Potential
Integration with existing systems

Rapid Technological Change
Risk of obsolescence

3.2 Natural Language Processing (NLP) Application in Healthcare Information System

NLP has become one of the most effective technologies in the healthcare field in the meaning that it helps the AI systems to mine the electronic health records, physician notes, and clinical reports. The problem of managing a large volume of unstructured data is especially pertinent in EHRs; nonetheless, AI NLP models ensure the organization of that data to facilitate analysis by quantified human fields. In general, NLP increases the effectiveness of disease detection and prediction based on the recognition of significant patterns in text information. Such applications of AI enable NLP technologically by identifying physicians accurately, extracting medical terms from the raw text of physician's notes and structuring the informal text into useful information for healthcare professionals. This allows for Ace EHR to provide automated suggestions to clinicians in regard to which patients should be categorized as high risk and properly monitored. Besides, NLP helps in documentation improvement through reducing the problem of clinical language inaccuracy and enriching medical records with the most consistent documentation (Zhou *et al.,* 2022).

In addition to diagnosing, NLP helps in the medical field to gather patient data from various studies conducted, thus assisting the researchers to identify various disease tendencies in different areas, results of treatments and any relation that may be present in between them. NLP also helps analyse the records and reports of contagious diseases or posts on social media or any epidemiological data to monitor and control the spread of diseases in real-time. In addition, NLP projects for clinical virtual assistants improve administrative workflow interference and decrease clinician's fatigue (Garadi *et al.,* 2022).

3.3 Improving Patient Care for Life-Threatening Diseases

It has revealed several possibilities in improving diagnostics, treatment, and management of cancers, cardiovascular diseases, and neurological diseases. In oncology, the imaging helps in using specialized radiology to analyze the images and identify the cancerous lesions at an earlier stage than it is done by a human. Artificial intelligence pathology slide helps oncologists to diagnose malignancies and determine the aggressiveness of the cancer and the likelihood of tumor progression. Machine learning deepens the use of genomic data to make screening and risk assessment of cancer enhanced by detection of hereditary cancer types such as BRCA1 and BRCA2. In cardiovascular medicine, there are machine learning algorithms that apply machine learning tools to diagnose data from ECG, lipid profile, and blood pressure (Shameer *et al.,* 2018). These models can identify signs of heart diseases early hence reduce cases of heart attacks or stroke since early solution can be sought. With the implementation of AI-tools, wearable gadgets in constant contact with the patient's body track HRV, arrhythmias and other cardiovascular biomarkers and immediately detect deviations from normal levels. Effectively, the use of AI in cardiology means that the cardiologists can assess a lot of data and make proper decisions which will help to improve the condition of the patients with the minimum incidence of heart diseases (Das., 2024).

The following are some of the neurologic disorders that involve the use of Artificial Intelligence in diagnosing and treatment; Alzheimer's disease, Parkinson's disease. Some of the artificial intelligence techniques predict even structural and functional changes in the brain through MRI and PET scans to diagnose declining cognition at its early stage. Sensors for speech and motion measure and record slight changes in motor dysfunctions and language impairments that are non-invasive ways of tracking disease progression. Further, analysis of brain waves through the use of AI is effective in the detection of epilepsy, especially by detecting the likely abnormal nerve activity that may lead to seizures so that necessary measures can be taken. The application of AI across these medical specialties is making progress in enhancing precision medicine in patient care, enhancing early management solutions, as well as management of patients characteristics. Due to improving the diagnostic capabilities of disease diagnosis and using AI for both diagnostic and preventative purposes, AI is helping to decrease the prevalence of diseases and advance patient longevity (Ali., 2022).

Table 2. AI's Impact on Early Diagnosis in Different Healthcare Specialties

Specialty	AI Application	Benefit
Oncology	Machine-learning based radiology and disease detection in slides.	Intelligent diagnostic devices for finding cancer in the early stage.
Cardiology	Smart cardiac monitoring devices for monitoring irregular heartbeats.	AI-assisted forecasting of cardiovascular disease and abnormal heartbeats.
Neurology	Deep learning patterns for brain scan and movement disease.	Early detection of Alzheimer's, Parkinson's.

4. RISK PREDICTION USING AI

AI improves risk estimation by analyzing large medical data to find out people who are prone to get diseases. Algorithms constructed for this purpose take into account the patient's age, previous illnesses, family history, and lifestyle to determine the possibilities of developing particular diseases with great accuracy. These tools assist healthcare workers in adopting early management strategies that contain the advancement of diseases and enhance cure performances. Further, it uses environmental and behavioral data for promoting improved disease models that are customized and detailed. Using the information derived from assessments of risk by artificial intelligence, the medical practitioners are in a position to prevent disease occurrence as well as prioritise when resources are scarce in the health facilities (Davis *et al.,* 2008).

4.1 AI in Patient-Specific Risk Evaluation

Machine learning and artificial intelligence algorithms predict various diseases relying on data big data to determine persons at greater risk of presenting with chronic and acute conditions. Such models use information from patients' characteristics, past history, behavior patterns, genetic profiles, or even current health status to accurately estimate the risk of diseases. The increased efficiency of patient data analysis with the help of machine learning techniques like logistic regressions, random forest, deep neural networks helps in early identification of individuals' who are liable to diseases like diabetes, cardiovascular disorders or neurodegenerative disorders. These survival prediction models identify the risk factors before the development of symptoms; therefore, they assist the healthcare providers in preventive measures that include lifestyle changes, screening programs, and early intercessions. This increases the health care benefits, cuts the costs, and relieves the medical structures from providing a cure after the emergence of a complication (Chattu., 2021).

Beyond individual risk assessment therefore, predictive analytics helps population health management to determine the occurrence of diseases in areas of a given population. Understanding the causal relationship between risk factors and diseases, therefore, can help epidemiologists and those involved in healthcare policies to formulate programs to be undertaken in the public domain, as well as distribute medical facilities and rise awareness to prevent the development of such diseases. These models shall continue to get enhanced where AI advances, with models being fed more details from other sources of data especially in enhancing risk prediction (Khalafi *et al.,* 2025).

4.2 Merging Biological, Personal, and Environmental Health Information

Both genetic, lifestyle as well as environmental factors plays a role in improving the disease prediction using AI. AI overcomes this exhibited weakness of conventional diagnosis techniques where diagnosis is usually reached after evaluating clinico-radiological findings and symptoms alone comparing to genetic sequencing data about patient's lifestyle and environmental factors. Genetic makeup serves as a main determinant that reveals how well someone might develop particular diseases. AI genomic analysis automatically detects hereditary genetic mutations which include BRCA mutations for breast cancer as well as APOE variants associated with Alzheimer's disease. AI, through genetic tests, differentiates patients' risks and suggests early screening of individual with such a potential (Choudhury and MacNee., 2017).

These lifestyle factors include diets, exercise, sleep, and substances that a person takes and can cause change in disease incidence. Wearable health sensors constantly measure these aspects and offer feedback as to what effects specific decisions about living can have on this individual's health profile. By that, AI models examine this information to provide health suggestions with an aim of altering the behavior of their clients in the process of avoiding falling ill. External and internal conditions of the body also exert significant impact on disease susceptibility. AI can predict the degree of health-relevant changes due to pollution exposure, hazardous working conditions, climate changes, and other socioeconomic factors. For instance, AI-driven air quality monitoring systems may figure out that increased pollution leads to asthmatic and chronic obstructive pulmonary disease (COPD) perpetrators. Because the environment affects one's likelihood of contracting a given disease, the algorithms make health improvement plans specific to an area that a person lives (Zhang *et al.,* 2020).

Figure 2.

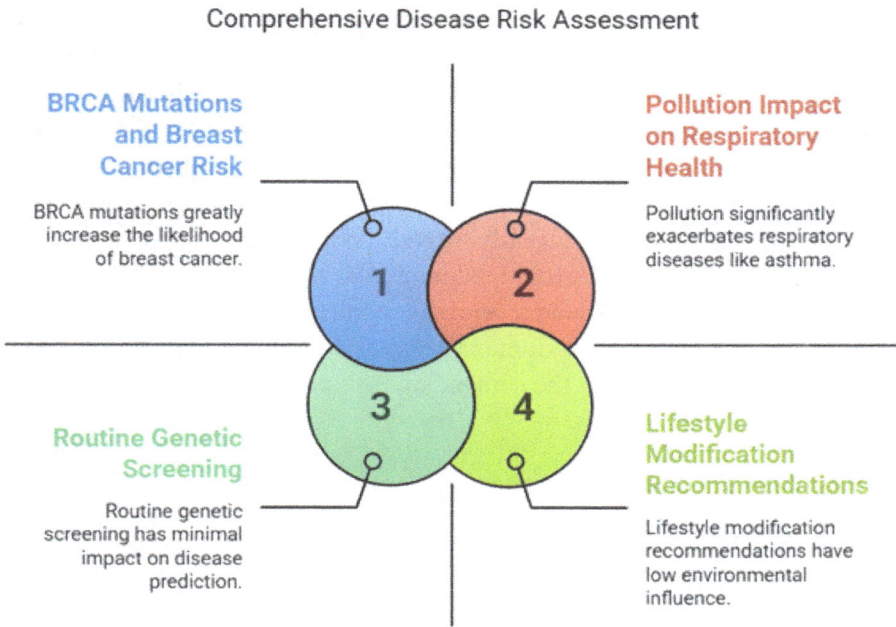

Comprehensive Disease Risk Assessment

BRCA Mutations and Breast Cancer Risk

BRCA mutations greatly increase the likelihood of breast cancer.

Pollution Impact on Respiratory Health

Pollution significantly exacerbates respiratory diseases like asthma.

1

2

3

4

Routine Genetic Screening

Routine genetic screening has minimal impact on disease prediction.

Lifestyle Modification Recommendations

Lifestyle modification recommendations have low environmental influence.

AI merges geneticisease and lifestyle and environmental information to form an extensive view of risk that helps healthcare providers develop advanced preventive healthcare solutions. The holistic method goes past basic risk measuring through individualized suggestion making which leads to enhanced patient health and extended longevity (Rane *et al.,* 2023).

4.3 Preventing Diseases by Analyzing Personal Health Factors

AI is a major aspect of personalized and preventive Healthcare since patient's treatment and prevention can be decided and administered based on their individual cases. Risk prediction makes it easier to choose the best treatment methods that will possess positive healing impacts while avoiding the negative ones. Artificial intelligence in drug discovery identifies medicines that will work best for your body type by checking the compatibility of the chemicals in the medication with the genetic attribute of the body and speeds up the process of inventing new drugs (Alowais et al., 2023).

In the realm of preventive medicine, AI constantly screens the patient data found in EHR and wearable devices to identify disease indicators that require preventive action taken by the doctors. Machine learning addresses trends in the patient records in an efficient manner to predict chronic diseases like Diabetic, Hypertension and Cardiovascular disorders before they occur. Virtual assistants in healthcare involve the use of artificial intelligence to diagnose patients' conditions and recommend a course of action to improve their health, consequently adopting a healthier lifestyle. Smart watches and biosensors, other appliances also allow AI to play a primary role of early diagnosis and prevention involving monitoring aspects like heart rate variability, blood oxygen levels, and the cycle of sleep. They help the centers to identify possible complications in early stages, and notify the healthcare workers to take the appropriate action or avoid readmission to the hospital. By incorporating the use of AI in personalized and preventive care more options and better solutions are put forward for medical practitioners besides improving the quality of life and enhancing efficiency reducing the demand on the system (Ye *et al.,* 2018).

5. AI'S BENEFITS FOR MEDICAL RISK ANALYSIS AND DIAGNOSIS ACCURACY

AI improves diagnostic outcomes, speeds up diagnosis, and refines the processes of making decisions in the treatment of patients, thus bringing change in healthcare. It works x million pieces of data by identifying various diseases' relation and thus minimizes the possibility of later diagnosis. AI allows for the reduction of some human innate traits such as errors and biases because it gets rid of subjectivism in diagnosing patients consistently across the different populations. With the help of real-time and data analysis it assists clinicians in decision-making, enhances the strategies of treatment, and patients' overall efficiency. This paper has discussed how AI can help with the implementation of the concept of personalized medicine with the help of predictive analytics in identifying risk factors to take proper measures to prevent them. In addition, the continuous adoption of innovative techniques, especially the Artificial Intelligence improve, the performance of the hospital in cutting unnecessary expenses, thereby improving on the work flow systems. The development of AI in the medical field will move to more accurate diagnosis, prognosis, and future individualized care of patients which will make the healthcare process more predictive and preventable (Johnson *et al.*, 2021).

5.1 Supporting Doctors with Accurate Medical Insights

It has increased the speed, reduced the human intervention and improved the accuracy of diagnosis techniques and patient analysis. The process of diagnosis in the current clinical environment has been carried out manually, and takes a lot of time, and may vary from one pathologist to another. Deep learning models especially CNNs have shown great effectiveness in identifying anomalies from the radiological images such as X-rays, MRI, and CT scan. Through these models, it is possible to detect some biomarkers that may not be easily detected by the human radiologists, given that this will boost early detection rates hence improving the patient's outcome. Similarly, artificial intelligence can also be used in the genetic analysis to determine the gene connection to hereditary illnesses and for estimating the propensity of health dangers inherent to the particular person. In the pathology aspect, the computing technology helps in digital image analysis for sample tissue, identifying malignancies accurately and urging the pathologists to arrive at a conclusion. Also, AI-driven automation helps to optimize lab operations; the analysis of test results is better and shorter compared to conventional diagnosis (Khalid *et al.*, 2020).

The application of AI within hospitals extends past diagnostic tools to achieve peak hospital resource efficiency through patient admission forecasting and medical supply control and staff scheduling methods. Healthcare facilities advance their operational performance while minimizing operational expenses and upgrading service quality by implementing AI management systems. AI scheduling tools help reduce waiting periods for patients because they allow healthcare providers to distribute their available time effectively for prompt medical services (Maleki Varnosfaderani and Forouzanfar., 2024).

5.2 Reduction in Human Errors and Bias

The major benefit of AI in healthcare practice exists in its capability to detect medical errors while decreasing decision-making biases. Traditional diagnostic systems base their evaluations on human judgments which result in inconsistent doctor-to-doctor analysis and possible wrong diagnoses. Standards in diagnostic criteria alongside patient data examination using accurate objective methods become possible through AI which helps reduce these diagnostic risks. Machine learning models integrate voluminous and divergent data during training to maintain objectivity of diagnosis and not be inclined towards the sentiment of the physician handling a given clinical data sample. With the help of artificial intelligence, tools may compare a patient's complaint, medical history, as well as imaging data with millions of documents containing valuable medical data and potential cases of missed or incorrect diagnosis. Each time AI systems are exposed to new data, they are able to learn from this data and increase the reliability in diagnosing since the accuracy of the prediction increases (Brown et al., 2023).

Another limitation that is closely connected to gender bias is that of the data itself and its capacity to contain samples of AI models that reflect the population of patients. If the AI models are trained particularly on one ethnic group, geographic region or socio-economic status, it may be inaccurate if readily applied to different ethnic, geographic or socio-economic groups of patients. To this end, methods such as adversarial debasing, re-weighting of samples, representation of sample, and other related methods are used to eliminate bias by the developers of AI. The firing of healthcare bias that stems from the use of Artificial Intelligence in patient care should be avoided in order to ensure quality outcomes are achieved in the healthcare department, and that patients do not get discriminated against based on the color of their skin or gender (Norori *et al.,* 2021).

Figure 3.

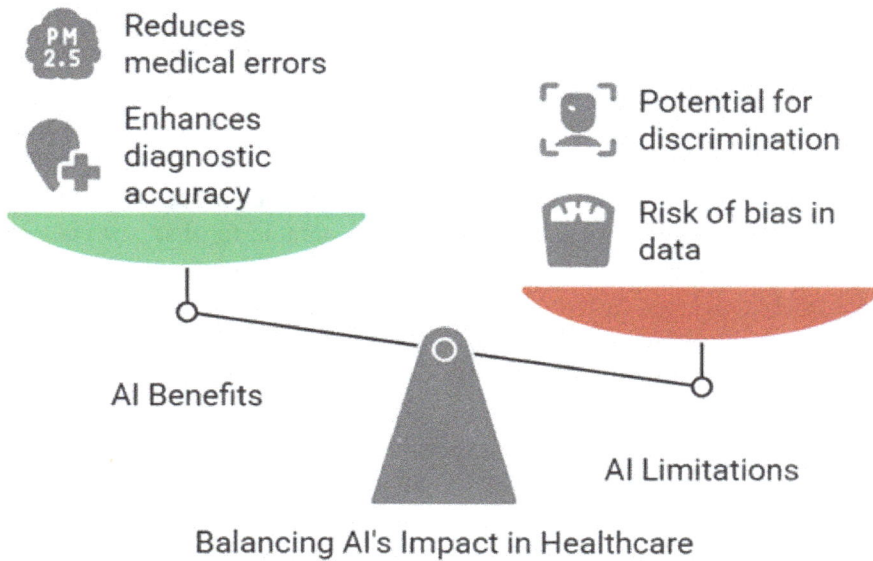

Balancing AI's Impact in Healthcare

5.3 Increased Decision Support for Clinicians

AI is beneficial to clinicians in that it will offer real time analysis and recommendations on patients' conditions hence facilitating accurate diagnosis and appropriate therapy plans. The Big Data thus construed, as highlighted prior, is used in MS decision-support systems concerning patient's characteristics such as medical history, lab test findings, genetic profile, imaging scans, etc to arrive at unique patient recommendations. By using this artificial intelligence, clinicians can be able to pick out on patients who are most likely to fall sick before the actual symptoms appear thereby being able to prevent the disease in the early stages. For example, the techniques that deal with deep analysis of signs that the patient's heart rhythm has forwarded ECG data for predictive models that helps doctors initiate prevention before adverse incidences such as heart attacks or strokes occur. Advanced algorithms assist in the identification of patients who may need immediate attention so benefiting the systems that are used in prioritizing the patients in the hospital (Alowais *et al.,* 2023).

Quite evident is the cross-disciplinary application of AI, which has been a significant revolution in this aspect. They include the use of a combination of big data technologies to manage big data from different specialties, hence making it easier for the different fields of medicine to work together in finding solutions to problems. For instance, actual smart tumor boards aggregate data regarding tumor diagnosis based on radiology, pathology, genetics, and oncology, in order to give oncologists an all-in-one insight of the state of the patient's disease and, therefore, help the final decision on the kind of treatment protocols most suitable for that particular case. Such models also enhances the accuracy of treatment procedures and the quality of decision-making sought through research. Apart from this, AI also plays a role in engaging patients through chat bots and virtual assistants. This technology avails information on their health status, book appointments and bare medical questions to the physicians thereby almost relieving the dearth burden from the side of the physicians and enhancing the level of patient satisfaction. Another area where AI applies innovations in administration also applies to the electronic health records (EHR), increasing efficiency of documentation process and relieving the burden from clinicians, in order for them to increase on their time with the patients (Khan et al., 2024).

More specifically, there is no doubt that as this technology advances, it will be impossible to imagine coordinating clinical expertise without the use of AI. Applying AI into healthcare system, the clinician gets more accurate analysis, prevents or minimizes errors, treat patients more effectively and make the hospital running more effectively to be patient-centric.

6. MANAGING AI'S LIMITATIONS IN CLINICAL PRACTICE

Some of the issues associated with the adoption of AI in healthcare include data privacy issues, issues with regard to the fairness and objectivity of the algorithms and legal requirements that need to be met. As earlier indicated, patients' information is a sensitive lot since AI seems to involve the manipulation of a lot of data. It is as a result of this that there has been issues on validation and fairness in assessing the model to avoid; proven biased on certain demography. Therefore, legal reforms should also be implemented to ensure that technologies developed through AI consider ethical appropriate use for medical aspirations by putting into consideration patient safety and liability. All of these issues are critical to address as a way of ensuring the continued trust of the public and good incorporation of AI into health care facilities (Albahri *et al.,* 2023).

Table 3. Challenges of Making AI Trustworthy and Reliable in Medicine

Challenge	Description	Potential Solution
Data Privacy	The problem of insecure storage of medical details.	Block chain for safe sharing of data, encryption techniques.
Algorithmic Bias	AI Models will prefer some populations.	Creating organized policies for controlling AI.
Regulatory Issues	Unclear laws regarding AI's role in patient care.	Formulating policies to manage AI application in hospitals.
Explain ability	It is challenging to explain why AI reaches certain medical conclusions.	Use of Explainable AI (XAI) for transparency.

6.1 Managing Risks Related to Health Information Security

That's why as the use of AI systems continue to rise, it is vital to protect the patient data from breaches of the HIPAA and GDPR acts. As technology advances, especially the inclusion of artificial intelligence within medical systems, various health organizations deal with large quantities of information about patients: this information is especially vulnerable to hacking and navigation by unauthorized personnel and modification in general. Kinds of risks range from ransomware attacks to phishing and even insider threats to healthcare institutions. To address these threats, data encryption methods, block chain approach, and the federated learning are being practiced to achieve secure and private sharing of the patient's data (Lee and Yoon., 2021).

In federated learning raw data does not need to be centralized therefore, it minimizes the risks of managing large databases. This gives security since it makes patient records to be decentralized and the records cannot be altered, manipulated or forged. Also, there is a process for developing differential privacy methods that would manage to scrub patient data before incorporating them into AI training away from claims of re-identification. The discussion is continued on patient permission for their data to be used for artificial intelligence, Type S problems such as data ownership, and how decisions based on artificial intelligence shall be made. The corporations need to introduce strict measures of data protection, security control, and management, security check-ups, and adjust the AI applications in health care to the legal and ethical requirements (Khatiwada *et al.,* 2024).

6.2 Standardizing AI Model Evaluation in Medicine

This will mean that such models will skewed and hence reflect an inherent bias skewing the health care delivery system against under privileged groups. This possibly leads to misdiagnosis and suboptimal treatment recommendation for the severity of the disease and this can be as a result of training AI systems on non-representative or skewed datasets. For example, the different AI models, which are primarily developed to carry out diagnostic tasks based on data from one particular community, may have poor diagnostic results for another whereby making health inequality worse (Paulus and Kent., 2020).

Bias and consequently unfair distribution also remain an important problem, especially if models are not validated using proper and credible datasets that cover the multiple profiles with different demographics and SES levels. This prerequisite makes it easier to apply bias-mitigation solutions like adversarial debasing, re-weighting training samples, and carrying algorithmic fairness testing for the healthcare field. A cultural synergy between data scientists, clinicians, ethicists, and other related professionals is essential in designing the fair and ethical AI. Moreover, more openness in the AI model or model building process such as open-source AI building methodologies and reviewed validation research studies will act as supportive measures. It is important for governmental authorities to come up with specific codes of practice and regulation which will compel developers of the artificial intelligence, to show, how fair and accurate their invented applications in the medical field will be (Paulus and Kent., 2020).

6.3 AI Healthcare Laws and Ethical Code of Conduct

This is why in the modern world, AI is used quite actively in the healthcare sector; that is why there is a great need for special regulation to protect the patient's rights and ensure the effectiveness of the chosen solution. National and supranational administrations and organizations are also engaging in an ongoing process of designing a legal framework regarding AI-based medical technology, primarily in the area of risk assessment of the models, model validation, and model interpretability. As with all diagnostic tools that employ advanced AI technology, these diagnostic tools must gain the permission of the FDA and EMA before they are deployed for clinical use due to their inherent risks and low performance. Regulatory standards need to handle all issues concerning explanation requirements as well as legal responsibilities and ethical dimensions. Healthcare professionals require explain ability in AI to comprehend and analyze diagnosing and treatment proposals from AI systems. Clinical staff and patients depend on clear understanding of AI decision processes for them to develop trust in the system. AI systems produce errors that generate legal and ethical dilemmas regarding accountability since the responsibility for those mistakes is difficult to establish (Mennella *et al., 2024)*.

Elements of patient's autonomy, consent, and clinician accountability should be encompassed in the policies over AI governance. It is crucial to note that such decisions made by AI-driven solutions should complement the internal decision making to enhance patient safety. It will be pertinent to note that regulatory policies should require-clinical trials for the AI-based tools as and when they require for presenting them to the market similar to that of drugs and affiliated medical instruments. It is recommended that post-market regulation should equally implemented to check on the safety and efficacy of AI in real clinical practice settings (Kothinti., 2024).

7. THE UPCOMING ADVANCEMENTS IN HEALTHCARE AND MEDICINE

AI is on the brink of changing the face of healthcare by promising great emergence of new technologies including federated learning for better patient data aggregation and Block chain for data exchange, real-time diagnostic and intervention AI. Explicable AI improves the credibility hence making clinical decisions reliable. The combination of AI with the IoT and wearable devices makes provides the continual and non-invasive monitoring of patient's health and early detection of complications that can be treated via the AI-recommended individual regimes to enhance the patients' state and increase the efficiency of healthcare systems (Adeniran *et al.,* 2024).

7.1 Revolutionary Ideas in Healthcare and Patient Care

Machine learning is becoming faster, and it is implementing new technologies that revolutionize diagnostics, treatment and healthcare management. Federated learning as an application of Artificial intelligence allows several hospitals or health care facilities to train separate models on decentralized data without ever sharing the data with other institutions; thus, enhancing the data privacy and model robustness. This is particularly important regarding data-sharing constraints to improve AI's predictive quality in various populations. Block chain has brought a big change in handling of secure data in the medical field in a way that it has paved a decentralized structure, while making sure it is unhampered, thus bringing down the probability of data breach, unauthorized access or simple fraud. This makes it possible to uphold the patient's right to privacy and, at the same time, integrating data sharing across various caregivers hence promoting continuity of care (Iqbal *et al.,* 2021).

Another marked improvement is real-time diagnostics generated from AI algorithms done through machine learning in which the latter interprets lots of data at real-time. This means that disease diagnosis is achieved in real time, clinical decisions as well as treatment is also quick. Application of artificial intelligence in hospital system means rationalization of resources, organization of patients' schedules and decrease of bureaucratic practices. This field is currently in the process of applying clinical treatment whereby specialized therapies can be adequately matched with patients based on their genetics, environment and complete lifestyles. Third, the application of robots in surgery departments has impacted on Paget's third element of delivering quality and efficient healthcare delivery as it has helped offer more accurate results with lower incidences of side effects hence increasing healing among patients (Ahmed *et al.,* 2020).

7.2 Role of Explainable AI in Clinical Decision-Making

The voice behind Artificial Intelligence (AI) systems is acceleratedly enhancing the healthcare sector through Explanatory AI (XAI). A major issue that concerns clinicians is the fact that traditional AI models are opaque or 'black box', and as such the clinicians may not be able to comprehend how the AI arrived at a certain decision. The lack of understanding of why the AI has arrived at a certain decision is mitigated by XAI, where the AI will provide understandable reasons for the Prediction, so that a healthcare professional can approve and almost immediately adopt its conclusions and recommendations into practice. The incorporation of XAI into healthcare systems helps clinicians grasp how AI technologies diagnose patients and develops treatments which in turn enhances safety protocols and reduces potential misdiagnoses. XAI ensures medical AI systems stay consistent with medical guidelines and ethical standards thus avoiding usage of subpar or prejudiced models. The evaluation process for implementation of AI healthcare tools by regulatory bodies becomes possible through XAI due to its ability to bring clarity to how these tools function while ensuring complete compliance with ethical rules (Albahri *et al.,* 2023).

The integration of explainable AI technologies helps medical workers and patients to accept AI-based medical solutions more easily. AI explanations serve to decrease doctors' medical risk exposure and elevate their trust in AI diagnostic systems. XAI integration in healthcare will serve as a crucial element to maintain innovation while deploying responsible patient-centered AI technologies which advance in their development (Patel *et al.,* 2024).

7.3 Role of AI- Based AoT Gadgets for Unceasing Tracking of Health

Morbidity, risk prevention, and individualized care: These are some of the areas where AI combined with the IoT and wearable health devices is revolutionizing the primarily patient surveillance. Smart watches and biosensors are the prominent examples of AI wearable that constantly monitor and record vital signs, pulse, blood oxygen saturation, sleep cycle, and other physiological information in real time. They are coupled with artificial intelligence that is used for identifying heart issues, changes and alert one on health complications such as arrhythmia, hypertension, and diabetes among others. Many studies have shown that the use of Artificial Intelligence for remote monitoring can help different healthcare practitioners monitor Chronic Diseases, manage treatments flexibly and hence prevent hospitalization. Also, integration with AI of IoT devices allows for early detection of diseases, providing the necessary interventions as well as giving the necessary recommendations to patients for their health to improve and become more efficient in the provision of health services (George *et al.,* 2023)

Figure 4.

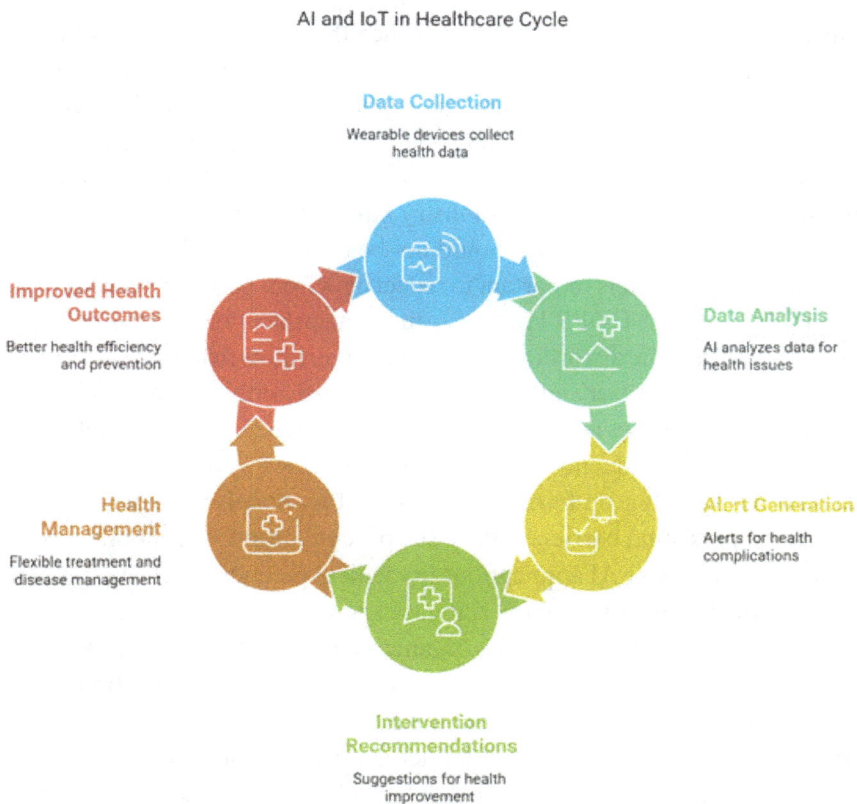

AI and IoT in Healthcare Cycle

Data Collection
Wearable devices collect health data

Data Analysis
AI analyzes data for health issues

Alert Generation
Alerts for health complications

Intervention Recommendations
Suggestions for health improvement

Health Management
Flexible treatment and disease management

Improved Health Outcomes
Better health efficiency and prevention

8. CONCLUSION

They have brought about a new technique in early stage disease diagnosis and about risk assessment in the field of medicine, replacing the ordinary methods of medical diagnosis with better precision, productivity and statistical accuracy. Combining of ML, DLs and big data analytics, AI helps the medical practitioners in diagnosing diseases at the initial stage and pursues effective treatment plans. Advance technologies such as artificial intelligence aided diagnosis systems that work through huge data such as scan, genetic makeup, and patient history have enhanced the proper decision making and have boosted the health outcomes. Perhaps the most significant application of AI is in the diagnosis of diseases through imaging by interpreting radiology scans as the algorithms are as accurate as human specialists. It further augments the electronic health records (EHR) by using NLP for analyzing semi-structured EHR to gain some important insights from unstructured data. However, without creativity, one may enhance cognitive ability through artificially intelligent assessed genetic, lifestyle, and environmental risks that will lead to specific disease diagnosis to enable preventive measures to be taken. However, the introduction of AI in the health industry has its challenges, which are revealed below. There are some issues that should not be overseen as AI systems work with significant patient data. It is important to redact data from patients' records to adhere with the HIPAA and the GDPR laws regarding data protection. Furthermore, the AI models also evidence the distortions in different algorithms that originate from using a non-representative dataset and come up with significantly different outputs in the health sector. These biases are possible if measures such as proper model validation are not put in place, uniqueness and ethical approaches in the development of AI models and the focusing on fairness in training the models are not implemented. Another of the persisting barriers is the issue of regulation for the application of AI. To standardize the use of AI applications in medical practice entails proper policies that would provide validation on the right accuracy of the model, safety of patients, and clinical responsibility. Currently, organizations like the FDA and EMA are in the process of regulation of artificial intelligence diagnostic applications based on the advancement in the technology and the effect that the same has on the society enactment of the same technology. Another significant concept under the current AI trend is the Explanatory AI (XAI), as it helps in the attainment of trust between patients, clinicians and artificial intelligence by providing clear and comprehensible results which can be explained and verified by clinicians. It is for the future that AI is advancing with such improvements such as federated learning where several institutions can train AI models without using patients' personal information. Block chain too has been noted to be used as a solution for secure and integrated medical records sharing and protection. The adoption of AI with IoT and wearable health appliances expands its uses to the areas of IoT and health advice, since patients' constant monitoring is possible with early signs detection. These advancements contribute to a more proactive one, patient centered approach towards treatment resulting in less hospitalization rates, and better patient care and health management in the long run.

Therefore, early disease diagnosis and risk prediction is area where artificial intelligence is revolutionizing the healthcare industry through better diagnostic accuracy, reduced errors than physicians and methods to integrate the use of these systems in clinical practice. Nevertheless, these issues cannot be ignored: privacy of data and patients' information, bias, and regulatory concerns yet, it is impossible to deny the benefits of applying AI and its impact on healthcare facilities. Depending on the cooperation between doctors, specialists in artificial intelligence, and politicians, AI should remain the leading factor of progress in the future of the healthcare system, making it more objective, better-organized, and available to the public. Therefore, the growth in AI is expected to improve the diagnosis of diseases, timely detection, treatment tailored for each person and enhance the functionality and productivity of the entire healthcare landscape.

REFERENCES

Aamir, A., Iqbal, A., Jawed, F., Ashfaque, F., Hafsa, H., Anas, Z., & Mansoor, T. (2024). Exploring the current and prospective role of artificial intelligence in disease diagnosis. *Annals of Medicine and Surgery (London)*, *86*(2), 943–949.

Adeniran, A. A., Onebunne, A. P., & William, P. (2024). Explainable AI (XAI) in healthcare: Enhancing trust and transparency in critical decision-making. *World J. Adv. Res. Rev*, *23*, 2647–2658.

Agrawal, S., & Jain, S. K. (2020). Medical text and image processing: applications, issues and challenges. *Machine Learning with Health Care Perspective: Machine Learning and Healthcare*, 237-262.

Ahmed, Z., Mohamed, K., Zeeshan, S., & Dong, X. (2020). Artificial intelligence with multi-functional machine learning platform development for better healthcare and precision medicine. *Database : The Journal of Biological Databases and Curation*, *2020*, baaa010.

Al-Garadi, M. A., Yang, Y. C., & Sarker, A. (2022, November). The role of natural language processing during the COVID-19 pandemic: Health applications, opportunities, and challenges. *Health Care*, *10*(11), 2270.

Albahri, A. S., Duhaim, A. M., Fadhel, M. A., Alnoor, A., Baqer, N. S., Alzubaidi, L., & Deveci, M. (2023). A systematic review of trustworthy and explainable artificial intelligence in healthcare: Assessment of quality, bias risk, and data fusion. *Information Fusion*, *96*, 156–191.

Albahri, A. S., Duhaim, A. M., Fadhel, M. A., Alnoor, A., Baqer, N. S., Alzubaidi, L., & Deveci, M. (2023). A systematic review of trustworthy and explainable artificial intelligence in healthcare: Assessment of quality, bias risk, and data fusion. *Information Fusion*, *96*, 156–191.

Ali, H. (2022). AI in neurodegenerative disease research: Early detection, cognitive decline prediction, and brain imaging biomarker identification. *Int J Eng Technol Res Manag*, *6*(10), 71.

Alowais, S. A., Alghamdi, S. S., Alsuhebany, N., Alqahtani, T., Alshaya, A. I., Almohareb, S. N., & Albekairy, A. M. (2023). Revolutionizing healthcare: The role of artificial intelligence in clinical practice. *BMC Medical Education*, *23*(1), 689.

Amann, J., Blasimme, A., Vayena, E., Frey, D., & Madai, V. I., & Precise4Q Consortium. (2020). Explainability for artificial intelligence in healthcare: A multidisciplinary perspective. *BMC Medical Informatics and Decision Making*, *20*, 1–9.

Aminizadeh, S., Heidari, A., Dehghan, M., Toumaj, S., Rezaei, M., Navimipour, N. J., & Unal, M. (2024). Opportunities and challenges of artificial intelligence and distributed systems to improve the quality of healthcare service. *Artificial Intelligence in Medicine, 149*, 102779.

Arinez, J. F., Chang, Q., Gao, R. X., Xu, C., & Zhang, J. (2020). Artificial intelligence in advanced manufacturing: Current status and future outlook. *Journal of Manufacturing Science and Engineering, 142*(11), 110804.

Ashiwaju, B. I., Orikpete, O. F., & Uzougbo, C. G. (2023). The intersection of artificial intelligence and big data in drug discovery: A review of current trends and future implications. *Matrix Science Pharma, 7*(2), 36–42.

Bi, W. L., Hosny, A., Schabath, M. B., Giger, M. L., Birkbak, N. J., Mehrtash, A., & Aerts, H. J. (2019). Artificial intelligence in cancer imaging: Clinical challenges and applications. *CA: a Cancer Journal for Clinicians, 69*(2), 127–157.

Brown, C., Nazeer, R., Gibbs, A., Le Page, P., Mitchell, A. R., & Mitchell, A. R. (2023). Breaking bias: The role of artificial intelligence in improving clinical decision-making. *Cureus, 15*(3).

Chattu, V. K. (2021). A review of artificial intelligence, big data, and blockchain technology applications in medicine and global health. *Big Data and Cognitive Computing, 5*(3), 41.

Choudhury, G., & MacNee, W. (2017). Role of inflammation and oxidative stress in the pathology of ageing in COPD: Potential therapeutic interventions. *COPD, 14*(1), 122–135.

Cui, M., & Zhang, D. Y. (2021). Artificial intelligence and computational pathology. *Laboratory Investigation, 101*(4), 412–422.

Das, S. (2024). Applications of Sensor Technology in Healthcare. In *Revolutionizing Healthcare Treatment with Sensor Technology* (pp. 79–99). IGI Global.

Dash, S., Shakyawar, S. K., Sharma, M., & Kaushik, S. (2019). Big data in healthcare: Management, analysis and future prospects. *Journal of Big Data, 6*(1), 1–25.

Davis, D. A., Chawla, N. V., Blumm, N., Christakis, N., & Barabási, A. L. (2008, October). Predicting individual disease risk based on medical history. In *Proceedings of the 17th ACM conference on Information and knowledge management* (pp. 769-778).

George, A. H., Shahul, A., & George, A. S. (2023). Wearable sensors: A new way to track health and wellness. *Partners Universal International Innovation Journal*, *1*(4), 15–34.

Ghaffar Nia, N., Kaplanoglu, E., & Nasab, A. (2023). Evaluation of artificial intelligence techniques in disease diagnosis and prediction. *Discover Artificial Intelligence*, *3*(1), 5.

Goel, A., Goel, A. K., & Kumar, A. (2023). The role of artificial neural network and machine learning in utilizing spatial information. *Spatial Information Research*, *31*(3), 275–285.

Gupta, P., & Pandey, M. K. (2024). Role of AI for smart health diagnosis and treatment. In *Smart Medical Imaging for Diagnosis and Treatment Planning* (pp. 23–45). Chapman and Hall/CRC.

Harry, A. (2023). Revolutionizing healthcare: How machine learning is transforming patient diagnoses-a comprehensive review of ai's impact on medical diagnosis. *BULLET: Jurnal Multidisiplin Ilmu*, *2*(4), 1259–1266.

Iqbal, M. J., Javed, Z., Sadia, H., Qureshi, I. A., Irshad, A., Ahmed, R., & Sharifi-Rad, J. (2021). Clinical applications of artificial intelligence and machine learning in cancer diagnosis: Looking into the future. *Cancer Cell International*, *21*(1), 270.

Javaid, M., Haleem, A., Singh, R. P., Suman, R., & Rab, S. (2022). Significance of machine learning in healthcare: Features, pillars and applications. *International Journal of Intelligent Networks*, *3*, 58–73.

Johnson, K. B., Wei, W. Q., Weeraratne, D., Frisse, M. E., Misulis, K., Rhee, K., & Snowdon, J. L. (2021). Precision medicine, AI, and the future of personalized health care. *Clinical and Translational Science*, *14*(1), 86–93.

Khalafi, P., Morsali, S., Hamidi, S., Ashayeri, H., Sobhi, N., Pedrammehr, S., & Jafarizadeh, A. (2025). Artificial intelligence in stroke risk assessment and management via retinal imaging. *Frontiers in Computational Neuroscience*, *19*, 1490603.

Khalid, H., Hussain, M., Al Ghamdi, M. A., Khalid, T., Khalid, K., Khan, M. A., & Ahmed, A. (2020). A comparative systematic literature review on knee bone reports from mri, x-rays and ct scans using deep learning and machine learning methodologies. *Diagnostics (Basel)*, *10*(8), 518.

Khan, M. M., Shah, N., Shaikh, N., Thabet, A., & Belkhair, S. (2024). Towards secure and trusted AI in healthcare: A systematic review of emerging innovations and ethical challenges. *International Journal of Medical Informatics*, 105780.

Khatiwada, P., Yang, B., Lin, J. C., & Blobel, B. (2024). Patient-generated health data (PGHD): Understanding, requirements, challenges, and existing techniques for data security and privacy. *Journal of Personalized Medicine*, *14*(3), 282.

Kothinti, R. R. (2024). Deep learning in healthcare: Transforming disease diagnosis, personalized treatment, and clinical decision-making through AI-driven innovations.

Lee, D., & Yoon, S. N. (2021). Application of artificial intelligence-based technologies in the healthcare industry: Opportunities and challenges. *International Journal of Environmental Research and Public Health*, *18*(1), 271.

Luo, Y. (2017). Recurrent neural networks for classifying relations in clinical notes. *Journal of Biomedical Informatics*, *72*, 85–95.

Maleki Varnosfaderani, S., & Forouzanfar, M. (2024). The role of AI in hospitals and clinics: Transforming healthcare in the 21st century. *Bioengineering (Basel, Switzerland)*, *11*(4), 337.

Mennella, C., Maniscalco, U., De Pietro, G., & Esposito, M. (2024). Ethical and regulatory challenges of AI technologies in healthcare: A narrative review. *Heliyon*, *10*(4).

Morid, M. A., Sheng, O. R. L., & Dunbar, J. (2023). Time series prediction using deep learning methods in healthcare. *ACM Transactions on Management Information Systems*, *14*(1), 1–29.

Munavalli, J. R., Boersma, H. J., Rao, S. V., & Van Merode, G. G. (2021). Real-time capacity management and patient flow optimization in hospitals using AI methods. *Artificial intelligence and Data mining in healthcare*, 55-69.

Nie, D., Trullo, R., Lian, J., Wang, L., Petitjean, C., Ruan, S., & Shen, D. (2018). Medical image synthesis with deep convolutional adversarial networks. *IEEE Transactions on Biomedical Engineering*, *65*(12), 2720–2730.

Norori, N., Hu, Q., Aellen, F. M., Faraci, F. D., & Tzovara, A. (2021). Addressing bias in big data and AI for health care: A call for open science. *Patterns (New York, N.Y.)*, *2*(10).

Patel, A. U., Gu, Q., Esper, R., Maeser, D., & Maeser, N. (2024). The crucial role of interdisciplinary conferences in advancing explainable AI in healthcare. *BioMedInformatics*, *4*(2), 1363–1383.

Paulus, J. K., & Kent, D. M. (2020). Predictably unequal: Understanding and addressing concerns that algorithmic clinical prediction may increase health disparities. *NPJ Digital Medicine*, *3*(1), 99.

Rane, N., Choudhary, S., & Rane, J. (2023). Towards Autonomous Healthcare: Integrating Artificial Intelligence (AI) for Personalized Medicine and Disease Prediction. *Available at SSRN* 4637894.

Rane, N., Choudhary, S., & Rane, J. (2023). Explainable artificial intelligence (XAI) in healthcare: Interpretable models for clinical decision support. *Available at SSRN* 4637897.

Shameer, K., Johnson, K. W., Glicksberg, B. S., Dudley, J. T., & Sengupta, P. P. (2018). Machine learning in cardiovascular medicine: Are we there yet? *Heart (British Cardiac Society)*, *104*(14), 1156–1164.

Sharma, A., Badea, M., Tiwari, S., & Marty, J. L. (2021). Wearable biosensors: An alternative and practical approach in healthcare and disease monitoring. *Molecules (Basel, Switzerland)*, *26*(3), 748.

Shehadeh, A., Alshboul, O., Al Mamlook, R. E., & Hamedat, O. (2021). Machine learning models for predicting the residual value of heavy construction equipment: An evaluation of modified decision tree, LightGBM, and XGBoost regression. *Automation in Construction*, *129*, 103827.

Singh, M., Kumar, A., Khanna, N. N., Laird, J. R., Nicolaides, A., Faa, G., & Suri, J. S. (2024). Artificial intelligence for cardiovascular disease risk assessment in personalised framework: A scoping review. *EClinicalMedicine*, 73.

Tsuneki, M. (2022). Deep learning models in medical image analysis. *Journal of Oral Biosciences*, *64*(3), 312–320.

Wu, J., Wang, J., Nicholas, S., Maitland, E., & Fan, Q. (2020). Application of big data technology for COVID-19 prevention and control in China: Lessons and recommendations. *Journal of Medical Internet Research*, *22*(10), e21980.

Ye, C., Fu, T., Hao, S., Zhang, Y., Wang, O., Jin, B., & Ling, X. (2018). Prediction of incident hypertension within the next year: Prospective study using statewide electronic health records and machine learning. *Journal of Medical Internet Research*, *20*(1), e22.

Yogeshappa, V. G. (2024). AI-driven Precision medicine: Revolutionizing personalized treatment plans. *International Journal of Computer Engineering and Technology*, *15*(5), 455–474.

Yu, H., Yang, L. T., Zhang, Q., Armstrong, D., & Deen, M. J. (2021). Convolutional neural networks for medical image analysis: State-of-the-art, comparisons, improvement and perspectives. *Neurocomputing*, *444*, 92–110.

Zhang, J., Oh, Y. J., Lange, P., Yu, Z., & Fukuoka, Y. (2020). Artificial intelligence chatbot behavior change model for designing artificial intelligence chatbots to promote physical activity and a healthy diet. *Journal of Medical Internet Research*, *22*(9), e22845.

Zhou, B., Yang, G., Shi, Z., & Ma, S. (2022). Natural language processing for smart healthcare. *IEEE Reviews in Biomedical Engineering*, *17*, 4–18.

Chapter 12
Securing Patient Data in Distributed Healthcare Systems

Vishal Jain

ⓘD https://orcid.org/0000-0003-1126-7424

Kuala Lumpur University of Science and Technology, Malaysia & Vivekananda Institute of Professional Studies, New Delhi, India

Sachin Jain

ⓘD https://orcid.org/0000-0002-2948-7858

Ajay Kumar Garg Engineering College, Ghaziabad, India

Danish Ather

ⓘD https://orcid.org/0000-0003-1596-5553

Amity University, Tashkent, Uzbekistan

Golnoosh Manteghi

Kuala Lumpur University of Science and Technology, Malaysia

Abu Bakar Abdul Hamid

ⓘD https://orcid.org/0009-0007-5177-8145

Kuala Lumpur University of Science and Technology, Malaysia

ABSTRACT

The healthcare industry is undergoing significant upheaval as more businesses use distributed edge computing. Better real-time data processing, simpler access, and more individualised patient care are just a few benefits of this shift. Security concerns with distributed edge-based healthcare systems are covered in this chapter. It looks at the bigger attack surface, the different kinds of features that devices can

DOI: 10.4018/979-8-3373-3196-6.ch012

offer, and how hard it is to manage data in all of its forms (in use, at rest, and in motion). It carefully talks about HIPAA, other countries' data protection laws, and industry standards. Behavioral analytics, edge-based breach detection, and incident response in distributed settings are also talked about in this chapter. It focuses on risk management and governance models such as threat modelling, managing vulnerabilities, and making security better. These security rules are shown in a detailed case study on safe telemedicine implementation. Post-quantum cryptography, AI-powered security, and blockchain make up the last part of the chapter.

I. INTRODUCTION

The coming together of healthcare and IT has opened up a world of new options for diagnosing, treating, and caring for patients. Edge computing and other types of distributed computing are key to this change because they bring computer power and data storage closer to where the data is being created in healthcare settings (Satyanarayanan, 2017). This decentralization makes real-time analytics possible, lowers latency, makes medical devices more responsive, and makes healthcare services easier to get to, especially in areas that aren't well covered or are far away (Liu et al., 2023). Wearable health trackers that constantly record vital signs are just a few examples. Smart medical devices that do diagnostics on-site and telemedicine platforms that let people have consultations from afar are also examples.

However, the shift to dispersed healthcare systems complicates and evolves security. A specified perimeter is the primary focus of security controls in conventional centralised healthcare IT infrastructures. However, distributed environments have a lot more devices, sensors, gateways, and edge servers that can be attacked because they are all linked to each other (Hassan, 2021). There are serious effects on healthcare security breaches that go beyond financial losses. Significant legal and regulatory repercussions, a possible risk to patient safety, and a drop in trust are some of these effects. Therefore, it is essential to keep patient health information (PHI) accurate, private, and accessible in these dynamic and distributed situations. When it comes to edge-based healthcare systems, traditional security approaches that depend on perimeter-based defences aren't performing well.

As a way to help researchers, medical professionals, and IT security experts build and keep safe distributed healthcare ecosystems that put patient data privacy and security first, this chapter talks about current security trends and gives a detailed case study.

The Security Landscape in Distributed Healthcare

Health care has always been a target of cyberattacks because patient data is valuable and easy to steal. These risks get worse as healthcare systems spread out and connect more network-edge devices and data sources. New security threats need to be carefully thought through (Bala et al., 2024).

Unique Challenges of Edge-Based Healthcare Systems

- **Expanded Attack Surface Across Distributed Nodes:** In contrast to centralised systems, edge settings don't have a perimeter. There are many sensors, devices, gateways, and edge servers spread out in different places. Bad actors might enter by any of these nodes, expanding the attack area significantly. Edge settings feature numerous devices, sensors, gateways, and edge servers dispersed throughout various locations, as opposed to centralised systems with a distinct perimeter. Every one of these nodes could be a way for bad people to get in, which greatly increases the attack area (Seshadri et al., 2005). It gets hard and takes a lot of time and resources to protect each gadget and the communication links between them.
- **Diverse Device Capabilities and Security Features:** Wearable sensors with limited computing power and security features are among the devices utilised in edge healthcare. More advanced medical devices and edge computers are also used. Because of this, it is hard to make sure that all parts of the environment follow the same security rules and policies. Many edge devices don't have enough resources to use standard security software and cryptographic algorithms (Hassan, 2021).
- **Data in Motion, At Rest, and In Use Considerations:** On edge devices and servers, patient data is at rest. It is also in motion as it is sent between devices and the cloud. It is also used at the edge for processing and analysis. Each of these states requires a different level of protection. Use encryption and secure communication to protect data in transit. It's hard to be sure that data stays safe and correct when it's in places you don't trust (Yuan & Li, 2019).
- **Limitations on resources for security implementations:** These include complicated ways to prove who you are, strong encryption, and full systems for finding intruders (Falayi et al., 2023). It is important to find security solutions that aren't too big and offer enough protection without slowing down devices or draining their batteries.

II. REGULATORY AND COMPLIANCE REQUIREMENTS

Many national, international, and industry-specific rules and laws must be followed by distributed healthcare systems (Satyanarayanan, 2017).

- **HIPAA and Other Regulations That Affect Healthcare:** The HIPAA Privacy, Security, and Breach Notification Rules protect the protected health information (PHI) of all American citizens. Since edge systems are spread out, it's harder to set up and keep up these security measures across devices and places. It takes careful planning and execution to send data over networks that aren't always reliable, control who can access edge devices, and create audit trails across faraway nodes (Yuan & Li, 2019).
- **Frameworks for international data protection:** Healthcare organisations that handle international data must follow international data protection frameworks. Data security laws in Canada and Asia-Pacific differ. Data security laws in Canada and Asia-Pacific differ. Data security laws in Canada and Asia-Pacific differ. The Canadian Personal Information Security and Electronic Documents Act (PIPEDA) and Asia-Pacific data security regulations differ. These rules can be very different in what they cover and how they are enforced (Yuan & Li, 2019).
- **Industry Medical Device Security Standards:** NIST and AAMI advise on medical device safety during design, development, deployment, and maintenance (Grassi et al., 2017). These standards address medical device-specific incident management, secure communication, vulnerability, and patch management. Since remote medical equipment is growing more complex and networked, these standards are crucial.
- **Healthcare Systems Certification Requirements:** Some medical equipment and healthcare IT systems need certification to fulfil safety and security criteria. As an illustration, consider the HITRUST Common Security Framework (CSF) approval, which offers a thorough method for handling the rules, guidelines, and business needs associated with the private and secure storage of health data. For distributed healthcare solutions to access the market and gain credibility, several accreditation requirements must be met.

III. SECURITY ARCHITECTURE FOR DISTRIBUTED HEALTHCARE

Standard models that concentrate on the perimeter must give way to ones that consider the entire system and the data in order to create a robust security architecture for distributed healthcare systems. The Zero Trust framework and defense-in-depth tactics are two important ideas that are especially useful in this situation (Rose et al., 2020).

Zero Trust Framework for Healthcare Edges

This is how the Zero Trust security model works: "never trust, always verify." It believes that no user, device, or part of the network can be trusted by itself, no matter where it is (inside or outside the traditional network perimeter). This framework works especially well with edge-based healthcare systems because they are spread out and change over time (Costan & Devadas, 2016).

- **Identity-Centric Security Models:** Identity is the new perimeter in a Zero Trust design. Security rules are followed based on the people, devices, and apps that are trying to get to resources. To make sure people are who they say they are before they can access patient data or important systems at the edge, you need strong authentication and authorization mechanisms shown in Figure 1. Multi-factor authentication (MFA) for users and strong login methods for devices are part of this.

Figure 1. Identity-Centric Security in a Distributed Healthcare System

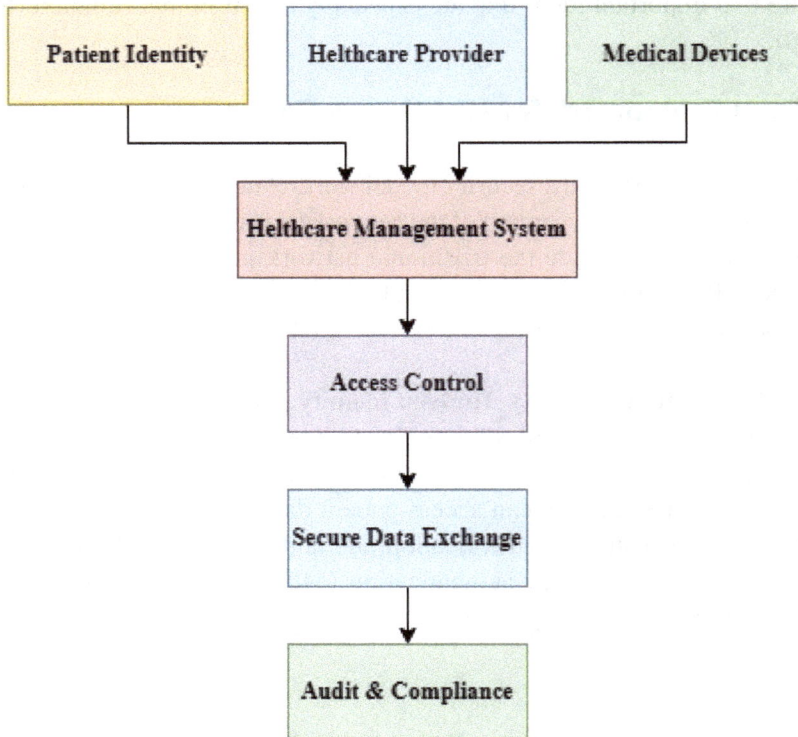

- **Continuous Verification and Attestation:** Zero Trust requires that the names of users and devices and their security posture are constantly checked. This includes continuous behaviour monitoring and adherence to security guidelines in addition to initial authentication. Device attestation is crucial for ensuring that only authorised and healthy devices have access to private data since it verifies the dependability and security of edge devices (Seshadri et al., 2005).

- **Least Privilege Access Control Implementation:** Only the bare minimum of access should be granted to users and devices so they can fulfil their legal obligations. This is known as the least privilege principle. This entails precisely establishing roles and permissions in distributed healthcare in order to access patient data and system operations at the edge. In this manner, the impact of a compromised account or device will be lessened.

- **Micro-segmentation Strategies for Medical Networks:** Micro-segmentation separates the network into smaller, separate parts so attackers can't move from one part to another. In a healthcare setting with many medical devices that are all linked to each other, dividing the network into sections based on device type, function, and risk level can make it much less likely that a security breach on one device will affect the whole network shown in Figure 2. Network security controls like firewalls and other types of controls make sure that traffic between these parts follows strict rules.

Figure 2. Micro-segmentation in a Distributed Healthcare Network

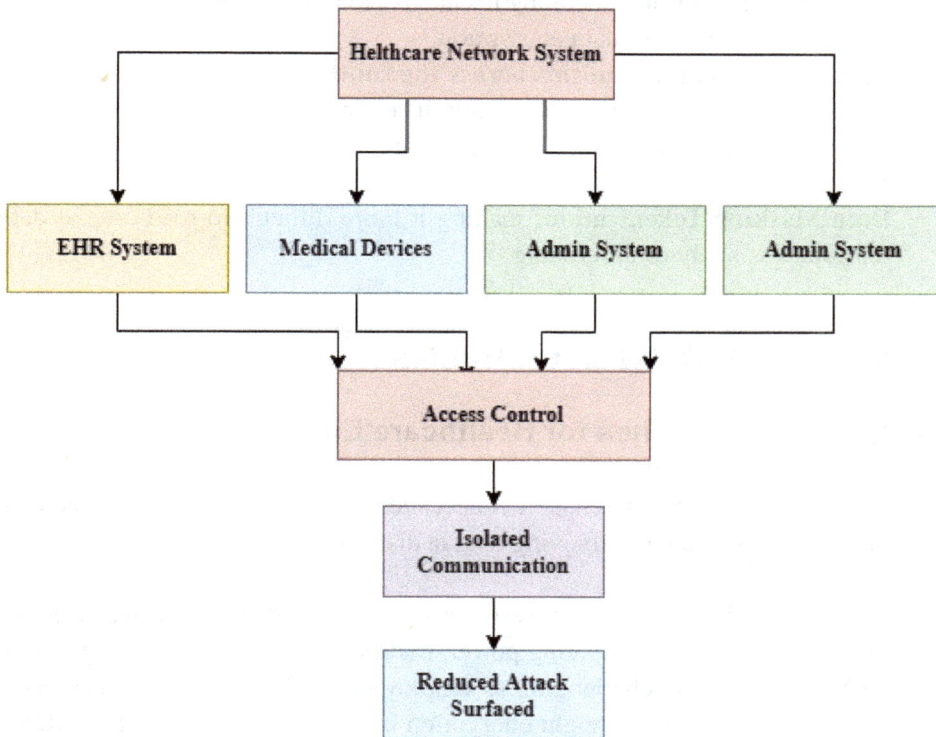

IV. DEFENSE-IN-DEPTH STRATEGIES

Defense-in-depth, which is also called "layered security," is a way to protect against different threats by using multiple security controls that work together. Because distributed healthcare systems are more complicated and have more possible failure points, this approach is even more important (Dash et al., 2021).

- **Layered Security Controls for Edge Devices:** To keep edge devices safe, you need to use a multi-layered method that includes:
- **Endpoint Protection:** Software that blocks malware, personal firewalls, and host-based intrusion protection systems (HIPS).
- **Device Hardening:** By turning off services that aren't needed, quickly fixing security holes, and using strong passwords.
- **Medical Network Security:** It is very important to protect the network infrastructure that sends patient data and connects edge devices. Some of these are:
- **IDS/IPS and firewalls:** Looking for bad behaviour in network data.
- **VPNs:** Public network data encryption.
- **Data protection mechanisms across the continuum:** To keep patient data safe in a distributed system throughout its entire lifetime, you must:
- **Encryption:** Data encryption during transmission and storage on edge devices and computers.
- **Data Masking/Tokenization:** making it more difficult to read crucial data for pointless study or processing.

V. DATA PROTECTION MECHANISMS

Encryption Approaches for Healthcare Edge

Data is encrypted into an unreadable code (called "ciphertext"). It is a basic security technique for moving and non-moving data in distributed healthcare environments.

- **Lightweight Encryption for Resource-Constrained Devices:** Because they may require a lot of computing power, traditional encryption techniques like AES-256 might be challenging to employ on devices with low resources. For these devices, lightweight encryption methods like PRESENT, SIMON, and SPECK are a good mix of security and speed (Robert et al., 2024). You should consider the device's performance, memory, and energy consumption when choosing an algorithm.
- **End-to-End Encryption for Patient Data:** When it is feasible, end-to-end encryption (E2EE) should be utilised to safeguard patient data privacy while it is being transferred across a distributed system. This implies that data is encrypted at the point of origin (such as a wearable sensor) and remains encrypted until it reaches its destination (such as a secure cloud server or a clinician's PC). E2EE prevents unauthorised users from accessing the data, even in the event that middle-level nodes or communication links are compromised.

- **Key Management in Distributed Environments:** For encryption to function, cryptographic keys must be securely stored. Due to the large number of devices and the constantly changing environment, key management in remote healthcare systems can be challenging. Encryption keys can be kept private and secure by using hardware security modules (HSMs) and secure key exchange protocols with centralised key management systems, if at all possible (Sabiri et al., 2025).
- **Secure Enclave Technologies for Sensitive Processing:** Secure enclaves are hardware-based, isolated work spaces that provide a highly private and secure environment for managing sensitive data. Two technologies that can be utilised to safeguard patient data even when it is being handled at the edge are Intel SGX and ARM TrustZone. Attacks on the operating system or other software components are less likely as a result (Costan & Devadas, 2016). This is especially helpful for uses that need to do analytics or machine learning on private data while it's on the device.

Privacy-Preserving Computation

You can process and analyse data using privacy-preserving computation (PPC) techniques while maintaining the highest level of confidentiality for sensitive information. These techniques are particularly effective in healthcare settings where it is necessary to collect and evaluate data from multiple sources for research or to assist physicians in making choices without jeopardising patient privacy (Brendan McMahan et al., 2017).

- **Homomorphic Encryption Applications:** Calculating encrypted data without decrypting it is possible using homomorphic encryption (HE). Only the secret keyholder can read these calculations because they are encrypted. HE has a lot of potential to make multi-party computation and privacy-preserving analytics possible in healthcare. For example, (Gentry, 2009) says that HE could be used to do statistical analysis on pooled patient data without showing individual records. But the HE schemes we have now still require a lot of computer power and might not work for all edge computing situations.
- **Secure Multi-Party Computation for Distributed Analysis:** Secure multi-party computation (SMPC) methods let several people work together to solve a problem using their own private data, but they don't tell each other about the data they are using. SMPC could be used in healthcare to allow researchers from different schools to work together on large datasets of patients without having to share raw data (Liu et al., 2023).

- **Differential Privacy Implementations for Aggregate Data:** Differential privacy, or DP, is a method for protecting the privacy of individual data providers by adding a carefully measured amount of noise to the results of a query. Even though the exact numbers for each patient are still secret, the noisy overall data can still be used to learn useful things about statistics. Wearable tech or other edge sensors can send data that can be analyzed using DP to find patterns and trends without putting people's privacy at risk (Dwork & Roth, 2014).
- **Privacy-Guaranteed Federated Computing:** Federated learning (FL) is a sort of distributed machine learning that permits models be learned on datasets from numerous edge devices or organisations without sharing raw data. When coupled with safe aggregation or differential privacy, federated learning can protect AI model training on remote healthcare data (Brendan McMahan et al., 2017).

Access and Identity Management

When combined with safe aggregation or differential privacy, federated learning can protect AI model training on dispersed healthcare data (Falayi et al., 2023).

Authentication and Authorization

Authorization governs a user or object's behaviour after authentication. Protecting confidential data demands robust authentication and fine-grained permission in remote healthcare.

- **Multi-Factor Authentication for Clinical Access:** Before gaining access to hospital systems and patient data, users using multi-factor authentication (MFA) are required to present two or more forms of identification. These proofs could be things they know, things they have, or things they are. Using MFA when healthcare professionals log in to shared systems can greatly lower the chance of unauthorized entry due to stolen passwords (Rose et al., 2020).
- **Context-Aware Access Control Policies:** User jobs are often the only thing that traditional access control models use. Context-aware access control (CAC) considers more than only the user's location, the device they are using, the time of access, and the kind of sensitive data they are requesting. This enables it to choose more precisely and flexibly who can access what. Depending on the details of the access attempt, CAC can be used to enforce

more stringent access constraints in dispersed healthcare. For example, a doctor should only be able to access a patient's data when they are in the hospital.

- **Role-Based Access for Clinical Personnel:** Role-based access control (RBAC) tells users what they can and can't do based on their jobs in the healthcare company. This makes managing access easier and makes sure that users can only see the information and use the tools they need to do their jobs. All edge devices and systems handling patient data in a dispersed environment must adhere to the same RBAC guidelines at all times. **Emergency Access Provisions and Break-Glass Procedures:** Emergency access and "break-glass" procedures are necessary in situations where you need to access patient data immediately in order to give care, even though regular access rules would often prevent you from doing so. To ensure that these procedures are not being misused and that people can easily reach them in an emergency, you should put them in writing, make sure they are clear, and review them frequently.

Device Identity and Trust

Distributed healthcare systems with numerous sensors and medical devices that connect to patient data must manage device identities and trust for security reasons.

- **Validation of Device Integrity:** Device validation verifies an edge device's identity and functionality. Cryptographically verifying the device's hardware and software configuration ensures that it hasn't been tampered with and is running reliable software. The security of dispersed devices can be continuously monitored via remote attestation (Seshadri et al., 2005).
- **Certificate Management for Medical Devices:** Digital certificates are useful for data security and medical device verification. A robust certificate management framework is required in order to generate, distribute, and delete certificates for every device in a distributed healthcare system.
- **Hardware Security Modules and Trusted Platform Modules:** The cryptographic keys that HSMs manage and store cannot be altered. TPMs, or Trusted Platform Modules, are tiny chips that ensure system integrity and safeguard keys. Edge devices are safer and give hardware trust when HSMs and TPMs are added (Seshadri et al., 2005).
- **Secure Boot and Runtime Verification:** Secure boot ensures that only known and digitally signed software is loaded when the device first boots up. Runtime verification techniques constantly check the software and firmware of the device for any changes that were not allowed or any other bad behavior.

These steps help keep hacked software from running on edge devices and getting to private patient info.

Threat Detection and Response

Distributed healthcare systems need strong threat detection and incident response tools because they have a bigger attack area and security incidents could be very bad.

Security Monitoring in Distributed Systems

To manage security well, you need to be able to gather, analyze, and connect information about security from many different sources.

- **Distributed Logging and Monitoring Architecture:** It is very important to have a centralized infrastructure for logging and tracking that can collect logs and security events from all edge devices, network components, and cloud services. This design should be able to grow as needed and handle the large amount of data that is created in a distributed healthcare setting shown in Figure 3.

Figure 3. Distributed Logging and Monitoring Architecture

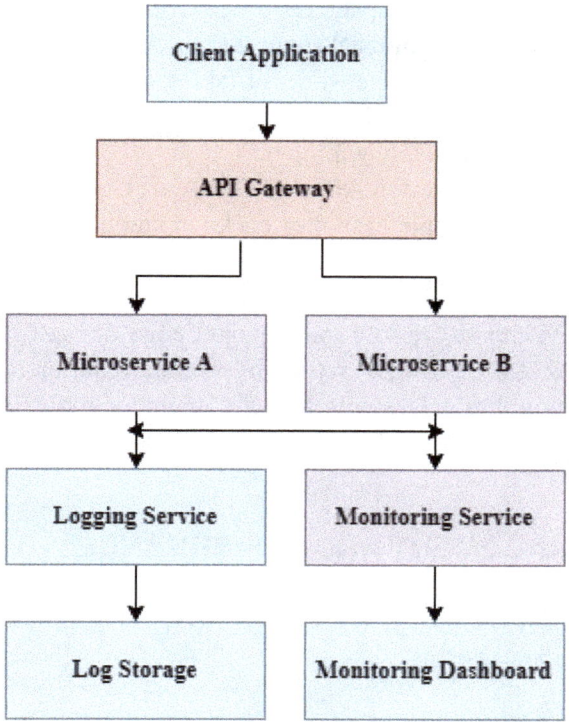

Behavioral Analytics for Anomaly Detection: Machine learning algorithms are used in behavioral analytics to find the normal patterns of activity for people, devices, and network traffic. If these baselines aren't met, it could mean that there are security risks or that the device has been hacked. Complex threats that could evade conventional signature-based security measures can be identified with the use of behavioural analytics in both the primary monitoring system and at the edge (Bala et al., 2024).

VI. INCIDENT RESPONSE CONSIDERATIONS

- Handling security issues in the healthcare industry is more difficult than in other industries due to the dispersed nature of assets. Patient care may be impacted by this. **Edge-Specific Danger Protocols:** Incident response plans must include edge device threats such physical tampering, device compromise, and connectivity loss. These steps should help identify affected devices, secure forensic evidence, and restore functionality.

- **How to contain compromised devices:** Quick action is needed to prevent hackers from entering into networks or taking data from vulnerable devices. Containment strategies include removing the device from the network, turning off features, or remotely wiping it.
- **Data Integrity Verification After an Incident:** Check patient data for security issues. Cryptographic hashes or backup comparisons can uncover unauthorised changes.
- **Recovery in Dispersed Environments:** Post-event recovery plans should include procedures to restore systems and edge devices. This may require building new device images, retrieving backup data, or reestablishing safe communication. For places with lots of computers, tools for automation and orchestration can help get things back up and running faster.

VII. RISK MANAGEMENT AND GOVERNANCE

Control and risk management must be proactive and comprehensive to protect distributed healthcare systems.

Security Risk Assessment Methodologies

Distributed healthcare facilities must frequently analyse security risks to discover weaknesses and install safeguards.

- **Modeling Threats to Cutting-Edge Healthcare Systems:** Threat models uncover system flaws. Distributed healthcare threat models should consider edge devices, network topologies, and data flows. STRIDE (Spoofing, Tampering, Repudiation, Information Disclosure, Denial of Service, Elevation of Privilege) or attack trees can help you assess threats (Yuan & Li, 2019).
- **Methods to quantify risk:** Risk quantification entails assessing the likelihood and severity of threats in order to determine the most effective approach to minimise them. Quantitative risk assessment approaches that quantify losses assist firms in determining security investments.
- **Vulnerability Management Across Distributed Assets:** It is difficult to keep track of flaws on a variety of edge devices. A good vulnerability management software should include vulnerability scanning, patch management, and configuration management to swiftly identify and fix security flaws. In

situations with a big number of staff, automation technologies can assist speed up these tasks.

- **Considerations in Supply Chain Security:** Distributed healthcare systems rely on hardware and software from different manufacturers. Businesses should consider supply chain security concerns and ensure vendors sign stringent contracts and undergo security tests to ensure third-party components can be trusted.

Security Governance Frameworks

To manage security, distributed healthcare companies require clear security policies, methods, roles, and responsibilities.

Dispersed Medical System Security Guidelines: When developing shared security laws, it is important to recognise the unique issues that the healthcare business faces. These standards should cover network segmentation, data encryption, access control, and security for edge devices. These guidelines should be reviewed and amended as needed to reflect the organization's architecture and evolving threats.

- **Mechanisms for auditing and ensuring compliance** In order to ensure that distributed healthcare systems are adhering to all applicable laws, regulations, and internal security standards, it is recommended that they undergo periodic audits and inspections. To help with the retrieval and analysis of security data from distant systems, automated audit solutions are available. This facilitates the process of verifying compliance.

- **Indicators of security and performance:** Setting up and monitoring key performance indicators (KPIs) and security metrics allows you to examine the overall security of the distributed healthcare system as well as the effectiveness of security measures. The quantity of security events discovered, the response time to an occurrence, and the proportion of users who apply patches are a few crucial indicators.

- **Constant Security Improvements:** Security is a continual process. Organizations should establish continuing security improvements. Regular risk assessments, teaching staff about security issues, and using what was learned from security events should all be part of these.

VIII. CASE STUDY: SECURE TELEMEDICINE IMPLEMENTATION

This is a case study of a healthcare organisation that conducts virtual consultations and remotely monitors patients using edge computing. This will show how the security principles we've talked about in this chapter can be used in real life.

- **Security Architecture and Control Implementation:**
- **Zero Trust:** The platform uses a "Zero Trust" model, which means that both patients and healthcare workers who want to access the system must use strong authentication (MFA). Device attestation checks the integrity of monitoring devices worn by patients and outcomes used by providers. Least privilege access is used based on the job of the user and the situation they are in. Microsegments separate patient data and contact channels on the telemedicine network.
- **Defense-in-Depth:** When data is at rest on patient-worn devices, it is encrypted lightly, and when data is moving to edge channels, it is encrypted securely using TLS protocols. Edge servers that work with local data encrypt the whole disk and do sensitive computations in safe areas. Firewalls and intrusion detection systems keep an eye on the data going between edge devices, the cloud platform, and provider networks.
- **Data Protection:** For both video and audio talks, end-to-end encryption is used. The cloud encrypts patient data both while it is being sent and while it is being kept. RBAC controls who can see patient information, and audit logs keep track of all attempts to get to the data.
- **IAM:** Users log in with a mobile app that uses biometric security and multifactor authentication (MFA). When they use MFA, healthcare workers use their organization's credentials. Access to patient data is limited by context-aware policies that take into account the provider's role and the present patient assignment.
- **Risk Assessment and Mitigation Strategies:**
- A full threat model found possible dangers like getting into patient data on edge devices without permission, listening in on communication lines, and hacking into edge servers.
- Strong encryption, secure boot and runtime verification on edge devices, secure key management, regular vulnerability scanning and patching, and strong incident response plans adapted to telemedicine-specific threats were some of the ways that threats were reduced.
- **Regulatory Compliance Approach:**
- The platform was made to follow HIPAA rules, GDPR (for patients in the EU), and other medical equipment security standards.

- Agreements were made with all third-party vendors to handle data. Regular checks are done to make sure that compliance stays high.
- **Performance Impact and Optimization Techniques:**
- The healthcare group carefully looked at how the new security controls affected performance, especially on edge devices that didn't have a lot of resources.
- For wearable sensors, encryption algorithms that are easy to use were picked. Edge computing was used to process data locally so that delay was kept to a minimum. The architecture of security was changed to get the best balance of speed, safety, and ease of use.

IX. FUTURE SECURITY TRENDS AND TECHNOLOGIES

The world of security is always changing because new threats and technologies are always coming out. Healthcare groups need to keep up with these changes to make sure their spread-out systems stay safe.

- **Post-Quantum Cryptography for Healthcare Data:** In the future, quantum computers might be able to break the public-key cryptography methods that are currently used. To keep patient data safe in the long term, healthcare organisations should look into and come up with plans for using post-quantum cryptographic algorithms.
- **AI-Based Security for Distributed Systems:** Machine learning (ML) and artificial intelligence (AI) can be used to make the sharing of healthcare safer. AI-powered behavioural analytics can facilitate threat detection, expedite incident response, and provide more intelligent security insights. (Jain et al., 2025).
- **Blockchain Applications for Data Integrity:** Due to its distributed ledger and inability to be changed, blockchain technology could improve the security and provenance of healthcare data. For instance, medical equipment can be detected, audit records maintained and shared, and patient health information communicated with consent. (Sabiri et al., 2025).
- **Features of Next-Generation Hardware Security:** Hardware security is improving to safeguard data and edge devices in distributed healthcare environments. New features like more secure enclaves, physically unclonable functions (PUFs) for device identification, and private computing techniques might be useful.

X. CONCLUSION

Patient data privacy in remote healthcare systems is complicated and necessitates a multifaceted approach. Compared to centralised security techniques, edge computing provides a broader attack surface, more devices capable of performing multiple tasks, and more complicated data flow difficulties.

Implementation Roadmap for Secure Edge Deployments:

- **Implement security monitoring tools and resolve concerns:** Create durable edge protocols to support distributed logging, incident response, and behavioural analytics. Establish compliance and security governance guidelines: Set security policies, audit periodically, and ensure compliance.
- **Strong management of identities and access:** Use strong mobile identity management, context-aware access controls, and multifactor authentication (MFA).
- **Implement data protection measures:** Use the right security and computing methods to protect your privacy.
- **Outline the steps you take to stay safe:** Ensure that all patient workers are aware of security and data protection procedures. Conduct a thorough risk assessment to identify and address healthcare-specific threats and vulnerabilities.
- **Set up an architecture for security:** Building a complete security system based on defense-in-depth and Zero Trust ideas is important.

Choosing the Ideal Security, Functionality, and Clinical Performance Balance:

By adhering to these principles and a defined execution roadmap, healthcare firms may develop and run safe distributed healthcare systems that maximise edge computing while protecting patient data. Distribution models are becoming increasingly significant in healthcare. To maintain patient trust and improve care, patient safety is essential. Understanding that security shouldn't hinder healthcare systems or professionals' work is crucial. Security and medical professionals must work together to achieve this balance.

REFERENCES

Bala, I., Pindoo, I. A., Mijwil, M. M., Abotaleb, M., & Yundong, W. (2024). Ensuring Security and Privacy in Healthcare Systems: A Review Exploring Challenges, Solutions, Future Trends, and the Practical Applications of Artificial Intelligence. *Jordan Medical Journal*, *58*(2), 250–270. DOI: 10.35516/jmj.v58i2.2527

Brendan McMahan, H., Moore, E., Ramage, D., Hampson, S., & Agüera y Arcas, B. (2017). Communication-efficient learning of deep networks from decentralized data. *Proceedings of the 20th International Conference on Artificial Intelligence and Statistics, AISTATS 2017*, 1273–1282.

Costan, V., & Devadas, S. (2016). Intel SGX Explained. In *IACR Cryptol, ePrint Arch.* (pp. 1–118).

Dash, S., Gantayat, P. K., & Das, R. K. (2021). Blockchain technology in healthcare: Opportunities and challenges. In *Intelligent Systems Reference Library* (Vol. 203, pp. 97–111). https://doi.org/DOI: 10.1007/978-3-030-69395-4_6

Dwork, C., & Roth, A. (2014). The algorithmic foundations of differential privacy. *Foundations and Trends®in Theoretical Computer Science, 9*(3--4), 211–407.

Falayi, A., Wang, Q., Liao, W., & Yu, W. (2023). Survey of Distributed and Decentralized IoT Securities: Approaches Using Deep Learning and Blockchain Technology. *Future Internet, 15*(5), 178. DOI: 10.3390/fi15050178

Gentry, C. (2009). A Fully Homomorphic Encryption Scheme [Stanford University]. In *Dissertation* (Issue September). https://cs.au.dk/~stm/local-cache/gentry-thesis.pdf

Grassi, P. A., Fenton, J. L., Lefkovitz, N. B., Danker, J. M., Choong, Y.-Y., Greene, K. K., & Theofanos, M. F. (2017). NIST Special Publication 800-63A - Digital identity guidelines: enrollment and identity proofing. In *National Institute of Standards and Technology Special Publication*. https://nvlpubs.nist.gov/nistpubs/SpecialPublications/NIST.SP.800-63a.pdf%0Ahttp://nvlpubs.nist.gov/nistpubs/SpecialPublications/NIST.SP.800-63a.pdf

Hassan, A. (2021). Lightweight Cryptography for the Internet of Things. *Advances in Intelligent Systems and Computing, 1290*, 780–795. DOI: 10.1007/978-3-030-63092-8_52

Jain, S., Jain, V., & Chatterjee, J. M. (2025). Ensemble based brain tumor classification technique from MRI based on K fold validation approach. *Journal of Integrated Science and Technology, 13*(5), 1114. DOI: 10.62110/sciencein.jist.2025.V13.1114

Liu, Y. Y., Zhang, Y., Wu, Y., & Feng, M. (2023). Healthcare and Fitness Services: A Comprehensive Assessment of Blockchain, IoT, and Edge Computing in Smart Cities. *Journal of Grid Computing*, *21*(4), 82. DOI: 10.1007/s10723-023-09712-8

Robert, W., Denis, A., Thomas, A., Samuel, A., Kabiito, S. P., Morish, Z., & Ali, G. (2024). A Comprehensive Review on Cryptographic Techniques for Securing Internet of Medical Things: A State-of-the-Art, Applications, Security Attacks, Mitigation Measures, and Future Research Direction. *Mesopotamian Journal of Artificial Intelligence in Healthcare*, *2024*, 135–169. DOI: 10.58496/mjaih/2024/016

Rose, S., Borchert, O., Mitchell, S., & Connelly, S. (2020). NIST Special Publication 807-207: Zero Trust Architecture. In *Controlling Privacy and the Use of Data Assets* (Issues 800–207). https://doi.org/DOI: 10.6028/NIST.SP.800-207%0Ahttps://nvlpubs.nist.gov/nistpubs/SpecialPublications/NIST.SP.800-207.pdf?TB_iframe=true&width=370.8&height=658.8

Sabiri, K., Sousa, F., & Rocha, T. (2025). A systematic review of privacy-preserving blockchain applications in healthcare. *Multimedia Tools and Applications*, *84*(32), 39925–39980. DOI: 10.1007/s11042-024-20541-z

Satyanarayanan, M. (2017). The emergence of edge computing. *Computer*, *50*(1), 30–39. DOI: 10.1109/MC.2017.9

Seshadri, A., Luk, M., Shi, E., Perrig, A., Van Doorn, L., & Khosla, P. (2005). Pioneer: Verifying code integrity and enforcing untampered code execution on legacy systems. *Proceedings of the 20th ACM Symposium on Operating Systems Principles, SOSP 2005*, 1–16. https://doi.org/DOI: 10.1145/1095810.1095812

Yuan, B., & Li, J. (2019). The policy effect of the general data protection regulation (GDPR) on the digital public health sector in the european union: An empirical investigation. *International Journal of Environmental Research and Public Health*, *16*(6), 1070. DOI: 10.3390/ijerph16061070 PMID: 30934648

Chapter 13
Integration of AI With Electronic Health Records

Dolly Yumnam
https://orcid.org/0009-0001-2089-3665

Department of Optometry, UIAHS, Chandigarh University, Mohali, India

Laxmi Oinam
https://orcid.org/0009-0003-1102-0832

Department of Optometry, UIAHS, Chandigarh University, Mohali, India

Sachitanand Singh
https://orcid.org/0000-0003-0713-3618

Department of Optometry, UIAHS, Chandigarh University, Mohali, India

Krishnasri Padamandala
https://orcid.org/0000-0002-2828-0302

Department of Optometry, School of Allied and Health Care Sciences, Malla Reddy University, Hyderabad, India

Sanskriti Singh
https://orcid.org/0009-0003-4341-1053

Department of Nursing, UIN, Chandigarh University, Mohali, India

ABSTRACT

Abstract Metabolic diseases, such as diabetes, obesity, and dyslipidemia, are growing in complexity, and are increasingly seen across the globe where they are demanding a significant burden on health systems. Traditional methods continue to under-utilize the vast amount of health information available in Electronic Health Records (EHRs). Artificial intelligence (AI) is a powerful solution as it can study complex amounts of data to identify patterns and generate actionable insights. This

DOI: 10.4018/979-8-3373-3196-6.ch013

AI-powered decision making benefits precision medicine because it creates opportunities for early diagnosis, tailored treatment, and long-term monitoring, when used with EHRs. This chapter explores the ways in which artificial intelligence (AI) can provide real-world guidance to clinicians making decisions in metabolic disease, specifically how it can use EHR sources of information to help with diagnosis, risk stratification and treatment decision making.

1 INTRODUCTION

Digitization of patient data gathering, storage, and evaluation has changed and improved the uniqueness of Electronic Health Records (EHRs) in the healthcare industry. It improves providers access to information, and works more extremely efficiently in health delivery systems, where the provider can assess and make well-informed decisions about care for the patient. AI is capable of making clinical workflows more efficient through the elimination of workflows by automating repetitive tasks(Gorrepati, 2024). The goal of embedding AI into EHR systems is to document care episodes, while enhancing patient results through more personalised and efficient care by providing healthcare personnel the ability to emphasise patient care and not shift their focus to paperwork. In other words, the health profiles of patients are considered so as to ensure that patients are receiving the right treatment, at the right time(Gorrepati, 2024).

The integration of cybersecurity and artificial intelligence (AI) into EHRs will undoubtedly transform the healthcare system. EHR promotes clinical decision making and improves patient outcomes by providing a complete, real-time record of a patient(Paraschiv et al., 2024). There are several key benefits and challenges of incorporating AI Technology. Artificial Intelligence (AI) can revolutionize the healthcare industry by enabling customized treatment plans, predictive analytics, and faster administrative functions. But it raises challenges regarding patient confidentiality, data privacy, objections, and ethics.(Paraschiv et al., 2024).

It is no longer accurate to refer to "electronic medical records" in light of the terminology changes to "electronic health records" or "patient records"; these electronic documents are now comprehensive electronic documents that integrate clinical data from various sources into a patient health record - that is, the complete view of a patient's health (Paraschiv et al., 2024). Electronic health records, or EHR, are the cornerstone of safe and effective care (Paraschiv et al., 2024)

1.1 Background

To improve the effectiveness and usefulness of electronic health records (EHRs), researchers have become interested in exploring the use of agent-based systems and artificial intelligence (AI) in the healthcare system. Privacy and security are an important factor of EHR adoption and/or implementation. A key component of EHR adoption and/or implementation is the privacy and security. When a patient goes to see a physician, each time the physicians update the patient's records, it is important since the records contain pertinent health and wellness details from the patient, as well as a timeline of the care received to date(Alruwaili, 2020). The concept of security and privacy is stressed in relation to collecting, managing and sharing EHR data. Such innovations provide a level of demand for securing medical records during use and transfer that had previously been unheard-of. The purpose of this EHR is to enhance the security of patient medical data monitoring and retention capabilities. This includes all of the patients' medical history, current health status, demographic information, etc. These records are required by research, hospitals, emergency departments, medical laboratories, and even health insurance companies.(Alruwaili, 2020).

1.2 Importance of EHR in Metabolic Medicines

EHRs, or electronic health records, are critical to metabolic medicine by improving the treatment, tracking and future outcomes of long-term metabolic diseases such as diabetes, metabolic syndrome, and dyslipidaemia. Artificial intelligence in medicine can help improve data precision and analysis. Traditional data management depends on human effort which is often prone to errors(Paraschiv et al., 2024). The information contained in EHRs is used not only to help guide management and health policy decisions; data contained in EHRs also supports decision-making for different areas of patient care (Kadambi et al., 2018).

- Enhanced Diabetes Quality of Care

EHR systems have been correlated to improved diabetes management and greater compliance with clinical guidelines. A study published in the "New England Journal of Medicine" showed that compared to practices using paper records, those using EHRs provided diabetic patients with improved treatment, greater percentage of recommended care processes were prescribed and improved outcomes(Cebul et al., 2011).

- Improved Tracking and Monitoring

It has been shown that incorporating clinical standards within EHRs improves monitoring of urgent health indicators in diabetic patients. The systematic review noted this association improved blood pressure and cholesterol management and increased screening for microvascular complications.(Shah et al., 2021).

- Facilitating Population Health Management and Research

The use of EHRs will provide significant advantages to clinical research and community health management. EHRs allow for the retrieval and analysis of large volumes of data, which will enhance the feasibility of examining disease trends, determining the level of treatment and efficacy of treatments for metabolic disorders. (Shen et al., 2020).

- Advancements in Personalized Medicine

EHRs will help advance personalized medicine by allowing the customization of genetic information, or other personalized information, to be available in a patient's care. This capability supports customized treatment plans for individuals with metabolic diseases (Cebul et al., 2011).

1.3 Role of Artificial Intelligence in Health Care

The field of healthcare continues to change as artificial intelligence (AI) improves efficiency, reduces costs, and improves diagnosis and personalised treatment. AI is influencing/had influenced human decisions in predictive analytics and telemedicine; this teams will provide better choices and better patient outcomes. The classic applications of AI in healthcare include precision medicine, robotic surgery, and chatbots(Padmavathi, 2022). Communicating with patients in the simplest way can be done using chatbots. They can be useful in some aspects of healthcare including scheduling appointments with specialists, and answering questions related to illness and prescriptions. However, in practice, they are not too useful because patients are still uncomfortable communicating with computers and find them to be unreliable(Padmavathi, 2022).

1.3.1 Medical Imaging and Diagnostic Services

Analyzing echocardiogram and ECG charts with tools like AI is a clever and promising way for cardiologists to help support their decision-making. AI using body imaging modalities has produced some promising results for the early diagnosis of pneumonia, eye disease, and skin and breast cancer. Similarly, there seems to be an effective use of AI for identifying and screening for neurological conditions such as Parkinson's disease, as well as predicting psychotic episodes using speech patterns(Al Kuwaiti et al., 2023). In a more recent study screened for heart patterns, machine learning algorithms were used to predict the onset of diabetes. In this study, it found that the most predictive model for predicting the various domains of diabetes was a two-class augmented decision tree.(Al Kuwaiti et al., 2023).

1.3.2 AI for Drug Discovery

Healthcare industries using AI technologies have made it possible for pharmaceutical companies to improve the drug research timeline. While it does automate the target identification process. AI has also made it possible to re-purpose drugs by analyzing the off-target compounds. Therefore AI-assisted discovery makes routine work faster and eliminates it in the areas of artificial intelligence and healthcare(Talati, 2023).

1.3.3 Precision Medicine

Using algorithm-based machine learning to accurately diagnose a medical issue is known as precision medicine. The majority of these diagnoses are based on collections of previously gathered datasets, including laboratory tests, signs and symptoms, and radiological and pathological pictures. Although AI diagnosis accuracy is comparatively high, patient data sharing remains a contentious medical ethical issue(Padmavathi, 2022).

1.3.4 Remote Patient Monitoring

Remote patient monitoring (RPM) is one form of telemedicine with the ability to track, assess and report on patients' status. RPM uses communications technologies and sensors to minimize the uncertainty surrounding medication actions. RPM creates a means for remote assessment of patient challenges and health records. The effectiveness of traditional patient monitoring system relies on how much time healthcare professionals (HCPs) take and the volume of work they have on-hand. (Al Kuwaiti et al., 2023).

1.3.5 Clinical Research

In clinical research, the participants are given newly created drugs to evaluate their effectiveness always this has taken a long time and expense to reach that step, however the success rates are very low. In summary, digitalization in clinical trials has been shown to benefit AI and Health Care. In addition, medical care and support from artificial intelligence. Clinical studies with AI can utilize huge datasets and generate very accurate results. Artificial intelligence may aid in the development of clinical outcomes and efficiency and may also reduce the length of clinical study cycles(Talati, 2023).

1.3.6 Patient Engagement

Patient engagement and adherence has always been the "final stretch" challenge of healthcare and represents the last barrier to improving health outcomes. Individuals clearly have better health outcomes, including healthcare utilization, cost, and patient experience when they are meaningfully engaged in their care (Al Kuwaiti et al., 2023). Healthcare practitioners develop treatment plans with the aid of their clinical judgment to improve health for patients with acute or chronic illnesses. In general, it doesn't much matter if a patient doesn't follow a treatment plan, or control their body weight, or follow up on an appointment(Al Kuwaiti et al., 2023).

1.4 Objectives of the Chapter

The potential for artificial intelligence (AI) to revolutionize electronic health records (EHRs) addresses how decisional support, predictive analytics, and predictive care will enhance clinical judgement and patient outcomes across multiple healthcare domains. This chapter summarizes relevant existing use cases in order to illuminate the potential of AI powered EHRs. Further, the chapter considers how these systems can improve care providers' administrative efficiencies, workflow optimization, and documentation accuracy in order to support system governance and even direct care. Finally, the chapter evaluates the interoperability and effectiveness of AI powered EHR systems with other digital health platforms, with implications for future strategies towards successful AI adoption and equity in healthcare delivery.

2 FUNDAMENTALS OF ELECTRONIC HEALTH RECORDS (EHRS)

The overall concepts and essential components that dictate how Electronic Health Records (EHRs) will function in a healthcare environment are defined as the EHR fundamentals. EHRs are basically a paper patient chart in digital form; stored and evaluated electronically. The fundamental aim and intention of EHRs are to enhance patient care, quality, safety, efficiency, care coordination and communication.

2.1 History and Evolution

Medical records have been around for as long as there has been health care. We can look back into history and see that, in the early days of medical records, physicians documented disease and likely aetiology. In the early 20th century, medical information was documented on three-by-five cards(Seymour et al., 2012). Through the auspices of federal legislative efforts to establish Medicare in the 1960s and 1970s, the healthcare industry was going through rapid and enthusiastic changes(Seymour et al., 2012). Simultaneously, stricter regulations for the healthcare industry were slowly becoming codified. Other third-party payers were also gaining traction, and disagreement about the course of action in healthcare began to emerge. While all of this was happening, patients began to care about the quality of healthcare they were to receive(Seymour et al., 2012). Healthcare providers were hesitant to embrace electronic health records.

When Congress passed the American Recovery and Investment Act of 2009, it was estimated that less than 8% of hospitals had electronic health records. Healthcare providers that were incentivized to migrate away from paper-based records and adopt EHR systems that are provided under this legislation. The federal government continues to offer incentives to all healthcare providers(Seymour et al., 2012).

EHRs became broadly adopted in the 2010s because of governmental incentives and the acknowledgement that EHRs could improve quality, safety, and efficiency in healthcare delivery. Interoperability, which is the ability of different EHR systems to exchange and analyse shared data, has been one of the central areas of focus (Shen et al., 2024).

2.2 Comparison of Traditional EHR and AI Enhanced EHR

Table 1. Traditional EHR vs AI Enhanced EHR

Feature	Traditional EHR	AI Enhanced EHR
Clinical Decision Support	Populated manually by healthcare personnel; slow and error-prone	AI can automate data entry through voice recognition, NLP, and intelligent forms.
Data Entry	Rule-based alerts and reminders (often encompassing)	AI provides predictive and personalized insights using real-time data sources.
Data Search and Retrieval	Basic searching; often keyword based	AI provides smart and context-aware search and summarizes the patient's history

continued on following page

Table 1. Continued

Feature	Traditional EHR	AI Enhanced EHR
Documentation	Typed or dictated notes; manual review and updates necessary	Automated documentation with real-time note development with suggestions.
Patient risk Prediction	Relies on limited, static data	AI provides real-time data-driven risk predictions (ex. sepsis, readmission).
Workflow Efficiency	Many disparate tasks; limited automation	Automates repetitive tasks, priorities actions, and remains aware of clinician workflows
Alert System	Many alerts, frequent generic alerts (alert fatigue common)	Alerts based on context (prioritized dimensionally as urgent and relevant)
Population Health Management	Static reports and historical data	Real-time trend analysis and cohort detection/ identification using machine learning
Patient engagement	Basic portals for appointments, record	Interactive, chatbots, and personalized health insights using artificial intelligence
Usability and User Experience	Often crowded interfaces; difficult to navigate	Intuitive interfaces with streamlined functionality while interacting and compounding knowledge with adaptive AI responsiveness

2.3 Components of EHRs

There are many types of information that comprise EHR data, including subjects of care identification, demographics, health history, clinical summaries, problem lists and diagnoses, diagnostic values and interpretation, care plans/decision support, treatments, consent, vital signs and alerts, provider identifiers, clinical documentation for chronic disease, encounters, vaccinations, primary care, community care, and quality and safety information.(Katehakis & Tsiknakis, 2006).

Key Components of EHRs

• Documentation of Patients

Every face-to-face interaction that occurs during a patient-physician encounter must be documented in the electronic health record. The documentation must efficient and simple because the physician has a community of patients to serve, and limited time. The integrated health record includes physician orders, prescription drug orders, laboratory results, x-ray and radiography reports and other care delivery(Seymour et al., 2012).

• Quality Assurance

By utilizing the EHR, hospitals and physicians will have the data they need to maintain compliance with various government and insurance company requirements. The EHR stores a singular source for all medical orders for lab, x-ray, and other tests.

Additionally, this data can be monitored to see if the physician is ordering appropriate tests for the patient.(Seymour et al., 2012).

- Regulatory Use and Safety Monitoring

Since active post-marketing safety surveillance and signal detection offer data on actual drug use and incidence rates (as opposed to spontaneous event reporting), they represent significant new applications for EHRs. The European Medicines Agency (EMA) is coordinating the European Network of Centres for Pharmacoepidemiology and Pharmacovigilance (ENCePP), which intends to do post marketing risk assessment using a variety of EHR source data(Cowie et al., 2017).

- Communication and telecommunication facilities

A technology infrastructure must be established before health information can be transferred among the various stakeholders involved in health care. Ensuring privacy, security, and confidentiality of health information while allowing appropriate use of that information is incumbent upon HICT leadership as well as state and federal governing authority(Moghaddasi et al., 2011).

- Coding and Billing

Accurate medical coding refers to the proper description of the patient's health issue (Seymour et al., 2012). Medical coding also determines the patient's bill. Improper billing stems directly from improper coding. Billing mistakes could put the healthcare provider at risk of fraud fines by creating problems with Medicare and the insurance companies. EHR technology solves for correct documentation and contains diagnosis databases to enable coders and billers to accurately create medical claims. (Seymour et al., 2012).

- Confidentiality

The Health Insurance Portability and Accountability Act (HIPPA) provided specific rules to protect the security and privacy of electronic health records in the US (Moghaddasi et al., 2011). HIPPA security standards identify three categories of protections: administrative controls, technical controls, and physical controls. In transit, data could be de-identified, encrypted, and re-identified for the correct authorized use; and information systems in compliance with confidentiality and security standards specified by various organizations include E1762, E1869, ISO27000, and ISO17799(Moghaddasi et al., 2011).

Figure 1. Various components of Electronic Health Records (EHRs)

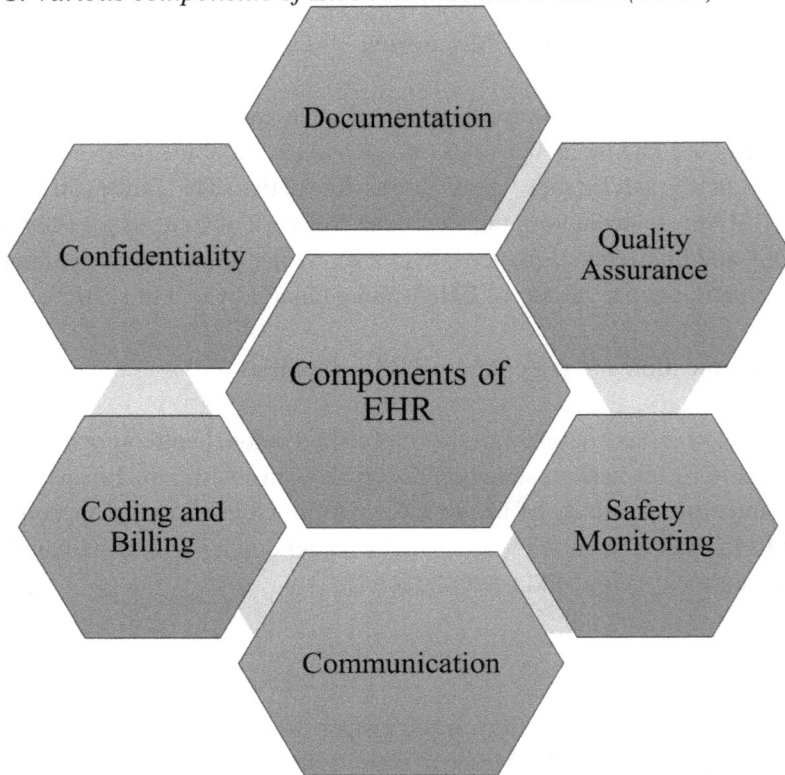

2.4 Challenges in Current EHR System

Many studies highlight how EHR may enhance the quality-of-care delivery in medicine, however there are a number of established downsides—including, inconsistent practices, ineffective work, less collaboration, additional cognitive burden, medical errors, and diminished quality of care. This highlights the need for robust quality EHR education (Kim et al., 2014). Healthcare professionals devoted a significant amount of time using EHR during work shifts based on the expansive adoption of EHR's across all components of the treatment process.(Tsai et al., 2020).

Efficiency was markedly impaired (i.e., surgical case turnover time increased) with the introduction of EHRs; this impairment continued for forty weeks. Workflow steps and efficiency were being costs due to not considering critical features that established usability and functionality of EHRs that support the care team's workflow efficiency related to valuable things like shared lab results, prescription lists, chronic illness and preventive health management etc.(Tsai et al., 2020). Clinicians were worried that doctors and nurses were going to be at arm's length or lose the opportunity for verbal communication of important details. There was also miscommunication mentioned when healthcare providers documented patient information, with complete attention paid to what they were writing in the EHRs to assume the information would be available to their colleagues, only to learn that their colleagues had not read the notes(Tsai et al., 2020). When workload is major, clinicians can make mistakes when submitting clinical observations. Also, since imputation methods can result in bias, it is important to consider that EHR data may be "missing not at random." Hence it may be prudent to use caution when dealing with EHR observations, because heuristic checks can obviously cause downstream bias(Honeyford et al., 2022).

2.5 EHRs in Metabolic Disease Management

Electronic Health Records (EHRs) are critical for managing metabolic diseases through better patient monitoring, personalized treatment, and improving data accessibility. Because they support better data collection and monitoring, electronic health records (EHRs), together with other digital tools, have become integral components of the management of metabolic disorders(Stanton et al., 2016). One key advantage of EHRs is their ability to aggregate relevant data in a standardised, centralised format for metabolic health. They speed up the process of treatment by converting paper-based methods and, therefore, allowing better tracking of important parameters associated with metabolic syndrome such as blood pressure, triglycerides, glucose levels, and waist circumference(Stanton et al., 2016). The usability and effectiveness of the system was established through iterative testing and showed high levels of user satisfaction and efficiency; two vital elements of continued patient participation on the management of chronic diseases(Farinango et al., 2018).

Beyond data management, eHealth platforms and EHRs offer clinical advantages. Patients with metabolic syndrome demonstrated notable improvements on anthropometric parameters such as body mass index, waist circumference, and systolic blood pressure, according to a meta-analysis of randomised controlled trials. These findings suggest that when properly implemented and created with patient/user needs in mind, eHealth tools—more especially, EHR-integrated tools—can significantly enhance health-promoting behaviours and clinical outcomes(D. Chen et al., 2020).

Electronic Health Records (EHRs) are helpful in the treatment of Metabolic Dysfunction-Associated Steatotic Liver Disease (MASLD). With non-invasive tests (NITs) supplanting invasive liver biopsies for diagnosis, EHRs enable the collection and processing of meaningful laboratory and imaging data. Digital platforms have also incorporated features such as the FIB-4 index to help identify patients who may be at risk for advanced fibrosis and to facilitate follow-up and referrals(Alkhouri & Noureddin, 2024).

3 OVERVIEW OF ARTIFICIAL INTELLIGENCE IN HEALTHCARE

3.1 Definitions and Subfields

Artificial Intelligence (AI) is when computers or machines act and learn like people. They can assist people and enable them to do things quicker and easier by helping to solve problems, develop choices, and even make sense of words or images. It includes several sub-fields such as:

● Expert Systems

Computer programs designed to act like human specialists. They use rule-based logic to evaluate information and provide recommendations or make decisions. Typically, in health care expert systems are used to diagnosis disease and/or plan treatment(Sigatapu et al., 2020).

● Networks of Neural System

Artificial Neural Networks (ANNs), which reflect various features of the human brain, have great value in detecting patterns and relationships in data. ANNs have been used for medical imaging processing, diagnosis, and risk prediction(Talati, 2023).

● Natural Language Processing (NLP)

Natural Language Processing (NLP) is a process by which a computer understands, interprets, and responds to human language. NLP provides great usefulness for clinical reasoning in health care by extracting meaningful information from research articles, clinical notes, and patient histories(Talati, 2023).

- Machine Learning (ML)

Machine Learning is referred to as creating an algorithm that allows machines to learn from data, to predict the outcome. ML has popular applications to predict patient outcomes, detect diseases early, and efficiencies in hospitals(Sigatapu et al., 2020).

- Deep Learning

Deep Learning is an approach that allows computers to learn to recognize patterns in data using a series of abstraction layers, or cognitive levels. It allows machines to learn to recognize for example, a face in a picture, the voice in a recording, or an illness in a medical image etc. In each of these types of recognition, there are example data used, like how humans progressively learn from experience.(Sigatapu et al., 2020)(Talati, 2023).

3.2 Machine Learning and Deep Learning

Predictive analytics, disease risk modelling, and treatment optimisation, are a fairly established area of the medical field using machine learning (ML). The ML concepts are very straightforward as summarised below:

- Supervised Learning: Learning algorithms that predict the future using labelled training data.
- Unsupervised Learning: Learning algorithms that find hidden patterns in unlabelled data.
- Reinforcement Learning: Learning algorithms that learn the best strategies using feedback mechanisms.

Deep Learning is an even more advanced algorithm that uses multi-layered neural networks to tackle very complex medical issues and medical problems such as diagnosis of radiological data and image recognition. Deep learning really improves performance in the following processes like radiology, oncology and drug discovery(Sigatapu et al., 2020; Padmavathi, 2022; Talati, 2023).

3.3 Natural Language of Processing

Through NLP, AI systems can take unstructured clinical text - like physician notes or discharge summaries - and find insights of meaning. Examples of applications include: Clinical decision support, Automated documentation, Patient sentiment analysis, Information retrieval from EHRs.

Healthcare is a large area of usage of NLP-based tools, especially as the processing of textual data supports applications for diagnosis, as well as administrative purposes(Sigatapu et al., 2020).

3.4 AI Application in Metabolic Medicine

AI has already shown active involvement in the identification, treatment, and tracking of metabolic diseases (as examples):

- Drug Discovery: AI speeds drug discovery of metabolic disease. Sanofi uses AI (through Exscientia) to find metabolic drugs(Talati, 2023).
- Precision Medicine: Using genetic and lifestyle data, machine learning tools are being developed to optimize treatment pathways.
- Clinical Trials: AIs help to enhance the logistics of planning and executing clinical studies for metabolic drugs, by maintaining a library of eligible participants and predicting responses to treatment(Talati, 2023).
- Robotic and Assistive Care: Robotics are supporting rehabilitation and care for chronic metabolic disorders due to obesity and diabetes(Padmavathi, 2022).

AI-SaMD's architecture is governed by quality standards, and follows a multi-layered approach. A multi-layered architecture can enable incremental development from a software-intensive systems perspective (Ebad et al., 2025). Once a layer is developed, its services will be available to users, and they can also be developed effectively to be exchanged and used by other layers of the system. Overall, we also have a highly reconfigurable and portable architecture. At a high level, our architecture segmentalizes the system into usable functional hierarchical layers. Layers provide services to their layers above, and we can think of some lower-level layers providing a core service to the system as a whole(Ebad et al., 2025).

Figure 2. AI-SaMD layers have additional complexity factors that should be implemented for aspects of the product development lifecycle such as explainability, continuous learning, inference, and model training while also respecting the underlying health software protocols. This additional complexity is what differentiates the architecture and adds sophisticated AI potential. AI significantly powers this architecture's ability to evaluate dynamic data-intense tasks.

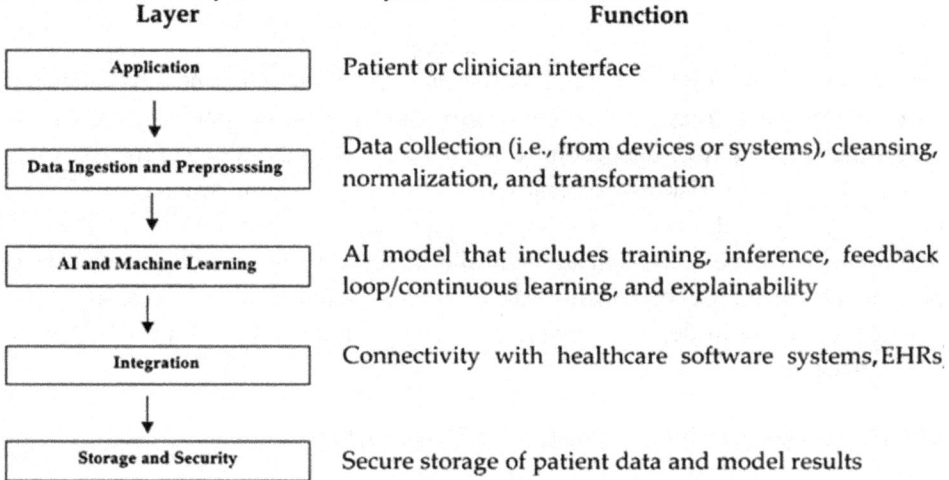

Layer	Function
Application	Patient or clinician interface
Data Ingestion and Preprosssssing	Data collection (i.e., from devices or systems), cleansing, normalization, and transformation
AI and Machine Learning	AI model that includes training, inference, feedback loop/continuous learning, and explainability
Integration	Connectivity with healthcare software systems, EHRs
Storage and Security	Secure storage of patient data and model results

Source: Ebad et al. (2025).

4 SYNERGY BETWEEN AI AND EHRS

The intersection of AI and Electronic Health Records (EHRs) supports health care innovation by converting big data of patients into novel solutions to real-world problems. Artificial Intelligence (AI) leverages EHR data to forecast risk, inform clinical decisions, deliver personalized medicine, and automate administrative tasks. Natural Language Processing (NLP) and Artificial Intelligence (AI) can also convert unstructured clinical notes into meaningful information that can help the efficiency and quality of patient treatment.

4.1 AI-Driven ERH Optimization

AI facilitates the transformation of EHRs from passive records to intelligent, evolving, and adaptive systems. EHR systems that leverage AI redefine EHRs by dynamically assessing intricate collaborative, clinical, behavioural, and demographic data to uncover patterns that promote improved care delivery and increased organizational efficiency, along with enhanced predictive and prescriptive insight. For instance, with embedded technology, AI helps EHRs seamlessly and continuously learn from clinical records so the decision support systems dynamically monitor conditions at the patient level(Reddy Kotha et al., 2024).

4.2 Predictive Analysis and Risk Stratification

Predictive analytics using machine learning and data mining can help clinicians identify potentially high-risk patients and predict patient outcomes. AI models incorporate multiple sources of data, including clinical results, socioeconomic status, etc., to provide a more in-depth contextualized view of a patient's risk profile(Bennett et al., 2012). These risk assessment tools allow for real-time stratification of risk to identify high-risk patients so they can receive prioritized clinical intervention, optimizing resource utilization and minimizing preventable harm. AI models incorporate multiple sources of data, including clinical results, socioeconomic status, etc., to provide a more in-depth contextualized view of a patient's risk profile (Bennett et al., 2012).

4.3 Real-Time Clinical Decision Support

Artificial intelligence (AI) is enabling electronic health records (EHRs) to deliver real-time clinical decision support (CDS) by changing recommendations for treatment based on patient data. Instead of static, rule-based systems, AI-enabled clinical decision support tools learn in real-time from ongoing clinical use and performance, continually changing algorithms without a delay between research and practice(Pantelis, n.d.). This "adaptive" clinical decision support attempts to minimize the deficiencies of generic treatment guidelines and increase clinical relevance. Real-time data integration facilitates feedback loops which allow AI systems to alert clinicians to changes to treatment, risks emerging, or care deviations. These systems can provide essential support in environments where rapid clinical response is required such as pandemic management or chronic disease follow-up(Haddad et al., 2022)

4.4 Personalization of Care Pathways

EHR systems can move from a one-size-fits-all approach to personalised care pathways by leveraging the analytical capabilities of AI. This is done with AI-selected multimodal data, including genetics, clinical, and socio-behavioral data, to develop treatment plans that take into account each patient's unique context and any comorbidities. The combination of blockchain and AI has the potential to create more individualized healthcare by securing patient data across decentralized networks that facilitate real time data updates and adaptive treatment recommendations without sacrificing confidentiality(Bennett et al., 2012; Haddad et al., 2022)

5 APPLICATION IN METABOLIC MEDICINE

5.1 Diabetes Mellitus

Artificial intelligence (AI) has played an important role in the management of "Type 2 Diabetes Mellitus" (T2DM) in predicting disease remission after bariatric surgery and identifying metabolic biomarkers. For example, Cao et al. utilized a Gaussian Bayesian Network (GBN) model to predict five-years of T2DM remission after bariatric surgery with an "Area under the curve" (AUC) of 0.942 which surpassed traditional models(Barberis et al., 2022). Furthermore, metabolomics coupled with machine learning (ML) has been used to differentiate among diabetes phenotypes. Complex computational algorithms similar to random forest (RF) and artificial neural networks (ANNs) have been used to assess type 2 diabetes (T2DM) outcomes using complex biological data, or omics data. These methodologies have proven to be highly accurate and assist healthcare providers to develop more individualized treatment plans for their patients.(Barberis et al., 2022).

5.2 Obesity and Metabolic Syndrome

Obesity and Metabolic Syndrome (MS) have emerged as significant targets for AI application due to the rapidly increasing of both the prevalence and the complexity of a multifactorial, evolving disease. In order to formulate association models between the MS and the Traditional Chinese Medicine (TCM) constitution and other clinical variables, specifically blood glucose, blood cholesterol and waist circumference, artificial intelligence (AI) techniques including logistic regression, decision trees and Bayesian networks were used(Ghosh et al., 2024). Machine learning models can also help physicians to quickly identify and prevent health issues. For instance, Random Forest and SVM are tools that have been used to discover specific indicators in the body, called biomarkers, that are associated with obesity and high cholesterol, and the models incorporate a significant amount of health data to build improved predictor models and facilitate initiating treatment sooner(Chien et al., 2021).

5.3 Non-Alcoholic Fatty Liver Disease (NAFLD)

Utilizing patient data and blood biomarkers, AI techniques, namely Random Forest (RF) and Support Vector Machine (SVM) algorithms, have been applied to evaluate liver fibrosis and diagnose non-alcoholic fatty liver disease (NAFLD). When serum measures (transaminases, hyaluronic acid, and markers of cell death) and RF were used to predict the degree of liver fibrosis in NAFLD patients prior to bariatric surgery, it was shown that individuals who had results from multiple tests exhibited better predictive values than those with only one test. Uehara et al. took this application one step further, by creating a rule-based AI model to diagnose Non-Alcoholic Steatohepatitis (NASH) non-invasively in obese Japanese patients. Their AI system was based on ALT, CRP, HOMA-IR, and albumin, and performed better than most traditional statistical models with regard to diagnostic sensitivity and specificity. Validation of metabolomic profiling with AI, specifically deep learning, have identified biomarkers of NAFLD based on visceral adipose tissue(Pantelis, 2022).

5.4 Dyslipidemia and Cardiometabolic Risk

Dyslipidemia means having too much fat (like triglycerides) or too little good cholesterol (HDL) in the blood. It is a critical component of a health issue called Metabolic Syndrome and can later lead to heart disease. AI tools such as SVM, ANN, and Decision Trees are used to help identify and manage fat-related issues as early as possible. Bayesian Network (BN) models are intelligent computer programs that can predict health outcomes(Ghosh et al., 2024). When the BN model is utilized with patient data, it can accurately predict whether a person's cholesterol problem (dyslipidemia) will improve following weight-loss surgery. Deep learning models coupled with wearable sensor data and electronic health records have enabled dynamic cardiometabolic risk assessment. For instance, researchers using feature fusion and ensemble DL models effectively predicted heart disease in obese patients with metabolic syndrome while highlighting the future applications of AI in health surveillance(Ghosh et al., 2024).

5.5 AI Models used in Metabolic Disease Prediction Using ERH Data

Table 2 provides a summary of how different AI models have been used to study different metabolic diseases using EHR data. For each condition, the table presents the AI methods used (e.g., logistic regression, neural networks), the EHR data investigated (e.g., lab tests, BMI, medications), and the relevant clinical purpose of the AI study including prediction, classification, or risk(J. H. Chen & Asch, 2017; Hossain et al., 2024; Miotto et al., 2016).

Table 2.

Metabolic Disease	AI Model Type	EHR Data Used	Purpose
Type 2 Diabetes	Logistic Regression, Random Forest, Neural Networks	Demographics, lab results (HbA1c, glucose), medications, BMI, diagnoses	Early prediction, risk scoring, patient stratification
Obesity	Decision Trees, Super Vector Machine (SVM), Deep Learning	Weight, body mass index (BMI), diet records, physical activity, comorbidities	Obesity risk classification, weight gain prediction
Hypertension	Random Forest, Gradient Boosting, Deep Neural Networks	Blood pressure readings, age, gender, lifestyle factors, medications	Early detection, treatment optimization
Cardiovascular disease	Logistic Regression, Echo Net-Dynamic, AI-ECG Platform	Lab data, ECG readings, medical history, cholesterol levels, smoking status	Prediction of events (e.g., stroke), risk stratification
Dyslipidemia	Logistic Regression, Ensemble Models	Lipid panel, age, gender, medications, diagnosis codes	Identification of high-risk individuals

6. CASE STUDIES AND IMPLEMENTATION MODELS

Models illustrate how Artificial Intelligence (AI) and Electronic Health Records (EHRs) could be combined, with attention to clinical care and chronic disease management such as metabolic disease:

6.1 Mayo Clinic AI EHR Integration

The health care industry is experiencing an enormous change in the current digital era due to the advances related to technology. Electronic health records (or EHR) are one of the earliest and most substantive technological developments that has changed how patient data is collected, stored, and accessed. They grant authorized healthcare professionals secure access to a patient's entire digital health record(Nelson R Saranya, 2024).

The Mayo Clinic suite includes complete custom solutions for clinicians, care teams, patients and consumers use. These solutions extend across patient engagement and to access, The acquisition will equip Agilon Health with a complete platform to deliver virtual care, care guidance platforms, and analytics.(Demaerschalk et al., 2023)

6.2 Kaiser Permanente Predictive Models

To reduce the clinical load on Clinicians, even when a high-risk patient had been identified based on the AAM score, a regional virtual quality nurse consultant (VQNC) was utilized to assist clinicians in the file review process. Based on standardised, dynamic criteria, which had been thoroughly validated by frontline input and oversight from front-line leadership, experienced nurses were also able to screen out patients for whom the appropriate treatment was already implemented when providing professional clinical assessments of patients at risk of declining(Martinez et al., 2022)

Medical vs surgical was determined by the department where the patient was admitted. The researchers first formed cohorts based upon diagnoses of interest, then used the cohort data to make models using a general method called logistic regression with special adjustments to allow for the impact of age, severity of illness, and chronic illnesses - including using a flexible method to model age.(van Walraven et al., 2010)

6.3 IBM Watson Health and Metabolic Care

In its long history, International Business Machine (IBM) has changed its identity many times, and now finds itself on a path towards the top cloud platform provider and cognitive solutions leader, with IBM Watson - a cognitive computing technology - paving the way. Way before Watson was a chess playing computer program called Deep Blue(Yang et al., 2020)

The proposed project incorporates IBM Auto AI services. Auto AI decreases the time for experimentation. There is so much research being conducted with Auto AI taking on problems such as classification, and other applications in seemingly every field. Auto AI does automation for the entire life cycle of AI i.e. from data prep to hyper-parameter optimization. Auto AI also does model building and feature engineering, etc. with one-click deployment.(Sumalata et al., 2024)

7 ETHICAL, LEGAL AND REGULATORY CONSIDERATIONS

7.1 Legal and Policy Framework

- The Rules and Act on Information Technology: Sensitive Personal Data or Information (SPDI) of a person is defined by the Data Protection Rules as such personal data, including information that relates to passwords; financial information; medical Records, Medical History and Biometric data; sexual orientation; and the physical, mental and psychological conditions of a person(D. Jain, 2023).

- DNA Technology (Use and Application) Regulation Bills: The main goal of the proposed legislation is "The extension of utilising DNA-based forensic technologies to facilitate and strengthen the justice delivery system of the country provide for the mandatory accreditation and the regulation of DNA laboratories throughout the country" (D. Jain, 2023).
- Health data management regulations: The proposed policy aimed to create a system for optional digital personal and medical records which would be based on individual informed consent and allow for secure transfer of health data while protecting information to adequate privacy level (D. Jain, 2023).
- Telemedicine Practice Guidelines: The guidelines require physicians to provide teleconsultations in the same way and with the same standard of care as they would an in-person consultation, and also impose a duty on patients to provide accurate information to medical professionals.(D. Jain, 2023).

7.2 Data Privacy and Security

When we are looking at security and privacy in the context of big data, we are looking at a very big discussion. The big data security model is not suggested due to the complexity of the applications, and will be turned off by default. Without a large data security model, data compromise is relatively easy. Therefore, throughout this section, the topics of privacy and security will be highlighted(P. Jain et al., 2016)

Assume that the supplier is an Internet user, and he is worried that he may to compromise his privacy through his online activities. The user can try to erase the data of his online activities by deleting cookies, clearing out the cache of his browser, deleting records of application usage, and other measures in order to protect his privacy. The provider may use a variety of security options specifically designed for the Internet environment to protect his data. For simplicity, a host of security options are made available as browser extensions(Lei Xu et al., 2014)

7.3 Regulatory Landscape (HIPAA, GDPR)

The functionality of HIPAA included robust penalties associated with non-compliance, the settlements and fines have demonstrated the federal oversight surrounding patient data protection. The implications of HIPAA and GDPR in terms of regulations, compliance, and accountability also provide insight into healthcare IT acquisitions and investments. Healthcare organizations across the globe have invested significant resources to improve cybersecurity and to comply with HIPPA and GDPR.(Gupta, 2020)

7.4 Future of AI Ethics in Health Data

It has been shown that most data breaches come from human error. Healthcare institutions must provide training and education to their personnel. Employees must be fully cognizant of whenever they process personal health data and the risks associated with security. Risk assessments should also be conducted on a regular basis, through which healthcare institutions could identify inherent limitations - such as any security breaches with data - and ultimately mitigate those limitations. There should be limited access of health records to patient's certified healthcare personnel, and access again restricted, for better confidentiality and security of data. Healthcare institutions could look at strengthening their authentication, looking at two-factor authentication as a best practice.(Bouderhem, 2024)

8 BARRIERS TO ADOPTION AND PRACTICAL CHALLENGES

There are various issues that make implementing AI in healthcare complicated. First, AI needs patient data so protecting that data must be made a priority. In addition, hospitals often have dim hits of data, which makes it impossible for AI tools to perform optimally. New AI technologies must rapidly interface with legacy healthcare systems to achieve interoperability. There are many reasons to point out that implementing healthcare AI is a complex endeavour.

8.1 Technical Interoperability

- Fragmented buying practices: All hospitals and clinics buy new digital devices in their own way so it is very hard for startups to plug their technology into many systems. A lack of understanding of the rules or process to get their products approved and operational in hospitals is the norm for many business owners(Olaye & Seixas, 2023).
- Difficulty in reaching decision makers: Finding and contacting the right people who are technology decision makers, is another challenge for startups that complicates the ability to integrate their products with hospital systems(Olaye & Seixas, 2023).
- Connecting With Decision Makers Can Be Challenging: Many new business owners are unsure of who to target in hospitals to get their equipment connected or approved. Due to this uncertainty, connecting their products to hospitals' systems becomes even more difficult(Olaye & Seixas, 2023).

EHRs, imaging archives, pathology databases, and insurance systems, all represent silos of healthcare data and makes the process of gathering data for AI acquisition and training, are a difficult proposition since it is very fragmented. In the study, even though interoperability, such as using standards like Fast Healthcare Interoperability Resources (FHIR), is mentioned as an advantage; interoperability, or even if a situation developed where there was semantic coding in EHRs that was more consistent, interoperability cannot go far enough to solve these issues(Kelly et al., 2019).

8.2 Infrastructure and Cost

- High Cost of Validation: Many start-ups lack the funds to publish data or conduct the expensive testing of RCTs due to proprietary constraints, which is what makes clinical buy-ins difficult(Olaye & Seixas, 2023). Once the AI system is in place, continuous updates and ongoing performance management are usually indicated, particularly for models that are learning and evolving. This will increase the complexity of updating and the long-term cost of maintaining an AI model. This will require healthcare organizations to change its operating procedures and develop its own infrastructure to continue to manage the monitoring, re-leveling, or retraining of models when the data changes(Kelly et al., 2019).
- Sales and Marketing Costs: The entrepreneur's thought process suggests that breaking into the health systems market often requires attending trade shows, industry conferences, and networking engagements, which are all very expensive and resource-heavy tasks(Olaye & Seixas, 2023).
- Regulatory compliance presents another challenge. A large number of AI systems are designed to learn continuously, or more practically, develop and change/product over time. This approach does not fit into traditional regulatory requirements in which assumptive behaviour is treated as fixed. The ongoing constraints of compliance mean repeat evaluations of performance and updates to the performance evaluation process and will incur costs beyond those referenced(Kelly et al., 2019).

8.3 Resistance from Clinicians

- Complexity and Unfamiliarity: Clinicians may struggle to accept and trust technologies because they do not fully understand how they work, especially because AI systems can make decisions that modify how clinicians provide care(Jena et al., 2024).

- Insufficient Trust and Explainability: The report indicate that AI systems are often inscrutable, particularly when it comes to the ways that decisions are made by AI systems. This fusion of complexity and uncertainty is at the heart of clinician resistance. In clinical situations, decisions must be interpretable and defensible (an obvious implication for informed consent); if a clinician cannot explain or defend a system's recommendation for an action, they are unlikely to act on the recommendation(Jena et al., 2024).
- AI systems based on deep learning can often function as "black boxes" with inscrutable internal decision-making logic, rendering them difficult to interpret. Clinicians may feel uncomfortable or suspicious about AI having a lack of transparency, especially when they are called to use AI outputs to inform important decisions about patient care(Kelly et al., 2019).
- Changes to Workflow: AI induction often disturbs clinical processes, and clinicians often feel uncomfortable altering work patterns or routines that they feel comfortable with. AI also misfires and creates a large number of alerts to users, often so many that the user simply ignores them or switches them off altogether. There is also a lack of formal training of clinicians on how to use and evaluate AI tools, contributing to a poor uptake and an overall lack of comfort with the technology(Rahimi et al., 2024).

8.4 Data Standardization Issues

AI systems, particularly in the health sciences, need many instances of clean, accurate, and uniformly formatted data to function properly. The most significant barrier mentioned in the document, is the standardization of data which poses a challenge to successful implementation of AI(Jena et al., 2024).

- Inconsistent and Disconnected Data Sources

Patient data is often found in multiple places (EHRs, lab systems, imaging devices) in different formats and disrupted organisation in real-world hospital systems. Due to this, collecting and analysing data is often challenging for AI. Poorly standardised data can produce, for instance, inaccurate predictions, data loss or misinterpretations(Jena et al., 2024).

- Impact on Scalability and Reliability of AI

Without data standardization, AI technologies are not applied effectively across institutions or patient groups. Variations in system design, labelling conventions, or data types preclude the function from one hospital being used in another. As a result, a great deal of the healthcare industry's ability to exploit AI technologies is impeded(Jena et al., 2024). AI requires good data and the data needs to be standardized. Poor standardization of inputs leads to biased, unreliable models that will work well in one setting but fail in another(Kelly et al., 2019).

- Poor Data Quality

Healthcare AI systems often underperform because the data they are trained on are messy; they are often incomplete, incorrectly labelled or not explicitly coded. The ability to develop AI models that work reliably across institutions is further limited by the fact that hospitals all use different systems and processes for the collection and storage of data. One additional obstacle that could affect model performance is "dataset shift"—where there are variations in patient characteristics or practice over time—making dated data less useful to future care decisions(Rahimi et al., 2024).

9. FUTURE PROSPECTS AND RESEARCH DIRECTIONS

9.1 AI-Enhanced Smart EHRs

Analysis of Medical Imaging: Convolutional Neural Networks (CNNs) are currently widely used in medical imaging and for segmentation, object classification, and image classification tasks. Examples of applications are:

- CNNs can be trained to detect patterns associated with a variety of medical abnormalities that help diagnose diseases, such as tumours or pneumonia, when using X-ray or CT scan imaging. CNNs perform histopathology image analysis on pathology slides to determine cancer type, assess grade and identify location.(Jhade et al., 2024).
- Example of an algorithm: DenseNet (Densely Connected Convolutional Networks) is one of the more unified architectures for medical image analysis that is less demanding as to input for training more efficiently and utilizing features from previous layers more well. CNNs are also a helpful approach to learning patterns and related information from medical images that will be used for clinical decisions through methods like diagnosis or public health interventions.(Jhade et al., 2024)

9.2 Federated Learning and Edge AI

The Federated Learning server can support one or more multiple dimensions and many sizes of populations. Round must be able to accommodate many different types of even fully distributed procedures since it may have thousands of participants or hundreds of millions. FL populations ranging from dozens of clients to hundreds of millions of devices should be feasible within an FL server. The updates can vary from kilobytes to gigabytes, and each cycle might be ten more megabytes; the volume of traffic that can move through a space might vary dramatically over the hours of the day depending on when devices are loading and not loading (Abreha et al., 2022)

9.3 Role of Digital Twins

Digital twins are being adopted to enhance productivity (i.e. reducing product quality failures), manage failures (i.e. predictive monitoring of machinery status in real-time), and reduce expenditure (i.e. optimizing processes) in manufacturing more and more. The health-related industries have only seen, however, tepid acceptance of the idea of a digital twin. They argue that because the results achieved in manufacturing and smart cities have been positive, the health-related sectors will achieve positive results with digital twins too(Kaul et al., 2023)

9.4 Role of AI in Public Health for Metabolic Disorders

Artificial intelligence (AI), defined as the use of computers and technology to emulate intelligent behaviour and higher order mental processes, has taken major steps toward improving precision medicine, clinical decision-making and predictably responding to therapy in a variety of illness management situations. In the past decade, advancements in AI have unlikely promise for improvements in Metabolic Syndrome due to its association with metabolic changes that increase the risk of future diabetes mellitus, cardiovascular disease, and ultimately death from future neoplasm risk. Furthermore, studies have shown that lifestyle change is an effective way to reverse Metabolic Syndrome(Choubey et al., 2024)

10. CONCLUSION

10.1 Summary of Key Points

- Increased Predictive Capabilities: Using EHR data in conjunction with AI algorithms helps improve the prediction and early detection of metabolic diseases (e.g., diabetes, obesity, and dyslipidaemia) based on structured and unstructured data.

- Precision and Personalized Care: AI enables the development of personalized treatment plans which account for genetic markers, lifestyle data, and longitudinal health records.
- Clinical Decision Support: Real-time advanced analytics embedded in EHR systems leverage clinicians' capabilities to do the best job possible in challenging healthcare environments.
- Operational Efficiency: AI to filter and streamline administrative tasks, documentation, and decrease clinician burdens improve health delivery.
- Imaging and Diagnostics: AI imaging analytics that enhance imaging analytics produce high-quality, timely diagnosis and assessment of diseases like diabetic retinopathy and metabolic liver disease.

10.2 Strategic Recommendations

- Invest in Multimodal Data Infrastructure: Integrating EHR data with genomic, environmental, behavioral, and imaging data will help create full care models.
- Encourage Interoperability and Data Standards: To be able to effectively deploy scalable AI systems across institutions, there must be standardized and interoperable systems.
- Ethical and Legal Frameworks: Steps must be taken to prioritize data privacy, algorithmic transparency and fairness.
- Augment Workforce Training: Clinicians and health workforce staff must be digitally literate in order to understand and use data-driven results of AI.
- Increased Predictive Capabilities: Using EHR data in conjunction with AI algorithms helps improve the prediction and early detection of metabolic diseases (e.g., diabetes, obesity, and dyslipidaemia) based on structured and unstructured data.

10.3 AI-EHR Roadmap for Metabolic Medicine

- Advanced Imaging analytics: AI models can aid in forecasting when a disease may develop and how. They take a broad look at a person's medical history, health scans, and lifestyle habits, making them particularly useful where healthcare capacity is reduced.
- Rosk Prediction Models: In the eye care area, machine learning can analyze combinations of eye scans and medical histories to detect early problems

with glaucoma and diabetic retinopathy, leading to improved diagnosis and treatment of ocular diseases.

- Screening Efficiency: Validated algorithms increase screening efficiency and resource allocation, identifying individuals at risk for a condition earlier and elevating care priority.
- Scalable Applications: AI applications can facilitate scalable, high surgery accuracy applications that add to the clinical judgment in post-travel assessment of chronic metabolic issues.

REFERENCES

Abreha, H. G., Hayajneh, M., & Serhani, M. A. (2022). Federated Learning in Edge Computing: A Systematic Survey. In *Sensors* (Vol. 22, Issue 2). MDPI. DOI: 10.3390/s22020450

Al Kuwaiti, A., Nazer, K., Al-Reedy, A., Al-Shehri, S., Al-Muhanna, A., Subbarayalu, A. V., Al Muhanna, D., & Al-Muhanna, F. A. (2023). A Review of the Role of Artificial Intelligence in Healthcare. In *Journal of Personalized Medicine* (Vol. 13, Issue 6). MDPI. DOI: 10.3390/jpm13060951

Alkhouri, N., & Noureddin, M. (2024). Management strategies for metabolic dysfunction-associated steatotic liver disease (MASLD). *The American Journal of Managed Care*, 30(9, Suppl), S159–S174. DOI: 10.37765/ajmc.2024.89635

Alruwaili, F. F. (2020). Artificial intelligence and multi agent based distributed ledger system for better privacy and security of electronic healthcare records. *PeerJ. Computer Science*, 6, 1–14. DOI: 10.7717/PEERJ-CS.323

Barberis, E., Khoso, S., Sica, A., Falasca, M., Gennari, A., Dondero, F., Afantitis, A., & Manfredi, M. (2022). Precision Medicine Approaches with Metabolomics and Artificial Intelligence. In *International Journal of Molecular Sciences* (Vol. 23, Issue 19). MDPI. DOI: 10.3390/ijms231911269

Bennett, C. C., Doub, T. W., & Selove, R. (2012). EHRs connect research and practice: Where predictive modeling, artificial intelligence, and clinical decision support intersect. *Health Policy and Technology*, 1(2), 105–114. DOI: 10.1016/j. hlpt.2012.03.001

Bouderhem, R. (2024). Shaping the future of AI in healthcare through ethics and governance. *Humanities & Social Sciences Communications*, 11(1). Advance online publication. DOI: 10.1057/s41599-024-02894-w

Cebul, R. D., Love, T. E., Jain, A. K., & Hebert, C. J. (2011). Electronic Health Records and Quality of Diabetes Care. *The New England Journal of Medicine*, 365(9), 825–833. DOI: 10.1056/nejmsa1102519

Chen, D., Ye, Z., Shao, J., Tang, L., Zhang, H., Wang, X., Qiu, R., & Zhang, Q. (2020). Effect of electronic health interventions on metabolic syndrome: A systematic review and meta-analysis. In *BMJ Open* (Vol. 10, Issue 10). BMJ Publishing Group. DOI: 10.1136/bmjopen-2020-036927

Chen, J. H., & Asch, S. M. (2017). Machine Learning and Prediction in Medicine — Beyond the Peak of Inflated Expectations. *The New England Journal of Medicine*, *376*(26), 2507–2509. DOI: 10.1056/nejmp1702071

Chien, P. L., Liu, C. F., Huang, H. T., Jou, H. J., Chen, S. M., Young, T. G., Wang, Y. F., & Liao, P. H. (2021). Application of Artificial Intelligence in the Establishment of an Association Model between Metabolic Syndrome, TCM Constitution, and the Guidance of Medicated Diet Care. *Evidence-Based Complementary and Alternative Medicine : eCAM*, *2021*. Advance online publication. DOI: 10.1155/2021/5530717

Choubey, U., Upadrasta, V. A., Kaur, I. P., Banker, H., Kanagala, S. G., Anamika, F. N. U., Virmani, M., & Jain, R. (2024). From prevention to management: exploring AI's role in metabolic syndrome management: a comprehensive review. *The Egyptian Journal of Internal Medicine*, *36*(1), 106. DOI: 10.1186/s43162-024-00373-x

Cowie, M. R., Blomster, J. I., Curtis, L. H., Duclaux, S., Ford, I., Fritz, F., Goldman, S., Janmohamed, S., Kreuzer, J., Leenay, M., Michel, A., Ong, S., Pell, J. P., Southworth, M. R., Stough, W. G., Thoenes, M., Zannad, F., & Zalewski, A. (2017). Electronic health records to facilitate clinical research. In *Clinical Research in Cardiology* (Vol. 106, Issue 1). Dr. Dietrich Steinkopff Verlag GmbH and Co. KG. DOI: 10.1007/s00392-016-1025-6

Demaerschalk, B. M., Coffey, J. D., Lunde, J. J., Speltz, B. L., Oyarzabal, B. A., & Copeland, B. J. (2023). Rationale for Establishing a Digital Health Research Center at Mayo Clinic. *Mayo Clinic Proceedings. Digital Health*, *1*(3), 343–348. DOI: 10.1016/j.mcpdig.2023.06.001

Ebad, S. A., Alhashmi, A., Amara, M., Ben Miled, A., & Saqib, M. (2025). Artificial Intelligence-Based Software as a Medical Device (AI-SaMD): A Systematic Review. In *Healthcare (Switzerland)* (Vol. 13, Issue 7). Multidisciplinary Digital Publishing Institute (MDPI). DOI: 10.3390/healthcare13070817

Farinango, C. D., Benavides, J. S., Cerón, J. D., López, D. M., & Álvarez, R. E. (2018). Human-centered design of a personal health record system for metabolic syndrome management based on the ISO 9241-210:2010 standard. *Journal of Multidisciplinary Healthcare*, *11*, 21–37. DOI: 10.2147/JMDH.S150976

Ghosh, J., Chaudhury, S. R., Singh, K., & Koner, S. (2024). Application of Machine Learning Algorithm and Artificial Intelligence in Improving Metabolic Syndrome related complications: A review. In *International Journal of Advancement in Life Sciences Research* (Vol. 7, Issue 2, pp. 59–85). Dr Tarak Nath Podder Memorial Foundation. DOI: 10.31632/ijalsr.2024.v07i02.004

Gorrepati, L. P. (2024). Integrating AI with Electronic Health Records (EHRs) to Enhance Patient Care. *International Journal of Health Sciences*, 7(8). www.carijournals

Gupta, R. (2020). Navigating Regulatory Landscapes in Healthcare IT: Upholding HIPAA and GDPR Compliance. In *Advances in Computer Sciences* (Vol. 3).

Haddad, A., Habaebi, M., Islam, M., Hasbullah, N., & Ahmad Zabidi, S. (2022). Systematic review on AI-blockchain-based e-healthcare records management systems. *IEEE Access : Practical Innovations, Open Solutions*, *10*, 1–1. DOI: 10.1109/ACCESS.2022.3201878

Honeyford, K., Expert, P., Mendelsohn, E. E., Post, B., Faisal, A. A., Glampson, B., Mayer, E. K., & Costelloe, C. E. (2022). Challenges and recommendations for high quality research using electronic health records. *Frontiers in Digital Health*, *4*. Advance online publication. DOI: 10.3389/fdgth.2022.940330

Hossain, S., Hasan, M. K., Faruk, M. O., Aktar, N., Hossain, R., & Hossain, K. (2024). Machine learning approach for predicting cardiovascular disease in Bangladesh: Evidence from a cross-sectional study in 2023. *BMC Cardiovascular Disorders*, *24*(1). Advance online publication. DOI: 10.1186/s12872-024-03883-2

Jain, D. (2023). Regulation of Digital Healthcare in India: Ethical and Legal Challenges. *Healthcare (Switzerland)*, *11*(6). Advance online publication. DOI: 10.3390/healthcare11060911

Jain, P., Gyanchandani, M., & Khare, N. (2016). Big data privacy: A technological perspective and review. *Journal of Big Data*, *3*(1). Advance online publication. DOI: 10.1186/s40537-016-0059-y

Jena, M. C., Mishra, S. K., & Moharana, H. S. (2024). The way forward to overcome challenges and drawbacks of AI. *Computers and Artificial Intelligence*, *1581*. Advance online publication. DOI: 10.59400/cai1581

Jhade, S., & Gangavarapu, S. P. Channabasamma, & Igorevich Rozhdestvenskiy, O. (2024). Smart Medicine: Exploring the Landscape of AI-Enhanced Clinical Decision Support Systems. *MATEC Web of Conferences, 392*, 01083. DOI: 10.1051/matecconf/202439201083

Kadambi, V., Kadambi, N., Bettgeri, S., Buddiga, P., Ramaswami, N., & Hegde, R. (2018). *Review of an Electronic Health Record model to facilitate Remote Patient Management in metabolic and lifestyle diseases.*

Katehakis, D. G., & Tsiknakis, M. (2006). *ELECTRONIC HEALTH RECORD.*

Kaul, R., Ossai, C., Forkan, A. R. M., Jayaraman, P. P., Zelcer, J., Vaughan, S., & Wickramasinghe, N. (2023). The role of AI for developing digital twins in health-care: The case of cancer care. *Wiley Interdisciplinary Reviews. Data Mining and Knowledge Discovery*, *13*(1). Advance online publication. DOI: 10.1002/widm.1480

Kelly, C. J., Karthikesalingam, A., Suleyman, M., Corrado, G., & King, D. (2019). Key challenges for delivering clinical impact with artificial intelligence. In *BMC Medicine* (Vol. 17, Issue 1). BioMed Central Ltd. DOI: 10.1186/s12916-019-1426-2

Kim, M. S., Clarke, M. A., Belden, J. L., & Hinton, E. (2014). Usability Challenges and Barriers in EHR Training of Primary Care Resident Physicians. In *LNCS* (Vol. 8529).

Martinez, V. A., Betts, R. K., Scruth, E. A., Buckley, J. D., Cadiz, V. R., Bertrand, L. D., Paulson, S. S., Dummett, B. A., Abhyankar, S. S., Reyes, V. M., Hatton, J. R., Sulit, R., & Liu, V. X. (2022). The Kaiser Permanente Northern California Advance Alert Monitor Program: An Automated Early Warning System for Adults at Risk for In-Hospital Clinical Deterioration. *Joint Commission Journal on Quality and Patient Safety*, *48*(8), 370–375. DOI: 10.1016/j.jcjq.2022.05.005

Miotto, R., Li, L., Kidd, B. A., & Dudley, J. T. (2016). Deep Patient: An Unsuper-vised Representation to Predict the Future of Patients from the Electronic Health Records. *Scientific Reports*, *6*. Advance online publication. DOI: 10.1038/srep26094

Moghaddasi, H., Hosseini, A., Asadi, F., & Ganjali, R. (2011). Infrastructures of the System for Developing Electronic Health Record. In *Journal of Paramedical Sciences (JPS) Spring* (Vol. 2, Issue 2).

Nelson, R., & Saranya, S. (2024). Revolutionizing Health Records: The AI Way. [IJSR]. *International Journal of Scientific Research*, *13*(4), 1310–1313. DOI: 10.21275/sr24417190214

Olaye, I. M., & Seixas, A. A. (2023). The Gap Between AI and Bedside: Partici-patory Workshop on the Barriers to the Integration, Translation, and Adoption of Digital Health Care and AI Startup Technology Into Clinical Practice. *Journal of Medical Internet Research, 25*. DOI: 10.2196/32962

Padmavathi, S. (2022). Artificial Intelligence in Health Care. *Annals of SBV*, *10*(2), 23–23. DOI: 10.5005/jp-journals-10085-9112

Pantelis, A. G. (2022). *Current and Potential Applications of Artificial Intelligence in Metabolic Bariatric Surgery*. www.intechopen.com

Paraschiv, E.-A., Cîrnu, C. E., & Vevera, A. V. (2024). *Integrating Artificial Intelligence and Cybersecurity in Electronic Health Records: Addressing Challenges and Optimizing Healthcare Systems*. www.intechopen.com

Rahimi, A. K., Pienaar, O., Ghadimi, M., Canfell, O. J., Pole, J. D., Shrapnel, S., van der Vegt, A. H., & Sullivan, C. (2024). Implementing AI in Hospitals to Achieve a Learning Health System: Systematic Review of Current Enablers and Barriers. In *Journal of Medical Internet Research* (Vol. 26). JMIR Publications Inc., DOI: 10.2196/49655

Reddy Kotha, K., Charan Tokachichu, S., & Padakanti, S. (2024). *Synergizing AI and ERP for Predictive Supply Chain Management and Quality Assurance in Healthcare*. www.ijfmr.com

Sigatapu, L., Sundar, S., Padmalatha, K., Sravya, K., Ooha, D., & Devi, P. U. (2023). Artificial intelligence in healthcare-An overview. *Asian Journal of Pharmacy and Technology*, *13*(3), 218–222.

Seymour, T., Frantsvog, D., & Graeber, T. (2012). Electronic Health Records (EHR). In *American Journal of Health Sciences-Third Quarter* (Vol. 3, Issue 3). https://www.cluteinstitute.com/

Shah, S., Yeheskel, A., Hossain, A., Kerr, J., Young, K., Shakik, S., Nichols, J., & Yu, C. (2021). The Impact of Guideline Integration into Electronic Medical Records on Outcomes for Patients with Diabetes: A Systematic Review. In *American Journal of Medicine* (Vol. 134, Issue 8, pp. 952-962.e4). Elsevier Inc. DOI: 10.1016/j.amjmed.2021.03.004

Shen, Y., Yu, J., Zhou, J., & Hu, G. (2024). Twenty-Five Years of Evolution and Hurdles in Electronic Health Records and Interoperability in Medical Research: Comprehensive Review *(Preprint)*. DOI: 10.2196/preprints.59024

Shen, Y., Zhou, J., & Hu, G. (2020). Practical use of electronic health records among patients with diabetes in scientific research. In *Chinese Medical Journal* (Vol. 133, Issue 10, pp. 1224–1230). Lippincott Williams and Wilkins. DOI: 10.1097/CM9.0000000000000784

Stanton, R., Platania-Phung, C., Gaskin, C. J., & Happell, B. (2016). Screening for metabolic syndrome in mental health consumers using an electronic metabolic monitoring form. *Issues in Mental Health Nursing*, *37*(4), 239–244. DOI: 10.3109/01612840.2015.1119221

Sumalata, G. L., Joshitha, C., & Meenaksh, K. (2024). Prediction of diabetes mellitus using artificial intelligence techniques. *Scalable Computing, 25*(4), 3200–3213. DOI: 10.12694/scpe.v25i4.2884

Talati, D. (2023). AI in healthcare domain. *Journal of Knowledge Learning and Science Technology ISSN: 2959-6386 (Online), 2*(3), 256–262. DOI: 10.60087/jklst.vol2.n3.p262

Tsai, C. H., Eghdam, A., Davoody, N., Wright, G., Flowerday, S., & Koch, S. (2020). Effects of electronic health record implementation and barriers to adoption and use: A scoping review and qualitative analysis of the content. *Life (Chicago, Ill.), 10*(12), 1–27. DOI: 10.3390/life10120327

van Walraven, C., Escobar, G. J., Greene, J. D., & Forster, A. J. (2010). The Kaiser Permanente inpatient risk adjustment methodology was valid in an external patient population. *Journal of Clinical Epidemiology, 63*(7), 798–803. DOI: 10.1016/j.jclinepi.2009.08.020

Xu, L., Jiang, C., Wang, J., Yuan, J., & Ren, Y. (2014). Information Security in Big Data: Privacy and Data Mining. *IEEE Access : Practical Innovations, Open Solutions, 2*, 1149–1176. DOI: 10.1109/access.2014.2362522

Yang, J., Chesbrough, H., & Hurmelinna-Laukkanen, P. (2020). *The rise, fall, and resurrection of IBM Watson Health*. UC Berkeley and University of Oulu, Research Project 2019 Fall.

Chapter 14
Challenges and Future Directions:
Case Studies and Real-Time Applications in AI-Based Metabolic Medicine

C. Selvamurugan
https://orcid.org/0000-0003-3447-1970
Dhaanish Ahmed Institute of Technology, India

K. G. Parthiban
Aalim Muhammed Salegh College of Engineering, India

J. Tharik Raja
Dhaanish Ahmed Institute of Technology, India

K. Lakshmikandhan
CMS College of Engineering and Technology, India

M. Santhiya
Dhaanish Ahmed Institute of Technology, India

A. Munirathinam
Dhaanish Ahmed Institute of Technology, India

ABSTRACT

Artificial Intelligence (AI) has emerged as a transformative force in the field of metabolic medicine, offering innovative solutions to complex challenges. This paper delves into the pivotal role of AI in advancing metabolic medicine by exploring case studies and real-time applications. It highlights the integration of machine learning models, predictive analytics, and personalized medicine in diagnosing, monitoring, and treating metabolic disorders. The study emphasizes the successes achieved in areas such as diabetes management, obesity control, and lipid metabolism disorders. However, it also addresses the challenges faced, including ethical considerations, data privacy concerns, and the need for robust validation methods. Furthermore,

DOI: 10.4018/979-8-3373-3196-6.ch014

this work envisions future directions, focusing on the potential of AI-driven precision medicine, enhanced patient care through real-time analytics, and interdisciplinary collaboration. By bridging existing gaps, this paper aims to foster innovation and provide a roadmap for the next phase of AI adoption in metabolic medicine.

INTRODUCTION

In recent years, Artificial Intelligence (AI) has emerged as a revolutionary force across diverse domains of medicine, offering new paradigms for tackling long-standing challenges. Metabolic medicine, which focuses on diagnosing and managing disorders related to metabolic processes such as diabetes, obesity, lipid imbalances, and inherited metabolic diseases, stands to benefit significantly from these advancements. These conditions often involve a complex interplay of genetic, environmental, and lifestyle factors, making them challenging to diagnose, monitor, and treat using conventional medical approaches.(Hirani R et al., 2024)

AI technologies, particularly those driven by machine learning, deep learning, and predictive analytics, have transformed the way clinicians and researchers approach metabolic disorders. By leveraging vast amounts of data from genomic sequencing, wearable devices, electronic health records, and even environmental datasets, AI can identify patterns and correlations that would be impossible for human cognition alone to discern. This capability not only aids in early diagnosis but also enables the development of personalized treatment plans tailored to the unique metabolic profiles of individual patients. (Hamet P et al., 2017)

Furthermore, AI-powered real-time monitoring systems, such as continuous glucose monitoring devices and AI-driven dietary management applications, have brought a new level of precision and convenience to patient care. These innovations empower patients to play an active role in managing their conditions while providing healthcare providers with actionable insights.

Despite its promising applications, the integration of AI in metabolic medicine is not without its challenges. Ethical concerns related to data privacy, the lack of diversity in training datasets, and the need for rigorous clinical validation are some of the critical barriers that need to be addressed. Additionally, the scalability and accessibility of AI technologies remain a concern, particularly in resource-limited settings.

This paper aims to explore the multifaceted role of AI in metabolic medicine through an analysis of case studies and real-time applications. It seeks to highlight the transformative potential of AI while providing a balanced perspective on the challenges and limitations that must be overcome. By examining both the successes and hurdles, this work endeavors to chart a path forward, envisioning a future where

AI-driven solutions contribute significantly to the advancement of metabolic healthcare. The emphasis is on fostering interdisciplinary collaboration and innovation to ensure that AI's benefits are equitably distributed and sustainably implemented.

DEFINITIONANDCONCEPT

Figure 1. Application of AI in Healthcare

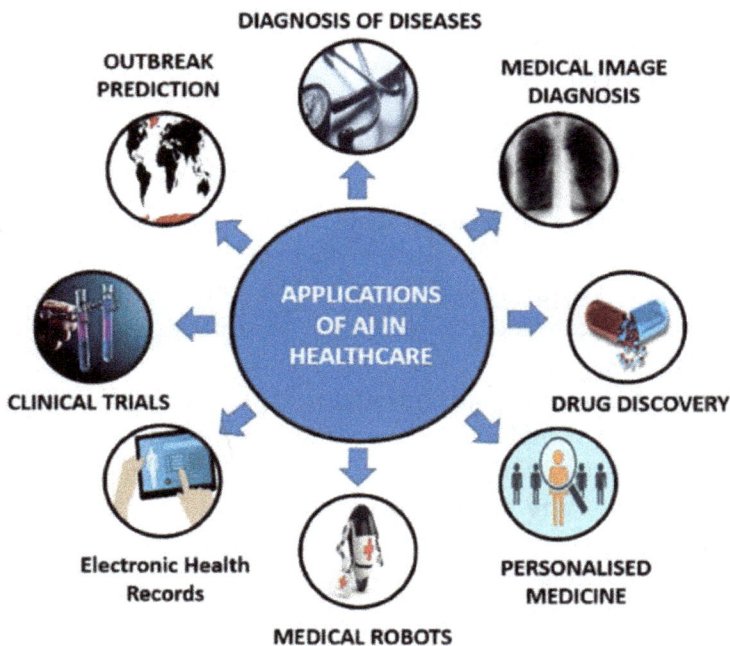

Definition

AI-based metabolic medicine is a specialized interdisciplinary domain that combines artificial intelligence (AI) technologies with metabolic healthcare practices. Metabolic disorders, which include conditions like diabetes mellitus, obesity, metabolic syndrome, dyslipidemia, and inherited metabolic diseases, are typically characterized by disruptions in the body's chemical processes that regulate energy production and utilization. AI-based metabolic medicine seeks to address these disruptions through sophisticated computational tools designed to analyze, predict, and intervene in metabolic health issues with unparalleled precision.

This field leverages a variety of AI methodologies such as machine learning, deep learning, neural networks, and natural language processing to sift through and make sense of large, complex datasets. These datasets may include information derived from genomics, proteomics, metabolomics, clinical records, environmental factors, and behavioral data. The ultimate objective of AI-based metabolic medicine is to improve healthcare outcomes by enabling more accurate diagnosis, effective treatment planning, and personalized care for patients suffering from metabolic disorders. (Anwar Aetal., 2025)

Concept

The concept of AI-based metabolic medicine is fundamentally rooted in the integration of computational intelligence into the study and management of metabolic health. Metabolic processes are vital for the body's energy production, growth, and repair. They are intricately linked to genetic predispositions, lifestyle choices, environmental exposures, and other multifaceted factors, often creating complex webs of interactions that are challenging to untangle using conventional medical methods.

AI addresses these complexities by offering advanced tools to analyze, model, and predict outcomes based on a variety of variables. For example, machine learning algorithms can identify biomarkers for early detection of metabolic diseases, while deep learning models can simulate metabolic pathways to understand disease progression. These insights help healthcare providers move beyond one-size-fits-all approaches, offering patient-specific solutions tailored to individual metabolic profiles.

The concept also emphasizes real-time data collection and analysis as a cornerstone of AI-based metabolic medicine. With the rise of wearable devices and biosensors, patients can continuously monitor critical metabolic parameters such as glucose levels, cholesterol levels, and even stress indicators. AI-powered analytics transform this data into actionable insights, providing timely feedback to patients and healthcare providers. This not only facilitates proactive disease management but also empowers patients to take an active role in their own health journeys.

Additionally, AI-based metabolic medicine involves developing predictive models that forecast disease trajectories and assess the potential impact of interventions. For instance, machine learning can predict how a diabetic patient's blood sugar levels will respond to specific dietary changes or medication adjustments, enabling clinicians to make informed decisions before implementing treatment plans. (Alexis Pengfei Zhao et al., 2024)

Despite these advancements, the concept is not without its challenges. Ethical issues such as data privacy and informed consent, technical barriers such as algorithmic bias, and logistical hurdles such as the accessibility of AI technologies in resource-limited settings require careful consideration. Addressing these challenges necessitates interdisciplinary collaboration among clinicians, AI experts, ethicists, policymakers, and patients themselves.

Overall, AI-based metabolic medicine represents a transformative shift in healthcare. By bridging the gap between research and clinical practice, it offers innovative solutions that not only enhance patient care but also advance scientific understanding of metabolic processes. This field holds the promise of redefining how metabolic disorders are diagnosed, monitored, and treated, paving the way for a future where healthcare is more efficient, precise, and personalized.

IMPACT

The integration of artificial intelligence (AI) into metabolic medicine has revolutionized the field, offering transformative solutions to longstanding challenges. Its impact spans across multiple dimensions, including clinical care, research, patient engagement, and global health initiatives. Below is a comprehensive analysis of its multifaceted impact:

1. Enhanced Diagnostic Accuracy

AI has significantly improved the precision of diagnosing metabolic disorders. Traditional diagnostic methods often rely on limited datasets and subjective interpretations, which can lead to delays or inaccuracies. AI algorithms, on the other hand, analyze vast datasets from genomic studies, proteomics, metabolomics, and electronic health records to identify subtle patterns and biomarkers. For example, machine learning models can detect early signs of diabetes or lipid metabolism disorders by analyzing genetic predispositions and lifestyle factors. This early detection enables timely intervention, reducing the risk of complications and improving patient outcomes.

2. Personalized Treatment Plans

One of the most profound impacts of AI in metabolic medicine is its ability to facilitate personalized healthcare. By leveraging patient-specific data, such as genetic profiles, metabolic rates, and lifestyle behaviors, AI systems can recommend tailored treatment plans. These plans optimize therapeutic efficacy by addressing the unique needs of each patient. For instance, AI can suggest dietary modifications, exercise regimens, and medication adjustments based on an individual's metabolic profile, minimizing trial-and-error approaches and enhancing patient satisfaction. (Simmons LA et al., 2016)

3. Real-Time Monitoring and Feedback

AI-powered wearable devices and biosensors have transformed the way metabolic parameters are monitored. These devices continuously track metrics such as glucose levels, cholesterol, body composition, and even stress indicators. AI algorithms process this data in real-time, providing actionable insights to both patients and healthcare providers. This dynamic feedback loop enables proactive disease management, allowing for timely adjustments to treatment plans and reducing the likelihood of adverse events.

4. Improved Patient Engagement

AI-driven applications and platforms have empowered patients to take an active role in managing their metabolic health. Interactive tools provide educational resources, track progress, and offer motivational support, fostering a sense of ownership and accountability. For example, AI-based apps can guide patients through lifestyle changes, such as adopting healthier eating habits or increasing physical activity, while providing positive reinforcement and personalized recommendations.

5. Advancements in Research

AI has accelerated research in metabolic medicine by enabling the analysis of complex datasets and simulating metabolic pathways. Researchers can use AI to identify novel biomarkers, therapeutic targets, and insights into disease mechanisms. For instance, deep learning models can predict the impact of genetic mutations on metabolic processes, paving the way for innovative treatments. AI also facilitates the integration of interdisciplinary research, bringing together experts from fields such as genomics, bioinformatics, and clinical medicine.

6. Cost Efficiency

The adoption of AI in metabolic medicine has contributed to cost savings in healthcare. By streamlining diagnostic processes and optimizing treatment plans, AI reduces the need for expensive and invasive procedures. Early detection and personalized interventions minimize hospitalizations and complications, making metabolic healthcare more accessible and affordable for patients and healthcare systems alike.

7. Global Health Impact

AI-based metabolic medicine has the potential to address global health challenges by improving access to quality care in underserved regions. Telemedicine platforms powered by AI can provide remote consultations, diagnostics, and monitoring, bridging gaps in healthcare delivery. This is particularly impactful in low-resource settings, where access to specialized metabolic care is limited. AI-driven solutions can democratize healthcare, ensuring that patients worldwide benefit from advancements in metabolic medicine. (Zuhair V et al., 2024)

8. Challenges and Ethical Considerations

While the impact of AI in metabolic medicine is overwhelmingly positive, it is essential to address challenges such as data privacy, algorithmic bias, and the need for robust validation. Ethical considerations must be prioritized to ensure equitable and responsible AI adoption. For example, ensuring diversity in training datasets can mitigate biases and improve the accuracy of AI models across different populations. Additionally, transparent and interpretable AI systems are crucial for building trust among patients and healthcare providers.

CHALLENGESANDETHICALCONSIDERATION

Challenges in AI-Based Metabolic Medicine

Data Privacy and Security AI systems rely on vast amounts of sensitive patient data, including genomic information, electronic health records, and wearable device metrics. Ensuring the privacy and security of this data is a significant challenge. Breaches or misuse of data can lead to ethical and legal repercussions, as well as a loss of trust among patients and healthcare providers.

Algorithmic Bias AI models are only as unbiased as the data they are trained on. If training datasets lack diversity or contain inherent biases, the resulting AI systems may produce skewed outcomes. For instance, an AI model trained predominantly on data from one demographic may fail to accurately diagnose or treat patients from other demographics, leading to disparities in healthcare.

Interpretability and Transparency Many AI algorithms, especially deep learning models, operate as "black boxes," making it difficult to understand how they arrive at specific conclusions. This lack of interpretability can hinder clinicians' ability to trust and validate AI-driven recommendations, posing challenges for integration into clinical practice.

Validation and Reliability AI systems must undergo rigorous validation to ensure their reliability and accuracy in real-world settings. The lack of standardized protocols for validating AI models in metabolic medicine can impede their adoption and effectiveness.

Integration into Clinical Workflow Integrating AI technologies into existing clinical workflows is a complex process that requires significant changes in infrastructure, training, and resource allocation. Resistance to change among healthcare providers and institutions can further complicate this integration.

Scalability and Accessibility While AI has the potential to democratize healthcare, its implementation often requires substantial resources, including advanced computing infrastructure and skilled personnel. This can limit its accessibility in resource-constrained settings, exacerbating healthcare disparities. (Jiang L et al., 2021)

Ethical Considerations in AI-Based Metabolic Medicine

Informed Consent Patients must be fully informed about how their data will be used, stored, and analyzed by AI systems. Ensuring that patients understand the implications of AI-driven healthcare is crucial for maintaining ethical standards.

Accountability and Liability Determining accountability in cases where AI systems make errors or fail to deliver accurate results is a complex ethical issue. Questions about whether the responsibility lies with the developers, clinicians, or institutions must be addressed.

Equity and Fairness AI systems must be designed to provide equitable healthcare outcomes for all patients, regardless of their demographic, socioeconomic, or geographic background. Addressing biases in AI models is essential to achieving fairness.

Patient-Physician Relationship The integration of AI into healthcare has the potential to alter the traditional patient-physician relationship. Ethical considerations must ensure that AI enhances, rather than diminishes, the human connection in healthcare.

Regulatory and Legal Frameworks The rapid advancement of AI technologies has outpaced the development of regulatory and legal frameworks. Establishing clear guidelines for the ethical use of AI in metabolic medicine is essential to ensure compliance and accountability.

Ethics by Design AI systems should be developed with ethical principles embedded in their design. This includes prioritizing transparency, fairness, and patient safety throughout the development and implementation process.

HISTORY OF AI-BASED METABOLIC MEDICINE

Figure 2. Timeline of AI in Healthcare

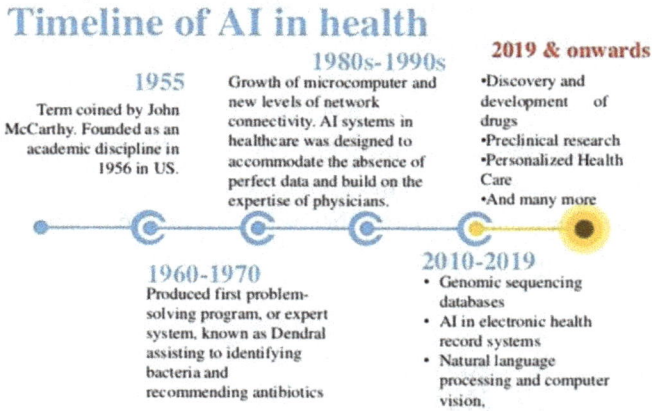

Timeline of AI in health

1955
Term coined by John McCarthy. Founded as an academic discipline in 1956 in US.

1980s-1990s
Growth of microcomputer and new levels of network connectivity. AI systems in healthcare was designed to accommodate the absence of perfect data and build on the expertise of physicians.

2019 & onwards
•Discovery and development of drugs
•Preclinical research
•Personalized Health Care
•And many more

1960-1970
Produced first problem-solving program, or expert system, known as Dendral assisting to identifying bacteria and recommending antibiotics

2010-2019
• Genomic sequencing databases
• AI in electronic health record systems
• Natural language processing and computer vision,

The evolution of AI-based metabolic medicine is deeply intertwined with the broader advancements in artificial intelligence and healthcare technologies. Its history can be traced through several key milestones:

Early Computational Tools in Medicine The foundation of AI in healthcare began in the mid-20th century with the development of early computational tools. These tools were primarily used for data analysis and statistical modeling, laying the groundwork for more sophisticated AI applications. In metabolic medicine, early efforts focused on using algorithms to analyze biochemical data and predict metabolic trends. (Ambinder EP2005)

Emergence of Machine Learning The advent of machine learning in the late 20th century marked a turning point. Machine learning algorithms, capable of learning from data and improving over time, were applied to metabolic research. For example, researchers began using these algorithms to identify risk factors for diabetes and obesity by analyzing patient data.

Integration of Big Data and Genomics The 21st century saw the rise of big data analytics and genomic technologies. The ability to sequence entire genomes and analyze vast datasets revolutionized metabolic medicine. AI played a crucial role in processing and interpreting this data, enabling the identification of genetic markers associated with metabolic disorders.

Development of Wearable Devices The introduction of wearable devices equipped with biosensors was a significant milestone. These devices allowed for continuous monitoring of metabolic parameters such as glucose levels and physical activity.

AI algorithms were integrated into these devices to provide real-time feedback and personalized recommendations.

Advancements in Deep Learning Deep learning, a subset of machine learning, brought unprecedented capabilities to AI-based metabolic medicine. Neural networks capable of processing complex data structures were used to model metabolic pathways and predict disease progression. This era also saw the development of AI-driven diagnostic tools and virtual health assistants.

Telemedicine and Remote Monitoring The COVID-19 pandemic accelerated the adoption of telemedicine and remote monitoring technologies. AI-based metabolic medicine became a cornerstone of these efforts, enabling remote consultations, diagnostics, and treatment planning for patients with metabolic disorders.

CULTURAL SIGNIFICANCE OF AI-BASED METABOLIC MEDICINE

The cultural significance of AI-based metabolic medicine lies in its transformative impact on healthcare practices, societal perceptions, and global health equity. Below are the key aspects of its cultural relevance:

Shift Toward Proactive Healthcare AI-based metabolic medicine has shifted the focus from reactive to proactive healthcare. By enabling early detection and personalized interventions, it has fostered a culture of prevention and self-management. Patients are now empowered to take an active role in their health, reflecting a broader societal emphasis on wellness and accountability

Democratization of Healthcare One of the most profound cultural impacts is the democratization of healthcare. AI technologies have made advanced diagnostic and treatment tools accessible to diverse populations, including those in underserved regions. This inclusivity aligns with cultural values of equity and justice, promoting a more holistic approach to healthcare.

Interdisciplinary Collaboration The integration of AI into metabolic medicine has fostered interdisciplinary collaboration. Experts from fields such as computer science, medicine, ethics, and public health work together to develop innovative solutions. This collaborative culture has enriched scientific understanding and accelerated advancements in metabolic healthcare.

Ethical Considerations and Public Discourse The adoption of AI in metabolic medicine has sparked important ethical discussions. Issues such as data privacy, algorithmic bias, and informed consent have highlighted the need for responsible practices. These conversations reflect broader societal values and underscore the importance of aligning technological advancements with ethical principles.

Global Health Impact AI-based metabolic medicine has the potential to address global health challenges by improving access to quality care. Telemedicine platforms powered by AI have bridged gaps in healthcare delivery, particularly in low-resource settings. This global reach underscores the cultural significance of AI as a tool for promoting health equity.

Integration into Daily Life Wearable devices and AI-driven health apps have become integral to daily life for many individuals. These technologies have not only improved health outcomes but also influenced cultural attitudes toward technology and health. The widespread adoption of these tools reflects a growing acceptance of AI as a trusted partner in healthcare. (Hamed Taherdoost 2024)

ROLE OF AI-BASED METABOLIC MEDICINE IN METABOLIC HEALTHCARE

AI-based metabolic medicine plays a transformative role in addressing the complexities of metabolic disorders, which are often multifactorial and involve intricate interactions between genetic, environmental, and lifestyle factors. Below are the key areas where AI has a significant impact:

1. Early Diagnosis and Risk Prediction

Metabolic disorders, such as diabetes, obesity, and metabolic syndrome, often develop gradually and may remain undetected until complications arise. AI algorithms excel at analyzing large datasets, including genetic information, clinical records, and lifestyle data, to identify early warning signs and predict an individual's risk of developing these conditions. For example:

Machine learning models can analyze patterns in blood glucose levels, body mass index (BMI), and lipid profiles to predict the onset of diabetes or cardiovascular diseases.

AI-driven risk assessment tools enable clinicians to stratify patients based on their likelihood of developing metabolic disorders, allowing for targeted preventive measures.

2. Personalized Treatment and Precision Medicine

AI has revolutionized the concept of personalized medicine in metabolic healthcare by tailoring treatment plans to individual patients. This is particularly important for metabolic disorders, where one-size-fits-all approaches often fall short. AI systems analyze patient-specific data, such as genetic predispositions, metabolic rates, and lifestyle factors, to recommend:

- Customized dietary plans and exercise regimens.
- Optimal medication dosages and combinations.
- Predictive models that forecast how a patient will respond to specific interventions, enabling clinicians to make informed decisions.

3. Real-Time Monitoring and Dynamic Management

Wearable devices and biosensors equipped with AI capabilities have become integral to the management of metabolic disorders. These devices continuously monitor key metabolic parameters, such as glucose levels, cholesterol, and physical activity, and provide real-time feedback. AI processes this data to:

- Detect anomalies and alert patients or healthcare providers to potential issues.
- Adjust treatment plans dynamically based on real-time insights.
- Empower patients to actively manage their conditions through user-friendly interfaces and actionable recommendations.

4. Advancing Research and Biomarker Discovery

AI has accelerated research in metabolic medicine by enabling the analysis of complex datasets and uncovering novel insights. For instance:

- AI-driven tools can identify biomarkers associated with metabolic disorders, facilitating early diagnosis and targeted therapies.
- Deep learning models simulate metabolic pathways to understand disease mechanisms and identify potential therapeutic targets.
- AI supports interdisciplinary research by integrating data from genomics, proteomics, and metabolomics, advancing the understanding of metabolic health.

5. Improving Healthcare Accessibility

AI-based metabolic medicine has the potential to bridge gaps in healthcare delivery, particularly in underserved regions. Telemedicine platforms powered by AI enable remote consultations, diagnostics, and treatment planning, making advanced metabolic care accessible to patients who might otherwise lack access to specialized services.

6. Enhancing Preventive Healthcare

Prevention is a cornerstone of metabolic medicine, and AI plays a pivotal role in promoting preventive measures. By analyzing lifestyle data and environmental factors, AI systems can

- Recommend lifestyle modifications to reduce the risk of metabolic disorders.
- Provide personalized health coaching through mobile applications and virtual assistants.
- Monitor adherence to preventive strategies and offer motivational support.

7. Streamlining Clinical Decision-Making

AI acts as a decision-support tool for clinicians, enhancing their ability to diagnose and treat metabolic disorders. For example:

- Natural language processing (NLP) algorithms extract relevant information from electronic health records to provide clinicians with a comprehensive view of a patient's health history.
- AI-powered decision-support systems suggest evidence-based treatment options, improving the quality and efficiency of care.

8. Addressing Global Health Challenges

Metabolic disorders are a growing global health concern, with rising prevalence in both developed and developing countries. AI-based metabolic medicine addresses these challenges by:

- Enabling large-scale population health management through predictive analytics.
- Supporting public health initiatives aimed at reducing the burden of metabolic disorders.
- Facilitating cross-border collaborations in research and healthcare delivery.

CASESTUDIESANDBEST PRACTICES INSOCIALDINING PLATFORMS

Case Study 1: AI in Diabetes Management

Diabetes is one of the most prevalent metabolic disorders globally, and AI has played a pivotal role in revolutionizing its management. Tools like the Guardian Connect system andDreaMed Diabetes have been developed to assist patients and healthcare providers in managing diabetes more effectively. These systems utilize machine learning algorithms to analyze continuous glucose monitoring (CGM) data, predict blood sugar fluctuations, and recommend insulin adjustments. For example:

- **Guardian Connect System:** This AI-powered tool provides real-time alerts to patients about impending hypo- or hyperglycemia, enabling timely interventions. It also offers personalized insights based on individual glucose patterns.
- **DreaMed Diabetes:** This platform uses AI to optimize insulin therapy by analyzing CGM data and patient-specific factors. It has been shown to improve glycemic control and reduce the burden on healthcare providers.

These tools have demonstrated significant improvements in patient outcomes, including better glycemic control, reduced risk of complications, and enhanced quality of life.

Case Study 2: AI in Metabolic Syndrome Prevention

Metabolic syndrome (MetS) is a cluster of conditions, including hypertension, dyslipidemia, and obesity, that pose a significant public health threat. AI has been integrated into the prevention and management of MetS through tools that monitor key health indices and facilitate lifestyle modifications. For instance:

AI-driven platforms analyze data from wearable devices to track blood pressure, glucose levels, and lipid profiles. These platforms provide personalized recommendations for dietary changes, physical activity, and stress management.(Swarup S et al.,2025)

Case Study 3: AI-Driven Biomarker Discovery

Biomarker discovery is critical for the early diagnosis and treatment of metabolic disorders. AI has been instrumental in identifying novel biomarkers by analyzing genomic, proteomic, and metabolomic data. For example:

- Researchers used AI to identify biomarkers associated with metabolic dysfunction-associated fatty liver disease (MAFLD). These biomarkers enable early diagnosis and targeted therapies, reducing the risk of complications such as liver fibrosis and hepatocellular carcinoma.
- AI algorithms have also been used to predict thyroid dysfunction by analyzing patterns in hormone levels and genetic data.

These discoveries have accelerated research and improved clinical outcomes by enabling more precise and personalized approaches to metabolic healthcare.

Case Study 4: AI in Personalized Nutrition

Personalized nutrition is a growing field within metabolic medicine, and AI has been at the forefront of its development. AI applications analyze data from wearable devices, electronic health records, and dietary logs to provide tailored nutrition plans. For example:

- AI-powered apps recommend dietary adjustments based on an individual's metabolic profile, including factors such as glucose tolerance, lipid levels, and gut microbiome composition.
- These apps also monitor adherence to dietary plans and provide motivational support to encourage healthy eating habits.

Studies have shown that personalized nutrition plans guided by AI can significantly improve metabolic health outcomes, including weight management and lipid control.

Case Study 5: AI in Obesity Management

Obesity is a complex metabolic disorder that requires multifaceted interventions. AI has been used to develop tools that assist in weight management and behavioral modification. For instance:

- AI-driven platforms analyze data from wearable devices to track physical activity, caloric intake, and sleep patterns. These platforms provide personalized recommendations for weight loss strategies.
- Virtual health coaches powered by AI offer real-time support and guidance, helping patients stay motivated and achieve their weight management goals.
- Clinical trials have demonstrated the effectiveness of these tools in reducing BMI and improving overall metabolic health.

Case Study 6: AI in Lipid Metabolism Disorders

AI has been applied to the management of lipid metabolism disorders, such as dyslipidemia. Tools like AI-powered lipid monitoring systems analyze lipid profiles and recommend interventions to optimize cholesterol levels. For example:

- AI algorithms predict the impact of dietary changes and medications on lipid levels, enabling clinicians to make informed decisions.
- Real-time monitoring systems track lipid levels and provide alerts for abnormal values, facilitating timely interventions.
- These tools have been shown to improve lipid control and reduce the risk of cardiovascular complications.

BEST PRACTICES

1. DATA COLLECTION AND MANAGEMENT

Ensure Data Privacy and Security: Protecting sensitive patient data is paramount. Robust encryption, secure storage systems, and access control measures should be implemented to safeguard genomic, clinical, and wearable device data. Compliance with data protection regulations, such as GDPR or HIPAA, is essential.

Standardize Data Formats: Standardized data formats facilitate interoperability across AI systems and healthcare platforms. This ensures seamless integration and enhances the accuracy of AI-driven insights.

Diverse and Representative Datasets: Training AI models on diverse datasets that represent various demographics, ethnicities, and geographic regions minimizes bias and improves the generalizability of AI systems.

2. ALGORITHM DEVELOPMENT AND VALIDATION

Transparent and Interpretable Models: AI algorithms should be designed to be interpretable, allowing clinicians to understand how recommendations are generated. This builds trust and facilitates adoption in clinical settings.

Rigorous Validation Protocols: AI systems must undergo extensive validation studies to ensure their reliability and accuracy in real-world applications. Validation should include clinical trials and peer-reviewed assessments.

Continuous Improvement: AI models should be regularly updated and refined based on new data, user feedback, and advancements in technology to maintain their effectiveness.

3. INTEGRATION INTO CLINICAL PRACTICE

Seamless Workflow Integration: AI tools should be designed to integrate seamlessly into existing clinical workflows, minimizing disruptions and enhancing efficiency. This includes compatibility with electronic health records (EHRs) and other healthcare systems.

Training for Healthcare Providers: Comprehensive training programs should be provided to clinicians and staff to ensure they can effectively use AI systems and interpret their outputs. This reduces resistance to adoption and enhances utilization.

Patient-Centric Design: AI applications should prioritize user-friendly interfaces and patient engagement. Tools that empower patients to actively participate in their healthcare foster better outcomes and adherence.

4. ETHICAL AND REGULATORY COMPLIANCE

Informed Consent: Patients must be fully informed about how their data will be used, stored, and analyzed by AI systems. Transparent communication and consent processes are critical.

Address Algorithmic Bias: Developers should actively identify and mitigate biases in AI models to ensure equitable healthcare outcomes for all patients, regardless of demographic or socioeconomic background.

Adherence to Regulations: Compliance with local and international regulations governing AI in healthcare, such as data protection laws and ethical guidelines, is essential for responsible implementation.

5. COLLABORATION AND INTERDISCIPLINARY APPROACH

Foster Collaboration: Interdisciplinary collaboration among AI developers, clinicians, ethicists, and policymakers is crucial for addressing challenges and improving outcomes. This ensures that AI systems are designed with clinical relevance and ethical considerations in mind.

Engage Stakeholders: Involving patients, caregivers, and community representatives in the development and implementation of AI systems ensures that their needs and concerns are addressed.

6. MONITORING AND FEEDBACK

Real-Time Monitoring: AI systems should continuously monitor patient health and provide dynamic feedback to healthcare providers. This enables proactive interventions and enhances patient care.

Feedback Loops: Establish mechanisms for collecting feedback from users to identify areas for improvement and refine AI tools. This iterative process ensures that AI systems remain effective and user-friendly.

7. FOCUS ON ACCESSIBILITY

Scalable Solutions: AI systems should be designed to be scalable and accessible, particularly in resource-constrained settings. This includes leveraging cloud-based platforms and cost-effective technologies.

Telemedicine Integration: AI-powered telemedicine platforms can provide remote consultations and care for patients in underserved regions, bridging gaps in healthcare delivery.

8. PROMOTE PREVENTIVE HEALTHCARE

Lifestyle Modification Tools: AI applications should emphasize preventive measures by providing personalized recommendations for dietary changes, physical activity, and stress management.

Educational Resources: AI-driven platforms can offer educational resources to patients, empowering them to make informed decisions about their health.

EXISTING RESEARCH

1. Artificial Intelligence in the Management of Metabolic Disorders

A comprehensive review published in the *Journal of Endocrinological Investigation* explores the significant role of AI in managing metabolic disorders such as diabetes, obesity, metabolic dysfunction-associated fatty liver disease (MAFLD), and thyroid dysfunction. The study highlights the use of AI-driven methodologies, including machine learning (ML), deep learning (DL), natural language processing (NLP), and reinforcement learning, to address challenges in early diagnosis, personalized treatment, risk assessment, and biomarker discovery. It also emphasizes the ethical considerations associated with AI implementation, such as data privacy and bias mitigation. The review discusses tools like Idx, Guardian Connect system, and DreaMed for diabetes management, showcasing their transformative potential in improving patient outcomes.

2. From Prevention to Management: Exploring AI's Role in Metabolic Syndrome

Metabolic syndrome, a cluster of risk factors that increase the likelihood of developing cardiovascular disease, diabetes, and stroke, is a growing global health concern. Affecting nearly one in four adults worldwide, its early detection, prevention, and management are critical to reducing the burden of chronic diseases. Traditionally, metabolic syndrome has been addressed through lifestyle interventions, such as diet and exercise, as well as medications to control individual risk factors like hypertension, high cholesterol, and insulin resistance. However, these approaches often fall short in terms of early intervention and personalized care. (Choubey et al., 2024)

Artificial Intelligence (AI) has the potential to revolutionize both the prevention and management of metabolic syndrome. By leveraging vast amounts of data, AI systems can uncover early warning signs, predict individual risk, and personalize treatment strategies. In this article, we explore the transformative role of AI in tackling metabolic syndrome from its early stages all the way through ongoing management.

What is Metabolic Syndrome?

Metabolic syndrome is a collection of five conditions that significantly increase the risk of developing serious health problems:
Abdominal obesity (excess fat around the waist)
High blood pressure
High blood sugar
Abnormal cholesterol levels (low HDL or high triglycerides)
Insulin resistance
When three or more of these factors are present, a person is considered to have metabolic syndrome. It is closely associated with obesity, physical inactivity, and an unhealthy diet, but genetic and environmental factors also play significant roles.

AI in Preventing Metabolic Syndrome

1. Early Detection of Risk Factors

AI's ability to analyze large datasets enables the identification of subtle patterns in patients' health data that may not be evident through traditional methods. Machine learning models trained on diverse clinical, genetic, and environmental data can predict the likelihood of metabolic syndrome long before overt symptoms manifest.

Predictive Modeling: By integrating data from electronic health records (EHRs), AI can spot early warning signs such as slight increases in blood pressure or glucose levels, or emerging patterns of insulin resistance. These models can help clinicians identify individuals at risk and recommend early interventions.

Wearables and Continuous Monitoring: Devices like smartwatches, continuous glucose monitors (CGMs), and fitness trackers provide real-time data on activity levels, heart rate, glucose fluctuations, and more. AI-powered algorithms can continuously analyze this data to detect early deviations from healthy norms, alerting both the user and their healthcare provider.

2. Tailored Lifestyle Recommendations

Prevention isn't just about monitoring medical parameters; it's also about addressing the root causes of metabolic syndrome. AI can analyze an individual's lifestyle, dietary habits, and genetic makeup to deliver highly personalized recommendations for prevention.

Personalized Nutrition and Fitness Plans: Companies like Noom and Lumen use AI to create diet plans and fitness regimens tailored to the user's metabolism, goals, and progress. These personalized interventions help prevent the onset of metabolic syndrome by adjusting to the individual's unique metabolic response.

Behavioral Insights: AI can also offer behavioral nudges, encouraging users to adopt healthier habits by integrating with mobile apps or smart devices. For example, AI algorithms in health apps can provide reminders for physical activity or suggest healthier food options based on real-time monitoring of the user's behavior. (Sumner J et al., 2023)

AI in Managing Metabolic Syndrome

1. Precision Medicine and Risk Stratification

AI's ability to integrate a wide range of data sources—from genomic and proteomic information to lifestyle factors—makes it invaluable in creating a comprehensive, personalized approach to managing metabolic syndrome.

Genomic and Multi-Omics Approaches: By analyzing a person's genetic predisposition to metabolic syndrome and other chronic conditions, AI can help identify specific risk factors and predict the most effective interventions. AI models can also analyze microbiome data, providing insights into how gut health influences metabolic processes and guiding personalized dietary or probiotic recommendations.

Predicting Disease Progression: AI models can track the progression of metabolic syndrome in real-time by analyzing biomarkers and clinical data. These models can predict the likelihood of a patient developing diabetes or cardiovascular diseases, allowing healthcare providers to adjust management plans accordingly.

2. Medication Management

Managing metabolic syndrome often involves multiple medications to control blood pressure, cholesterol, blood sugar, and insulin sensitivity. AI can help optimize this multi-drug management approach by suggesting the most effective treatment regimens based on individual profiles.

Drug Interaction and Optimization: AI can predict drug interactions and adjust dosages for maximum efficacy and minimal side effects. For example, AI systems can integrate data from a patient's history of drug responses to recommend the most suitable treatment for conditions like insulin resistance or hypertension.

Monitoring and Adaptive Dosing: AI-powered tools that integrate with wearable devices or home monitoring systems can track real-time data and adjust treatment plans dynamically. For example, AI in insulin pumps can continuously adjust insulin delivery based on glucose readings, ensuring better blood sugar control.

3. Real-Time Monitoring for Better Outcomes

AI-powered monitoring tools are especially valuable in managing metabolic syndrome because they allow for continuous tracking of key metrics such as glucose levels, blood pressure, and weight. These real-time insights enable both patients and healthcare providers to make proactive adjustments to treatment plans.

Continuous Glucose Monitoring (CGM): AI-enhanced CGM devices can predict glucose fluctuations hours or even days in advance, allowing patients to adjust their diet or medication before significant changes occur.

Smart Wearables for Early Intervention: AI-powered smartwatches or fitness trackers can detect physiological changes such as elevated heart rate, blood pressure, or abnormal movement patterns, alerting the user or their healthcare provider when intervention is needed.

Challenges and Future Directions

While the potential of AI in metabolic syndrome management is immense, several challenges remain:

Data Privacy and Security: The use of personal health data raises significant concerns about privacy and security. Ensuring that AI tools comply with regulations like GDPR or HIPAA is crucial to maintaining patient trust.

Health Equity: AI systems must be trained on diverse datasets to avoid biases that could exacerbate health disparities. Ensuring that these tools are accessible and effective across all demographics is key to their widespread success.

Integration with Traditional Healthcare: AI systems must be integrated seamlessly with existing healthcare infrastructure. This includes ensuring that AI tools complement the clinical decision-making process without replacing human judgment or oversight.

3. Revolutionizing Metabolic Medicine with Artificial Intelligence

Metabolic disorders such as obesity, type 2 diabetes, and metabolic syndrome represent some of the most widespread and costly health challenges globally. Despite significant progress in understanding their biological underpinnings, current approaches to prevention, diagnosis, and treatment often fall short—largely due to the immense complexity and variability in metabolic processes across individuals.

Artificial Intelligence (AI) is now emerging as a game-changing force in metabolic medicine. By harnessing vast datasets—from genomics and electronic health records to continuous glucose monitors and wearable devices—AI enables a deeper, more dynamic understanding of human metabolism. What once took years of longitudinal research can now be modeled in minutes, revealing hidden patterns and making accurate predictions that can inform clinical decisions in real time.

Understanding the Challenges in Metabolic Medicine

Metabolic medicine is inherently complex due to the multifactorial nature of conditions it seeks to address. Challenges include:

Early Detection: Symptoms of metabolic disorders often manifest late, when disease progression is advanced.

Inter-Individual Variability: Genetic, epigenetic, lifestyle, and environmental differences influence disease onset and progression.

Lack of Personalization: Standardized treatment regimens fail to account for individual metabolic profiles and responses.

Data Overload: While patient data is more abundant than ever, making sense of it remains a challenge.

AI as a Catalyst for Precision Metabolic Medicine

Artificial Intelligence offers solutions that were previously out of reach:

1. Predictive Diagnostics

AI models trained on diverse datasets can detect subtle signs of metabolic dysfunction long before clinical symptoms appear. For instance, machine learning algorithms analyzing continuous glucose monitoring (CGM) data can identify pre-diabetic states or predict hypoglycemic episodes with high accuracy. (Iftikhar M et al., 2024)

2. Personalized Treatment Plans

With AI, it's possible to tailor therapies based on individual patient profiles. AI systems can analyze genetic data, microbiome composition, dietary habits, and medication history to recommend optimal interventions—from pharmaceutical options to lifestyle changes.

3. Real-Time Monitoring and Feedback

Wearable technologies integrated with AI can provide continuous insights into a patient's metabolic state. Systems such as AI-powered insulin pumps or digital twin models simulate metabolic responses, enabling fine-tuned, real-time therapeutic adjustments.

4. Drug Discovery and Repurposing

AI accelerates the identification of novel drug targets and the repurposing of existing compounds for metabolic diseases. Deep learning tools can scan molecular databases, predict interactions, and identify candidates that would otherwise be overlooked. (Pushpakom, S et al., 2019)

Case Studies and Innovations

Diabetes Management: Platforms like Google's DeepMind and Medtronic's Guardian Connect use AI to forecast blood glucose trends and adjust insulin dosing automatically.

Obesity Interventions: Companies like Noom and Lumen leverage AI to deliver personalized nutrition and behavioral coaching based on real-time metabolic data.

Genomic Integration: AI models can analyze polygenic risk scores to forecast metabolic disease likelihood and guide early interventions.

Ethical, Regulatory, and Practical Considerations

As with all AI applications in healthcare, caution is critical:

Bias and Equity: AI models trained on non-diverse datasets risk perpetuating health disparities.

Privacy and Data Security: Protecting sensitive health information, especially in wearable and mobile health applications, is paramount.

Regulatory Oversight: Transparent, explainable AI models must be developed in accordance with evolving medical standards and regulatory frameworks.

The Road Ahead: Integrative, Intelligent, and Inclusive

The future of metabolic medicine lies at the intersection of biology, technology, and data science. AI-driven platforms will increasingly integrate multi-omic data (genomics, proteomics, metabolomics), environmental sensors, and even digital phenotyping to build holistic, dynamic health profiles. With the right infrastructure, these tools can extend advanced metabolic care beyond hospital walls—into communities, homes, and underserved regions.

4. Precision Medicine in the Era of Artificial Intelligence

Research on precision medicine highlights the transformative role of AI in chronic disease management, including metabolic disorders. AI-driven tools are used to analyze genomic, proteomic, and metabolomic data, enabling personalized treatment strategies and biomarker discovery. Studies emphasize the importance of interdisciplinary collaboration and ethical considerations in advancing AI-based precision medicine.

5. Artificial Intelligence in Diabetes Management

This study explores the role of AI in diabetes care, focusing on tools like continuous glucose monitoring (CGM) systems and AI-driven insulin therapy optimization platforms. It highlights the transformative potential of AI in improving glycemic control and reducing complications while addressing challenges such as data privacy and algorithmic bias.

6. Precision Medicine in the Era of Artificial Intelligence

This research emphasizes the integration of AI in precision medicine, particularly for chronic diseases like diabetes and obesity. It discusses the use of AI in biomarker discovery, personalized treatment plans, and predictive modeling, showcasing its impact on improving patient outcomes.

7. AI-Driven Biomarker Discovery for Metabolic Dysfunction-Associated Fatty Liver Disease (MAFLD)

This study focuses on the application of AI in identifying novel biomarkers for MAFLD. By analyzing genomic and proteomic data, AI systems have enabled early diagnosis and targeted therapies, reducing the risk of complications such as liver fibrosis and hepatocellular carcinoma.

8. AI in Obesity Management: Personalized Interventions and Behavioral Modification

Obesity is a core component of metabolic syndrome and a key driver of its associated complications. Effective obesity management requires long-term behavioral changes and individualized care — areas where artificial intelligence (AI) is increasingly demonstrating value. AI-driven tools are being utilized to deliver personalized interventions, predict weight-loss outcomes, and enhance patient adherence through real-time feedback and coaching. (Huang L et al., 2025)

1. Personalized Interventions through Data-Driven Insights

AI models can analyze vast and diverse datasets — including electronic health records (EHRs), genetic profiles, lifestyle habits, and wearable sensor data — to tailor intervention strategies for individual patients. Machine learning algorithms can identify the most effective combinations of diet, physical activity, and behavioral therapies based on patient-specific variables such as age, metabolic profile, psychological state, and social context. For example, AI can predict which individuals are more likely to benefit from low-carbohydrate diets versus low-fat diets or whether a patient would respond better to intermittent fasting or continuous calorie restriction.

2. Digital Coaching and Behavioral Nudges

Digital health platforms powered by AI provide behavioral modification support through virtual coaching, reminders, and motivational messaging. These platforms use natural language processing (NLP) and reinforcement learning to interact with users in a conversational and adaptive manner. Chatbots and virtual health assistants help users set goals, track progress, and maintain accountability — all crucial for sustainable weight loss. Some systems are capable of adjusting recommendations in real time based on user input, mood detection, or engagement patterns. (Aishwarya et al., 2025)

3. Predicting Risk of Weight Regain

One of the biggest challenges in obesity management is maintaining long-term weight loss. AI algorithms can help identify early signs of relapse by monitoring patterns in dietary intake, physical activity, sleep quality, and even emotional states. By analyzing continuous data from smart devices and wearables, AI systems can detect deviations and deliver timely interventions, such as alerting healthcare providers or suggesting behavioral adjustments.

4. Enhancing Patient Engagement and Outcomes

By making interventions more interactive, personalized, and convenient, AI contributes to greater patient engagement — a key predictor of success in obesity treatment. Gamification elements, real-time progress dashboards, and customized encouragement foster a sense of ownership and motivation in users. These technologies not only improve health outcomes but also reduce the burden on healthcare providers by automating routine monitoring and support tasks.

9. From Prevention to Management: Exploring AI's Role in Metabolic Syndrome Management

Metabolic syndrome (MetS) represents a growing global health challenge, characterized by a cluster of conditions such as abdominal obesity, hypertension, dyslipidemia, and insulin resistance, all of which significantly increase the risk of cardiovascular disease and type 2 diabetes. Traditional management strategies have relied heavily on reactive approaches, often addressing symptoms only after they manifest. However, the integration of artificial intelligence (AI) into healthcare systems is paving the way for a paradigm shift — from reactive treatment to proactive prevention and personalized management. By leveraging large datasets and advanced machine learning algorithms, AI has the potential to identify at-risk individuals, guide lifestyle interventions, optimize clinical decision-making, and enable continuous monitoring, thereby transforming the entire trajectory of metabolic syndrome care.

CONCLUSION

AI-based metabolic medicine represents a groundbreaking convergence of technology and healthcare, offering innovative solutions to some of the most pressing challenges in managing metabolic disorders. By leveraging advanced computational tools such as machine learning, deep learning, and predictive analytics, this field has transformed the way metabolic disorders are diagnosed, monitored, and treated. The integration of AI into metabolic medicine has not only enhanced clinical precision but also empowered patients through personalized care and real-time monitoring.

Through case studies and real-time applications, the transformative potential of AI in metabolic medicine has been demonstrated across various domains, including diabetes management, obesity control, lipid metabolism, and metabolic syndrome prevention. AI-driven tools have enabled early diagnosis, personalized treatment plans, and dynamic disease management, significantly improving patient outcomes and quality of life. Moreover, AI has accelerated research by uncovering novel biomarkers and therapeutic targets, paving the way for precision medicine.

However, the journey of AI-based metabolic medicine is not without its challenges. Ethical considerations such as data privacy, algorithmic bias, and informed consent remain critical issues that must be addressed to ensure equitable and responsible implementation. Technical barriers, including the need for diverse datasets, model interpretability, and rigorous validation, also pose significant hurdles. Additionally, the scalability and accessibility of AI technologies in resource-limited settings require focused efforts to bridge healthcare disparities.

Looking ahead, the future of AI-based metabolic medicine lies in fostering interdisciplinary collaboration among clinicians, researchers, technologists, and policymakers. By addressing existing challenges and embracing innovative approaches, the field can unlock the full potential of AI to revolutionize metabolic healthcare. Ethical frameworks and regulatory guidelines must evolve alongside technological advancements to ensure that AI-driven solutions are safe, transparent, and inclusive.

The ultimate vision for AI-based metabolic medicine is to create a healthcare ecosystem that is efficient, patient-centered, and globally accessible. By integrating AI into clinical practice and public health initiatives, we can move closer to a future where metabolic disorders are managed with unparalleled precision and care. This transformative journey underscores the importance of innovation, collaboration, and ethical responsibility in shaping the future of healthcare.

REFERENCES

Aishwarya, S., Selvamurugan, C., Parthiban, K. G., Nathan, B., Manoj Prabhakar, J., & Mohamed Noordeen, A. (2024, December). Generative AI in Focus: A Comprehensive Review of Leading Models Across Modalities. In 2024 4th International Conference on Ubiquitous Computing and Intelligent Information Systems (ICUIS) (pp. 1-9). IEEE.

Ambinder, E. P. (2005, July). A history of the shift toward full computerization of medicine. *Journal of Oncology Practice / American Society of Clinical Oncology*, *1*(2), 54–56. DOI: 10.1200/JOP.2005.1.2.54 PMID: 20871680

Anwar, A., Rana, S., & Pathak, P. (2025, February 19). Artificial intelligence in the management of metabolic disorders: A comprehensive review. *Journal of Endocrinological Investigation*, ●●●. Advance online publication. DOI: 10.1007/s40618-025-02548-x PMID: 39969797

Choubey, U., Upadrasta, V. A., Kaur, I. P., Banker, H., Kanagala, S. G., Anamika, F. N. U., & Jain, R. (2024). From prevention to management: exploring AI's role in metabolic syndrome management: a comprehensive review. *The Egyptian Journal of Internal Medicine*, *36*(1), 106.

Hamet, P., & Tremblay, J. (2017). Artificial intelligence in medicine. *Metabolism: Clinical and Experimental*, *69*, S36–S40. DOI: 10.1016/j.metabol.2017.01.011 PMID: 28126242

Hirani, R., Noruzi, K., Khuram, H., Hussaini, A. S., Aifuwa, E. I., Ely, K. E., Lewis, J. M., Gabr, A. E., Smiley, A., Tiwari, R. K., & Etienne, M. (2024, April 26). Artificial Intelligence and Healthcare: A Journey through History, Present Innovations, and Future Possibilities. *Life (Basel, Switzerland)*, *14*(5), 557. DOI: 10.3390/life14050557 PMID: 38792579

Huang, L., Huhulea, E. N., Abraham, E., Bienenstock, R., Aifuwa, E., Hirani, R., Schulhof, A., Tiwari, R. K., & Etienne, M. (2025, February 19). The Role of Artificial Intelligence in Obesity Risk Prediction and Management: Approaches, Insights, and Recommendations. *Medicina (Kaunas, Lithuania)*, *61*(2), 358. DOI: 10.3390/medicina61020358 PMID: 40005474

Iftikhar, M., Saqib, M., Qayyum, S. N., Asmat, R., Mumtaz, H., Rehan, M., Ullah, I., Ud-Din, I., Noori, S., Khan, M., Rehman, E., & Ejaz, Z. (2024, July 23). Artificial intelligence-driven transformations in diabetes care: A comprehensive literature review. *Annals of Medicine and Surgery (London)*, *86*(9), 5334–5342. DOI: 10.1097/MS9.0000000000002369 PMID: 39238969

Jiang, L., Wu, Z., Xu, X., Zhan, Y., Jin, X., Wang, L., & Qiu, Y. (2021, March). Opportunities and challenges of artificial intelligence in the medical field: Current application, emerging problems, and problem-solving strategies. *The Journal of International Medical Research*, *49*(3), 3000605211000157. DOI: 10.1177/03000605211000157 PMID: 33771068

Pushpakom, S., Iorio, F., & Eyers, P.. (2019). Drug repurposing: Progress, challenges and recommendations. *Nature Reviews. Drug Discovery*, *18*, 41–58. DOI: 10.1038/nrd.2018.168 PMID: 30310233

Simmons, L. A., Drake, C. D., Gaudet, T. W., & Snyderman, R. (2016, January). Personalized Health Planning in Primary Care Settings. *Federal Practitioner : for the Health Care Professionals of the VA, DoD, and PHS*, *33*(1), 27–34. PMID: 30766135

Sumner, J., Bundele, A., Lim, H. W., Phan, P., Motani, M., & Mukhopadhyay, A. (2023, December 8). Developing an Artificial Intelligence-Driven Nudge Intervention to Improve Medication Adherence: A Human-Centred Design Approach. *Journal of Medical Systems*, *48*(1), 3. DOI: 10.1007/s10916-023-02024-0 PMID: 38063940

Swarup, S., Ahmed, I., & Grigorova, Y.. (2025 Jan). Metabolic Syndrome. [Updated 2024 Mar 7] In *StatPearls* [Internet]. StatPearls Publishing., Available from https://www.ncbi.nlm.nih.gov/books/NBK459248/

Taherdoost, H., & Ghofrani, A. (2024). AI's role in revolutionizing personalized medicine by reshaping pharmacogenomics and drug therapy. *Intelligent Pharmacy*, *2*(5), 643–650. DOI: 10.1016/j.ipha.2024.08.005

Zhao, A. P., Li, S., Cao, Z., Hu, P. J.-H., Wang, J., Xiang, Y., & Da Xie, X. L. (2024). AI for science: Predicting infectious diseases. *Journal of Safety Science and Resilience = An Quan Ke Xue Yu Ren Xing (Ying Wen)*, *5*(2), 130–146. DOI: 10.1016/j.jnlssr.2024.02.002

Zuhair, V., Babar, A., Ali, R., Oduoye, M. O., Noor, Z., Chris, K., Okon, I. I., & Rehman, L. U. (2024, January-December). Exploring the Impact of Artificial Intelligence on Global Health and Enhancing Healthcare in Developing Nations. *Journal of Primary Care & Community Health*, *15*, 21501319241245847. DOI: 10.1177/21501319241245847 PMID: 38605668

Compilation of References

Aamir, A., Iqbal, A., Jawed, F., Ashfaque, F., Hafsa, H., Anas, Z., & Mansoor, T. (2024). Exploring the current and prospective role of artificial intelligence in disease diagnosis. *Annals of Medicine and Surgery (London)*, *86*(2), 943–949.

Aas, A. M., Axelsen, M., Churuangsuk, C., Hermansen, K., Kendall, C. W. C., Kahleova, H., Khan, T., Lean, M. E. J., Mann, J. I., Pedersen, E., Pfeiffer, A., Rahelić, D., Reynolds, A. N., Risérus, U., Rivellese, A. A., Salas-Salvadó, J., Schwab, U., Sievenpiper, J. L., Thanopoulou, A., & Uusitupa, E. M. (2023). Evidence-based European recommendations for the dietary management of diabetes. *Diabetologia*, *66*(6). Advance online publication. DOI: 10.1007/s00125-023-05894-8

Abbasi, N., Fnu, N., & Zeb, S. (2023). *AI in Healthcare: Integrating Advanced Technologies with Traditional Practices for Enhanced Patient Care. 2*(03).

Abdollahi, M., Jafarizadeh, A., Asbagh, A. G., Sobhi, N., Pourmoghtader, K., Pedrammehr, S., . . . Acharya, U. R. (2023). Artificial intelligence in assessing cardiovascular diseases and risk factors via retinal fundus images: A review of the last decade. *arXiv*. https://doi.org//arXiv.2311.07609DOI: 10.48550

Aberle, D. R., Adams, A. M., Berg, C. D., Black, W. C., Clapp, J. D., Fagerstrom, R. M., Gareen, I. F., Gatsonis, C., Marcus, P. M., & Sicks, J. R. D. (2011). Reduced lung-cancer mortality with low-dose computed tomographic screening. *The New England Journal of Medicine*, *365*, 395–409. DOI: 10.1056/nejmoa1102873 PMID: 21714641

Abràmoff, M. D., Lavin, P. T., Birch, M., Shah, N., & Folk, J. C. (2018). Pivotal trial of an autonomous AI-based diagnostic system for detection of diabetic retinopathy in primary care offices. npj. *Digital Medicine*, *1*(1), 1–8. DOI: 10.1038/s41746-018-0040-6 PMID: 31304320

Abreha, H. G., Hayajneh, M., & Serhani, M. A. (2022). Federated Learning in Edge Computing: A Systematic Survey. In *Sensors* (Vol. 22, Issue 2). MDPI. DOI: 10.3390/s22020450

Abut, F., Akça, E., Akay, M. F., Irmak, M., Irmak, M., & Adigüzel, Y. (2024). Harnessing AI for health: Optimized neural network models for resting metabolic rate prediction. *IEEE Access: Practical Innovations, Open Solutions*, *12*, 156050–156064.

Adeniran, A. A., Onebunne, A. P., & William, P. (2024). Explainable AI (XAI) in healthcare: Enhancing trust and transparency in critical decision-making. *World J. Adv. Res. Rev*, *23*, 2647–2658.

Adesina, N., Dogan, H., Green, S., & Tsofliou, F. (2022). Effectiveness and usability of digital tools to support dietary self-management of gestational diabetes mellitus: A systematic review. In *Nutrients* (Vol. 14, Issue 1). https://doi.org/DOI: 10.3390/nu14010010

Aggarwal, N., Saini, B. S., & Gupta, S. (2023). Role of artificial intelligence techniques and neuroimaging modalities in detection of Parkinson's Disease: A Systematic review. *Cognitive Computation*, *16*(4), 2078–2115. DOI: 10.1007/s12559-023-10175-y

Aggoun, Y. (2007). Obesity, metabolic syndrome, and cardiovascular disease. *Pediatric Research*, *61*(6), 653–659. DOI: 10.1203/pdr.0b013e31805d8a8c PMID: 17426660

Agrawal, S., & Jain, S. K. (2020). Medical text and image processing: applications, issues and challenges. *Machine Learning with Health Care Perspective: Machine Learning and Healthcare*, 237-262.

Ahmad, A., & Mehfuz, S. (2022). *Explainable AI-based early detection of diabetes for smart healthcare*. https://doi.org/DOI: 10.1049/icp.2022.0608

Ahmad, A., Uddin, S., & Steinhoff, M. (2020). CAR-T cell therapies: An overview of clinical studies supporting their approved use against acute lymphoblastic leukemia and large B-cell lymphomas. *International Journal of Molecular Sciences*, *21*(11). Advance online publication. DOI: 10.3390/ijms21113906 PMID: 32486160

Ahmed, A., Aziz, S., Abd-alrazaq, A., Farooq, F., & Sheikh, J. (2022). Overview of artificial intelligence–driven wearable devices for diabetes: Scoping review. *Journal of Medical Internet Research*, *24*(8), e36010. https://www.jmir.org/2022/8/e36010 PMID: 35943772

Ahmed, Z., Mohamed, K., Zeeshan, S., & Dong, X. (2020). Artificial intelligence with multi-functional machine learning platform development for better healthcare and precision medicine. *Database : The Journal of Biological Databases and Curation*, *2020*, baaa010.

Aishwarya, S., Selvamurugan, C., Parthiban, K. G., Nathan, B., Manoj Prabhakar, J., & Mohamed Noordeen, A. (2024, December). Generative AI in Focus: A Comprehensive Review of Leading Models Across Modalities. In 2024 4th International Conference on Ubiquitous Computing and Intelligent Information Systems (ICUIS) (pp. 1-9). IEEE.

Al Kuwaiti, A., Nazer, K., Al-Reedy, A., Al-Shehri, S., Al-Muhanna, A., Subbarayalu, A. V., Al Muhanna, D., & Al-Muhanna, F. A. (2023). A Review of the Role of Artificial Intelligence in Healthcare. In *Journal of Personalized Medicine* (Vol. 13, Issue 6). MDPI. DOI: 10.3390/jpm13060951

Alam, M. A., Sohel, A., Hasan, K. M., & Islam, M. A. (2024). Machine Learning And Artificial Intelligence in Diabetes Prediction And Management: A Comprehensive Review of Models. Journal of Next-Gen Engineering Systems.

Albahri, A. S., Duhaim, A. M., Fadhel, M. A., Alnoor, A., Baqer, N. S., Alzubaidi, L., & Deveci, M. (2023). A systematic review of trustworthy and explainable artificial intelligence in healthcare: Assessment of quality, bias risk, and data fusion. *Information Fusion*, *96*, 156–191.

Alberti, K. G. M. M., Eckel, R. H., Grundy, S. M., Zimmet, P. Z., Cleeman, J. I., Donato, K. A., & Smith, S. C. (2009). Harmonizing the metabolic syndrome: A joint interim statement of the international diabetes federation task force on epidemiology and prevention; National heart, lung, and blood institute; American heart association; World heart federation; International. *Circulation*, *120*(16), 1640–1645. DOI: 10.1161/CIRCULATIONAHA.109.192644 PMID: 19805654

Al-Dekah, A. M., & Sweileh, W. (2025). Role of artificial intelligence in early identification and risk evaluation of non-communicable diseases: A bibliometric analysis of global research trends. *BMJ Open*, *15*(5). Advance online publication. DOI: 10.1136/bmjopen-2025-101169 PMID: 40316361

Al-Garadi, M. A., Yang, Y. C., & Sarker, A. (2022, November). The role of natural language processing during the COVID-19 pandemic: Health applications, opportunities, and challenges. *Health Care*, *10*(11), 2270.

Ali, H. (2022). AI in neurodegenerative disease research: Early detection, cognitive decline prediction, and brain imaging biomarker identification. *Int J Eng Technol Res Manag*, *6*(10), 71.

Ali, O., Abdelbaki, W., Shrestha, A., Elbasi, E., Alryalat, M. A., & Dwivedi, Y. K. (2023). A systematic literature review of artificial intelligence in the healthcare sector: Benefits, challenges, methodologies, and functionalities. *Journal of Innovation & Knowledge*, *8*(1), 100333. DOI: 10.1016/j.jik.2023.100333

Alkhatib, A. (2020). Personalising Exercise and Nutrition Behaviours in Diabetes Lifestyle Prevention. *European Medical Journal*. Advance online publication. DOI: 10.33590/emj/19-00139

Alkhouri, N., & Noureddin, M. (2024). Management strategies for metabolic dysfunction-associated steatotic liver disease (MASLD). *The American Journal of Managed Care*, *30*(9, Suppl), S159–S174. DOI: 10.37765/ajmc.2024.89635

Almaiah, M. A., Yelisetti, S., & Arya, L., CNKB, B., Kaliappan, K., Vellaisamy, P., Hajjej, F., & Alkdour, T. (2023). A novel approach for improving the security of IoT–medical data systems using an enhanced dynamic Bayesian network. *Electronics (Basel)*, *12*(20), 1–15. DOI: 10.3390/en16010008

Almeida, A., Nayfach, S., Boland, M., Strozzi, F., Beracochea, M., Shi, Z. J., Pollard, K. S., Sakharova, E., Parks, D. H., & Hugenholtz, P. (2021). A unified catalog of 204,938 reference genomes from the human gut microbiome. *Nature Biotechnology*, *39*, 105–114. PMID: 32690973

Alowais, S. A., Alghamdi, S. S., Alsuhebany, N., Alqahtani, T., Alshaya, A. I., Almohareb, S. N., Aldairem, A., Alrashed, M., Bin Saleh, K., Badreldin, H. A., Al Yami, M. S., Al Harbi, S., & Albekairy, A. M. (2023). Revolutionizing healthcare: the role of artificial intelligence in clinical practice. In *BMC Medical Education* (Vol. 23, Issue 1). BioMed Central Ltd. https://doi.org/DOI: 10.1186/s12909-023-04698-z

Alowais, S. A., Alghamdi, S. S., Alsuhebany, N., Alqahtani, T., Alshaya, A. I., Almohareb, S. N., & Albekairy, A. M. (2023). Revolutionizing healthcare: The role of artificial intelligence in clinical practice. *BMC Medical Education*, *23*(1), 689.

Alruwaili, F. F. (2020). Artificial intelligence and multi agent based distributed ledger system for better privacy and security of electronic healthcare records. *PeerJ. Computer Science*, *6*, 1–14. DOI: 10.7717/PEERJ-CS.323

Al-Waisy, A. S., Mohammed, M. A., Al-Fahdawi, S., Maashi, M. S., Garcia-Zapirain, B., Abdulkareem, K. H., Mostafa, S. A., Kumar, N. M., & Le, D. (2021). COVID-DeepNet: Hybrid multimodal deep learning system for improving COVID-19 pneumonia detection in chest x-ray images. *Computers, Materials & Continua/Computers. Materials & Continua (Print)*, *67*(2), 2409–2429. DOI: 10.32604/cmc.2021.012955

Amann, J., Blasimme, A., Vayena, E., Frey, D., & Madai, V. I., & Precise4Q Consortium. (2020). Explainability for artificial intelligence in healthcare: A multidisciplinary perspective. *BMC Medical Informatics and Decision Making*, *20*, 1–9.

Ambinder, E. P. (2005, July). A history of the shift toward full computerization of medicine. *Journal of Oncology Practice / American Society of Clinical Oncology*, *1*(2), 54–56. DOI: 10.1200/JOP.2005.1.2.54 PMID: 20871680

American Diabetes Association. (2018). Economic costs of diabetes in the U.S. in 2017. *Diabetes Care*, *41*, 917–928. PMID: 29567642

Aminizadeh, S., Heidari, A., Dehghan, M., Toumaj, S., Rezaei, M., Navimipour, N. J., & Unal, M. (2024). Opportunities and challenges of artificial intelligence and distributed systems to improve the quality of healthcare service. *Artificial Intelligence in Medicine*, *149*, 102779.

Andrès, E., Meyer, L., Zulfiqar, A. A., Hajjam, M., Talha, S., Bahougne, T., Ervé, S., Hajjam, J., Doucet, J., Jeandidier, N., & El Hassani, A. H. (2019). Telemonitoring in diabetes: evolution of concepts and technologies, with a focus on results of the more recent studies. *Journal of Medicine and Life, 2019*(3). https://doi.org/DOI: 10.25122/jml-2019-0006

Anwar, S. M., Majid, M., Qayyum, A., Awais, M., Alnowami, M., & Khan, M. K. (2018). Medical Image Analysis using Convolutional Neural Networks: A Review. In *Journal of Medical Systems* (Vol. 42, Issue 11). Springer New York LLC. https://doi.org/DOI: 10.1007/s10916-018-1088-1

Anwar, A., Rana, S., & Pathak, P. (2025). *Artificial intelligence in the management of metabolic disorders: a comprehensive review*. Springer., DOI: 10.1007/S40618-025-02548-X

Anwar, A., Rana, S., & Pathak, P. (2025, February 19). Artificial intelligence in the management of metabolic disorders: A comprehensive review. *Journal of Endocrinological Investigation*, ●●●. Advance online publication. DOI: 10.1007/s40618-025-02548-x PMID: 39969797

Ardila, D., Kiraly, A. P., Bharadwaj, S., Choi, B., Reicher, J. J., Peng, L., Tse, D., Etemadi, M., Ye, W., & Corrado, G.. (2019). End-to-end lung cancer screening with three-dimensional deep learning on low-dose chest computed tomography. *Nature Medicine*, *25*, 954–961. DOI: 10.1038/s41591-019-0447-x PMID: 31110349

Arefeen, A., Fessler, S., Mostafavi, S. M., Johnston, C. S., & Ghasemzadeh, H. (2025). MealMeter: Using multimodal sensing and machine learning for automatically estimating nutrition intake. *arXiv preprint* arXiv:2503.11683.

Arimura, H., Soufi, M., Ninomiya, K., Kamezawa, H., & Yamada, M. (2018). Potentials of radiomics for cancer diagnosis and treatment in comparison with computer-aided diagnosis. In *Radiological Physics and Technology* (Vol. 11, Issue 4, pp. 365–374). Springer Tokyo. https://doi.org/DOI: 10.1007/s12194-018-0486-x

Arinez, J. F., Chang, Q., Gao, R. X., Xu, C., & Zhang, J. (2020). Artificial intelligence in advanced manufacturing: Current status and future outlook. *Journal of Manufacturing Science and Engineering*, *142*(11), 110804.

Arslan, S. (2023). Exploring the potential of Chat GPT in personalized obesity treatment. *Annals of Biomedical Engineering*, *51*, 1887–1888. PMID: 37145177

Arumugam, N., Kalavathi, P., & Mahalingam, P. U. (2014). Lignin database for diversity of lignin-degrading microbial enzymes (LD2L). *Research in Biotechnology*, *5*, 13–18.

Arya, L. (2024). Securing Healthcare Data and Cybersecurity Innovations in the Era of Industry 5.0. In Cybersecurity and Data Management Innovations for Revolutionizing Healthcare (pp. 132–147).

Arya, L., Lavudiya, N. S., Sateesh, G., Padmanaban, H., Srinivasulu, B. V., & Rastogi, R. (2024). Fuzzy logic-driven machine learning algorithms for improved early disease diagnosis. *International Journal of Advanced Computer Science and Applications*, *15*(11).

Arya, L., Sharma, Y. K., Nayak, S., & Sivakumar, J. (2025). Comparative evaluation of deep learning models in Alzheimer's disease diagnosis. *Procedia Computer Science*, *258*, 2352–2361. DOI: 10.1016/j.procs.2025.04.498

Arya, L., Singh, L., & Yadav, S.. (2024). Investigation of machine learning algorithms and plasmonic waveguide-based Fano resonance sensor for diagnosis of estrogen. *Plasmonics*. Advance online publication. DOI: 10.1007/s11468-024-02680-z

Ashiwaju, B. I., Orikpete, O. F., & Uzougbo, C. G. (2023). The intersection of artificial intelligence and big data in drug discovery: A review of current trends and future implications. *Matrix Science Pharma*, *7*(2), 36–42.

Astaraki, M., Zakko, Y., Toma Dasu, I., Smedby, Ö., & Wang, C. (2021). Benign-malignant pulmonary nodule classification in low-dose CT with convolutional features. *Physica Medica*, *83*, 146–153. DOI: 10.1016/j.ejmp.2021.03.013 PMID: 33774339

Awari, A., Kaushik, D., Kumar, A., Oz, E., Çadırcı, K., Brennan, C., Proestos, C., Kumar, M., & Oz, F. (2025). Obesity Biomarkers: Exploring Factors, Ramification, Machine Learning, and AI-Unveiling Insights in Health Research. *Wiley Online Library*, *6*(7). Advance online publication. DOI: 10.1002/MCO2.70169 PMID: 40551726

Baccouche, A., Garcia-Zapirain, B., Castillo Olea, C., & Elmaghraby, A. S. (2021). Connected-UNets: A deep learning architecture for breast mass segmentation. *NPJ Breast Cancer*, *7*, 1–12. DOI: 10.1038/s41523-021-00358-x PMID: 34857755

Bagheri, F., Kamran, R. R., & Darvishi, M. (2024). A Comparative Study of Data Science Techniques based on Ensemble Classification Algorithms in Healthcare Systems (Case study: Diabetic patients).

Bak-Sosnowska, M. (2018). The level of anxiety in women seeking professional support in reduction of excessive weight. *Obesity Facts*, ●●●, 11.

Bala, I., Pindoo, I. A., Mijwil, M. M., Abotaleb, M., & Yundong, W. (2024). Ensuring Security and Privacy in Healthcare Systems: A Review Exploring Challenges, Solutions, Future Trends, and the Practical Applications of Artificial Intelligence. *Jordan Medical Journal*, *58*(2), 250–270. DOI: 10.35516/jmj.v58i2.2527

Baldwin, D. R., Gustafson, J., Pickup, L., Arteta, C., Novotny, P., Declerck, J., Kadir, T., Figueiras, C., Sterba, A., & Exell, A.. (2020). External validation of a convolutional neural network artificial intelligence tool to predict malignancy in pulmonary nodules. *Thorax*, *75*(4), 306–312. DOI: 10.1136/thoraxjnl-2019-214104 PMID: 32139611

BALFOUR, C. (2021). OBESITY IN AVIATION MEDICINE. *The Journal of the Australasian Society of Aerospace Medicine*, *12*(1). Advance online publication. DOI: 10.21307/asam-2020-001

Bansal, H., Bondhopadhyay, B., Santoshi, S., Himansu, & Mazumder, R. (2025). Transformative Insights: Integrating IoMT With Generative AI for Personalized Medicine and Drug Discovery. *Igi-Global.ComH Bansal, B Bondhopadhyay, S Santoshi, R MazumderConvergence of Internet of Medical Things (IoMT) and Generative AI, 2025●igi-Global.Com*, 535–564. https://doi.org/DOI: 10.4018/979-8-3693-6180-1.CH023

Bao, D., Liu, Z., Geng, Y., Li, L., Xu, H., Zhang, Y., Hu, L., Zhao, X., Zhao, Y., & Luo, D. (2022). Baseline MRI-based radiomics model assisted predicting disease progression in nasopharyngeal carcinoma patients with complete response after treatment. *Cancer Imaging; the Official Publication of the International Cancer Imaging Society*, *22*(1). Advance online publication. DOI: 10.1186/s40644-022-00448-4 PMID: 35090572

Barberis, E., Khoso, S., Sica, A., Falasca, M., Gennari, A., Dondero, F., Afantitis, A., & Manfredi, M. (2022). Precision Medicine Approaches with Metabolomics and Artificial Intelligence. In *International Journal of Molecular Sciences* (Vol. 23, Issue 19). MDPI. DOI: 10.3390/ijms231911269

Barratt, M. J., Lebrilla, C., Shapiro, H.-Y., & Gordon, J. I. (2017). The gut microbiota, food science, and human nutrition: A timely marriage. *Cell Host & Microbe*, *22*(2), 134–141. DOI: 10.1016/j.chom.2017.07.006 PMID: 28799899

Barturen, G., Babaei, S., & Catala-Moll, F. (2020). Integrative analysis reveals a molecular stratification of systemic autoimmune diseases. *Arthritis and Rheumatism*. Advance online publication. DOI: 10.1002/art.41610 PMID: 33497037

Bauer, E., Zimmermann, J., Baldini, F., Thiele, I., & Kaleta, C. (2017). BacArena: Individual-based metabolic modeling of heterogeneous microbes in complex communities. *PLoS Computational Biology*, *13*(5), e1005544. DOI: 10.1371/journal.pcbi.1005544 PMID: 28531184

Becker, J., Decker, J. A., Römmele, C., Kahn, M., Messmann, H., Wehler, M., Schwarz, F., Kroencke, T., & Scheurig-Muenkler, C. (2022). Artificial Intelligence-Based Detection of Pneumonia in Chest Radiographs. *Diagnostics (Basel)*, *12*(6). Advance online publication. DOI: 10.3390/diagnostics12061465 PMID: 35741276

Beer, L., Sahin, H., Bateman, N. W., Blazic, I., Vargas, H. A., Veeraraghavan, H., Kirby, J., Fevrier-Sullivan, B., Freymann, J. B., Jaffe, C. C., Brenton, J., Miccó, M., Nougaret, S., Darcy, K. M., Maxwell, G. L., Conrads, T. P., Huang, E., & Sala, E. (2020). Integration of proteomics with CT-based qualitative and radiomic features in high-grade serous ovarian cancer patients: An exploratory analysis. *European Radiology*, *30*(8), 4306–4316. DOI: 10.1007/s00330-020-06755-3 PMID: 32253542

Beig, N., Khorrami, M., Alilou, M., Prasanna, P., Braman, N., Orooji, M., Rakshit, S., Bera, K., Rajiah, P., & Ginsberg, J.. (2019). Perinodular and intranodular radiomic features on lung CT images distinguish adenocarcinomas from granulomas. *Radiology*, *290*(3), 783–792. DOI: 10.1148/radiol.2018180910 PMID: 30561278

Belazi, A., El-Latif, A. A. A., & Belghith, S. (2016). A novel image encryption scheme based on substitution-permutation network and chaos. *Signal Processing Image Communication*, *28*(3), 292–300. DOI: 10.1016/j.sigpro.2016.03.021

Bello, B., Bundey, Y. N., Bhave, R., Khotimchenko, M., Baran, S. W., Chakravarty, K., & Varshney, J. (2023). Integrating AI/ML Models for Patient Stratification Leveraging Omics Dataset and Clinical Biomarkers from COVID-19 Patients: A Promising Approach to Personalized Medicine. *International Journal of Molecular Sciences*, *24*(7), 7. Advance online publication. DOI: 10.3390/ijms24076250 PMID: 37047222

Benke, K., & Benke, G. (2018). Artificial intelligence and big data in public health. *International Journal of Environmental Research and Public Health*, *15*(12), 2796. DOI: 10.3390/ijerph15122796 PMID: 30544648

Bennett, C. C., Doub, T. W., & Selove, R. (2012). EHRs connect research and practice: Where predictive modeling, artificial intelligence, and clinical decision support intersect. *Health Policy and Technology*, *1*(2), 105–114. DOI: 10.1016/j.hlpt.2012.03.001

Bera, K., Katz, I., & Madabhushi, A. (2020). Reimagining T staging through artificial intelligence and machine learning image processing approaches in digital pathology. *JCO Clinical Cancer Informatics*, *4*, 1039–1050. DOI: 10.1200/CCI.20.00110 PMID: 33166198

Bera, K., Schalper, K. A., Rimm, D. L., Velcheti, V., & Madabhushi, A. (2019). Artificial intelligence in digital pathology—New tools for diagnosis and precision oncology. *Nature Reviews. Clinical Oncology*, *16*, 703–715. DOI: 10.1038/s41571-019-0252-y PMID: 31399699

Berry, S. E., Valdes, A., Drew, G., Asnicar, C., Mazidi, H., Wolf, T. A., & Chan, E. (2020). Human postprandial responses to food and potential for precision nutrition. *Nature Medicine*, *26*(6), 964–973. PMID: 32528151

Beyeler, M., Légeret, C., Kiwitz, F., & van der Horst, K. (2023). Usability and overall perception of a health bot for nutrition-related questions for patients receiving bariatric care: Mixed methods study. *JMIR Human Factors*, *10*, e47913. PMID: 37938894

Beyer, S. E., McKee, B. J., Regis, S. M., McKee, A. B., Flacke, S., Saadawi, G., & El Wald, C. (2017). Automatic Lung-RADSTM classification with a natural language processing system. *Journal of Thoracic Disease*, *9*(12), 3114–3124. DOI: 10.21037/jtd.2017.08.13 PMID: 29221286

Biswas, N., & Chakrabarti, S. (2020). Artificial intelligence (AI)-based systems biology approaches in multi-omics data analysis of cancer. *Frontiers in Oncology*, *10*, 588221. PMID: 33154949

Bi, W. L., Hosny, A., Schabath, M. B., Giger, M. L., Birkbak, N. J., Mehrtash, A., & Aerts, H. J. (2019). Artificial intelligence in cancer imaging: Clinical challenges and applications. *CA: a Cancer Journal for Clinicians*, *69*(2), 127–157.

Bouderhem, R. (2024). Shaping the future of AI in healthcare through ethics and governance. *Humanities & Social Sciences Communications*, *11*(1). Advance online publication. DOI: 10.1057/s41599-024-02894-w

Bozyel, S., Şimşek, E., Koçyiğit, D., Güler, A., Korkmaz, Y., Şeker, M., & Keser, N. (2024). Artificial intelligence-based clinical decision support systems in cardiovascular diseases. *The Anatolian Journal of Cardiology*, *28*(2), 74. PMID: 38168009

Bradley, P. H., Nayfach, S., & Pollard, K. S. (2018). Phylogeny-corrected identification of microbial gene families relevant to human gut colonization. *PLoS Computational Biology*, *14*(8), e1006242. DOI: 10.1371/journal.pcbi.1006242 PMID: 30091981

Brendan McMahan, H., Moore, E., Ramage, D., Hampson, S., & Agüera y Arcas, B. (2017). Communication-efficient learning of deep networks from decentralized data. *Proceedings of the 20th International Conference on Artificial Intelligence and Statistics, AISTATS 2017*, 1273–1282.

Brennan, L., & de Roos, B. (2023). Role of metabolomics in the delivery of precision nutrition. *Redox Biology*, *65*, 102808. PMID: 37423161

Brończyk-Puzoń, A., Piecha, D., Nowak, J., Koszowska, A., Kulik-Kupka, K., Dittfeld, A., & Zubelewicz-Szkodzińska, B. (2015). Guidelines for dietary management of menopausal women with simple obesity. In *Przeglad Menopauzalny* (Vol. 14, Issue 1). https://doi.org/DOI: 10.5114/pm.2015.48678

Brown, C., Nazeer, R., Gibbs, A., Le Page, P., Mitchell, A. R., & Mitchell, A. R. (2023). Breaking bias: The role of artificial intelligence in improving clinical decision-making. *Cureus*, *15*(3).

Browning, L., Colling, R., Rakha, E., Rajpoot, N., Rittscher, J., James, J. A., Salto-Tellez, M., Snead, D. R. J., & Verrill, C. (2021). Digital pathology and artificial intelligence will be key to supporting clinical and academic cellular pathology through COVID-19 and future crises: The PathLAKE consortium perspective. *Journal of Clinical Pathology*, *74*, 443–447. DOI: 10.1136/jclinpath-2020-206854 PMID: 32620678

Bul, K., Holliday, N., Bhuiyan, M. R. A., Clark, C. C. T., Allen, J., & Wark, P. A. (2023). Usability and Preliminary Efficacy of an Artificial Intelligence-Driven Platform Supporting Dietary Management in Diabetes: Mixed Methods Study. *JMIR Human Factors*, *10*. Advance online publication. DOI: 10.2196/43959

Bulusu, G., Vidyasagar, K. E. C., & Mudigonda, M.. (2025). Cancer detection using artificial intelligence: A paradigm in early diagnosis. *Archives of Computational Methods in Engineering*. Advance online publication. DOI: 10.1007/s11831-025-10045-3

Campanella, G., Hanna, M. G., Geneslaw, L., Miraflor, A., Werneck Krauss Silva, V., Busam, K. J., Brogi, E., Reuter, V. E., Klimstra, D. S., & Fuchs, T. J. (2019). Clinical-grade computational pathology using weakly supervised deep learning on whole slide images. *Nature Medicine*, *25*, 1301–1309. DOI: 10.1038/s41591-019-0508-1 PMID: 31308507

Cao, W., Zhou, Y., Chen, C. L. P., & Xia, L. (2017). Medical image encryption using edge maps. *Signal Processing*, *132*, 96–109. DOI: 10.1016/j.sigpro.2016.10.003

Cao, X., Wang, X., Song, J., Su, Y., Wang, L., & Yin, Y. (2024). Pretreatment multiparametric MRI radiomics-integrated clinical hematological biomarkers can predict early rapid metastasis in patients with nasopharyngeal carcinoma. *BMC Cancer*, *24*(1). Advance online publication. DOI: 10.1186/s12885-024-12209-6 PMID: 38589858

Castaner, O., Goday, A., Park, Y.-M., Lee, S.-H., Magkos, F., & Shiow, S.-A. T. E.. (2018). The gut microbiome profile in obesity: A systematic review. *International Journal of Endocrinology*, *2018*, 1–9.

Cebul, R. D., Love, T. E., Jain, A. K., & Hebert, C. J. (2011). Electronic Health Records and Quality of Diabetes Care. *The New England Journal of Medicine*, *365*(9), 825–833. DOI: 10.1056/nejmsa1102519

Cè, M., Chiriac, M. D., Cozzi, A., Macrì, L., Rabaiotti, F. L., Irmici, G., Fazzini, D., Carrafiello, G., & Cellina, M. (2024). Decoding Radiomics: A Step-by-Step Guide to Machine Learning Workflow in Hand-Crafted and Deep Learning Radiomics Studies. *Diagnostics (Basel)*, *14*(22), 2473. DOI: 10.3390/diagnostics14222473 PMID: 39594139

Cepeda, S., Esteban-Sinovas, O., Singh, V., Moiyadi, A., Zemmoura, I., Del Bene, M., Barbotti, A., DiMeco, F., West, T. R., Nahed, B. V., Giammalva, G. R., Arrese, I., & Sarabia, R. (2025). Prognostic Modeling of Overall Survival in Glioblastoma Using Radiomic Features Derived from Intraoperative Ultrasound: A Multi-Institutional Study. *Cancers (Basel)*, *17*(2). Advance online publication. DOI: 10.3390/cancers17020280 PMID: 39858063

Chang, D., Gupta, V. K., & Hur, B.. (2024). Gut Microbiome Wellness Index 2 enhances health status prediction from gut microbiome taxonomic profiles. *Nature Communications*, *15*, 7447. DOI: 10.1038/s41467-024-51651-9 PMID: 39198444

Chang, D., Gupta, V. K., Hur, B., Cunningham, K. Y., & Sung, J. (2023). GMWI-webtool: A user-friendly browser application for assessing health through metagenomic gut microbiome profiling. *Bioinformatics (Oxford, England)*, *39*, btad061. PMID: 36707995

Chan, P. Z., Jin, E., Jansson, M., & Chew, H. S. J. (2024). AI-based noninvasive blood glucose monitoring: Scoping review. *Journal of Medical Internet Research*, *26*, e58892. DOI: 10.2196/58892 PMID: 39561353

Charalampopoulos, G., Bale, R., Filippiadis, D., Odisio, B. C., Wood, B., & Solbiati, L. (2024). Navigation and robotics in interventional oncology: Current status and future roadmap. *Mdpi.ComG Charalampopoulos, R Bale, D Filippiadis, BC Odisio, B Wood, L SolbiatiDiagnostics, 2023•mdpi. Com*, *14*(1). Advance online publication. DOI: 10.3390/DIAGNOSTICS14010098 PMID: 38201407

Chatelan, A., Clerc, A., & Fonta, P. A. (2023). ChatGPT and future artificial intelligence chatbots: What may be the influence on credentialed nutrition and dietetics practitioners? *Journal of the Academy of Nutrition and Dietetics*, *123*, 1525–1531. PMID: 37544375

Chattu, V. K. (2021). A review of artificial intelligence, big data, and blockchain technology applications in medicine and global health. *Big Data and Cognitive Computing*, *5*(3), 41.

Chen, D., Ye, Z., Shao, J., Tang, L., Zhang, H., Wang, X., Qiu, R., & Zhang, Q. (2020). Effect of electronic health interventions on metabolic syndrome: A systematic review and meta-analysis. In *BMJ Open* (Vol. 10, Issue 10). BMJ Publishing Group. DOI: 10.1136/bmjopen-2020-036927

Chen, B. Y., Xie, H., Li, Y., Jiang, X. H., Xiong, L., Tang, X. F., Lin, X. F., Li, L., & Cai, P. Q. (2022). MRI-Based Radiomics Features to Predict Treatment Response to Neoadjuvant Chemotherapy in Locally Advanced Rectal Cancer: A Single Center, Prospective Study. *Frontiers in Oncology, 12*. Advance online publication. DOI: 10.3389/fonc.2022.801743 PMID: 35646677

Chen, C. K., Lai, J. L., & Chang, C. C. (2008). Efficient watermarking method based on significant difference of wavelet coefficient quantization. *IEEE Transactions on Multimedia, 10*(5), 746–757. DOI: 10.1109/TMM.2008.922839

Cheng, L., Zhou, J., Zhao, Y., Wang, N., Jin, M., Mao, W., Zhu, G., Wang, D., Liang, J., Shen, B., & Zheng, Y. (2024). The associations of insulin resistance, obesity, and lifestyle with the risk of developing hyperuricaemia in adolescents. *Springer, 24*(1). https://doi.org/DOI: 10.1186/S12902-024-01757-4

Chen, G., Ma, M., Tang, C., & Lei, Z. (2020). Generalized optical encryption framework based on shearlets for medical image. *Optics and Lasers in Engineering, 128*, 106026. Advance online publication. DOI: 10.1016/j.optlaseng.2020.106026

Chen, J. H., & Asch, S. M. (2017). Machine Learning and Prediction in Medicine — Beyond the Peak of Inflated Expectations. *The New England Journal of Medicine, 376*(26), 2507–2509. DOI: 10.1056/nejmp1702071

Chen, J., Gu, H., Fan, W., Wang, Y., Chen, S., Chen, X., & Wang, Z. (2020). MRI-based radiomic model for preoperative risk stratification in stage I endometrial cancer. *Journal of Cancer, 12*(3), 726–734. DOI: 10.7150/jca.50872 PMID: 33403030

Chen, T., & Guestrin, C. (2016). XGBoost: A scalable tree boosting system. *Proceedings of the ACM SIGKDD International Conference on Knowledge Discovery and Data Mining, 13-17-Augu*, 785–794. DOI: 10.1145/2939672.2939785

Chen, X., Feng, B., Chen, Y., Liu, K., Li, K., Duan, X., Hao, Y., Cui, E., Liu, Z., & Zhang, C.. (2020). A CT-based radiomics nomogram for prediction of lung adenocarcinomas and granulomatous lesions in patients with solitary sub-centimeter solid nodules. *Cancer Imaging; the Official Publication of the International Cancer Imaging Society, 20*(1), 1–13. DOI: 10.1186/s40644-020-00320-3 PMID: 32641166

Chen, Y., Wang, Z., Yin, G., Sui, C., Liu, Z., Li, X., & Chen, W. (2022). Prediction of HER2 expression in breast cancer by combining PET/CT radiomic analysis and machine learning. *Annals of Nuclear Medicine, 36*(2), 172–182. DOI: 10.1007/s12149-021-01688-3 PMID: 34716873

Chicco, D., & Jurman, G. (2020). Machine learning can predict survival of patients with heart failure from serum creatinine and ejection fraction alone. *BMC Medical Informatics and Decision Making*, *20*(1), 1–16. DOI: 10.1186/s12911-020-1023-5 PMID: 32013925

Chien, P. L., Liu, C. F., Huang, H. T., Jou, H. J., Chen, S. M., Young, T. G., Wang, Y. F., & Liao, P. H. (2021). Application of Artificial Intelligence in the Establishment of an Association Model between Metabolic Syndrome, TCM Constitution, and the Guidance of Medicated Diet Care. *Evidence-Based Complementary and Alternative Medicine : eCAM*, *2021*. Advance online publication. DOI: 10.1155/2021/5530717

Choe, E. K., Rhee, H., Lee, S., Shin, E., Oh, S.-W., Lee, J.-E., & Choi, S. H. (2018). Metabolic Syndrome Prediction Using Machine Learning Models with Genetic and Clinical Information from a Nonobese Healthy Population. *Genomics & Informatics*, *16*(4), e31. DOI: 10.5808/gi.2018.16.4.e31 PMID: 30602092

Choi, S. W., Mak, T. S.-H., & O'Reilly, P. F. (2020). Tutorial: A guide to performing polygenic risk score analyses. *Nature Protocols*, *15*, 2759–2772. PMID: 32709988

Choubey, U., Upadrasta, V. A., Kaur, I. P., Banker, H., Kanagala, S. G., & Anamika, F. N. U.. (2024). From prevention to management: exploring AI's role in metabolic syndrome management: a comprehensive review. *The Egyptian Journal of Internal Medicine*, *36*(1), 106.

Choudhury, G., & MacNee, W. (2017). Role of inflammation and oxidative stress in the pathology of ageing in COPD: Potential therapeutic interventions. *COPD*, *14*(1), 122–135.

Clarke, E. D., Rollo, M. E., Pezdirc, K., Collins, C. E., & Haslam, R. L. (2020). Urinary biomarkers of dietary intake: A review. *Nutrition Reviews*, *78*, 364–381. PMID: 31670796

Costan, V., & Devadas, S. (2016). Intel SGX Explained. In *IACR Cryptol, ePrint Arch.* (pp. 1–118).

Côté, M., & Lamarche, B. (2021). Artificial intelligence in nutrition research: Perspectives on current and future applications. *Applied Physiology, Nutrition, and Metabolism*, *46*(9), 1–8. PMID: 34525321

Coudray, N., Ocampo, P. S., Sakellaropoulos, T., Narula, N., Snuderl, M., Fenyö, D., Moreira, A. L., Razavian, N., & Tsirigos, A. (2018). Classification and mutation prediction from non–small cell lung cancer histopathology images using deep learning. *Nature Medicine*, *24*, 1559–1567. DOI: 10.1038/s41591-018-0177-5 PMID: 30224757

Cowie, M. R., Blomster, J. I., Curtis, L. H., Duclaux, S., Ford, I., Fritz, F., Goldman, S., Janmohamed, S., Kreuzer, J., Leenay, M., Michel, A., Ong, S., Pell, J. P., Southworth, M. R., Stough, W. G., Thoenes, M., Zannad, F., & Zalewski, A. (2017). Electronic health records to facilitate clinical research. In *Clinical Research in Cardiology* (Vol. 106, Issue 1). Dr. Dietrich Steinkopff Verlag GmbH and Co. KG. DOI: 10.1007/s00392-016-1025-6

Crompvoets, P. I., Nieboer, A. P., van Rossum, E. F. C., & Cramm, J. M. (2024). Perceived weight stigma in healthcare settings among adults living with obesity: A cross-sectional investigation of the relationship with patient characteristics and person-centred care. *Health Expectations*, *27*(1). Advance online publication. DOI: 10.1111/hex.13954

Cui, M., & Zhang, D. Y. (2021). Artificial intelligence and computational pathology. *Laboratory Investigation*, *101*(4), 412–422.

Cushley, L. N., Krezel, A., Curran, K., Parker, K., Millar, S., & Peto, T. (2023). Influences on technology use and interpretation among young people living with type 1 diabetes. *Lifestyle Medicine*, *4*(1). Advance online publication. DOI: 10.1002/lim2.73

D'Adderio, L., & Bates, D. W. (2025). Transforming diagnosis through artificial intelligence. In *npj Digital Medicine* (Vol. 8, Issue 1). Nature Research. https://doi.org/DOI: 10.1038/s41746-025-01460-1

D'Urso, F., & Broccolo, F. (2024). Applications of artificial intelligence in microbiome analysis and probiotic interventions—An overview and perspective based on the current state of the art. *Applied Sciences (Basel, Switzerland)*, *14*(19), 8627. DOI: 10.3390/app14198627

da Silva, L. M., Pereira, E. M., Salles, P. G. O., Godrich, R., Ceballos, R., Kunz, J. D., Casson, A., Viret, J., Chandarlapaty, S., & Ferreira, C. G.. (2021). Independent real-world application of a clinical-grade automated prostate cancer detection system. *The Journal of Pathology*, *254*, 147–158. DOI: 10.1002/path.5662 PMID: 33904171

Da'Costa, A., Teke, J., Origbo, J. E., Osonuga, A., Egbon, E., & Olawade, D. B. (2025). AI-driven triage in emergency departments: A review of benefits, challenges, and future directions. *International Journal of Medical Informatics*, *197*, 105838. DOI: 10.1016/j.ijmedinf.2025.105838 PMID: 39965433

Danforth, K. N., Early, M. I., Ngan, S., Kosco, A. E., Zheng, C., & Gould, M. K. (2012). Automated identification of patients with pulmonary nodules in an integrated health system using administrative health plan data, radiology reports, and natural language processing. *Journal of Thoracic Oncology*, *7*(8), 1257–1262. DOI: 10.1097/JTO.0b013e31825bd9f5 PMID: 22627647

Dang, V. N., Campello, V. M., Hernández-González, J., & Lekadir, K. (2025). *Empirical comparison of post-processing debiasing methods for machine learning classifiers in healthcare*. Springer., DOI: 10.1007/S41666-025-00196-7

Dankwa-Mullan, I., Rivo, M., Sepulveda, M., Park, Y., Snowdon, J., & Rhee, K. (2019). Transforming Diabetes Care Through Artificial Intelligence: The Future Is Here. *Population Health Management*, *22*(3). Advance online publication. DOI: 10.1089/pop.2018.0129

Dash, S., Gantayat, P. K., & Das, R. K. (2021). Blockchain technology in healthcare: Opportunities and challenges. In *Intelligent Systems Reference Library* (Vol. 203, pp. 97–111). https://doi.org/DOI: 10.1007/978-3-030-69395-4_6

Dash, R. C., Jones, N., Merrick, R., Haroske, G., Harrison, J., Sayers, C., Haarselhorst, N., Wintell, M., Herrmann, M. D., & Macary, F. (2021). Integrating the Health-care Enterprise Pathology and Laboratory Medicine guideline for digital pathology interoperability. *Journal of Pathology Informatics*, *12*, 16. DOI: 10.4103/jpi.jpi_98_20 PMID: 34221632

Dash, S., Shakyawar, S. K., Sharma, M., & Kaushik, S. (2019). Big data in healthcare: Management, analysis and future prospects. *Journal of Big Data*, *6*(1), 1–25.

Das, P., Banka, R., Ghosh, J., Singh, K., Choudhury, S. R., & Koner, S. (2024). Synergism of diet, genetics, and microbiome on health. In *Nutrition controversies and advances in autoimmune disease* (pp. 131–189). IGI Global.

Das, S. (2024). Applications of Sensor Technology in Healthcare. In *Revolutionizing Healthcare Treatment with Sensor Technology* (pp. 79–99). IGI Global.

DATA-CAN. Health Data Research Hub for Cancer | UCLPartners. (n.d.). Retrieved October 18, 2021, from https://www.data-can.org

Davis, C. R., Murphy, K. J., Curtis, R. G., & Maher, C. A. (2020). A process evaluation examining the performance, adherence, and acceptability of a physical activity and diet artificial intelligence virtual health assistant. *International Journal of Environmental Research and Public Health*, *17*, 9137. PMID: 33297456

Davis, D. A., Chawla, N. V., Blumm, N., Christakis, N., & Barabási, A. L. (2008, October). Predicting individual disease risk based on medical history. In *Proceedings of the 17th ACM conference on Information and knowledge management* (pp. 769-778).

De Filippis, F., Pellegrini, N., Vannini, L., Jeffery, I. B., La Storia, A., & Laghi, L.. (2016). High-level adherence to a Mediterranean diet beneficially impacts the gut microbiota and associated metabolome. *Gut*, *65*, 1812–1821. DOI: 10.1136/gutjnl-2015-309957 PMID: 26416813

de Koning, H. J., van der Aalst, C. M., de Jong, P. A., Scholten, E. T., Nackaerts, K., Heuvelmans, M. A., Lammers, J.-W. J., Weenink, C., Yousaf-Khan, U., & Horeweg, N.. (2020). Reduced lung-cancer mortality with volume CT screening in a randomized trial. *The New England Journal of Medicine*, *382*, 503–513. DOI: 10.1056/NEJMoa1911793 PMID: 31995683

Delzenne, N. M., Olivares, M., Neyrinck, A. M., Beaumont, M., Kjølbæk, L., & Larsen, T. M.. (2019). Nutritional interest of dietary fiber and prebiotics in obesity: Lessons from the MyNewGut consortium. *Clinical Nutrition (Edinburgh, Lothian)*, *39*, 414–424. DOI: 10.1016/j.clnu.2019.03.002 PMID: 30904186

Demaerschalk, B. M., Coffey, J. D., Lunde, J. J., Speltz, B. L., Oyarzabal, B. A., & Copeland, B. J. (2023). Rationale for Establishing a Digital Health Research Center at Mayo Clinic. *Mayo Clinic Proceedings. Digital Health*, *1*(3), 343–348. DOI: 10.1016/j.mcpdig.2023.06.001

Demircioğlu, A. (2022). The effect of preprocessing filters on predictive performance in radiomics. *European Radiology Experimental*, *6*(1). Advance online publication. DOI: 10.1186/s41747-022-00294-w PMID: 36045274

Detopoulou, P., Voulgaridou, G., Moschos, P., Levidi, D., Anastasiou, T., Dedes, V., & Papadopoulou, S. K. (2023). Artificial intelligence, nutrition, and ethical issues: A mini-review. *Clinical Nutrition Open Science*, *50*, 46–56.

Dewi Yudhani, R., Nurwening Sholikhah, E., Aris Agung Nugrahaningsih, D., & Primaningtyas, W. (2022). The bidirectional interaction between climate change and type 2 diabetes burden. *IOP Conference Series. Earth and Environmental Science*, *1016*(1). Advance online publication. DOI: 10.1088/1755-1315/1016/1/012054

Dimitriades, M. E., & Pillay, K. (2021). Dietary management practices for type 1 diabetes mellitus by dietitians in Kwazulu-Natal. *Health SA Gesondheid*, *26*. Advance online publication. DOI: 10.4102/hsag.v26i0.1506

Dinov, I. D. (2018). *Data science and predictive analytics*. Springer.

Dipro, S. H., Islam, M., Al, N. A., Sharmita, A. M., Chakrabarty, A., & Reza, T. (2022). A federated learning based privacy preserving approach for detecting Parkinson's disease using deep learning. International Conference on Computer and Information Technology (ICCIT), 139 144.https://doi.org/DOI: 10.1109/IC-CIT57492.2022.10055787

Dromain, C., Boyer, B., Ferré, R., Canale, S., Delaloge, S., & Balleyguier, C. (2013). Computed-aided diagnosis (CAD) in the detection of breast cancer. *European Journal of Radiology*, *82*(3), 417–423. DOI: 10.1016/j.ejrad.2012.03.005 PMID: 22939365

Du, R., Lee, V. H., Yuan, H., Lam, K. O., Pang, H. H., Chen, Y., Lam, E. Y., Khong, P. L., Lee, A. W., Kwong, D. L., & Vardhanabhuti, V. (2019). Radiomics model to predict early progression of nonmetastatic nasopharyngeal carcinoma after intensity modulation radiation therapy: A multicenter study. *Radiology. Artificial Intelligence*, *1*(4). Advance online publication. DOI: 10.1148/ryai.2019180075 PMID: 33937796

Dwork, C., & Roth, A. (2014). The algorithmic foundations of differential privacy. *Foundations and Trends®in Theoretical Computer Science, 9*(3--4), 211–407.

Dyer, O. (2021). US task force recommends extending lung cancer screenings to over 50s. *BMJ (Clinical Research Ed.), 372*(698). Advance online publication. DOI: 10.1136/bmj.n698 PMID: 33707175

Ebad, S. A., Alhashmi, A., Amara, M., Ben Miled, A., & Saqib, M. (2025). Artificial Intelligence-Based Software as a Medical Device (AI-SaMD): A Systematic Review. In *Healthcare (Switzerland)* (Vol. 13, Issue 7). Multidisciplinary Digital Publishing Institute (MDPI). DOI: 10.3390/healthcare13070817

Eguia, H., Sánchez-Bocanegra, C. L., Vinciarelli, F., Alvarez-Lopez, F., & Saigí-Rubió, F. (2024). Clinical decision support and natural language processing in medicine: Systematic literature review. *Journal of Medical Internet Research, 26*, e55315. PMID: 39348889

Ehteshami Bejnordi, B., Mullooly, M., Pfeiffer, R. M., Fan, S., Vacek, P. M., Weaver, D. L., Herschorn, S., Brinton, L. A., van Ginneken, B., & Karssemeijer, N.. (2018). Using deep convolutional neural networks to identify and classify tumor-associated stroma in diagnostic breast biopsies. *Modern Pathology, 31*, 1502–1512. DOI: 10.1038/s41379-018-0073-z PMID: 29899550

Esteva, A., Kuprel, B., Novoa, R. A., Ko, J., Swetter, S. M., Blau, H. M., & Thrun, S. (2017). Dermatologist-level classification of skin cancer with deep neural networks. *Nature, 542*(7639), 115–118. DOI: 10.1038/nature21056 PMID: 28117445

Eyvazlou, M., Hosseinpouri, M., Mokarami, H., Gharibi, V., Jahangiri, M., Cousins, R., Nikbakht, H.-A., & Barkhordari, A. (2020). Prediction of metabolic syndrome based on sleep and work-related risk factors using an artificial neural network. *SpringerM Eyvazlou, M Hosseinpouri, H Mokarami, V Gharibi, M Jahangiri, R Cousins, HA NikbakhtBMC Endocrine Disorders, 2020•Springer*. https://doi.org/ DOI: 10.1186/S12902-024-01498-6

Falayi, A., Wang, Q., Liao, W., & Yu, W. (2023). Survey of Distributed and Decentralized IoT Securities: Approaches Using Deep Learning and Blockchain Technology. *Future Internet*, *15*(5), 178. DOI: 10.3390/fi15050178

Farhud, D., & Shalileh, M. (2008). Phenylketonuria and its dietary therapy in children. *Iranian Journal of Pediatrics*, *18*, 88–98.

Farinango, C. D., Benavides, J. S., Cerón, J. D., López, D. M., & Álvarez, R. E. (2018). Human-centered design of a personal health record system for metabolic syndrome management based on the ISO 9241-210:2010 standard. *Journal of Multidisciplinary Healthcare*, *11*, 21–37. DOI: 10.2147/JMDH.S150976

Farjah, F., Halgrim, S., Buist, D. S. M., Gould, M. K., Zeliadt, S. B., Loggers, E. T., & Carrell, D. S. (2016). An automated method for identifying individuals with a lung nodule can be feasibly implemented across health systems. *EGEMS (Washington, DC)*, *4*(1), 15. DOI: 10.13063/2327-9214.1254 PMID: 27668266

Fassler, D. J., Abousamra, S., Gupta, R., Chen, C., Zhao, M., Paredes, D., Batool, S. A., Knudsen, B. S., Escobar-Hoyos, L., & Shroyer, K. R.. (2020). Deep learning–based image analysis methods for brightfield-acquired multiplex immunohistochemistry images. *Diagnostic Pathology*, *15*, 1–11. DOI: 10.1186/S13000-020-01003-0 PMID: 32723384

Ferguson, L. R. (2009). Nutrigenomics approaches to functional foods. *Journal of the American Dietetic Association*, *109*, 452–458. PMID: 19248861

Ferreira, D. D., Ferreira, L. G., Amorim, K. A., Delfino, D. C. T., Ferreira, A. C. B. H., & Souza, L. P. C. E. (2025). Assessing the links between artificial intelligence and precision nutrition. *Current Nutrition Reports*, *14*(1), 47. DOI: 10.1007/s13668-025-00635-2 PMID: 40087237

Franco, E. F., Rana, P., Cruz, A., Calderón, V. V., Azevedo, V., Ramos, R. T. J., & Ghosh, P. (2021). Performance comparison of deep learning autoencoders for cancer subtype detection using multi-omics data. *Cancers (Basel)*, *13*, 2013. DOI: 10.3390/cancers13092013 PMID: 33921978

Fregoso-Aparicio, L., Noguez, J., Montesinos, L., & García-García, J. A. (2021). Machine learning and deep learning predictive models for type 2 diabetes: A systematic review. *Diabetology & Metabolic Syndrome*, *13*(1), 148.

Fridrich, J. (1998). Symmetric ciphers based on two-dimensional chaotic maps. *International Journal of Bifurcation and Chaos in Applied Sciences and Engineering*, *8*(6), 1259–1284. DOI: 10.1142/S021812749800098X

Fu, C., Meng, W., Zhan, Y., & Qi, C. (2013). An efficient and secure medical image protection scheme based on chaotic maps. *Computers & Electrical Engineering*, *39*(5), 1606–1622. DOI: 10.1016/j.compeleceng.2013.05.005

Fukuzawa, F.. (2024). Importance of patient history in artificial intelligence-assisted medical diagnosis: Comparison study. *JMIR Medical Education*, *10*, e52674. PMID: 38602313

Galal, A., Talal, M., & Moustafa, A. (2022). Applications of machine learning in metabolomics: Disease modeling and classification. *Frontiersin.OrgA Galal, M Talal, A MoustafaFrontiers in Genetics, 2022•frontiersin. Org*, *13*. Advance online publication. DOI: 10.3389/FGENE.2022.1017340/FULL

Galarregui, C., Navas-Carretero, S., Zulet, M. A., González-Navarro, C. J., Martínez, J. A., & de Cuevillas, B.. (2024). Precision nutrition impact on metabolic health and quality of life in an aging population after a 3-month intervention: A randomized intervention. *The Journal of Nutrition, Health & Aging*, *28*(7), 100289. PMID: 38865737

Gali, R. L., Manne, P., & Veeramalla, S. K. (2023). Structuring hybrid model using bilateral and guided filters for image denoising. In *2023 International Conference on Next Generation Electronics (NEleX)*. IEEE. https://doi.org/DOI: 10.1109/NEleX59773.2023.10421518

Gardner, S., Das, S., Taylor, K., Gardner, S., Das, S., & Taylor, K. (2020). AI Enabled Precision Medicine: Patient Stratification, Drug Repurposing and Combination Therapies. In *Artificial Intelligence in Oncology Drug Discovery and Development*. IntechOpen. https://doi.org/DOI: 10.5772/intechopen.92594

Genomics, D. S.-B. M., & 2024, undefined. (2024). Prediction of metabolic syndrome using machine learning approaches based on genetic and nutritional factors: a 14-year prospective-based cohort study. *SpringerD ShinBMC Medical Genomics, 2024•Springer, 17*(1). https://doi.org/DOI: 10.1186/S12920-024-01998-1

Gentry, C. (2009). A Fully Homomorphic Encryption Scheme [Stanford University]. In *Dissertation* (Issue September). https://cs.au.dk/~stm/local-cache/gentry-thesis.pdf

George, A. H., Shahul, A., & George, A. S. (2023). Wearable sensors: A new way to track health and wellness. *Partners Universal International Innovation Journal, 1*(4), 15–34.

Ghaffar Nia, N., Kaplanoglu, E., & Nasab, A. (2023). Evaluation of artificial intelligence techniques in disease diagnosis and prediction. *Discover Artificial Intelligence, 3*(1), 5.

Ghosh, J., Chaudhury, S. R., Singh, K., & Koner, S. (2024). Application of Machine Learning Algorithm and Artificial Intelligence in Improving Metabolic Syndrome related complications: A review. In *International Journal of Advancement in Life Sciences Research* (Vol. 7, Issue 2, pp. 59–85). Dr Tarak Nath Podder Memorial Foundation. DOI: 10.31632/ijalsr.2024.v07i02.004

Ghosh, J., Roy Choudhury, S., & Koner, S. (2023). Nutraceuticals and bone health. In D. Sharma, M.M. Gupta, A.K. Sharma, R.K. Keservani, & R.K. Kesharwani (Eds.), *AAP Advances in Nutraceuticals Series* (in production). Academic Press. doi: DOI: 10.1201/9781003415084-13

Ghosh, J. (2023). A review on understanding the risk factors for coronary heart disease in Indian college students. *International Journal of Noncommunicable Diseases, 8,* 117–128.

Ghosh, J. (2024b). Recognizing and predicting the risk of malnutrition in the elderly using artificial intelligence: A systematic review. *International Journal of Advancement in Life Sciences Research, 7*(3). Advance online publication. DOI: 10.31632/ijalsr.2024.v07i03.001

Ghosh, J., Chaudhuri, D., Saha, I., & Nag Chaudhuri, A. (2020). Prevalence of metabolic syndrome, vitamin D level, and their association among elderly women in a rural community of West Bengal, India. *Medical Journal of Dr. D.Y. Patil Vidyapeeth, 13*(4), 315–320.

Ghosh, J., Choudhury, S. R., Singh, K., & Koner, S. (2024). Application of machine learning algorithm and artificial intelligence in improving metabolic syndrome related complications: A review. *International Journal of Advancement in Life Sciences Research, 7*(2), 41–67.

Ghosh, J., Choudhury, S. R., Singh, K., & Koner, S. (2025, February). Development and performance analysis of machine learning methods for predicting metabolic syndrome among postmenopausal women of India. *International Journal of Advancement in Life Sciences Research, 8*(1), 006. Advance online publication. DOI: 10.31632/ijalsr.2025.v08i01.006

Ghosh, J., & Sanyal, P. (2024). Development and evaluation of machine learning models for predicting constipation and its risk factors among college-aged females. *Nutrition & Food Science*, *12*(3). https://bit.ly/3MPo6eH

Ghosh, J., Shakil, S., Singh, K., & Mandal, S. (2024). Depression and cognitive function in accordance with the nutritional status of elderly women residing in Rajarhat-Newtown area of Kolkata, India. *Medical Journal of Dr. D.Y. Patil Vidyapeeth*, *17*(5), 951–956. DOI: 10.4103/mjdrdypu.mjdrdypu_423_23

GII Research. (2024). Global precision nutrition market size study, by technology, application, service type, end use, supplement, and regional forecasts 2022–2032. Global Info Research.

Gillies, R. J., Kinahan, P. E., & Hricak, H. (2016). Radiomics: Images are more than pictures, they are data. *Radiology*, *278*(2), 563–577. DOI: 10.1148/radiol.2015151169 PMID: 26579733

Gillum, R. F. (2013). From papyrus to the electronic tablet: A brief history of the clinical medical record with lessons for the digital age. *The American Journal of Medicine*, *126*(10), 853–857. DOI: 10.1016/j.amjmed.2013.03.024 PMID: 24054954

Glaser, A. P., Jordan, B. J., Cohen, J., Desai, A., Silberman, P., & Meeks, J. J. (2018). Automated extraction of grade, stage, and quality information from transurethral resection of bladder tumor pathology reports using natural language processing. *JCO Clinical Cancer Informatics*, *2*, 1–8. DOI: 10.1200/CCI.17.00128 PMID: 30652586

Gloyn, A. L., & Drucker, D. J. (2018). Precision medicine in the management of type 2 diabetes. *The Lancet. Diabetes & Endocrinology*, *6*(11), 891–900. DOI: 10.1016/S2213-8587(18)30052-4 PMID: 29699867

Goel, A., Goel, A. K., & Kumar, A. (2023). The role of artificial neural network and machine learning in utilizing spatial information. *Spatial Information Research*, *31*(3), 275–285.

Goh, K. I.. (2007). The human disease network. *Proceedings of the National Academy of Sciences of the United States of America*, *104*, 8685–8690. PMID: 17502601

Gomez-Cabello, C. A., Borna, S., Pressman, S., Haider, S. A., Haider, C. R., & Forte, A. J. (2024). Artificial-intelligence-based clinical decision support systems in primary care: A scoping review of current clinical implementations. *European Journal of Investigation in Health, Psychology and Education*, *14*(3), 685–698. PMID: 38534906

Gorrepati, L. P. (2024). Integrating AI with Electronic Health Records (EHRs) to Enhance Patient Care. *International Journal of Health Sciences*, 7(8), 8. Advance online publication. DOI: 10.47941/ijhs.2368

Grassi, P. A., Fenton, J. L., Lefkovitz, N. B., Danker, J. M., Choong, Y.-Y., Greene, K. K., & Theofanos, M. F. (2017). NIST Special Publication 800-63A - Digital identity guidelines: enrollment and identity proofing. In *National Institute of Standards and Technology Special Publication*. https://nvlpubs.nist.gov/nistpubs/SpecialPublications/NIST.SP.800-63a.pdf%0Ahttp://nvlpubs.nist.gov/nistpubs/SpecialPublications/NIST.SP.800-63a.pdf

Guan, Y., Aamir, M., Rahman, Z., Ali, A., Abro, W. A., Dayo, Z. A., Bhutta, M. S., Hu, Z., Guan, Y., & Aamir, M.. (2021). A framework for efficient brain tumor classification using MRI images. *Mathematical Biosciences and Engineering*, 18, 5790–5815. DOI: 10.3934/mbe.2021292 PMID: 34517512

Guarducci, S., Jayousi, S., Caputo, S., & Mucchi, L. (2025). Key Fundamentals and Examples of Sensors for Human Health: Wearable, Non-Continuous, and Non-Contact Monitoring Devices. *Mdpi.ComS Guarducci, S Jayousi, S Caputo, L MucchiSensors, 2025•mdpi. Com, 25*(2). Advance online publication. DOI: 10.3390/S25020556 PMID: 39860927

Gupta, R. (2020). Navigating Regulatory Landscapes in Healthcare IT: Upholding HIPAA and GDPR Compliance. In *Advances in Computer Sciences* (Vol. 3).

Gupta, P., & Pandey, M. K. (2024). Role of AI for smart health diagnosis and treatment. In *Smart Medical Imaging for Diagnosis and Treatment Planning* (pp. 23–45). Chapman and Hall/CRC.

Gupta, R., Srivastava, D., Sahu, M., Tiwari, S., Ambasta, R. K., & Kumar, P. (2021). Artificial intelligence to deep learning: Machine intelligence approach for drug discovery. *Molecular Diversity*, 25(3), 1315–1360. DOI: 10.1007/s11030-021-10217-3 PMID: 33844136

Gutiérrez-Esparza, G. O., Vázquez, O. I., Vallejo, M., & Hernández-Torruco, J. (2020). Prediction of metabolic syndrome in a Mexican population applying machine learning algorithms. *Symmetry*, 12(4), 1–16. DOI: 10.3390/SYM12040581

Haak, T.. (2017). Flash glucose-sensing technology as a replacement for blood glucose monitoring for the management of insulin-treated type 2 diabetes: A multicenter, open-label randomized controlled trial. *Diabetes Therapy : Research, Treatment and Education of Diabetes and Related Disorders*, 8, 55–73. PMID: 28000140

Haddad, A., Habaebi, M., Islam, M., Hasbullah, N., & Ahmad Zabidi, S. (2022). Systematic review on AI-blockchain-based e-healthcare records management systems. *IEEE Access : Practical Innovations, Open Solutions*, *10*, 1–1. DOI: 10.1109/ ACCESS.2022.3201878

Halse, H., Colebatch, A. J., Petrone, P., Henderson, M. A., Mills, J. K., Snow, H., Westwood, J. A., Sandhu, S., Raleigh, J. M., & Behren, A.. (2018). Multiplex immunohistochemistry accurately defines the immune context of metastatic melanoma. *Scientific Reports*, *8*, 11158. DOI: 10.1038/s41598-018-28944-3 PMID: 30042403

Hamamoto, R., Komatsu, M., Takasawa, K., Asada, K., & Kaneko, S. (2019). Epigenetics analysis and integrated analysis of multiomics data, including epigenetic data, using artificial intelligence in the era of precision medicine. *Biomolecules*, *10*(1), 62. PMID: 31905969

Hamet, P., & Tremblay, J. (2017). Artificial intelligence in medicine. *Metabolism: Clinical and Experimental*, *69*, S36–S40. DOI: 10.1016/j.metabol.2017.01.011 PMID: 28126242

Hanna, M. G., Pantanowitz, L., Dash, R., Harrison, J. H., Deebajah, M., Pantanowitz, J., & Rashidi, H. H. (2025). Future of Artificial Intelligence—Machine Learning Trends in Pathology and Medicine. In *Modern Pathology* (Vol. 38, Issue 4). Elsevier B.V. https://doi.org/DOI: 10.1016/j.modpat.2025.100705

Harry, A. (2023). Revolutionizing healthcare: How machine learning is transforming patient diagnoses-a comprehensive review of ai's impact on medical diagnosis. *BULLET: Jurnal Multidisiplin Ilmu*, *2*(4), 1259–1266.

Hassan, A. (2021). Lightweight Cryptography for the Internet of Things. *Advances in Intelligent Systems and Computing*, *1290*, 780–795. DOI: 10.1007/978-3-030-63092-8_52

He, K., Zhang, X., Ren, S., & Sun, J. (2016). Deep residual learning for image recognition. In *Proceedings of the IEEE Conference on Computer Vision and Pattern Recognition* (pp. 770–778). Las Vegas, NV, USA. https://doi.org/DOI: 10.1109/ CVPR.2016.90

Henderson, J., & Alexander, S. (2012). e-Learning – The future of child and adolescent obesity! *Obesity Research & Clinical Practice*, *6*. Advance online publication. DOI: 10.1016/j.orcp.2012.08.153

Hernández-Mijares, A., Bañuls, C., Gómez-Balaguer, M., Bergoglio, M., Víctor, V. M., & Rocha, M. (2013). Influence of obesity on atherogenic dyslipidemia in women with polycystic ovary syndrome. *European Journal of Clinical Investigation*, *43*(6). Advance online publication. DOI: 10.1111/eci.12080

Hetzel, D. J.. (1992). HER-2/neu expression: A major prognostic factor in endometrial cancer. *Gynecologic Oncology*, *47*(2), 179–185. DOI: 10.1016/0090-8258(92)90103-p PMID: 1361478

Hillesheim, E., Ryan, M. F., Gibney, E., Roche, H. M., & Brennan, L. (2020). Optimization of a metabotype approach to deliver targeted dietary advice. *Nutrition & Metabolism*, *17*, 1–12. PMID: 33005208

Hirani, R., Noruzi, K., Khuram, H., Hussaini, A. S., Aifuwa, E. I., Ely, K. E., Lewis, J. M., Gabr, A. E., Smiley, A., Tiwari, R. K., & Etienne, M. (2024, April 26). Artificial Intelligence and Healthcare: A Journey through History, Present Innovations, and Future Possibilities. *Life (Basel, Switzerland)*, *14*(5), 557. DOI: 10.3390/life14050557 PMID: 38792579

Honeyford, K., Expert, P., Mendelsohn, E. E., Post, B., Faisal, A. A., Glampson, B., Mayer, E. K., & Costelloe, C. E. (2022). Challenges and recommendations for high quality research using electronic health records. *Frontiers in Digital Health*, *4*. Advance online publication. DOI: 10.3389/fdgth.2022.940330

Hossain, S., Hasan, M. K., Faruk, M. O., Aktar, N., Hossain, R., & Hossain, K. (2024). Machine learning approach for predicting cardiovascular disease in Bangladesh: Evidence from a cross-sectional study in 2023. *BMC Cardiovascular Disorders*, *24*(1). Advance online publication. DOI: 10.1186/s12872-024-03883-2

Hosseini-Esfahani, F., Alafchi, B., Cheraghi, Z., Doosti-Irani, A., Mirmiran, P., Khalili, D., & Azizi, F. (2021). Using machine learning techniques to predict factors contributing to the incidence of metabolic syndrome in tehran: Cohort study. *JMIR Public Health and Surveillance*, *7*(9), 1–12. DOI: 10.2196/27304 PMID: 34473070

Huang, G., Liu, Z., Van Der Maaten, L., & Weinberger, K. Q. (2017). Densely connected convolutional networks. In *Proceedings of the IEEE Conference on Computer Vision and Pattern Recognition (CVPR 2017)* (pp. 2261–2269). Honolulu, HI, USA. https://doi.org/DOI: 10.1109/CVPR.2017.243

Huang, L., Huhulea, E. N., Abraham, E., Bienenstock, R., Aifuwa, E., Hirani, R., Schulhof, A., Tiwari, R. K., & Etienne, M. (2025, February 19). The Role of Artificial Intelligence in Obesity Risk Prediction and Management: Approaches, Insights, and Recommendations. *Medicina (Kaunas, Lithuania)*, *61*(2), 358. DOI: 10.3390/medicina61020358 PMID: 40005474

Huang, L., Jiang, S., & Shi, Y. (2020). Tyrosine kinase inhibitors for solid tumors in the past 20 years (2001–2020). *Journal of Hematology & Oncology, 13*(1), 143. DOI: 10.1186/s13045-020-00977-0 PMID: 33109256

Hua, Z., Yi, S., & Zhou, Y. (2018). Medical image encryption using high-speed scrambling and pixel adaptive diffusion. *Signal Processing, 144*, 134–144. DOI: 10.1016/j.sigpro.2017.10.004

Hunter, B., Reis, S., Campbell, D., Matharu, S., Ratnakumar, P., & Mercuri, L.. (2021). Development of a structured query language and natural language processing algorithm to identify lung nodules in a cancer centre. *Frontiers in Medicine, 8*, 748168. DOI: 10.3389/fmed.2021.748168 PMID: 34805217

Hwalla, N., & Jaafar, Z. (2021). Dietary management of obesity: A review of the evidence. In *Diagnostics* (Vol. 11, Issue 1). https://doi.org/DOI: 10.3390/diagnostics11010024

Hwalla, N., Jaafar, Z., & Sawaya, S. (2021). Dietary management of type 2 diabetes in the mena region: A review of the evidence. In *Nutrients* (Vol. 13, Issue 4). https://doi.org/DOI: 10.3390/nu13041060

Iftikhar, M., Saqib, M., Qayyum, S. N., Asmat, R., Mumtaz, H., Rehan, M., Ullah, I., Ud-Din, I., Noori, S., Khan, M., Rehman, E., & Ejaz, Z. (2024, July 23). Artificial intelligence-driven transformations in diabetes care: A comprehensive literature review. *Annals of Medicine and Surgery (London), 86*(9), 5334–5342. DOI: 10.1097/MS9.0000000000002369 PMID: 39238969

iMSMS Consortium. (2022). Gut microbiome of multiple sclerosis patients and paired household healthy controls reveal associations with disease risk and course. Cell, 185, 3467–3486.e16.

Informatics Education. (2019). *Metabolic Syndrome Prediction* [Dataset]. data.world. Retrieved October 28, 2025, https://data.world/informatics-edu/metabolic-syndrome-prediction

Iqbal, M. J., Javed, Z., Sadia, H., Qureshi, I. A., Irshad, A., Ahmed, R., & Sharifi-Rad, J. (2021). Clinical applications of artificial intelligence and machine learning in cancer diagnosis: Looking into the future. *Cancer Cell International, 21*(1), 270.

Jain, D. (2023). Regulation of Digital Healthcare in India: Ethical and Legal Challenges. *Healthcare (Switzerland), 11*(6). Advance online publication. DOI: 10.3390/healthcare11060911

Jain, P., Gyanchandani, M., & Khare, N. (2016). Big data privacy: A technological perspective and review. *Journal of Big Data*, *3*(1). Advance online publication. DOI: 10.1186/s40537-016-0059-y

Jain, S., Jain, V., & Chatterjee, J. M. (2025). Ensemble based brain tumor classification technique from MRI based on K fold validation approach. *Journal of Integrated Science and Technology*, *13*(5), 1114. DOI: 10.62110/sciencein.jist.2025.V13.1114

Jansson, M., Ohtonen, P., Alalääkkölä, T., Heikkinen, J., Mäkiniemi, M., Lahtinen, S., Lahtela, R., Ahonen, M., Jämsä, S., & Liisantti, J. (2022). Artificial intelligence-enhanced care pathway planning and scheduling system: Content validity assessment of required functionalities. *BMC Health Services Research*, *22*(1). Advance online publication. DOI: 10.1186/s12913-022-08780-y PMID: 36510176

Jan, Z., El Assadi, F., Abd-alrazaq, A., & Jithesh, P. V. (2023). Artificial intelligence for the prediction and early diagnosis of pancreatic cancer: Scoping review. *Journal of Medical Internet Research*, *25*, e44248. DOI: 10.2196/44248 PMID: 37000507

Javaid, M., Haleem, A., Singh, R. P., Suman, R., & Rab, S. (2022). Significance of machine learning in healthcare: Features, pillars and applications. *International Journal of Intelligent Networks*, *3*, 58–73. DOI: 10.1016/j.ijin.2022.05.002

Javidi, H., Mariam, A., Alkhaled, L., Pantalone, K. M., & Rotroff, D. M. (2024). An interpretable predictive deep learning platform for pediatric metabolic diseases. *Academic.Oup.ComH Javidi, A Mariam, L Alkhaled, KM Pantalone, DM RotroffJournal of the American Medical Informatics Association, 2024•academic. Oup. Com*, *31*(6), 1227–1238. DOI: 10.1093/JAMIA/OCAE049 PMID: 38497983

Jena, M. C., Mishra, S. K., & Moharana, H. S. (2024). The way forward to overcome challenges and drawbacks of AI. *Computers and Artificial Intelligence*, *1581*. Advance online publication. DOI: 10.59400/cai1581

Jhade, S., & Gangavarapu, S. P. Channabasamma, & Igorevich Rozhdestvenskiy, O. (2024). Smart Medicine: Exploring the Landscape of AI-Enhanced Clinical Decision Support Systems. *MATEC Web of Conferences, 392*, 01083. DOI: 10.1051/matecconf/202439201083

Jiang, F., Fu, X., Kuang, K., & Fan, D. (2022). Artificial Intelligence Algorithm-Based Differential Diagnosis of Crohn's disease and Ulcerative colitis by CT Image. *Computational and Mathematical Methods in Medicine*, 1–12. DOI: 10.1155/2022/3871994 PMID: 35419083

Jiang, L., Wu, Z., Xu, X., Zhan, Y., Jin, X., Wang, L., & Qiu, Y. (2021, March). Opportunities and challenges of artificial intelligence in the medical field: Current application, emerging problems, and problem-solving strategies. *The Journal of International Medical Research*, *49*(3), 3000605211000157. DOI: 10.1177/03000605211000157 PMID: 33771068

Ji, C., Ge, W., Zhu, C., Shen, F., Yu, Y., Pang, G., Li, Q., Zhu, M., Ma, Z., Zhu, X., Fu, Y., Gong, L., Wang, T., Du, L., Jin, G., & Zhu, M. (2025). Family history and genetic risk score combined to guide cancer risk stratification: A prospective cohort study. *International Journal of Cancer*, *156*(3), 505–517. DOI: 10.1002/ijc.35187 PMID: 39291673

Jo, G. D., Ahn, C., Hong, J. H., Kim, D. S., Park, J., Kim, H., Kim, J. H., Goo, J. M., & Nam, J. G. (2023). 75% radiation dose reduction using deep learning reconstruction on low-dose chest CT. *BMC Medical Imaging*, *23*(1). Advance online publication. DOI: 10.1186/s12880-023-01081-8 PMID: 37697262

Johnson, K. B., Wei, W. Q., Weeraratne, D., Frisse, M. E., Misulis, K., Rhee, K., & Snowdon, J. L. (2021). Precision medicine, AI, and the future of personalized health care. *Clinical and Translational Science*, *14*(1), 86–93.

Juluru, K., Shih, H.-H., Keshava Murthy, K. N., Elnajjar, P., El-Rowmeim, A., Roth, C., Genereaux, B., Fox, J., Siegel, E., & Rubin, D. L. (2021). Integrating Al Algorithms into the Clinical Workflow. *Radiology. Artificial Intelligence*, *3*(6), e210013. DOI: 10.1148/ryai.2021210013 PMID: 34870216

Jyothi, N. M. (2023). AI-Enabled Genomic Biomarkers: The Future of Pharmaceutical Industry and Personalized Medicine. *Seybold Report Journal*, *18*(08), 54–72.

Kadambi, V., Kadambi, N., Bettgeri, S., Buddiga, P., Ramaswami, N., & Hegde, R. (2018). *Review of an Electronic Health Record model to facilitate Remote Patient Management in metabolic and lifestyle diseases.*

Kamal, S. T., Hosny, K. M., Elgindy, T. M., Darwish, M. M., & Fouda, M. M. (2021). A new image encryption algorithm for grey and color medical images. *IEEE Access : Practical Innovations, Open Solutions*, *9*, 37855–37865. DOI: 10.1109/ACCESS.2021.3063237

Kamoun, A., Idbaih, A., Dehais, C., Elarouci, N., Carpentier, C., Letouzé, E., Colin, C., Mokhtari, K., Jouvet, A., & Uro-Coste, E.. (2016). Integrated multi-omics analysis of oligodendroglial tumours identifies three subgroups of 1p/19q co-deleted gliomas. *Nature Communications*, *7*, 11263. DOI: 10.1038/ncomms11263 PMID: 27090007

Kang, Y. K., Ha, S., Jeong, J. B., & Oh, S. W. (2024). The value of PET/CT radiomics for predicting survival outcomes in patients with pancreatic ductal adenocarcinoma. *Scientific Reports*, *14*(1). Advance online publication. DOI: 10.1038/s41598-024-77022-4 PMID: 39578496

Kanso, A., & Smaoui, N. (2009). Logistic chaotic maps for binary numbers generations. *Chaos, Solitons, and Fractals*, *40*(5), 2557–2568. DOI: 10.1016/j.chaos.2007.10.049

Karakan, T., Gundogdu, A., Alagözlü, H., Ekmen, N., Ozgul, S., Tunali, V., & Nalbantoglu, O. U. (2022). Artificial intelligence-based personalized diet: A pilot clinical study for irritable bowel syndrome. *Gut Microbes*, *14*(1). Advance online publication. DOI: 10.1080/19490976.2022.2138672 PMID: 36318623

Katehakis, D. G., & Tsiknakis, M. (2006). *ELECTRONIC HEALTH RECORD*.

Kaul, R., Ossai, C., Forkan, A. R. M., Jayaraman, P. P., Zelcer, J., Vaughan, S., & Wickramasinghe, N. (2023). The role of AI for developing digital twins in healthcare: The case of cancer care. *Wiley Interdisciplinary Reviews. Data Mining and Knowledge Discovery*, *13*(1). Advance online publication. DOI: 10.1002/widm.1480

Kaul, V., Enslin, S., & Gross, S. A. (2020). History of artificial intelligence in medicine. *Gastrointestinal Endoscopy*, *92*(4), 807–812. DOI: 10.1016/j.gie.2020.06.040 PMID: 32565184

Kaur, M., & Kaur, R. (2011). Image encryption techniques: A selected review. *Journal of Theoretical and Applied Information Technology*, *30*(1), 1–12.

Kaur, R., Kumar, R., & Gupta, M. (2022). Predicting risk of obesity and meal planning to reduce the obese in adulthood using artificial intelligence. *Endocrine*, *78*(3). Advance online publication. DOI: 10.1007/s12020-022-03215-4

Kawakami, E., Tabata, J., Yanaihara, N., Ishikawa, T., Koseki, K., Iida, Y., Saito, M., Komazaki, H., Shapiro, J. S., & Goto, C.. (2019). Application of artificial intelligence for preoperative diagnostic and prognostic prediction in epithelial ovarian cancer based on blood biomarkers. *Clinical Cancer Research*, *25*, 3006–3015. DOI: 10.1158/1078-0432.CCR-18-3378 PMID: 30979733

Ke, G., Wang, H., Zhou, S., & Zhang, H. (2019). Encryption of medical image with most significant bit and high capacity in piecewise linear chaos graphics. *Measurement*, *135*, 385–391. DOI: 10.1016/j.measurement.2018.11.074

Kelly, C. J., Karthikesalingam, A., Suleyman, M., Corrado, G., & King, D. (2019). Key challenges for delivering clinical impact with artificial intelligence. In *BMC Medicine* (Vol. 17, Issue 1). BioMed Central Ltd. DOI: 10.1186/s12916-019-1426-2

Khalafi, P., Morsali, S., Hamidi, S., Ashayeri, H., Sobhi, N., Pedrammehr, S., & Jafarizadeh, A. (2025). Artificial intelligence in stroke risk assessment and management via retinal imaging. *Frontiers in Computational Neuroscience, 19*, 1490603.

Khalid, H., Hussain, M., Al Ghamdi, M. A., Khalid, T., Khalid, K., Khan, M. A., & Ahmed, A. (2020). A comparative systematic literature review on knee bone reports from mri, x-rays and ct scans using deep learning and machine learning methodologies. *Diagnostics (Basel), 10*(8), 518.

Khalifa, M., & Albadawy, M. (2024). Artificial Intelligence for Clinical Prediction: Exploring Key Domains and Essential Functions. In *Computer Methods and Programs in Biomedicine Update* (Vol. 5). Elsevier B.V. https://doi.org/DOI: 10.1016/j.cmpbup.2024.100148

Khalifa, M., & Albadawy, M. (2024). AI in diagnostic imaging: Revolutionising accuracy and efficiency. *Computer Methods and Programs in Biomedicine Update, 5*, 100146. DOI: 10.1016/j.cmpbup.2024.100146

Khan, M., & Shah, T. (2014). A literature review on image encryption techniques. *3D Research, 5*(4), Article 29. https://doi.org/DOI: 10.1007/s13319-014-0029-0

Khan, M. M., Shah, N., Shaikh, N., Thabet, A., & Belkhair, S. (2024). Towards secure and trusted AI in healthcare: A systematic review of emerging innovations and ethical challenges. *International Journal of Medical Informatics*, 105780.

Khatiwada, P., Yang, B., Lin, J. C., & Blobel, B. (2024). Patient-generated health data (PGHD): Understanding, requirements, challenges, and existing techniques for data security and privacy. *Journal of Personalized Medicine, 14*(3), 282.

Khattak, M., & Rehman, A. ur, Muqaddas, T., Hussain, R., Rasool, M. F., Saleem, Z., Almalki, M. S., Alturkistani, S. A., Firash, S. Z., Alzahrani, O. M., Bahauddin, A. A., Abuhussain, S. A., Najjar, M. F., Elsabaa, H. M. A., & Haseeb, A. (2024). Tuberculosis (TB) treatment challenges in TB-diabetes comorbid patients: A systematic review and meta-analysis. *Annals of Medicine, 56*(1). Advance online publication. DOI: 10.1080/07853890.2024.2313683

Kim, J., Mun, S., Lee, S., Jeong, K., Health, Y. B.-B. P., & 2022, undefined. (2021). Prediction of metabolic and pre-metabolic syndromes using machine learning models with anthropometric, lifestyle, and biochemical factors from a middle-aged. *SpringerJ Kim, S Mun, S Lee, K Jeong, Y BaekBMC Public Health, 2022•Springer*. https://doi.org/DOI: 10.1186/S12889-024-16248-3

Kim, M. S., Clarke, M. A., Belden, J. L., & Hinton, E. (2014). Usability Challenges and Barriers in EHR Training of Primary Care Resident Physicians. In *LNCS* (Vol. 8529).

Kim, H., & Rebholz, C. M. (2021). Metabolomic biomarkers of healthy dietary patterns and cardiovascular outcomes. *Current Atherosclerosis Reports*, *23*, 1–12. PMID: 33782776

Kim, J., Mun, S., Lee, S., Jeong, K., & Baek, Y. (2022). Prediction of metabolic and pre-metabolic syndromes using machine learning models with anthropometric, lifestyle, and biochemical factors from a middle-aged population in Korea. *BMC Public Health*, *22*(1), 1–11. DOI: 10.1186/s12889-022-13131-x PMID: 35387629

Kings Research. (2024). Precision nutrition market [2031] – Share, trends & growth. Kings Research & Analytics.

Kirk, D., Kok, E., Tufano, M., Tekinerdogan, B., Feskens, E. J. M., & Camps, G. (2022). Machine learning in nutrition research. *Advances in Nutrition*, *13*, 2573–2589. PMID: 36166846

Knijnenburg, T. A., Wang, L., Zimmermann, M. T., Chambwe, N., Gao, G. F., Cherniack, A. D., Fan, H., Shen, H., Way, G. P., & Greene, C. S.. (2018). Genomic and molecular landscape of DNA damage repair deficiency across The Cancer Genome Atlas. *Cell Reports*, *23*, 239–254. DOI: 10.1016/j.celrep.2018.03.076 PMID: 29617664

Kocak, B., Akinci D'Antonoli, T., Mercaldo, N., Alberich-Bayarri, A., Baessler, B., Ambrosini, I., Andreychenko, A. E., Bakas, S., Beets-Tan, R. G. H., Bressem, K., Buvat, I., Cannella, R., Cappellini, L. A., Cavallo, A. U., Chepelev, L. L., Chu, L. C. H., Demircioglu, A., deSouza, N. M., Dietzel, M., & Cuocolo, R. (2024). METhodological RadiomICs Score (METRICS): A quality scoring tool for radiomics research endorsed by EuSoMII. *Insights Into Imaging*, *15*(1). Advance online publication. DOI: 10.1186/s13244-023-01572-w PMID: 38228979

Konishi, K., Nakagawa, H., Asaoka, T., Kasamatsu, Y., Goto, T., & Shirano, M. (2024). Brief communication: Body composition and hidden obesity in people living with HIV on antiretroviral therapy. *AIDS Research and Therapy*, *21*(1). Advance online publication. DOI: 10.1186/s12981-024-00599-3

Kothinti, R. R. (2024). Deep learning in healthcare: Transforming disease diagnosis, personalized treatment, and clinical decision-making through AI-driven innovations.

Kreimeyer, K., Foster, M., Pandey, A., Arya, N., Halford, G., Jones, S. F., & Botsis, T. (2017). Natural language processing systems for capturing and standardizing unstructured clinical information: A systematic review. *Journal of Biomedical Informatics*, *73*, 14–29. DOI: 10.1016/j.jbi.2017.07.012 PMID: 28729030

Krist, A. H., Davidson, K. W., Mangione, C. M., Barry, M. J., Cabana, M., Caughey, A. B., Davis, E. M., Donahue, K. E., Doubeni, C. A., & Kubik, M.. (2021). Screening for lung cancer: US Preventive Services Task Force recommendation statement. *Journal of the American Medical Association*, *325*, 962–970. DOI: 10.1001/jama.2021.1117 PMID: 33687470

Krizhevsky, A., Sutskever, I., & Hinton, G. E. (2017). ImageNet classification with deep convolutional neural networks. *Communications of the ACM*, *60*, 84–90. DOI: 10.1145/3065386

Kshatri, S. S., & Singh, D. (2023). Convolutional neural network in medical image analysis: A review. *Archives of Computational Methods in Engineering*, *30*(4), 2793–2810.

Kumar, B. P. P., & Manoj, H. M. (2024). Comparative assessment of machine learning models for predicting glucose intolerance risk. *Springer, 5*(7). https://doi.org/DOI: 10.1007/S42979-024-03259-5

Kumar, D. N., Chowdhary, D. L., Pathuri, T., Katta, P., & Arya, L. (2024). AI enhanced-smart genome editing: Integration of CRISPR-Cas9 with artificial intelligence for cancer treatment. In 2024 5th International Conference for Emerging Technology (INCET) (pp. 1–6). https://doi.org/DOI: 10.1109/INCET61516.2024.10592877

Kumar, P., Chauhan, S., & Awasthi, L. K. (2023). Artificial Intelligence in Healthcare: Review, Ethics, Trust Challenges & Future Research Directions. *Engineering Applications of Artificial Intelligence*, *120*, 105894. DOI: 10.1016/j.engappai.2023.105894

Kumar, V., Gu, Y., Basu, S., Berglund, A., Eschrich, S. A., Schabath, M. B., Forster, K., Aerts, H. J. W. L., Dekker, A., Fenstermacher, D., Goldgof, D. B., Hall, L. O., Lambin, P., Balagurunathan, Y., Gatenby, R. A., & Gillies, R. J. (2012). Radiomics: The process and the challenges. *Magnetic Resonance Imaging*, *30*(9), 1234–1248. DOI: 10.1016/j.mri.2012.06.010 PMID: 22898692

Kuruvilla, M. E., Lee, F. E., & Lee, G. B. (2019). Understanding asthma phenotypes, endotypes, and mechanisms of disease. *Clinical Reviews in Allergy & Immunology*, *56*(2), 219–233. DOI: 10.1007/s12016-018-8712-1 PMID: 30206782

Lakey, J. R., Casazza, K., Lernhardt, W., Mathur, E. J., & Jenkins, I. (2024). Machine Learning and Augmented Intelligence Enables Prognosis of Type 2 Diabetes Prior to Clinical Manifestation. *Current Diabetes Reviews*, *20*. Advance online publication. DOI: 10.2174/0115733998276990240117113408

LaValley, M. P. (2008). Logistic regression. *Circulation*, *117*(18), 2395–2399. DOI: 10.1161/CIRCULATIONAHA.106.682658 PMID: 18458181

Lebeaud, A., Antoun, L., Paccard, J. R., Edeline, J., Bourien, H., Fares, N., Tournigand, C., Lecomte, T., Tougeron, D., Hautefeuille, V., Viénot, A., Henriques, J., Williet, N., Bachet, J. B., Smolenschi, C., Hollebecque, A., Macarulla, T., Castet, F., Malka, D., … Turpin, A. (2024). Management of biliary tract cancers in early-onset patients: A nested multicenter retrospective study of the ACABI GERCOR PRONOBIL cohort. *Wiley Online LibraryA Lebeaud, L Antoun, JR Paccard, J Edeline, H Bourien, N Fares, C Tournigand, T LecomteLiver International, 2024•Wiley Online Library*, *44*(8), 1886–1899. https://doi.org/DOI: 10.1111/LIV.15922

Lecun, Y., Bengio, Y., & Hinton, G. (2015). Deep learning. In *Nature* (Vol. 521, Issue 7553, pp. 436–444). Nature Publishing Group. https://doi.org/DOI: 10.1038/nature14539

Lee, M. H., Zea, R., Garrett, J. W., Summers, R. M., & Pickhardt, P. J. (2024). AI-based abdominal CT measurements of orthotopic and ectopic fat predict mortality and cardiometabolic disease risk in adults. *SpringerMH Lee, R Zea, JW Garrett, RM Summers, PJ PickhardtEuropean Radiology, 2025•Springer*. https://doi.org/DOI: 10.1007/S00330-024-10935-W

Lee, D., & Yoon, S. N. (2021). Application of artificial intelligence-based technologies in the healthcare industry: Opportunities and challenges. *International Journal of Environmental Research and Public Health*, *18*(1), 271.

Lee, H. A., Huang, T. T., Yen, L. H., Wu, P. H., Chen, K. W., & Kung, H. H.. (2022). Precision nutrient management using artificial intelligence based on digital data collection framework. *Applied Sciences (Basel, Switzerland)*, *12*(9), 4167.

Lee, J. Y., & Lee, K. sig, Seo, B. K., Cho, K. R., Woo, O. H., Song, S. E., Kim, E. K., Lee, H. Y., Kim, J. S., & Cha, J. (2022). Radiomic machine learning for predicting prognostic biomarkers and molecular subtypes of breast cancer using tumor heterogeneity and angiogenesis properties on MRI. *European Radiology*, *32*(1), 650–660. DOI: 10.1007/s00330-021-08146-8 PMID: 34226990

Lee, J., Kim, S. H., Kim, Y., Park, J., Park, G. E., & Kang, B. J. (2022). Radiomics Nomogram: Prediction of 2-Year Disease-Free Survival in Young Age Breast Cancer. *Cancers (Basel)*, *14*(18). Advance online publication. DOI: 10.3390/cancers14184461 PMID: 36139620

Lee, S. J., & Rho, M. (2022). Multimodal deep learning applied to classify healthy and disease states of human microbiome. *Scientific Reports*, *12*, 824. DOI: 10.1038/s41598-022-04773-3 PMID: 35039534

Liao, X., Yin, J., Guo, S., Li, X., & Sangaiah, A. K. (2018). Medical JPEG image steganography based on preserving inter-block dependencies. *Computers & Electrical Engineering*, *67*, 320–329. DOI: 10.1016/j.compeleceng.2017.08.020

Liew, X. Y., Hameed, N., & Clos, J. (2021). An investigation of XGBoost-based algorithm for breast cancer classification. *Machine Learning with Applications*, *6*, 100154. DOI: 10.1016/j.mlwa.2021.100154

Li, J.. (2020). The Mediterranean diet, plasma metabolome, and cardiovascular disease risk. *European Heart Journal*, *41*, 2645–2656. PMID: 32406924

Limketkai, B. N.. (2021). The age of artificial intelligence: Use of digital technology in clinical nutrition. *Current Surgery Reports*, *9*, 20. PMID: 34123579

Lin, X.-X., Li, M.-D., Ruan, S.-M., Ke, W.-P., Zhang, H.-R., Huang, H., Wu, S.-H., Cheng, M.-Q., Tong, W.-J., Hu, H.-T., He, D.-N., Lu, R.-F., Lin, Y.-D., Kuang, M., Lu, M.-D., Chen, L.-D., Huang, Q.-H., & Wang, W. (2025). Autonomous robotic ultrasound scanning system: A key to enhancing image analysis reproducibility and observer consistency in ultrasound imaging. *Frontiers in Robotics and AI*, *12*. Advance online publication. DOI: 10.3389/frobt.2025.1527686 PMID: 39975565

Lin, Y., Wu, R. C., Lin, Y. C., Huang, Y. L., Lin, C. Y., Lo, C. J., Lu, H. Y., Lu, K. Y., Tsai, S. Y., Hsieh, C. Y., Yang, L. Y., Cheng, M. L., Chao, A., Lai, C. H., & Lin, G. (2024). Endometrial cancer risk stratification using MRI radiomics: Corroborating with choline metabolism. *Cancer Imaging; the Official Publication of the International Cancer Imaging Society*, *24*(1). Advance online publication. DOI: 10.1186/s40644-024-00756-x PMID: 39182135

Li, P., Luo, H., & Ji, B.. (2022). Machine learning for data integration in human gut microbiome. *Microbial Cell Factories*, *21*, 241. DOI: 10.1186/s12934-022-01973-4 PMID: 36419034

Liu, Z., Duan, T., Zhang, Y., Weng, S., Xu, H., Ren, Y., Zhang, Z., & Han, X. (2023). Radiogenomics: a key component of precision cancer medicine. In *British Journal of Cancer* (Vol. 129, Issue 5, pp. 741–753). Springer Nature. https://doi.org/DOI: 10.1038/s41416-023-02317-8

Liu, B., Liu, Y., Pan, X., Li, M., Yang, S., & Li, S. C. (2019). DNA methylation markers for pan-cancer prediction by deep learning. *Genes*, *10*, 778. DOI: 10.3390/genes10100778 PMID: 31590287

Liu, H., & Wang, X. (2011). Color image encryption using spatial bit-level permutation and high-dimension chaotic system. *Optics Communications*, *284*(16–17), 3895–3903. DOI: 10.1016/j.optcom.2011.04.001

Liu, J., Liu, Z., Liu, C., Sun, H., Li, X., & Yang, Y. (2025). Integrating Artificial Intelligence in the Diagnosis and Management of Metabolic Syndrome: A Comprehensive Review. *Wiley Online Library*, *41*(4). Advance online publication. DOI: 10.1002/DMRR.70039 PMID: 40145661

Liu, J., Xia, C., & Wang, G. (2020). Multi-omics analysis in initiation and progression of meningiomas: From pathogenesis to diagnosis. *Frontiers in Oncology*, *10*, 1491. DOI: 10.3389/fonc.2020.01491 PMID: 32983987

Liu, R., Wang, M., & Zheng, T.. (2022). An artificial intelligence-based risk prediction model of myocardial infarction. *BMC Bioinformatics*, *23*, 217. DOI: 10.1186/s12859-022-04845-3 PMID: 35672659

Liu, S., Wang, X., Xiang, Y., Xu, H., Wang, H., & Tang, B. (2022). Multi-channel fusion LSTM for medical event prediction using EHRs. *Journal of Biomedical Informatics*, *127*, 104011. DOI: 10.1016/j.jbi.2022.104011 PMID: 35176451

Liu, Y. Y., Zhang, Y., Wu, Y., & Feng, M. (2023). Healthcare and Fitness Services: A Comprehensive Assessment of Blockchain, IoT, and Edge Computing in Smart Cities. *Journal of Grid Computing*, *21*(4), 82. DOI: 10.1007/s10723-023-09712-8

Liu, Y., Yu, D., Luo, J., Cai, S., Ye, P., Yao, Z., Luo, M., & Zhao, L. (2022). Self-Reported Dietary Management Behaviors and Dietary Intake among Chinese Adults with Diabetes: A Population-Based Study. *Nutrients*, *14*(23). Advance online publication. DOI: 10.3390/nu14235178

Liu, Z., & Xiao, D. (2020). Medical image encryption using a novel chaos-based encryption algorithm. *IEEE Access : Practical Innovations, Open Solutions*, *8*, 172894–172905. DOI: 10.1109/ACCESS.2020.2991420

Li, Z., Wu, W., & Kang, H. (2024). Machine Learning-Driven Metabolic Syndrome Prediction: An International Cohort Validation Study. *Mdpi.ComZ Li, W Wu, H KangHealthcare, 2024•mdpi. Com, 12*(24). Advance online publication. DOI: 10.3390/HEALTHCARE12242527 PMID: 39765954

Lloyd-Price, J., Arze, C., Ananthakrishnan, A. N., Schirmer, M., Avila-Pacheco, J., Poon, T. W., Andrews, E., Ajami, N. J., Bonham, K. S., & Brislawn, C. J.. (2019). Multi-omics of the gut microbial ecosystem in inflammatory bowel diseases. *Nature, 569*, 655–662. PMID: 31142855

Lokhande, A., Bonthu, S., & Singhal, N. (2020). Carcino-Net: A deep learning framework for automated Gleason grading of prostate biopsies. In *Proceedings of the Annual International Conference of the IEEE Engineering in Medicine and Biology Society (EMBS)* (pp. 1380–1383). Montreal, QC, Canada. https://doi.org/DOI: 10.1109/EMBC44109.2020.9176011

Louis, T., Lucia, F., Cousin, F., Mievis, C., Jansen, N., Duysinx, B., Le Pennec, R., Visvikis, D., Nebbache, M., Rehn, M., Hamya, M., Geier, M., Salaun, P. Y., Schick, U., Hatt, M., Coucke, P., Lovinfosse, P., & Hustinx, R. (2024). Identification of CT radiomic features robust to acquisition and segmentation variations for improved prediction of radiotherapy-treated lung cancer patient recurrence. *Scientific Reports, 14*(1). Advance online publication. DOI: 10.1038/s41598-024-58551-4 PMID: 38641673

Lu, C. F., Liao, C. Y., Chao, H. S., Chiu, H. Y., Wang, T. W., Lee, Y., Chen, J. R., Shiao, T. H., Chen, Y. M., & Te Wu, Y. (2023). A radiomics-based deep learning approach to predict progression free-survival after tyrosine kinase inhibitor therapy in non-small cell lung cancer. *Cancer Imaging; the Official Publication of the International Cancer Imaging Society, 23*(1). Advance online publication. DOI: 10.1186/s40644-023-00522-5 PMID: 36670497

Lu, H., Arshad, M., Thornton, A., Avesani, G., Cunnea, P., Curry, E., Kanavati, F., Liang, J., Nixon, K., & Williams, S. T.. (2019). A mathematical-descriptor of tumor-mesoscopic-structure from computed-tomography images annotates prognostic- and molecular-phenotypes of epithelial ovarian cancer. *Nature Communications, 10*, 764. DOI: 10.1038/s41467-019-08718-9 PMID: 30770825

Lundberg, S. M., & Lee, S. I. (2017). A unified approach to interpreting model predictions. *Advances in Neural Information Processing Systems*, 4766–4775.

Luo, Y. (2017). Recurrent neural networks for classifying relations in clinical notes. *Journal of Biomedical Informatics, 72*, 85–95.

Lu, Y. (2019). Artificial intelligence: A survey on evolution, models, applications and future trends. *Journal of Management Analytics*, *6*(1), 1–29. DOI: 10.1080/23270012.2019.1570365

Madabhushi, A., Feldman, M. D., & Leo, P. (2020). Deep-learning approaches for Gleason grading of prostate biopsies. *The Lancet. Oncology*, *21*, 187–189. DOI: 10.1016/S1470-2045(19)30793-4 PMID: 31926804

Maharjan, B., Li, J., Kong, J., & Tao, C. (2019). Alexa, what should I eat?: A personalized virtual nutrition coach for Native American diabetes patients using Amazon's smart speaker technology. In *Proceedings of the 2019 IEEE International Conference on E-Health Networking, Application & Services (HealthCom)* (pp. 1–6).

Mahendran, M., Karthika, B., Verma, M. K., & Krishnaja, U. (2024). *AI innovations in nutrition: A critical analysis*. Department of Community Science, College of Agriculture Vellayani.

Maher, C. A., Davis, C. R., Curtis, R. G., Short, C. E., & Murphy, K. J. (2020). A physical activity and diet program delivered by artificially intelligent virtual health coach: Proof-of-concept study. *JMIR mHealth and uHealth*, *8*, e17558. PMID: 32673246

Malakar, S., Sutaoney, P., Madhyastha, H., Shah, K., Chauhan, N. S., & Banerjee, P. (2024). Understanding gut microbiome-based machine learning platforms: A review on therapeutic approaches using deep learning. *Chemistry & Biodiversity Drug Design*, *103*(3), e14505. DOI: 10.1111/cbdd.14505 PMID: 38491814

Maleki Varnosfaderani, S., & Forouzanfar, M. (2024). The role of AI in hospitals and clinics: Transforming healthcare in the 21st century. *Bioengineering (Basel, Switzerland)*, *11*(4), 337.

Maleki Varnosfaderani, S., & Forouzanfar, M. (2024). The Role of AI in Hospitals and Clinics: Transforming Healthcare in the 21st Century. *Bioengineering (Basel, Switzerland)*, *11*(4), 337. DOI: 10.3390/bioengineering11040337 PMID: 38671759

Malik, S., Das, R., Thongtan, T., Thompson, K., & Dbouk, N. (2024). AI in Hepatology: Revolutionizing the Diagnosis and Management of Liver Disease. *Mdpi.ComS Malik, R Das, T Thongtan, K Thompson, N DboukJournal of Clinical Medicine, 2024•mdpi. Com*, *13*(24). Advance online publication. DOI: 10.3390/JCM13247833 PMID: 39768756

Mannava, M., Nangineni, S. M., Birru, S. K., & Arya, L. (2025). Innovative patient care: The transformative role of artificial intelligence and IoT in remote patient monitoring. *AIP Conference Proceedings*, *3237*, 020007. DOI: 10.1063/5.0247075

Mansouri, Z., Salimi, Y., Amini, M., Hajianfar, G., Oveisi, M., Shiri, I., & Zaidi, H. (2024). Development and validation of survival prognostic models for head and neck cancer patients using machine learning and dosiomics and CT radiomics features: A multicentric study. *Radiation Oncology (London, England)*, *19*(1). Advance online publication. DOI: 10.1186/s13014-024-02409-6 PMID: 38254203

MarketsandMarkets. (2024). Precision nutrition market worth $12.89 billion by 2029 – Exclusive report by MarketsandMarkets.

Martinez, V. A., Betts, R. K., Scruth, E. A., Buckley, J. D., Cadiz, V. R., Bertrand, L. D., Paulson, S. S., Dummett, B. A., Abhyankar, S. S., Reyes, V. M., Hatton, J. R., Sulit, R., & Liu, V. X. (2022). The Kaiser Permanente Northern California Advance Alert Monitor Program: An Automated Early Warning System for Adults at Risk for In-Hospital Clinical Deterioration. *Joint Commission Journal on Quality and Patient Safety*, *48*(8), 370–375. DOI: 10.1016/j.jcjq.2022.05.005

Ma, S., Li, X., & Wang, X. (2019). Current progress in CAR-T cell therapy for solid tumors. *International Journal of Biological Sciences*, *15*(12), 2548–2560. DOI: 10.7150/ijbs.34213 PMID: 31754328

Mayerhoefer, M. E., Materka, A., Langs, G., Häggström, I., Szczypiński, P., Gibbs, P., & Cook, G. (2020). Introduction to radiomics. *Journal of Nuclear Medicine*, *61*(4), 488–495. DOI: 10.2967/jnumed.118.222893 PMID: 32060219

McCoubrey, L. E., Elbadawi, M., Orlu, M., Gaisford, S., & Basit, A. W. (2021). Harnessing machine learning for development of microbiome therapeutics. *Gut Microbes*, *13*(1). Advance online publication. DOI: 10.1080/19490976.2021.1872323 PMID: 33522391

McKinney, S. M., Sieniek, M., Godbole, V., Godwin, J., Antropova, N., Ashrafian, H., & Suleyman, M. (2020). International evaluation of an AI system for breast cancer screening. *Nature*, *577*(7788), 89–94. DOI: 10.1038/s41586-019-1799-6 PMID: 31894144

Medina Inojosa, B. J., Somers, V. K., Lara-Breitinger, K., Johnson, L. A., Medina-Inojosa, J. R., & Lopez-Jimenez, F. (2024). PREDICTION OF METABOLIC SYNDROME USING REGIONAL BODY VOLUMES MEASURED USING A MULTISENSORY WHITE-LIGHT 3-D SCANNER. *Jacc. Org*, *5*, 582–590. DOI: 10.1093/EHJDH/ZTAD093

Meena, K. B., & Tyagi, V. (2021). A deep learning based method for image splicing detection. In *Journal of Physics: Conference Series* (Vol. 1714). IOP Publishing Ltd. DOI: 10.1088/1742-6596/1714/1/012038

Meena, K. B., & Tyagi, V. (2020). A copy-move image forgery detection technique based on tetrolet transform. *Journal of Information Security and Applications*, *52*. Advance online publication. DOI: 10.1016/j.jisa.2020.102481

Mehta, N., Ahlawat, J., & Arya, L. (2023). Framework for blockchain in healthcare. In *Blockchain Applications in Healthcare*. Innovations and Practices.

Mennella, C., Maniscalco, U., De Pietro, G., & Esposito, M. (2024). Ethical and regulatory challenges of AI technologies in healthcare: A narrative review. *Heliyon*, *10*(4).

Menzies, S. W., Sinz, C., Menzies, M., Lo, S. N., Yolland, W., Lingohr, J., Razmara, M., Tschandl, P., Guitera, P., Scolyer, R. A., Boltz, F., Borik-Heil, L., Chan, H. H., Chromy, D., Coker, D. J., Collgros, H., Eghtedari, M., Forteza, M. C., Forward, E., & Kittler, H. (2023). Comparison of humans versus mobile phone-powered artificial intelligence for the diagnosis and management of pigmented skin cancer in secondary care: A multicentre, prospective, diagnostic, clinical trial. *The Lancet. Digital Health*, *5*(10), e679–e691. DOI: 10.1016/s2589-7500(23)00130-9 PMID: 37775188

Meyers, D. E., & Banerji, S. (2020). Biomarkers of immune checkpoint inhibitor efficacy in cancer. *Current Oncology (Toronto, Ont.)*, *27*(suppl. 2), S106–S114. DOI: 10.3747/co.27.5549 PMID: 32368180

Mickelson, B., Herfel, T. M., Booth, J., & Wilson, R. P. (2019). Nutrition. In *The Laboratory Rat* (3rd ed., pp. 243–347). Academic Press.

Miller, R. J. H., Huang, C., Liang, J. X., & Slomka, P. J. (2022). Artificial intelligence for disease diagnosis and risk prediction in nuclear cardiology. *Journal of Nuclear Cardiology*, *29*(5), 1754–1762. DOI: 10.1007/s12350-021-02839-5 PMID: 35508795

Milletari, F., Navab, N., & Ahmadi, S. A. (2016). V-Net: Fully convolutional neural networks for volumetric medical image segmentation. In *Proceedings of the 2016 4th International Conference on 3D Vision (3DV)* (pp. 565–571). Stanford, CA, USA. https://doi.org/DOI: 10.1109/3DV.2016.79

Mills, S., Stanton, C., Lane, J. A., Smith, G. J., & Ross, R. P. (2019). Precision nutrition and the microbiome, part I: Current state of the science. *Nutrients*, *11*, 923. PMID: 31022973

Miotto, R., Li, L., Kidd, B. A., & Dudley, J. T. (2016). Deep Patient: An Unsupervised Representation to Predict the Future of Patients from the Electronic Health Records. *Scientific Reports*, *6*. Advance online publication. DOI: 10.1038/srep26094

Miotto, R., Wang, F., Wang, S., Jiang, X., & Dudley, J. T. (2017). Deep learning for healthcare: Review, opportunities and challenges. *Briefings in Bioinformatics*, *19*(6), 1236–1246. DOI: 10.1093/bib/bbx044 PMID: 28481991

Mishro, P. K., Agrawal, S., Panda, R., & Abraham, A. (2020). Novel fuzzy clustering-based bias field correction technique for brain magnetic resonance images. *IET Image Processing*, *14*(9), 1701–1709. DOI: 10.1049/iet-ipr.2019.0942

Moghaddasi, H., Hosseini, A., Asadi, F., & Ganjali, R. (2011). Infrastructures of the System for Developing Electronic Health Record. In *Journal of Paramedical Sciences (JPS) Spring* (Vol. 2, Issue 2).

Mohsen, F., Ali, H., El Hajj, N., & Shah, Z. (2022). Artificial intelligence-based methods for fusion of electronic health records and imaging data. *Scientific Reports*, *12*(1). Advance online publication. DOI: 10.1038/s41598-022-22514-4 PMID: 36289266

Mohsen, F., & Shah, Z. (2025). *Improving Early Prediction of Type 2 Diabetes Mellitus with ECG-DiaNet: A Multimodal Neural Network Leveraging Electrocardiogram and Clinical Risk Factors*. https://arxiv.org/abs/2504.05338

Moons, K. G. M., Altman, D. G., Reitsma, J. B., Ioannidis, J. P. A., Macaskill, P., Steyerberg, E. W., Vickers, A. J., Ransohoff, D. F., & Collins, G. S. (2015). Transparent reporting of a multivariable prediction model for individual prognosis or diagnosis (TRIPOD): Explanation and elaboration. *Annals of Internal Medicine*, *162*(1), W1–W73. DOI: 10.7326/M14-0698 PMID: 25560730

Moore, C. R., Farrag, A., & Ashkin, E. (2017). Using natural language processing to extract abnormal results from cancer screening reports. *Journal of Patient Safety*, *13*(3), 138–143. DOI: 10.1097/PTS.0000000000000127 PMID: 25025472

Mordor Intelligence. (2024). *Personalized nutrition market size & share analysis – Industry research report – Growth trends*. Mordor Intelligence Pvt. Ltd.

Morid, M. A., Sheng, O. R. L., & Dunbar, J. (2023). Time series prediction using deep learning methods in healthcare. *ACM Transactions on Management Information Systems*, *14*(1), 1–29.

Morin, O., Vallières, M., Braunstein, S., Ginart, J. B., Upadhaya, T., Woodruff, H. C., & Zwanenburg, A.. (2021). An artificial intelligence framework integrating longitudinal electronic health records with real-world data enables continuous pan-cancer prognostication. *Nature Cancer*, *2*(6), 709–722. DOI: 10.1038/s43018-021-00236-2 PMID: 35121948

Muhammad, W., Hart, G. R., Nartowt, B., Farrell, J. J., Johung, K., Liang, Y., & Deng, J. (2019). Pancreatic cancer prediction through an artificial neural network. *Frontiers in Artificial Intelligence*, *2*, 2. DOI: 10.3389/frai.2019.00002 PMID: 33733091

Munavalli, J. R., Boersma, H. J., Rao, S. V., & Van Merode, G. G. (2021). Real-time capacity management and patient flow optimization in hospitals using AI methods. *Artificial intelligence and Data mining in healthcare*, 55-69.

Naik, N., Madani, A., Esteva, A., Keskar, N. S., Press, M. F., Ruderman, D., Agus, D. B., & Socher, R. (2020). Deep learning–enabled breast cancer hormonal receptor status determination from base-level H&E stains. *Nature Communications*, *11*, 5727. DOI: 10.1038/s41467-020-19334-3 PMID: 33199723

Naithani, N., Atal, A. T., Tilak, T. V. S. V. G. K., Vasudevan, B., Misra, P., & Sinha, S. (2021). Precision medicine: Uses and challenges. *Medical Journal, Armed Forces India*, *77*(3), 258–265. DOI: 10.1016/j.mjafi.2021.06.020 PMID: 34305277

Nam, J. G., Hwang, E. J., Kim, J., Park, N., Lee, E. H., Kim, H. J., Nam, M., Lee, J. H., Park, C. M., & Goo, J. M. (2023). AI improves nodule detection on chest radiographs in a health screening population: A randomized controlled trial. *Radiology*, *307*(2). Advance online publication. DOI: 10.1148/radiol.221894 PMID: 36749213

Nandakumar, S., Khan, S. A., Ganesan, P., Sweety, P., Francis, A. P., Sekar, M., ... & Meenakshi, D. U. (2022). Deep Learning and Precision Medicine: Lessons to Learn for the Preeminent Treatment for Malignant Tumors. *Deep Learning for Targeted Treatments: Transformation in Healthcare*, 127-169.

National Cholesterol Education Program. (2001). Third Report of the NCEP Expert Panel on Detection, Evaluation, and Treatment of High Blood Cholesterol in Adults (Adult Treatment Panel III). *Circulation*, *106*(25), 3143–3421. PMID: 12485966

Nayor, J., Borges, L. F., Goryachev, S., Gainer, V. S., & Saltzman, J. R. (2018). Natural language processing accurately calculates adenoma and sessile serrated polyp detection rates. *Digestive Diseases and Sciences*, *63*(7), 1794–1800. DOI: 10.1007/s10620-018-5078-4 PMID: 29696479

Neblett, D. A., & Kennedy-Malone, L. (2024). Establishing and Affirming Social Connections: Recruiting Non-Hispanic Black Adults with Type 2 Diabetes. *Clinical Nursing Research*, *33*(5). Advance online publication. DOI: 10.1177/10547738231216530

Nelson, R., & Saranya, S. (2024). Revolutionizing Health Records: The AI Way. [IJSR]. *International Journal of Scientific Research*, *13*(4), 1310–1313. DOI: 10.21275/SR24417190214

NHS Digital. (n.d.). Benefits of the new NHS cervical screening management system. Retrieved January 24, 2022, from https://digital.nhs.uk

NHS Digital. (n.d.). Cancer waiting times data collection (CWT). Retrieved October 18, 2021, from https://digital.nhs.uk/data-and-information/data-collections/cancer-waiting-times

NHSX. (n.d.). Digital transformation of screening. Retrieved January 24, 2022, from https://www.nhsx.nhs.uk

Nicoletti, G., Mazzetti, S., Maimone, G., Cignini, V., Cuocolo, R., Faletti, R., Gatti, M., Imbriaco, M., Longo, N., Ponsiglione, A., Russo, F., Serafini, A., Stanzione, A., Regge, D., & Giannini, V. (2024). Development and Validation of an Explainable Radiomics Model to Predict High-Aggressive Prostate Cancer: A Multicenter Radiomics Study Based on Biparametric MRI. *Cancers (Basel)*, *16*(1). Advance online publication. DOI: 10.3390/cancers16010203 PMID: 38201630

Nie, D., Trullo, R., Lian, J., Wang, L., Petitjean, C., Ruan, S., & Shen, D. (2018). Medical image synthesis with deep convolutional adversarial networks. *IEEE Transactions on Biomedical Engineering*, *65*(12), 2720–2730.

Nielsen, D. (2016). Tree Boosting With XGBoost Why Does XGBoost Win "Every" Machine Learning Competition? *Master of Science in Physics and Mathematics*, *3*(1), 24–34. DOI: 10.1111/j.1758-5899.2011.00096.x

Niszczota, P., & Rybicka, I. (2023). The credibility of dietary advice formulated by ChatGPT: Robo-diets for people with food allergies. *Nutrition (Burbank, Los Angeles County, Calif.)*, *112*, 112076. PMID: 37269717

Nittas, V., Daniore, P., Landers, C., Gille, F., Amann, J., Hubbs, S., & Blasimme, A. (2023). Beyond high hopes: A scoping review of the 2019–2021 scientific discourse on machine learning in medical imaging. *PLOS Digital Health*, *2*(1), e0000189. PMID: 36812620

Ni, Y., Wright, J., Perentesis, J., Lingren, T., Deleger, L., Kaiser, M., Kohane, I., & Solti, I. (2015). Increasing the efficiency of trial-patient matching: Automated clinical trial eligibility pre-screening for pediatric oncology patients. *BMC Medical Informatics and Decision Making*, *15*, 28. DOI: 10.1186/s12911-015-0149-3 PMID: 25881112

Norori, N., Hu, Q., Aellen, F. M., Faraci, F. D., & Tzovara, A. (2021). Addressing bias in big data and AI for health care: A call for open science. *Patterns (New York, N.Y.)*, *2*(10).

Ntantiso, L., Bagula, A., Ajayi, O., & Kahenga-Ngongo, F. (2023). A Review of Federated Learning: Algorithms, Frameworks and Applications. In *Lecture Notes of the Institute for Computer Sciences* (pp. 341–357). Social Informatics and Telecommunications Engineering., DOI: 10.1007/978-3-031-34896-9_20

Oh, Y. J., Zhang, J., Fang, M.-L., & Fukuoka, Y. (2021). A systematic review of artificial intelligence chatbots for promoting physical activity, healthy diet, and weight loss. *The International Journal of Behavioral Nutrition and Physical Activity*, *18*, 160. PMID: 34895247

Olatunji, S. O., Alotaibi, S., Almutairi, E., Alrabae, Z., Almajid, Y., Altabee, R., & Alhiyafi, J. (2021). Early diagnosis of thyroid cancer diseases using computational intelligence techniques: A case study of a Saudi Arabian dataset. *Computers in Biology and Medicine*, *131*, 104267. DOI: 10.1016/j.compbiomed.2021.104267 PMID: 33647831

Olaye, I. M., & Seixas, A. A. (2023). The Gap Between AI and Bedside: Participatory Workshop on the Barriers to the Integration, Translation, and Adoption of Digital Health Care and AI Startup Technology Into Clinical Practice. *Journal of Medical Internet Research, 25*. DOI: 10.2196/32962

Padmavathi, S. (2022). Artificial Intelligence in Health Care. *Annals of SBV, 10*(2), 23–23. DOI: 10.5005/jp-journals-10085-9112

Palacios, G., Druce, J., & Du, L. (2008). A new arenavirus in a cluster of fatal transplant-associated diseases. *The New England Journal of Medicine*, *358*, 991–998. DOI: 10.1056/NEJMoa073785 PMID: 18256387

Palmnäs, M.. (2020). Perspective: Metabotyping—a potential personalized nutrition strategy for precision prevention of cardiometabolic disease. *Advances in Nutrition*, *11*, 524–532. PMID: 31782487

Pantelis, A. G. (2022). *Current and Potential Applications of Artificial Intelligence in Metabolic Bariatric Surgery.* www.intechopen.com

Panza, G. A., Armstrong, L. E., Taylor, B. A., Puhl, R. M., Livingston, J., & Pescatello, L. S. (2018). Weight bias among exercise and nutrition professionals: a systematic review. In *Obesity Reviews* (Vol. 19, Issue 11). https://doi.org/DOI: 10.1111/obr.12743

Papadimitroulas, P., Brocki, L., Christopher Chung, N., Marchadour, W., Vermet, F., Gaubert, L., Eleftheriadis, V., Plachouris, D., Visvikis, D., & Kagadis, G. C.. (2021). Artificial intelligence: Deep learning in oncological radiomics and challenges of interpretability and data harmonization. *Physica Medica*, *83*, 108–121. DOI: 10.1016/j.ejmp.2021.03.009 PMID: 33765601

Paplomatas, P., Rigas, D., Sergounioti, A., & Vrahatis, A. (2024). Enhancing metabolic syndrome detection through blood tests using advanced machine learning. *Eng*, *5*(3), 1422–1434.

Paraschiv, E.-A., Cîrnu, C. E., & Vevera, A. V. (2024). *Integrating Artificial Intelligence and Cybersecurity in Electronic Health Records: Addressing Challenges and Optimizing Healthcare Systems*. www.intechopen.com

Pareek, N. K., Patidar, V., & Sud, K. K. (2006). Image encryption using chaotic logistic map. *Image and Vision Computing*, *24*(9), 926–934. DOI: 10.1016/j.imavis.2006.02.021

Park, I. G., Yoon, S. J., & Won, S. M.. (2024). Gut microbiota-based machine-learning signature for the diagnosis of alcohol-associated and metabolic dysfunction-associated steatotic liver disease. *Scientific Reports*, *14*, 16122. DOI: 10.1038/s41598-024-60768-2 PMID: 38997279

Parmar, C., Grossmann, P., Bussink, J., Lambin, P., & Aerts, H. J. W. L. (2015). Machine Learning methods for Quantitative Radiomic Biomarkers. *Scientific Reports*, *5*. Advance online publication. DOI: 10.1038/srep13087 PMID: 26278466

Patel, A. U., Gu, Q., Esper, R., Maeser, D., & Maeser, N. (2024). The crucial role of interdisciplinary conferences in advancing explainable AI in healthcare. *BioMedInformatics*, *4*(2), 1363–1383.

Paulus, J. K., & Kent, D. M. (2020). Predictably unequal: Understanding and addressing concerns that algorithmic clinical prediction may increase health disparities. *NPJ Digital Medicine*, *3*(1), 99.

Pawade, D., Bakhai, D., Admane, T., Arya, R., Salunke, Y., & Pawade, Y. (2024). Evaluating the Performance of Different Machine Learning Models for Metabolic Syndrome Prediction. *Procedia Computer Science*, *235*, 2932–2941.

Perveen, S., Shahbaz, M., Keshavjee, K., & Guergachi, A. (2019). Metabolic Syndrome and Development of Diabetes Mellitus: Predictive Modeling Based on Machine Learning Techniques. *IEEE Access : Practical Innovations, Open Solutions*, *7*, 1365–1375. DOI: 10.1109/ACCESS.2018.2884249

Philip, M. M., Watts, J., McKiddie, F., Welch, A., & Nath, M. (2024). Development and Validation of Prognostic Models Using Radiomic Features from Pre-Treatment Positron Emission Tomography (PET) Images in Head and Neck Squamous Cell Carcinoma (HNSCC) Patients. *Cancers (Basel)*, *16*(12). Advance online publication. DOI: 10.3390/cancers16122195 PMID: 38927901

Piccialli, F., Di Somma, V., Giampaolo, F., Cuomo, S., & Fortino, G. (2020). A survey on deep learning in medicine: Why, how and when? *Information Fusion*, *66*, 111–137. DOI: 10.1016/j.inffus.2020.09.006

Piette, J. D., Newman, S., Krein, S. L., Marinec, N., Chen, J., Williams, D. A., Edmond, S. N., Driscoll, M., LaChappelle, K. M., Kerns, R. D., Maly, M., Kim, H. M., Farris, K. B., Higgins, D. M., Buta, E., & Heapy, A. A. (2022). Patient-Centered pain care using artificial intelligence and mobile health tools. *JAMA Internal Medicine*, *182*(9), 975. DOI: 10.1001/jamainternmed.2022.3178 PMID: 35939288

Pindi, V. (2019). *A AI-ASSISTED CLINICAL DECISION SUPPORT SYSTEMS: ENHANCING DIAGNOSTIC ACCURACY AND TREATMENT RECOMMENDATIONS | International Journal of Innovations in Engineering Research and Technology.* *6*(10). https://doi.org/DOI: 10.26662/ijiert.v6i10.pp1-10

Pinto-Coelho, L. (2023). How Artificial intelligence is shaping medical Imaging Technology: A survey of Innovations and applications. *Bioengineering (Basel, Switzerland)*, *10*(12), 1435. DOI: 10.3390/bioengineering10121435 PMID: 38136026

Pongrac Barlovic, D., Harjutsalo, V., & Groop, P. H. (2022). Exercise and nutrition in type 1 diabetes: Insights from the FinnDiane cohort. In *Frontiers in Endocrinology* (Vol. 13). https://doi.org/DOI: 10.3389/fendo.2022.1064185

Porri, D., Morabito, L. A., Cavallaro, P., La Rosa, E., & Li, P. A., Pepe, G., & Wasniewska, M. (2024). Time to act on childhood obesity: the use of technology. In *Frontiers in Pediatrics* (Vol. 12). https://doi.org/DOI: 10.3389/fped.2024.1359484

Power, T. G., Baker, S. S., Barale, K. V., Aragón, M. C., Lanigan, J. D., Parker, L., Garcia, K. S., Auld, G., Micheli, N., & Hughes, S. O. (2024). Using Mobile Technology for Family-Based Prevention in Families with Low Incomes: Lessons from a Randomized Controlled Trial of a Childhood Obesity Prevention Program. *Prevention Science*, *25*(2). Advance online publication. DOI: 10.1007/s11121-023-01637-8

Pushpakom, S., Iorio, F., & Eyers, P.. (2019). Drug repurposing: Progress, challenges and recommendations. *Nature Reviews. Drug Discovery*, *18*, 41–58. DOI: 10.1038/nrd.2018.168 PMID: 30310233

Qin, J., Li, Y., Cai, Z., Li, S., Zhu, J., Zhang, F., Liang, S., Zhang, W., Guan, Y., & Shen, D.. (2012). A metagenome-wide association study of gut microbiota in type 2 diabetes. *Nature*, *490*, 55–60. PMID: 23023125

Rahimi, A. K., Pienaar, O., Ghadimi, M., Canfell, O. J., Pole, J. D., Shrapnel, S., van der Vegt, A. H., & Sullivan, C. (2024). Implementing AI in Hospitals to Achieve a Learning Health System: Systematic Review of Current Enablers and Barriers. In *Journal of Medical Internet Research* (Vol. 26). JMIR Publications Inc., DOI: 10.2196/49655

Rajkomar, A., Oren, E., Chen, K., Dai, A. M., Hajaj, N., Hardt, M., & Dean, J. (2018). Scalable and accurate deep learning with electronic health records. *Digital Medicine*, *1*(1), 1–10. DOI: 10.1038/s41746-018-0029-1 PMID: 31304302

Rajpurkar, P., Chen, E., Banerjee, O., & Topol, E. J. (2022). AI in health and medicine. *Nature Medicine*, *28*(1), 31–38.

Rane, N., Choudhary, S., & Rane, J. (2023). Explainable artificial intelligence (XAI) in healthcare: Interpretable models for clinical decision support. *Available at SSRN* 4637897.

Rane, N., Choudhary, S., & Rane, J. (2023). Towards Autonomous Healthcare: Integrating Artificial Intelligence (AI) for Personalized Medicine and Disease Prediction. *Available at SSRN* 4637894.

Raza, A., Guzzo, A., Ianni, M., Lappano, R., Zanolini, A., Maggiolini, M., & Fortino, G. (2025). Federated Learning in radiomics: A comprehensive meta-survey on medical image analysis. In *Computer Methods and Programs in Biomedicine* (Vol. 267). Elsevier Ireland Ltd., DOI: 10.1016/j.cmpb.2025.108768

Reddy Kotha, K., Charan Tokachichu, S., & Padakanti, S. (2024). *Synergizing AI and ERP for Predictive Supply Chain Management and Quality Assurance in Healthcare*. www.ijfmr.com

Richards, T. B., Doria-Rose, V. P., Soman, A., Klabunde, C. N., Caraballo, R. S., Gray, S. C., Houston, K. A., & White, M. C. (2019). Lung cancer screening inconsistent with U.S. Preventive Services Task Force recommendations. *American Journal of Preventive Medicine*, *56*, 66–73. DOI: 10.1016/j.amepre.2018.07.030 PMID: 30467092

Rizzo, S., Botta, F., Raimondi, S., Origgi, D., Fanciullo, C., Morganti, A. G., & Bellomi, M. (2018). Radiomics: the facts and the challenges of image analysis. In *European Radiology Experimental* (Vol. 2, Issue 1). Springer. https://doi.org/DOI: 10.1186/s41747-018-0068-z

Robert, W., Denis, A., Thomas, A., Samuel, A., Kabiito, S. P., Morish, Z., & Ali, G. (2024). A Comprehensive Review on Cryptographic Techniques for Securing Internet of Medical Things: A State-of-the-Art, Applications, Security Attacks, Mitigation Measures, and Future Research Direction. *Mesopotamian Journal of Artificial Intelligence in Healthcare*, *2024*, 135–169. DOI: 10.58496/mjaih/2024/016

Roch, A. M., Mehrabi, S., Krishnan, A., Schmidt, H. E., Kesterson, J., Beesley, C., Dexter, P. R., & Palakal, M. (2015). Automated pancreatic cyst screening using natural language processing: A new tool in the early detection of pancreatic cancer. *HPB : The Official Journal of the International Hepato Pancreato Biliary Association*, *17*(5), 447–453. DOI: 10.1111/hpb.12375 PMID: 25537257

Rodrigues, R. (2020). Legal and human rights issues of AI: Gaps, challenges and vulnerabilities. *Journal of Responsible Technology*, *4*, 100005. DOI: 10.1016/j.jrt.2020.100005

Rodríguez, N. R., Cote, L., Fuentes, C., Jaramillo, E., Arana, S., Castro, A., Behrens, E., Ramos, A., & Zerrweck, C. (2023). First National Consensus on the Safe Practice of Medical Tourism for Bariatric Surgery in Mexico. *Obesity Surgery*, *33*(4). Advance online publication. DOI: 10.1007/s11695-023-06468-8

Ronneberger, O., Fischer, P., & Brox, T. (2015). U-Net: Convolutional networks for biomedical image segmentation. In *Lecture Notes in Computer Science, 9351*, 234–241. https://doi.org/DOI: 10.1007/978-3-319-24574-4_28

Rose, S., Borchert, O., Mitchell, S., & Connelly, S. (2020). NIST Special Publication 807-207: Zero Trust Architecture. In *Controlling Privacy and the Use of Data Assets* (Issues 800–207). https://doi.org/DOI: 10.6028/NIST.SP.800-207%0Ahttps://nvlpubs.nist.gov/nistpubs/SpecialPublications/NIST.SP.800-207.pdf?TB_iframe=true&width=370.8&height=658.8

Rossi, G., Barabino, E., Fedeli, A., Ficarra, G., Coco, S., Russo, A., Adamo, V., Buemi, F., Zullo, L., Dono, M., de Luca, G., Longo, L., Dal Bello, M. G., Tagliamento, M., Alama, A., Cittadini, G., Pronzato, P., & Genova, C. (2021). Radiomic Detection of EGFR Mutations in NSCLC. *Cancer Research*, *81*(3), 724–731. DOI: 10.1158/0008-5472.CAN-20-0999 PMID: 33148663

Rouskas, K., Guela, M., Pantoura, M., Pagkalos, I., Hassapidou, M., Lalama, E., Pfeiffer, A. F. H., Decorte, E., Cornelissen, V., Wilson-Barnes, S., Hart, K., Mantovani, E., Dias, S. B., Hadjileontiadis, L., Gymnopoulos, L. P., Dimitropoulos, K., & Argiriou, A. (2025). The influence of an AI-driven personalized nutrition program on the human gut microbiome and its health implications. *Nutrients*, *17*(7), 1260. DOI: 10.3390/nu17071260 PMID: 40219016

Sabiri, K., Sousa, F., & Rocha, T. (2025). A systematic review of privacy-preserving blockchain applications in healthcare. *Multimedia Tools and Applications*, *84*(32), 39925–39980. DOI: 10.1007/s11042-024-20541-z

Saha, A., Dabic-Miletic, S., Senapati, T., Simic, V., Pamucar, D., Ala, A., & Arya, L. (2024). Fermatean fuzzy Dombi generalized Maclaurin symmetric mean operators for prioritizing bulk material handling technologies. *Cognitive Computation*. Advance online publication. DOI: 10.1007/s12559-024-10323-y

Saha, A., Senapati, T., Akram, M., Kahraman, C., Mesiar, R., & Arya, L. (2024). Dual Probabilistic Linguistic Consensus Reaching Method for Group Decision-Making. *Granular Computing*, *9*(35). Advance online publication. DOI: 10.1007/s41066-024-00458-6

Salinas Martínez, A. M., Juárez Montes, A. G., Ramírez Morado, Y., Cordero Franco, H. F., Guzmán de la Garza, F. J., Hernández Oyervides, L. C., & Núñez Rocha, G. M. (2023). Idealistic, realistic, and unrealistic expectations of pharmacological treatment in persons with type 2 diabetes in primary care. *Frontiers in Public Health*, *11*. Advance online publication. DOI: 10.3389/fpubh.2023.1058828

Sarker, I. H. (2021a). Machine learning: Algorithms, Real-World applications and research directions. *SN Computer Science*, *2*(3). Advance online publication. DOI: 10.1007/s42979-021-00592-x PMID: 33778771

Sarker, I. H. (2021b). Deep Learning: A comprehensive overview on techniques, taxonomy, applications and research directions. *SN Computer Science*, *2*(6). Advance online publication. DOI: 10.1007/s42979-021-00815-1 PMID: 34426802

Sarker, I. H. (2022). AI-Based modeling: Techniques, applications and research issues towards automation, intelligent and smart systems. *SN Computer Science*, *3*(2). Advance online publication. DOI: 10.1007/s42979-022-01043-x PMID: 35194580

Satyanarayanan, M. (2017). The emergence of edge computing. *Computer*, *50*(1), 30–39. DOI: 10.1109/MC.2017.9

Saunders, C. J., Miller, N. A., & Soden, S. E. (2012). Rapid whole-genome sequencing for genetic disease diagnosis in neonatal intensive care units. *Science Translational Medicine*, *4*, 154ra135. Advance online publication. DOI: 10.1126/scitranslmed.3004041 PMID: 23035047

Saw, S. N., & Ng, K. H. (2022). Current challenges of implementing artificial intelligence in medical imaging. *Physica Medica*, *100*, 12–17. DOI: 10.1016/j.ejmp.2022.06.003 PMID: 35714523

Scapicchio, C., Gabelloni, M., Barucci, A., Cioni, D., Saba, L., & Neri, E. (2021). A deep look into radiomics. In *Radiologia Medica* (Vol. 126, Issue 10, pp. 1296–1311). Springer-Verlag Italia s.r.l. https://doi.org/DOI: 10.1007/s11547-021-01389-x

Schlenger, J. (2024). Random Forest. *Computer Science in Sport*, 201–207. DOI: 10.1007/978-3-662-68313-2_24

Schüffler, P. J., Geneslaw, L., Yarlagadda, D. V. K., Hanna, M. G., Samboy, J., Stamelos, E., Vanderbilt, C., Philip, J., Jean, M.-H., & Corsale, L.. (2021). Integrated digital pathology at scale: A solution for clinical diagnostics and cancer research at a large academic medical center. *Journal of the American Medical Informatics Association : JAMIA*, 28, 1874–1886. DOI: 10.1093/jamia/ocab085 PMID: 34260720

Sefa-Yeboah, S. M., Osei Annor, K., Koomson, V. J., Saalia, F. K., Steiner-Asiedu, M., & Mills, G. A. (2021). Development of a Mobile Application Platform for Self-Management of Obesity Using Artificial Intelligence Techniques. *International Journal of Telemedicine and Applications*, 2021. Advance online publication. DOI: 10.1155/2021/6624057

Seshadri, A., Luk, M., Shi, E., Perrig, A., Van Doorn, L., & Khosla, P. (2005). Pioneer: Verifying code integrity and enforcing untampered code execution on legacy systems. *Proceedings of the 20th ACM Symposium on Operating Systems Principles, SOSP 2005*, 1–16. https://doi.org/DOI: 10.1145/1095810.1095812

Seymour, T., Frantsvog, D., & Graeber, T. (2012). Electronic Health Records (EHR). In *American Journal of Health Sciences-Third Quarter* (Vol. 3, Issue 3). https://www.cluteinstitute.com/

Sghaireen, M. G., Al-Smadi, Y., Al-Qerem, A., Srivastava, K. C., Ganji, K. K., Alam, M. K., Nashwan, S., & Khader, Y. (2022). Machine learning approach for metabolic syndrome diagnosis using explainable data-augmentation-based classification. *Mdpi. ComMG Sghaireen, Y Al-Smadi, A Al-Qerem, KC Srivastava, KK Ganji, MK Alam, S NashwanDiagnostics, 2022•mdpi. Com*, 12(12). Advance online publication. DOI: 10.3390/DIAGNOSTICS12123117 PMID: 36553124

Shah, N., Milstein, A., Jama, S. B.-, & 2019, undefined. (n.d.). Making machine learning models clinically useful. *Jamanetwork.Com*. https://doi.org/DOI: 10.1001/JAMA.2024.2456

Shah, S., Yeheskel, A., Hossain, A., Kerr, J., Young, K., Shakik, S., Nichols, J., & Yu, C. (2021). The Impact of Guideline Integration into Electronic Medical Records on Outcomes for Patients with Diabetes: A Systematic Review. In *American Journal of Medicine* (Vol. 134, Issue 8, pp. 952-962.e4). Elsevier Inc. DOI: 10.1016/j.amjmed.2021.03.004

Shah, S., Slaney, E., VerHage, E., Chen, J., Dias, R., Abdelmalik, B., & Neu, J. (2023). Application of artificial intelligence in the early detection of retinopathy of prematurity: Review of the literature. *Neonatology, 120*(5), 558–565. DOI: 10.1159/000530832 PMID: 37490881

Shakir, H., Deng, Y., & Rasheed, H. (2019). Radiomics based likelihood functions for cancer diagnosis. *Scientific Reports, 9*, 9501. DOI: 10.1038/s41598-019-45053-x PMID: 31263186

Shamanna, P., Saboo, B., Damodharan, S., Mohammed, J., Mohamed, M., Poon, T., Kleinman, N., & Thajudeen, M. (2020). Reducing HbA1c in Type 2 Diabetes Using Digital Twin Technology-Enabled Precision Nutrition: A Retrospective Analysis. *Diabetes Therapy : Research, Treatment and Education of Diabetes and Related Disorders, 11*(11). Advance online publication. DOI: 10.1007/s13300-020-00931-w

Shameer, K., Johnson, K. W., Glicksberg, B. S., Dudley, J. T., & Sengupta, P. P. (2018). Machine learning in cardiovascular medicine: Are we there yet? *Heart (British Cardiac Society), 104*(14), 1156–1164.

ShareMe Global. (2024). *Precision nutrition market expansion: Key drivers and emerging opportunities.* ShareMe Global Insights.

Sharma, A., Badea, M., Tiwari, S., & Marty, J. L. (2021). Wearable biosensors: An alternative and practical approach in healthcare and disease monitoring. *Molecules (Basel, Switzerland), 26*(3), 748.

Sharma, S., & Chaturvedi, R. (2020). AI-driven predictive modelling for early disease detection and prevention. *International Journal on Recent and Innovation Trends in Computing and Communication, 8*(12), 27–36. DOI: 10.17762/ijritcc.v8i12.3381

Sharma, V., Davies, A., & Ainsworth, J. (2021). Clinical risk prediction models: The canary in the coalmine for artificial intelligence in healthcare? *BMJ Health & Care Informatics, 28*(1), e100421. DOI: 10.1136/bmjhci-2021-100421 PMID: 34607819

Shehab, M., Abualigah, L., Shambour, Q., Abu-Hashem, M. A., Shambour, M. K. Y., Alsalibi, A. I., & Gandomi, A. H. (2022). Machine learning in medical applications: A review of state-of-the-art methods. *Computers in Biology and Medicine, 145*. Advance online publication. DOI: 10.1016/j.compbiomed.2022.105458 PMID: 35364311

Shehadeh, A., Alshboul, O., Al Mamlook, R. E., & Hamedat, O. (2021). Machine learning models for predicting the residual value of heavy construction equipment: An evaluation of modified decision tree, LightGBM, and XGBoost regression. *Automation in Construction, 129*, 103827.

Shen, Y., Zhou, J., & Hu, G. (2020). Practical use of electronic health records among patients with diabetes in scientific research. In *Chinese Medical Journal* (Vol. 133, Issue 10, pp. 1224–1230). Lippincott Williams and Wilkins. DOI: 10.1097/CM9.0000000000000784

Shen, H., Wang, Y., Liu, D., Lv, R., Huang, Y., Peng, C., Jiang, S., Wang, Y., He, Y., Lan, X., Huang, H., Sun, J., & Zhang, J. (2020). Predicting Progression-Free Survival Using MRI-Based Radiomics for Patients With Nonmetastatic Nasopharyngeal Carcinoma. *Frontiers in Oncology, 10*. Advance online publication. DOI: 10.3389/fonc.2020.00618 PMID: 32477932

Shen, Y., Yu, J., Zhou, J., & Hu, G. (2024). Twenty-Five Years of Evolution and Hurdles in Electronic Health Records and Interoperability in Medical Research: Comprehensive Review *(Preprint)*. DOI: 10.2196/preprints.59024

Sherminie, L. P. G., Jayatilake, M. L., Hewavithana, B., Weerakoon, B. S., & Vijithananda, S. M. (2023). Morphometry-based radiomics for predicting therapeutic response in patients with gliomas following radiotherapy. *Frontiers in Oncology, 13*. Advance online publication. DOI: 10.3389/fonc.2023.1139902 PMID: 37664038

Shin, H., Shim, S., & Oh, S. (2023). Machine learning-based predictive model for prevention of metabolic syndrome. *PLoS ONE, 18*(6 June), 1–28. DOI: 10.1371/journal.pone.0286635

Shui, L., Ren, H., Yang, X., Li, J., Chen, Z., Yi, C., Zhu, H., & Shui, P. (2021). The Era of Radiogenomics in Precision Medicine: An Emerging Approach to Support Diagnosis, Treatment Decisions, and Prognostication in Oncology. In *Frontiers in Oncology* (Vol. 10). Frontiers Media S.A., DOI: 10.3389/fonc.2020.570465

Sigatapu, L., Sundar, S., Padmalatha, K., Sravya, K., Ooha, D., & Devi, P. U. (2023). Artificial intelligence in healthcare-An overview. *Asian Journal of Pharmacy and Technology, 13*(3), 218–222.

Simmons, L. A., Drake, C. D., Gaudet, T. W., & Snyderman, R. (2016, January). Personalized Health Planning in Primary Care Settings. *Federal Practitioner : for the Health Care Professionals of the VA, DoD, and PHS, 33*(1), 27–34. PMID: 30766135

Singh, M., Kumar, A., Khanna, N. N., Laird, J. R., Nicolaides, A., Faa, G., & Suri, J. S. (2024). Artificial intelligence for cardiovascular disease risk assessment in personalised framework: A scoping review. *EClinicalMedicine, 73*.

Sosa-Holwerda, A., Park, O. H., Albracht-Schulte, K., Niraula, S., Thompson, L., & Oldewage-Theron, W. (2024). The role of artificial intelligence in nutrition research: A scoping review. *Nutrients, 16*(13), 2066. PMID: 38999814

Sozutok, S., Piskin, F. C., Balli, H. T., Yucel, S. P., & Aikimbaev, K. (2024). Predicting treatment responses using magnetic resonance imaging-based radiomics in hepatocellular carcinoma patients undergoing transarterial radioembolization. *Revista da Associação Médica Brasileira, 70*(11). Advance online publication. DOI: 10.1590/1806-9282.20240721 PMID: 39630762

Stanton, R., Platania-Phung, C., Gaskin, C. J., & Happell, B. (2016). Screening for metabolic syndrome in mental health consumers using an electronic metabolic monitoring form. *Issues in Mental Health Nursing, 37*(4), 239–244. DOI: 10.3109/01612840.2015.1119221

Stefano, A., Leal, A., Richiusa, S., Trang, P., Comelli, A., Benfante, V., Cosentino, S., Sabini, M. G., Tuttolomondo, A., Altieri, R., Certo, F., Barbagallo, G. M. V., Ippolito, M., & Russo, G. (2021). Robustness of pet radiomics features: Impact of co-registration with mri. *Applied Sciences (Switzerland), 11*(21). Advance online publication. DOI: 10.3390/app112110170

Steiner, G., Geissler, B., & Schernhammer, E. S. (2019). Hunger and obesity as symptoms of non-sustainable food systems and malnutrition. In *Applied Sciences (Switzerland)* (Vol. 9, Issue 6). https://doi.org/DOI: 10.3390/app9061062

Ström, P., Kartasalo, K., Olsson, H., Solorzano, L., Delahunt, B., Berney, D. M., Bostwick, D. G., Evans, A. J., Grignon, D. J., & Humphrey, P. A.. (2020). Artificial intelligence for diagnosis and grading of prostate cancer in biopsies: A population-based, diagnostic study. *The Lancet. Oncology, 21*, 222–232. DOI: 10.1016/S1470-2045(19)30738-7 PMID: 31926806

Suh, Y. J., Jung, J., & Cho, B. J. (2020). Automated breast cancer detection in digital mammograms of various densities via deep learning. *Journal of Personalized Medicine, 10*, 211. DOI: 10.3390/jpm10040211 PMID: 33172076

Sui, D., Liu, W., Chen, J., Zhao, C., Ma, X., Guo, M., & Tian, Z. (2021). A pyramid architecture-based deep learning framework for breast cancer detection. *BioMed Research International, 2021*, 1–10. DOI: 10.1155/2021/2567202 PMID: 34631877

Sumalata, G. L., Joshitha, C., & Meenaksh, K. (2024). Prediction of diabetes mellitus using artificial intelligence techniques. *Scalable Computing, 25*(4), 3200–3213. DOI: 10.12694/scpe.v25i4.2884

Sumner, J., Bundele, A., Lim, H. W., Phan, P., Motani, M., & Mukhopadhyay, A. (2023, December 8). Developing an Artificial Intelligence-Driven Nudge Intervention to Improve Medication Adherence: A Human-Centred Design Approach. *Journal of Medical Systems, 48*(1), 3. DOI: 10.1007/s10916-023-02024-0 PMID: 38063940

Sundar, R., Kumarakulasinghe, N. B., Chan, Y. H., Yoshida, K., Yoshikawa, T., Miyagi, Y., Rino, Y., Masuda, M., Guan, J., Sakamoto, J., Tanaka, S., Tan, A. L., Hoppe, M. M., Jeyasekharan, A. D., Ng, C. C. Y., De Simone, M., Grabsch, H. I., Lee, J., Oshima, T., & Tan, P. (2021). Machine-learning model derived gene signature predictive of paclitaxel survival benefit in gastric cancer: Results from the randomised phase III SAMIT trial. *Gut*, *71*(4), 676–685. DOI: 10.1136/gutjnl-2021-324060 PMID: 33980610

Sun, L., Zhang, H., Yang, Y., & Wang, X. (2023). Exploration of the influence of early rehabilitation training on circulating endothelial progenitor cell mobilization in patients with acute ischemic stroke and its related mechanism under a lightweight artificial intelligence algorithm. *PubMed*, *27*(12), 5338–5355. DOI: 10.26355/eurrev_202306_32768 PMID: 37401269

Swarup, S., Ahmed, I., & Grigorova, Y.. (2025 Jan). Metabolic Syndrome. [Updated 2024 Mar 7] In *StatPearls* [Internet]. StatPearls Publishing., Available from https://www.ncbi.nlm.nih.gov/books/NBK459248/

Szegedy, C., Liu, W., Jia, Y., Sermanet, P., Reed, S., Anguelov, D., Erhan, D., Vanhoucke, V., & Rabinovich, A. (2015). Going deeper with convolutions. In *Proceedings of the IEEE Conference on Computer Vision and Pattern Recognition* (pp. 1–9). Boston, MA, USA. https://doi.org/DOI: 10.1109/CVPR.2015.7298594

Taherdoost, H., & Ghofrani, A. (2024). AI's role in revolutionizing personalized medicine by reshaping pharmacogenomics and drug therapy. *Intelligent Pharmacy*, *2*(5), 643–650. DOI: 10.1016/j.ipha.2024.08.005

Takahashi, S., Takahashi, M., Tanaka, S., Takayanagi, S., Takami, H., Yamazawa, E., Nambu, S., Miyake, M., Satomi, K., & Ichimura, K.. (2021). A new era of neuro-oncology research pioneered by multi-omics analysis and machine learning. *Biomolecules*, *11*, 565. DOI: 10.3390/biom11040565 PMID: 33921457

Talati, D. (2023). AI in healthcare domain. *Journal of Knowledge Learning and Science Technology ISSN: 2959-6386 (Online)*, *2*(3), 256–262. DOI: 10.60087/jklst.vol2.n3.p262

Tan, M., & Le, Q. V. (2019). EfficientNet: Rethinking model scaling for convolutional neural networks. In *Proceedings of the 36th International Conference on Machine Learning* (pp. 10691–10700). Long Beach, CA, USA. https://proceedings.mlr.press/v97/tan19a.html

Tang, F. H., Fong, Y. W., Yung, S. H., Wong, C. K., Tu, C. L., & Chan, M. T. (2023). Radiomics-Clinical AI Model with Probability Weighted Strategy for Prognosis Prediction in Non-Small Cell Lung Cancer. *Biomedicines*, *11*(8). Advance online publication. DOI: 10.3390/biomedicines11082093 PMID: 37626590

Tang, T., Seddigh, S., Halbe, E., & Vesco, A. (2023). IDF2022-0929 TRIFECTA: Examining three digital health strategies to improve mental health outcomes in adults with type 1 diabetes. *Diabetes Research and Clinical Practice*, *197*. Advance online publication. DOI: 10.1016/j.diabres.2023.110357

Tavares, L. D., Manoel, A., Donato, T. H. R., Cesena, F., Minanni, C. A., Kashiwagi, N. M., & Szlejf, C. (2022). Prediction of metabolic syndrome: A machine learning approach to help primary prevention. *Diabetes Research and Clinical Practice*, *191*, 110047.

Taye, M. M. (2023). Understanding of Machine Learning with Deep Learning: Architectures, Workflow, Applications and Future Directions. *Computers*, *12*(5), 91. DOI: 10.3390/computers12050091

Thomas, J. AI in public health: Need to balance innovation with accountability.

Tian, J., Dong, D., Liu, Z., Zang, Y., Wei, J., Song, J., ... & Zhou, M. (2018). Radiomics in medical imaging—detection, extraction and segmentation. Artificial intelligence in decision support systems for diagnosis in medical imaging, 267-333.

Tian, Q., Li, X., Li, J., Cheng, Y., Niu, X., Zhu, S., Xu, W., & Guo, J. (2022). Image quality improvement in low-dose chest CT with deep learning image reconstruction. *Journal of Applied Clinical Medical Physics*, *23*(12). Advance online publication. DOI: 10.1002/acm2.13796 PMID: 36210060

Tixier, F., Cheze-le-Rest, C., Schick, U., Simon, B., Dufour, X., Key, S., Pradier, O., Aubry, M., Hatt, M., Corcos, L., & Visvikis, D. (2020). Transcriptomics in cancer revealed by Positron Emission Tomography radiomics. *Scientific Reports*, *10*(1). Advance online publication. DOI: 10.1038/s41598-020-62414-z PMID: 32221360

Tomar, J. S., Mishra, P., Gupta, A., Meena, K. B., & Tyagi, V. (2022). A Proposed Model for Precision Agriculture. *Communications in Computer and Information Science, 1614 CCIS*, 430–441. DOI: 10.1007/978-3-031-12641-3_35

Trigka, M., & Dritsas, E. (2023). Predicting the occurrence of metabolic syndrome using machine learning models. *Computation (Basel, Switzerland)*, *11*(9), 170.

Trouwborst, I., Verreijen, A., Memelink, R., Massanet, P., Boirie, Y., Weijs, P., & Tieland, M. (2018). Exercise and nutrition strategies to counteract sarcopenic obesity. In *Nutrients* (Vol. 10, Issue 5). https://doi.org/DOI: 10.3390/nu10050605

Trujillo, E., Davis, C., & Milner, J. (2006). Nutrigenomics, proteomics, metabolomics, and the practice of dietetics. *Journal of the American Dietetic Association, 106*, 403–413. PMID: 16503231

Tsai, C. H., Eghdam, A., Davoody, N., Wright, G., Flowerday, S., & Koch, S. (2020). Effects of electronic health record implementation and barriers to adoption and use: A scoping review and qualitative analysis of the content. *Life (Chicago, Ill.), 10*(12), 1–27. DOI: 10.3390/life10120327

Tsuneki, M. (2022). Deep learning models in medical image analysis. *Journal of Oral Biosciences, 64*(3), 312–320.

Tupsakhare, P. (2023). Improving Clinical Decision Support in Health Care Through AIs. *Progress in Medical Sciences, 1–4*. Advance online publication. DOI: 10.47363/PMS/2023(7)E118

Tyler, S., Olis, M., Aust, N., Patel, L., Simon, L., Triantafyllidis, C., & Jacobs, R. J. (2024). Use of artificial intelligence in triage in hospital emergency departments: A scoping review. *Cureus, 16*(5). PMID: 38854295

Udogadi, N. S., Onyenibe, N. S., & Abdullahi, M. K. (2019). Dietary Management of Diabetes Mellitus with Focus on Nigeria. *International Journal of Diabetes Research, 2*(1).

Usman, M. A., & Usman, M. R. (2018). Using image steganography for providing enhanced medical data security. In *Proceedings of the 2018 15th IEEE Annual Consumer Communications & Networking Conference (CCNC)* (pp. 1–4). IEEE. https://doi.org/DOI: 10.1109/CCNC.2018.8319263

van Smeden, M., Reitsma, J. B., Riley, R. D., Collins, G. S., & Moons, K. G. (2021). Clinical prediction models: Diagnosis versus prognosis. *Journal of Clinical Epidemiology, 132*, 142–145. DOI: 10.1016/j.jclinepi.2021.01.009 PMID: 33775387

van Timmeren, J. E., Cester, D., Tanadini-Lang, S., Alkadhi, H., & Baessler, B. (2020). Radiomics in medical imaging—"how-to" guide and critical reflection. In *Insights into Imaging* (Vol. 11, Issue 1). Springer. https://doi.org/DOI: 10.1186/s13244-020-00887-2

van Walraven, C., Escobar, G. J., Greene, J. D., & Forster, A. J. (2010). The Kaiser Permanente inpatient risk adjustment methodology was valid in an external patient population. *Journal of Clinical Epidemiology, 63*(7), 798–803. DOI: 10.1016/j.jclinepi.2009.08.020

Vasaikar, S. V., Straub, P., Wang, J., & Zhang, B. (2018). LinkedOmics: Analyzing multi-omics data within and across 32 cancer types. *Nucleic Acids Research, 46*, D956–D963. DOI: 10.1093/nar/gkx1090 PMID: 29136207

Vasiloglou, M. (2021). Comparison of novel and traditional dietary assessment methods in diabetes patients. *Diabetes Technology and Therapeutics, 23*(SUPPL 2).

Veeramalla, S. K., & Kumar, S. (2023). Segmentation of MRI images using a combination of active contour modeling and morphological processing. *Journal of Mechanics in Medicine and Biology, 23*(4), 2340002. Advance online publication. DOI: 10.1142/S021951942340002X

Vengadapurvaja, A. M., Nisha, G., Aarthy, R., & Sasikaladevi, N. (2017). An efficient homomorphic medical image encryption algorithm for cloud storage security. *Procedia Computer Science, 115*, 643–650. DOI: 10.1016/j.procs.2017.09.150

Venkataramani, M., Pollack, C. E., Yeh, H. C., & Maruthur, N. M. (2019). Prevalence and Correlates of Diabetes Prevention Program Referral and Participation. *American Journal of Preventive Medicine, 56*, 452–457. PMID: 30661888

Verified Market Research. (2024). Precision nutrition market size, share, trends, analysis & forecast.

Vettoretti, M., Cappon, G., Facchinetti, A., & Sparacino, G. (2020). Advanced diabetes management using artificial intelligence and continuous glucose monitoring sensors. *Sensors (Basel), 20*(14), 3870. DOI: 10.3390/s20143870 PMID: 32664432

Vijayalakshmi, K., Al-Otaibi, S., Arya, L., Almaiah, M. A., Anithaashri, T. P., Karthik, S. S., & Shishakly, R. (2023). Smart agricultural–industrial crop-monitoring system using unmanned aerial vehicle–Internet of Things classification techniques. *Sustainability, 15*(14), 11242. DOI: 10.3390/su151411242

Wahl, B., Cossy-Gantner, A., Germann, S., & Schwalbe, N. R. (2018). Artificial intelligence (AI) and global health: How can AI contribute to health in resource-poor settings? *BMJ Global Health, 3*(4), e000798. PMID: 30233828

Wang, L., Zhu, L., Yan, J., Qin, W., Wang, C., Xi, W., Xu, Z., Chen, Y., Jiang, J., Huang, S., Yan, C., Zhang, H., Pan, Z., & Zhang, J. (2023). CT-Based Radiomic Score: A Risk Stratifier in Far-Advanced Gastric Cancer Patients. *Academic Radiology, 30*, S220–S229. DOI: 10.1016/j.acra.2022.12.034 PMID: 36610930

Wang, P., Luo, Z., Luo, C., & Wang, T. (2024). Application of a Comprehensive Model Based on CT Radiomics and Clinical Features for Postoperative Recurrence Risk Prediction in Non-small Cell Lung Cancer. *Academic Radiology, 31*(6), 2579–2590. DOI: 10.1016/j.acra.2023.11.028 PMID: 38172022

Wang, T., Holscher, H. D., & Maslov, S.. (2025). Predicting metabolite response to dietary intervention using deep learning. *Nature Communications*, *16*, 815. DOI: 10.1038/s41467-025-56165-6 PMID: 39827177

Wang, T., She, Y., Yang, Y., Liu, X., Chen, S., Zhong, Y., Deng, J., Zhao, M., Sun, X., Xie, D., & Chen, C. (2022). Radiomics for Survival Risk Stratification of Clinical and Pathologic Stage IA Pure-Solid Non-Small Cell Lung Cancer. *Radiology*, *302*(2), 425–434. DOI: 10.1148/radiol.2021210109 PMID: 34726531

Wang, X., Zhang, Y., & Bao, X. (2015). A novel chaotic block image encryption algorithm based on dynamic random growth technique. *Optics and Lasers in Engineering*, *66*, 10–18. DOI: 10.1016/j.optlaseng.2014.08.005

Wei, L., Liu, H., Xu, J., Shi, L., Shan, Z., Zhao, B., & Gao, Y. (2023). Quantum machine learning in medical image analysis: A survey. *Neurocomputing*, *525*, 42–53. DOI: 10.1016/j.neucom.2023.01.049

Wei, Z.-Y., Zhang, Z., Zhao, D.-L., Zhao, W.-M., & Meng, Y.-G. (2024). Magnetic resonance imaging-based radiomics model for preoperative assessment of risk stratification in endometrial cancer. *World Journal of Clinical Cases*, *12*(26), 5908–5921. DOI: 10.12998/wjcc.v12.i26.5908 PMID: 39286374

Williams, B. J., Lee, J., Oien, K. A., & Treanor, D. (2018). Digital pathology access and usage in the UK: Results from a national survey on behalf of the National Cancer Research Institute's CM-Path initiative. *Journal of Clinical Pathology*, *71*, 463–468. DOI: 10.1136/jclinpath-2017-204808 PMID: 29317516

Wilson, C. A., Newham, J., Rankin, J., Ismail, K., Simonoff, E., Reynolds, R. M., Stoll, N., & Howard, L. M. (2022). Systematic review and meta-analysis of risk of gestational diabetes in women with preconception mental disorders. In *Journal of Psychiatric Research* (Vol. 149). https://doi.org/DOI: 10.1016/j.jpsychires.2022.03.013

Woerl, A. C., Eckstein, M., Geiger, J., Wagner, D. C., Daher, T., Stenzel, P., Fernandez, A., Hartmann, A., Wand, M., & Roth, W.. (2020). Deep learning predicts molecular subtype of muscle-invasive bladder cancer from conventional histopathological slides. *European Urology*, *78*, 256–264. DOI: 10.1016/j.eururo.2020.04.023 PMID: 32354610

Worachartcheewan, A., Shoombuatong, W., Pidetcha, P., Nopnithipat, W., Prachayasittikul, V., & Nantasenamat, C. (2015). Predicting metabolic syndrome using the random forest method. *The Scientific World Journal*, *2015*. Advance online publication. DOI: 10.1155/2015/581501 PMID: 26290899

World Health Organization. (1999). *Definition, Diagnosis and Classification of Diabetes Mellitus and its Complications*. WHO.

Wubineh, B. Z., Deriba, F. G., & Woldeyohannis, M. M. (2023). Exploring the opportunities and challenges of implementing artificial intelligence in healthcare: A systematic literature review. *Urologic Oncology Seminars and Original Investigations*, *42*(3), 48–56. DOI: 10.1016/j.urolonc.2023.11.019 PMID: 38101991

Wu, J., Wang, J., Nicholas, S., Maitland, E., & Fan, Q. (2020). Application of big data technology for COVID-19 prevention and control in China: Lessons and recommendations. *Journal of Medical Internet Research*, *22*(10), e21980.

Xiao, L. H., Chen, P. R., Gou, Z. P., Li, Y. Z., Li, M., Xiang, L. C., & Feng, P. (2017). Prostate cancer prediction using the random forest algorithm that takes into account transrectal ultrasound findings, age, and serum levels of prostate-specific antigen. *Asian Journal of Andrology*, *19*, 586–591. DOI: 10.4103/1008-682X.186884 PMID: 27586028

Xiaoxue, W., Zijun, W., Shichen, C., Mukun, Y., Yi, C., Linqing, M., & Wenpei, B. (2024). Risk prediction model of metabolic syndrome in perimenopausal women based on machine learning. *ElsevierW Xiaoxue, W Zijun, C Shichen, Y Mukun, C Yi, M Linqing, B WenpeiInternational Journal of Medical Informatics, 2024•Elsevier, 188*. https://doi.org/DOI: 10.1016/J.IJMEDINF.2024.105480

Xie, F., Zhao, Q., Li, S., Wu, S., Li, J., Li, H., Chen, S., Jiang, W., Dong, A., Wu, L., Liu, L., Huang, H., Xu, S., Shao, Y., Liu, L., Li, L., & Cai, P. (2022). Establishment and validation of novel MRI radiomic feature-based prognostic models to predict progression-free survival in locally advanced rectal cancer. *Frontiers in Oncology*, *12*. Advance online publication. DOI: 10.3389/fonc.2022.901287 PMID: 36408187

Xu, J., Li, J., Wang, T., Luo, X., Zhu, Z., Wang, Y., Wang, Y., Zhang, Z., Song, R., Yang, L. Z., Wang, H., Wong, S. T. C., & Li, H. (2025). Predicting treatment response and prognosis of immune checkpoint inhibitors-based combination therapy in advanced hepatocellular carcinoma using a longitudinal CT-based radiomics model: A multicenter study. *BMC Cancer*, *25*(1). Advance online publication. DOI: 10.1186/s12885-025-13978-4 PMID: 40181337

Xu, L., Jiang, C., Wang, J., Yuan, J., & Ren, Y. (2014). Information Security in Big Data: Privacy and Data Mining. *IEEE Access : Practical Innovations, Open Solutions*, *2*, 1149–1176. DOI: 10.1109/access.2014.2362522

Yang, J., Chesbrough, H., & Hurmelinna-Laukkanen, P. (2020). *The rise, fall, and resurrection of IBM Watson Health*. UC Berkeley and University of Oulu, Research Project 2019 Fall.

Yang, H., Wang, L., Shao, G., Dong, B., Wang, F., Wei, Y., Li, P., Chen, H., Chen, W., Zheng, Y., He, Y., Zhao, Y., Du, X., Sun, X., Wang, Z., Wang, Y., Zhou, X., Lai, X., Feng, W., & Xu, Y. (2022). A combined predictive model based on radiomics features and clinical factors for disease progression in early-stage non-small cell lung cancer treated with stereotactic ablative radiotherapy. *Frontiers in Oncology*, *12*. Advance online publication. DOI: 10.3389/fonc.2022.967360 PMID: 35982975

Yang, H., & Yu, B., OUYang, P., Li, X., Lai, X., Zhang, G., & Zhang, H. (2022). Machine learning-aided risk prediction for metabolic syndrome based on 3 years study. *Scientific Reports*, *12*(1), 1–11. DOI: 10.1038/s41598-022-06235-2 PMID: 34992227

Yang, Z., Shi, X., Wang, S., Du, L., Zhang, X., Zhang, K., Zhang, Y., Ma, J., & Zheng, R. (2025). *An early prediction model for gestational diabetes mellitus created using machine learning algorithms*. Wiley Online Library., DOI: 10.1002/IJGO.70055

Yao, M., Lin, K., Fan, J., Ji, X., Wang, Y., Dong, A., Han, X., Qi, J., Chi, C., Haroon, S., Jackson, D., Cheng, K. K., & Lehman, R. (2024). Design and Development of Communication Skills Training in Diabetes Care for General Practitioners in China. *Chinese General Practice*, *27*(7). Advance online publication. DOI: 10.12114/j.issn.1007-9572.2022.0900

Ye, C., Fu, T., Hao, S., Zhang, Y., Wang, O., Jin, B., & Ling, X. (2018). Prediction of incident hypertension within the next year: Prospective study using statewide electronic health records and machine learning. *Journal of Medical Internet Research*, *20*(1), e22.

Ye, G., & Huang, K. (2017). An efficient symmetric image encryption algorithm based on an intertwining logistic map. *Neurocomputing*, *251*, 45–53. DOI: 10.1016/j.neucom.2017.04.016

Yin, H., Jiang, Y., Xu, Z., Jia, H., & Lin, G. (2022). Combined diagnosis of multiparametric MRI-based deep learning models facilitates differentiating triple-negative breast cancer from fibroadenoma magnetic resonance BI-RADS 4 lesions. *Journal of Cancer Research and Clinical Oncology*, *149*(6), 2575–2584. DOI: 10.1007/s00432-022-04142-7 PMID: 35771263

Yogeshappa, V. G. (2024). AI-driven Precision medicine: Revolutionizing personalized treatment plans. *International Journal of Computer Engineering and Technology*, *15*(5), 455–474.

Yolchuyeva, S., Giacomazzi, E., Tonneau, M., Ebrahimpour, L., Lamaze, F. C., Orain, M., Coulombe, F., Malo, J., Belkaid, W., Routy, B., Joubert, P., & Manem, V. S. K. (2023). A Radiomics-Clinical Model Predicts Overall Survival of Non-Small Cell Lung Cancer Patients Treated with Immunotherapy: A Multicenter Study. *Cancers (Basel)*, *15*(15). Advance online publication. DOI: 10.3390/cancers15153829 PMID: 37568646

Yu, K. H., & Kohane, I. S. (2019). Framing the challenges of artificial intelligence in medicine. In *BMJ Quality and Safety* (Vol. 28, Issue 3, pp. 238–241). BMJ Publishing Group. https://doi.org/DOI: 10.1136/bmjqs-2018-008551

Yu, K. H., Beam, A. L., & Kohane, I. S. (2018). Artificial intelligence in healthcare. In *Nature Biomedical Engineering* (Vol. 2, Issue 10, pp. 719–731). Nature Publishing Group. https://doi.org/DOI: 10.1038/s41551-018-0305-z

Yuan, B., & Li, J. (2019). The policy effect of the general data protection regulation (GDPR) on the digital public health sector in the european union: An empirical investigation. *International Journal of Environmental Research and Public Health*, *16*(6), 1070. DOI: 10.3390/ijerph16061070 PMID: 30934648

Yu, C. S., Lin, Y. J., Lin, C. H., Te Wang, S., Lin, S. Y., Lin, S. H., & Chang, S. S. (2020). Predicting metabolic syndrome with machine learning models using a decision tree algorithm: Retrospective cohort study. *JMIR Medical Informatics*, *8*(3), 1–18. DOI: 10.2196/17110 PMID: 32202504

Yu, H., Yang, L. T., Zhang, Q., Armstrong, D., & Deen, M. J. (2021). Convolutional neural networks for medical image analysis: State-of-the-art, comparisons, improvement and perspectives. *Neurocomputing*, *444*, 92–110.

Zahedani, A. D., McLaughlin, T., & Veluvali, A.. (2023). Digital health application integrating wearable data and behavioral patterns improves metabolic health. *NPJ Digital Medicine*, *6*, 216. DOI: 10.1038/s41746-023-00956-y PMID: 38001287

Zarkogianni, K., Athanasiou, M., Mitsis, K., Chatzidaki, E., Polychronaki, N., Perakis, K., Vergeti, D., Antonopoulou, D., Papachristou, E., Chioti, V., Voutetakis, A., Kalafatis, E., Pervanidou, P., Kanaka-Gantenbein, C., & Nikita, K. (2021). A comprehensive approach to empower self-management of health in childhood obesity based on gamification mechanisms and biofeedback. *Diabetes Technology and Therapeutics, 23*(SUPPL 2).

Zhang, B., Lian, Z., Zhong, L., Zhang, X., Dong, Y., Chen, Q., Zhang, L., Mo, X., Huang, W., Yang, W., & Zhang, S. (2020). Machine-learning based MRI radiomics models for early detection of radiation-induced brain injury in nasopharyngeal carcinoma. *BMC Cancer*, *20*(1). Advance online publication. DOI: 10.1186/s12885-020-06957-4 PMID: 32487085

Zhang, C., & Lu, Y. (2021). Study on artificial intelligence: The state of the art and future prospects. *Journal of Industrial Information Integration*, *23*, 100224. DOI: 10.1016/j.jii.2021.100224

Zhang, F., Kaufman, H. L., Deng, Y., & Drabier, R. (2013). Recursive SVM biomarker selection for early detection of breast cancer in peripheral blood. *BMC Medical Genomics*, *6*(Suppl. 1), S4. DOI: 10.1186/1755-8794-6-S1-S4 PMID: 23369435

Zhang, J., Oh, Y. J., Lange, P., Yu, Z., & Fukuoka, Y. (2020). Artificial intelligence chatbot behavior change model for designing artificial intelligence chatbots to promote physical activity and a healthy diet. *Journal of Medical Internet Research*, *22*(9), e22845.

Zhang, X., Lu, B., Yang, X., Lan, D., Lin, S., Zhou, Z., Li, K., Deng, D., Peng, P., Zeng, Z., & Long, L. (2022). Prognostic analysis and risk stratification of lung adenocarcinoma undergoing EGFR-TKI therapy with time-serial CT-based radiomics signature. *European Radiology*, *33*, 825–835. DOI: 10.1007/s00330-022-09123-5/ Published PMID: 36166088

Zhang, X., Wang, Y., & Gu, Z. (2016). A novel image encryption scheme based on a linear hyperbolic chaotic system of partial differential equations. *Journal of Electronic Imaging*, *25*(2), 023014. Advance online publication. DOI: 10.1117/1.JEI.25.2.023014

Zhang, X., Yang, H., & Zhang, R. (2019). Challenges and future of precision medicine strategies for breast cancer based on a database on drug reactions. *Bioscience Reports*, ●●●, 39. PMID: 31387972

Zhao, A. P., Li, S., Cao, Z., Hu, P. J.-H., Wang, J., Xiang, Y., & Da Xie, X. L. (2024). AI for science: Predicting infectious diseases. *Journal of Safety Science and Resilience = An Quan Ke Xue Yu Ren Xing (Ying Wen)*, *5*(2), 130–146. DOI: 10.1016/j.jnlssr.2024.02.002

Zheng, Y., Campbell Rice, B., Melkus, G. D., Sun, M., Zweig, S., Jia, W., Parekh, N., He, H., Zhang, Y. L., & Wylie-Rosett, J. (2023). Dietary Self-Management Using Mobile Health Technology for Adults With Type 2 Diabetes: A Scoping Review. In *Journal of Diabetes Science and Technology* (Vol. 17, Issue 5). https://doi.org/ DOI: 10.1177/19322968231174038

Zhou, B., Yang, G., Shi, Z., & Ma, S. (2022). Natural language processing for smart healthcare. *IEEE Reviews in Biomedical Engineering, 17*, 4–18.

Zhou, B., Yang, G., Shi, Z., & Ma, S. (2024). Natural Language Processing for Smart Healthcare. *IEEE Reviews in Biomedical Engineering, 17*, 4–18. DOI: 10.1109/RBME.2022.3210270 PMID: 36170385

Zhou, T., Yang, M., Xiong, W., Zhu, F., Li, Q., Zhao, L., & Zhao, Z. (2024). The value of intratumoral and peritumoral radiomics features in differentiating early-stage lung invasive adenocarcinoma (≤3 cm) subtypes. *Translational Cancer Research, 13*(1), 202–216. DOI: 10.21037/tcr-23-1324 PMID: 38410219

Zhu, Y., Salowe, R., Chow, C., Li, S., Bastani, O., & O'Brien, J. M. (2024). Advancing Glaucoma Care: Integrating Artificial Intelligence in Diagnosis, Management, and Progression Detection. In *Bioengineering* (Vol. 11, Issue 2). Multidisciplinary Digital Publishing Institute (MDPI). https://doi.org/DOI: 10.3390/bioengineering11020122

Zhuang, Z., Liu, Z., Li, J., Wang, X., Xie, P., Xiong, F., Hu, J., Meng, X., Huang, M., Deng, Y., Lan, P., Yu, H., & Luo, Y. (2021). Radiomic signature of the FOWARC trial predicts pathological response to neoadjuvant treatment in rectal cancer. *Journal of Translational Medicine, 19*(1). Advance online publication. DOI: 10.1186/s12967-021-02919-x PMID: 34112180

Zschaubitz, E., Schröder, H., Glackin, C. C., Vogel, L., Labrenz, M., & Sperlea, T. (2025). A benchmark analysis of feature selection and machine learning methods for environmental metabarcoding datasets. *ElsevierE Zschaubitz, H Schröder, CC Glackin, L Vogel, M Labrenz, T SperleaComputational and Structural Biotechnology Journal, 2025•Elsevier, 27*, 1636–1647. https://doi.org/DOI: 10.1016/J.CSBJ.2025.04.017

Zuhair, V., Babar, A., Ali, R., Oduoye, M. O., Noor, Z., Chris, K., Okon, I. I., & Rehman, L. U. (2024, January-December). Exploring the Impact of Artificial Intelligence on Global Health and Enhancing Healthcare in Developing Nations. *Journal of Primary Care & Community Health, 15*, 21501319241245847. DOI: 10.1177/21501319241245847 PMID: 38605668

Zwanenburg, A., Vallières, M., Abdalah, M. A., Aerts, H. J. W. L., Andrearczyk, V., Apte, A., Ashrafinia, S., Bakas, S., Beukinga, R. J., Boellaard, R., Bogowicz, M., Boldrini, L., Buvat, I., Cook, G. J. R., Davatzikos, C., Depeursinge, A., Desseroit, M.-C., Dinapoli, N., Dinh, C. V., & Löck, S. (2020). The Image Biomarker Standardization Initiative: Standardized Quantitative Radiomics for High-Throughput Image-based Phenotyping. *Radiology, 295*(2), 328–338. DOI: 10.1148/radiol.2020191145 PMID: 32154773

About the Contributors

Pranav Kumar Prabhakar is currently working as a Deputy Director of, the Research and Development Cell, and Professor of Research Cadre at Parul University, Gujarat, India. He is among the World's Top 2% Scientists (list published by Stanford University, USA, 2021, 2022, and 2023). He has completed his PhD in Biotechnology from IIT Madras. His main area of research interest focuses on elucidating molecular Mechanisms and Strategies for Oral Insulin Delivery, Mimicking the signaling pathways in Metabolic Disorders (diabetes) with Natural Products. He is a member of the Royal Society of Chemistry, and the Asia-Pacific Chemical, Biological& Environmental Engineering Society. He is also serving as an editorial board member and reviewer for many reputed national and International Journals. Dr. Pranav received honors including the recipient of a travel grant towards attending ATTD 2009 in Greece from the Indian Institute of Technology Madras & Council for Scientific and Industrial Research (CSIR) and approved by the Department of Science and Technology (DST). He has published 100+ research articles in journals, authored 8 books, and 25 book chapters. He also delivered 9 oral and poster presentations in scientific meetings.

Ashok K Sah is working as an Assistant Professor in the Department of Medical Laboratory Sciences, College of Allied & Health Sciences, A' Sharqyiah University, Ibra Oman. I was a professor & Program Chair for Postgraduate Research at the Department of Medical Laboratory Technology, School of Allied Health Science, Galgotias University (GU), India, Before joining A' Sharqyiah University. Before GU, I worked as an associate professor and Head at The Neotia University, WB, India. I worked at the School of Allied Medical Sciences, IIMT University, Meerut, Uttar Pradesh from 2021 to Aug-2022. Since Oct 2016, I was an assistant professor at the Department of Medical Laboratory Technology, Amity Medical School, Amity University Haryana. Before joining Amity, I was an Assistant professor of medical laboratory technology at the School of Life & Allied Health Sciences, the

Glocal University, Saharanpur from 2015-2016. He has published 55 peer-reviewed research articles in renowned national and international journals, alongside 10 books and 8 book chapters, with notable publications in journals such as The Lancet, NPJ Clean Water (Nature), Biomarker Research, Molecular and Cellular Biology, Life, Biomedicines, Diagnostics, Obesity Surgery, etc. Dr. Sah has also shared his research at numerous national and international conferences, workshops, and symposia. With over 15 years of experience in both academia and industry at the national and international levels, Dr. Sah continues to be an active contributor to the field. Outside of his professional work, he enjoys reading, traveling, meeting new people, and exploring different communities and cultures. He is deeply committed to global public health and advocates for the principles of global citizenship.

***

Leena Arya is working as a Professor at the Department of Computer Science and Engineering at Koneru Lakshmaiah Education Foundation Deemed to be University, Vaddeswaram, 22nd NIRF Ranking University, Guntur, AP, India. She completed her Ph.D. from IIT Roorkee in 2012. She has published over 60 research papers in Scopus and SCI-indexed international journals. She handled a research project for the Department of Science and Technology, DST, New Delhi, as Principal Investigator under the Women Scientists Scheme (WOS-A). She has been granted a UK design and Australian Government Innovation patents. She has been a reviewer of many prestigious international journals and conferences. Her research area includes wireless communication, the Internet of Things (IoT), network security, and artificial intelligence.

Latha Banda, working as an Associate Professor CSE, in ABESEC, Ghaziabad, Uttar Pradesh. I have done my Ph.D from Jawaharlal Nehru University, New Delhi. I have more than 15 years' experience in teaching and research. I have published more than 30 journals and nferences, submitted 2 projects in DeiTY and DST, 4 patents. I have much experience in administration and organized more than 80+ seminars, workshops, Industrial visits etc. I have organized 5 International conferences and 2 National conferences. My research interests are Recommender Systems, Machine Learning and ArtificialIntelligence. I am the reviewer of many springer and ACM journals and PC member of various International conferences.I have guided thesis of 8+ M.Tech Students and Editor of Book series of Machine Learning in Security. I have collaborations with Jawaharlal Nehru University and National University of Malaysia.

Hina Bansal is an inspirational teacher and researcher with 16+ years of experience specializing in Bioinformatics/Computational Biology, working as an Assistant Professor in the centre for Bioinformatics and Computational Biology, Amity Institute of Biotechnology, Amity University, Noida since January 2008. Her research interest includes Network pharmacology, functional Genomics and Genome informatics, NGS, functional Proteomics, Molecular docking and simulation, Python, Artificial intelligence, and Machine learning. She has more than forty research publications in reputable peer reviewed journals, book, and book chapters. She has presented numerous papers in various national and international conferences. She has been an active member in organising several workshops and conferences. She is a dynamic reviewer for various peer reviewed journals including BMC Computational Biology and Scientific Reports. She is very proficient in programming languages like C, C++, Java and Python. With her perseverance, academic excellence, research capabilities, and leadership abilities, Dr. Hina a very potential candidate.

Shreyash Dhande is a B.Tech student in Computer Science and Engineering Technology at Jaypee University of Engineering and Technology, Guna. He has a keen interest in artificial intelligence and its application in healthcare. Skilled in Python, C++, SQL, and JavaScript, and familiar with tools like Flask, MySQL, and OpenCV. With strong problem-solving abilities and a solid grasp of data structures and algorithms, he continues to expand his knowledge in machine learning and AI. Driven by a desire to contribute to impactful and innovative solutions, especially in areas where technology can improve lives.

Mourad Elloumi received an Undergraduate Degree in Mathematics and Physics in 1984, and a Master's Degree in Computer Engineering in 1988, from the Faculty of Sciences of Tunis, Tunisia. He also received a Master's Degree in Computer Science in 1989, and a PhD Degree in Computer Science in 1994, from the University of Aix-Marseilles III, France. Then, he received a Habilitation for conducting research in Computer Science in 2003, from the National School of Computer Science, Tunis, Tunisia. He is currently a Full Professor in Computer Science, College of Computing and Information Technology, University of Bisha, Saudi Arabia. Professor Mourad Elloumi is the author/co-author of more than 80 publications in international journals, books and conference proceedings. He was a Guest Editor of a special issue on biological knowledge discovery and data mining, Knowledge Based Systems Journal (Elsevier 2002), a Guest Editor of a special issue on pattern finding in Computational Molecular Biology, Recent Patents on DNA and Gene Sequence Journal (Bentham Science 2012), a Co-Editor of the proceedings of two international conferences and Editor/Co-Editor of five books, respectively, on Algorithms in Computational Molecular Biology (Wiley 2011), Biological Knowledge Discovery (Wiley 2014), Pattern Recognition in Computational Molecular Biology (Wiley 2015), Algorithms for Next-Generation Sequencing Data (Springer 2017), Deep Learning for Biomedical Data Analysis (Springer 2021). His research interests include Algorithmics, Computational Molecular Biology, Knowledge Discovery and Data Mining, and Deep Learning."

Devendra Gautam PhD in CSE awarded in May 2024. Total academic experience exceeds 18 years. Currently working as an Assistant Professor in the Department of CSE, JIMS Engineering Management Technical Campus, Greater Noida, Uttar Pradesh, India

Joyeta Ghosh is a dedicated faculty member and researcher with a passion for exploring diverse aspects of Nutrition and Dietetics. Her expertise spans areas including Metabolic Syndrome, Cancer Biology, Genomics, Neurophysiology, and Stress Physiology. With a Ph.D. in Nutritional Biochemistry from the University of Calcutta (DST-INSPIRE Fellow)(2021), a Masters in Applied Nutrition from AIIPH, Kolkata, and a Bachelor's in Food and Nutrition (Honors) from the University of Calcutta, Dr. Ghosh has built a strong academic foundation. She further expanded her skillset with an M.Sc. in Data Science from Liverpool John Moores University, UK. Her core skills encompass experimental design with human subjects, fieldwork, statistical data analysis, and a wide range of laboratory techniques. As a consultant and data scientist in Nutrition Artificial Intelligence, Dr. Ghosh continues to push the boundaries of innovation in the field. Her commitment to excellence in teaching and research, coupled with a relentless pursuit of knowledge, drives her contributions to the advancement of science and nutrition.

Shubham Gupta Currently Working as an Associate and Head, Department of Medical Radiology, Imaging and Therapeutic Technology, Parul Institute of Allied and Healthcare Sciences, Faculty of Medicine, Parul University. Expert in the field of Radio-Imaging with an experiences of 8 years

Manan Jain is a B.Tech student in Computer Science and Engineering at Jaypee University of Engineering and Technology, Guna. He is passionate about artificial intelligence and its applications in healthcare and real-world problem-solving. With a strong foundation in data structures and algorithms (350+ problems solved on LeetCode, rated 1593), Manan consistently enhances his problem-solving skills. He is certified in Postman API Fundamentals and JSON Power DB, and actively explores backend development and full-stack applications. Manan is driven by a desire to create impactful, tech-based solutions that contribute positively to society, particularly in domains where innovation can directly improve lives.

Sachin Jain is working as an Associate Professor in the Department of Computer Science and Engineering at Ajay Kumar Garg Engineering College, Ghaziabad. He completed his B.Tech in Computer Science and Engineering in 2007 from UPTU, Lucknow and M.Tech in Computer Science and Engineering in 2010 from GGSIPU, Delhi. He has completed his Ph.D in Computer Science and Engineering from Sharda University Greater Noida in 2025. He is a UGC-NET qualified teacher and has total 16 years of teaching experience. His research interests lie in Artificial Intelligence, Deep Learning and Machine Learning. He has published several research papers in Peer-Reviewed Journals and Conference proceedings. Dr. Jain has filed several patents for his work.

Vishal Jain is pursuing Postdoc from Kuala Lumpur University of Science & Technology (KLUST) (formerly known as Infrastructure University Kuala Lumpur (IUKL)), Malaysia. He is presently working as a Professor at the School of Engineering & Technology, Vivekananda Institute of Professional Studies - Technical Campus, New Delhi, India Before that, he worked as Professor at Sharda University, Greater Noida and Associate Professor at Bharati Vidyapeeth's Institute of Computer Applications and Management (BVICAM), New Delhi. He has associated as a member of the Faculty Board, Board of Planning and Management, Executive Council, Academic Council, Curriculum Development and Review Committee and Academic Audit of various higher education Institutions. His research areas include machine learning, information retrieval, semantic web, ontology engineering, data mining, ad hoc networks, sensor networks and network security.

K. V. Rajani is an Associate Professor in CSE Department with 25+ years of work experience in teaching. Currently working at Keshav Memorial Institute of Technology, Narayanaguda, Hyderabad, Did M.C.A. from Andhra University, M.Tech from Acharya Nagarjuna University and Ph.D in Computer Science from JJTU. Her current research interests are in Data Science, Cybersecurity and Artificial Intelligence Applications in Medical field. She has published more than 23 papers in these areas. She has guided more than 100 projects in UG.

Harmanpreet Kaur is currently working as Assistant Professor with Chandigarh University. She received her Ph. D. degree in the field of Medical Imaging from Panjab University, Chandigarh, India in 2024. Further, she attained M.E and B.Tech degree in the field of Electronics and Communication Engineering in 2009 and 2007 respectively. She has more than 10 years of teaching experience and has various papers published in SCIE/Scopus journals, IEEE/Springer national and international conferences. Her research interest includes Image Processing, Digital Signal Processing and Medical Imaging.

Kunj Bihari Meena is a faculty and researcher in Computer Science and Engineering with a Ph.D. from Jaypee University of Engineering and Technology (JUET), Guna, an M.Tech from IIT Kharagpur, and a B.E. from Samrat Ashok Technological Institute (SATI), Vidisha. He has been associated with JUET, Guna since 2013 and has amassed over 12 years of teaching experience. Dr. Meena has extensive expertise in subjects including Data Structures, Object-Oriented Programming, Introduction to Computers and Programming, Machine Learning, and Microprocessors and Controllers. He has successfully guided numerous undergraduate and postgraduate students in their projects and dissertations, fostering research-oriented learning and innovation. An active researcher, Dr. Meena has published multiple papers in reputed international journals and conferences, including SCI and Scopus-indexed publications, with over five SCI-indexed articles to his credit. He has received Best Paper Awards for his research contributions and serves as a reviewer for prestigious SCI/Scopus journals and conferences. He is also a member of the Technical Program Committee (TPC) for several international conferences, reflecting his engagement with the global academic community.

Krishnasri Padamandala, PhD, is an accomplished Assistant Professor and Research & Development lead at CU, with extensive experience in teaching, research, academic coordination, and technological innovation. She holds a PhD in Health Sciences and also serves as a PhD Coordinator. A recipient of the prestigious Best Paper Award from the Indian Journal of Ophthalmology (IJO), Dr. Padamandala has represented her research internationally, traveling to Africa and Seattle. Her dynamic career includes hands-on involvement in healthtech incubation projects and proposal writing most notably for the "NeuroDrishti" initiative. She has also contributed as a technology consultant with Orbees, UB MedTech Market, and has demonstrated excellence in grant writing and interdisciplinary research. With a passion for academia and innovation, she brings expertise in Learning Management Systems (LMS), SHL question banking systems, and educational technology. Multitalented and deeply enthusiastic, Dr. Padamandala thrives at the intersection of healthcare, education, and research, continuously pushing boundaries as a professor, researcher, and thought leader.

Ravi Rastogi received his Ph.D. in Computer Science and Engineering in December 2011 from Uttarakhand Technical University, Dehradun, Uttarakhand, India. MS in Computer Science degree in September 2005 from Fairleigh Dickinson University, Teaneck, New Jersey, USA. He is working as a Professor in the Department of Computer Science and Engineering, JIMS Engineering Management Technical Campus, Greater Noida, India. He had worked at various Universities, Koneru Lakshmaiah Education Foundation Deemed to be a university, Andhra

Pradesh, India and Bisha University, KSA and Galgotias University, Greater Noida, India and Sharda University, Greater Noida, India and Jaypee University of Information and Technology, Solan, India. He was a database developer for Microsoft, Seattle, USA, and ING, Philadelphia, USA. His research interests are interconnection networks, stable matching problems, data mining and intelligence in systems, the Internet of Things, and cloud computing. Refereed International Journal publications are 23 and Refereed International Conference Publications are 8.

Wasswa Shafik (Member, IEEE) received a Bachelor of Science degree in information technology from Ndejje University, Uganda, a Master of Engineering degree in Information Technology (Computer and Communication Networks) from Yazd University, Iran, and a PhD in Computer Science with the School of Digital Science, Universiti Brunei Darussalam, Brunei Darussalam. He is also the Founder and Research Director of the Dig Connectivity Research Laboratory (DCRLab) after serving as a Research Associate at the Network Interconnectivity Research Laboratory at Yazd University. Prior to this, he worked as a Community Data Analyst at Population Services International (PSI-Uganda), a Community Data Officer at the Programme for Accessible Health Communication (PACE-Uganda), a Research Assistant at the Socio-Economic Data Centre (SEDC-Uganda), Uganda, an Assistant Data Officer at TechnoServe, Kampala, Uganda, and Asmaah Charity Organization as Cheif Executive Officer. He has hundreds of publications with renowned publishers. His research interests include Artificial Intelligence, Neural Networks, Computer Vision, Smart Agriculture, Digital Health, and Green Computing.

Anshu Singh is currently working as Associate Professor, Department of Medical Laboratory Sciences, Subharti College of Allied and Healthcare, Swami Vivekanand Subharti University, and Meerut. Before joining here he worked as Lecturer and Assistant Professor for 09 years into Disha Group of Institutions, Delhi and Haldwani, Uttarakhand. He has 07 years of research experience and 11 years of teaching experience and his specialization is Microbiology. He has completed their DMLT and BSCMLT from Punjab Technical University, M.Sc. Microbiology from NIMS University and PhD in Microbiology from Noida International University. He has authored or co-authored 30 Technical Papers,16 Books and Manuals, 35 Book chapters, has filed four copyrights and one patent application. He holds lifetime membership of several societies of health and biological sciences. He is in the editorial board of the various indexed journals.

Gurwinder Singh received his Ph. D. degree in Mechanical Engineering from Panjab University, Chandigarh, India in 2022. He completed his M.Tech and B.Tech degree in the field of Mechanical Engineering in 2013 and 2008 respectively. He worked on reversible modified PEM fuel cell and has various papers published in SCIE journals, national and international conferences. He has more than 10 years of teaching experience and his research interests are multidisciplinary.

Kunal Kumar Singh is currently pursuing Bachelor of Technology (B.Tech) in Computer Science and Engineering from Jaypee University of Engineering and Technology, Guna, Madhya Pradesh, India. He has a keen interest in the field of Artificial Intelligence and Machine Learning, with a special focus on healthcare data analytics. He is passionate about exploring the intersection of healthcare and technology to develop impactful solutions for real-world problems.

Salender Singh is a dedicated academician and researcher in the field of Medical Biochemistry, with over 10 years of teaching and clinical laboratory experience. He obtained his Master's degree in Medical Biochemistry from Shri Guru Ram Rai Institute of Medical and Health Sciences, Dehradun, and subsequently earned his Doctorate (Ph.D.) under the Faculty of Medicine from Malwanchal University, Indore. Throughout his academic journey, Dr. Singh has made significant contributions to biomedical research, having published four research papers in reputed journals, authored six book chapters, and secured one patent reflecting his innovative approach in the field. He has actively participated in the scientific community by presenting papers and posters at more than five international conferences, showcasing his commitment to continuous learning and advancement in medical science.

Nimisha Tiwari is pursuing PhD. in Power Electronics from Rajiv Gandhi Proudhyogiki Vishwavidalaya, (Bhopal). My research focuses on the development and optimization of low-cost technologies for use in developing economies. She has a strong background in Machine learning and Modern Electronics.

Shalaka Tyagi is PhD. in AI/ML from Bennett University, Gr. Noida. Her research focuses on the development and optimization of low-cost technologies for use in developing economies. She has a strong background in Machine learning and Deep Learning.

Vipin Tyagi is a distinguished academician, researcher and author, currently serving as Dean (Academics and Research) at Jaypee University of Engineering and Technology in Guna, Madhya Pradesh. With a rich background in Computer Science, his expertise spans across Image Processing, Cyber Forensics, and Speech Recognition. He is also Director – IQAC of JUET Guna. Prof. Tyagi has a prolific publication record, contributing significantly to his fields of interest. His scholarly work includes numerous journal articles, conference papers, and books. Some of his notable publications are in the areas of image forgery detection, image denoising, and content-based image retrieval. He has authored and edited several books and papers in the field of computing and data sciences, such as "Predictive Computing and Information Security" and "Content-Based Image Retrieval: Ideas, Influences, and Current Trends" published by Springer Singapore. His book "Understanding Digital Image Processing" using MATLAB, published by Taylor and Francis is highlighted by Mathworks. His scholarly work has earned him a respectable h-index and numerous citations in the academic community

Ankur Vashishtha Presently working as Assistant Professor in the Department of Medical Laboratory Technology at the School of Allied Health Sciences, Sharda University. He specializes in microbiology, with a strong emphasis on both teaching and research. With nearly six years of academic and professional experience across esteemed institutions and universities, he has actively contributed to the growth and advancement of the organizations he has been associated with. His research expertise includes infectious disease diagnostics, particularly in the molecular detection of enteric pathogens. He has been extensively involved in projects related to microbiological analysis and diagnostic methodologies. Committed to fostering academic excellence, he employs innovative teaching strategies while simultaneously contributing to scientific research, publications, and advancements in laboratory diagnostics.

Santhosh Kumar Veeramalla received the B.Tech. degree in electronics and communication engineering from the Jawaharlal Nehru Technological University, Hyderabad, India, in 2005 and the M.E. degree in electronics and communications from the University Visvesvaraya College of Engineering (UVCE), Bangalore, India in 2008. He received a Ph.D. in electronics and communication engineering from the National Institute of Technology, Warangal, India. Presently he is working as an associate professor at BVRIT Hyderabad College of Engineering for Women, Hyderabad. His research interests are in the area of biomedical signal processing and its implementation.

Rajesh Babu Yallamanda is working as a Assistant Professor at the Department of Computer Science and Engineering at Koneru Lakshmaiah Education Foundation Deemed to be University, Vaddeswaram, 22nd NIRF Ranking University, Guntur, AP, India. He completed his Ph.D. from Annamalai University, Tamil Nadu in 2024. He has published over 6 research papers in Scopus and SCI-indexed international journals.

Index